Cardiovascular Imaging: Modern Methods and Technologies

Cardiovascular Imaging: Modern Methods and Technologies

Editor: Mckinsey Harper

FOSTER ACADEMICS

www.fosteracademics.com

www.fosteracademics.com

FOSTER ACADEMICS

Cataloging-in-Publication Data

Cardiovascular imaging : modern methods and technologies / edited by Mckinsey Harper.
p. cm.
Includes bibliographical references and index.
ISBN 978-1-63242-530-0
1. Cardiovascular system--Imaging. 2. Cardiovascular system--Diseases--Diagnosis.
3. Heart--Imaging. I. Harper, Mckinsey.
RC670 .C37 2018
616.107 5--dc23

Foster Academics,
118-35 Queens Blvd., Suite 400,
Forest Hills, NY 11375, USA

ISBN 978-1-63242-530-0 (Hardback)

Printed and bound in China.

Contents

Preface

In my initial years as a student, I used to run to the library at every possible instance to grab a book and learn something new. Books were my primary source of knowledge and I would not have come such a long way without all that I learnt from them. Thus, when I was approached to edit this book; I became understandably nostalgic. It was an absolute honor to be considered worthy of guiding the current generation as well as those to come. I put all my knowledge and hard work into making this book most beneficial for its readers.

Cardiovascular imaging uses the most advanced technology to take images of the heart. It helps in diagnosing and treating a patient with any cardiovascular disease. Echocardiography and cardiac magnetic resonance imaging are the most popular methods of cardiovascular imaging. This book presents the complex subject of cardiovascular imaging in the most comprehensible and easy to understand language. While understanding the long-term perspectives of the topics, the book makes an effort in highlighting their impact as a modern tool for the growth of the discipline. It will provide comprehensive knowledge to the readers.

I wish to thank my publisher for supporting me at every step. I would also like to thank all the authors who have contributed their researches in this book. I hope this book will be a valuable contribution to the progress of the field.

Editor

1

Non-Enhanced T1-Weighted Liver Vessel Imaging at 7 Tesla

Anja Fischer[1,2]*, Oliver Kraff[2], Stefan Maderwald[2], Karsten Beiderwellen[1,2], Mark E. Ladd[1,2,3], Michael Forsting[1], Thomas C. Lauenstein[1], Lale Umutlu[1,2]

1 Department of Diagnostic and Interventional Radiology and Neuroradiology, University Hospital Essen, Essen, Germany, **2** Erwin L. Hahn Institute for Magnetic Resonance Imaging, University Duisburg-Essen, Essen, Germany, **3** German Cancer Research Center (DKFZ), Heidelberg, Germany

Abstract

Objectives: Aim of the study was to assess the feasibility and to compare three non-enhanced T1-weighted (w) sequences for liver vessel imaging at 7 Tesla (T).

Material and Methods: 12 healthy volunteers were examined on a 7 T whole-body MR-system. The following non-enhanced sequences were acquired: T1w 2D FLASH, T1w 3D FLASH and Time of flight (TOF)-MRA. Qualitative image analysis was performed by two radiologists including over all image quality as well as vessel delineation of the liver arteries, liver veins and portal vein and the presence of artifacts using a five-point scale (5 = excellent vessel delineation to 1 = non-diagnostic). Contrast ratios (CR), SNR und CNR of the above named vessels in correlation to adjacent liver tissue were calculated for quantitative assessment. For statistical analysis, a Wilcoxon Rank Test was applied.

Results: All three sequences provided a homogenous hyperintense delineation of the assessed liver vessels. Qualitative image analysis demonstrated the superiority of TOF-MRA, providing best overall image quality (TOF 4.17, 2D FLASH 3.42, 3D FLASH 3.46; $p<0.01$) as well as highest image quality values for all analyzed liver vessel segments. TOF-MRA was least impaired by B_1 inhomogeneity (4.13) and susceptibility artifacts (4.63) out of all three sequences ($p<0.01$). Quantitative image analysis confirmed the superiority of TOF MRA showing significant higher CR values for all liver vessels (e.g. right hepatic artery TOF 0.47, 2D FLASH 0.09, 3D FLASH 0.11 with $p = 0.02$ and 0.01, respectively). Providing the lowest standard deviation in noise, TOF showed highest values for SNR and CNR.

Conclusions: Non-enhanced T1w imaging in general and TOF MRA in particular, appear to be promising techniques for high quality non-enhanced liver vessel assessment at 7 T.

Editor: Jeroen Hendrikse, University Medical Center (UMC) Utrecht, Netherlands

Funding: The authors have no support or funding to report.

Competing Interests: The authors have declared that no competing interests exist.

* E-mail: anja.fischer@uk-essen.de

Introduction

Over the last decades, contrast-enhanced (ce) CT angiography and MR angiography (MRA) have been established as the imaging techniques of choice to assess liver vessel anatomy prior to hepatectomy or liver transplantation [1,2]. As CT angiography deploys ionizing radiation and the application of contrast agent in general bears the potential of side effects and is restricted in case of renal insufficiency [3], the focus of scientific research has shifted towards non-enhanced MRA techniques within the last few years. Several studies at lower field strength (1.5 Tesla) have demonstrated the diagnostic potential of non-contrast-enhanced liver vessel imaging, utilizing true steady-state free-precession sequences and time-spatial labeling inversion pulses. Shimada et al. reported initial results of 3D true SSFP imaging utilizing a spatial labeling inversion pulse to visualize hepatic arterial and venous vasculature, selectively achieving high arterial and venous vessel contrast and good suppression of the portal veins and surrounding static tissue [4–6].

In clinical routine, the standard magnetic field strength for imaging of hepatic vessels lies in 1.5 T MRI. The increase of the magnetic field strength to 3 T has been proven beneficial in terms of achieving higher spatiotemporal resolution, as well as enabling comparable or improved delineation of vessel structures [7]. With recent development in multi-channel transmit/receive RF (radiofrequency) body coil technology, the feasibility of ultra-high field imaging (7 T) of abdominal organs and vessel structures could be demonstrated [8–10]. A successful transformation of the increased signal-to-noise ratio into imaging at high spatiotemporal resolution could be observed, displaying highly defined anatomical details of parenchymatous organs and arterial vasculature [11,12]. Nevertheless, MR imaging at higher field strength also entails challenges, dealing with limitations based on increasing signal heterogeneities due to RF wavelength effects and restrictions due to increasing SAR (specific absorption rate) [13–15]. With SSFP and T2 TSE imaging being restricted at ultra-high-field strength, most studies on 7 Tesla non-enhanced MRA have focused on T1-weighted imaging, utilizing the inherently hyperintense vessel signal at 7 T.

Thus, non-enhanced MRA at 7 T has been successfully demonstrated for imaging of the intracranial and renal vasculature as well as vessels of the lower extremities [16–19].

The aim of this study was to investigate the feasibility of non-enhanced MR imaging of the arterial, venous and portal liver vessels comparing three T1w sequences at 7 Tesla.

Materials and Methods

Study Population

12 healthy volunteers were enrolled in this trial, including seven female and five male subjects. The average age was 31.2 years with a range of 23 to 44 years. The study was conducted in conformance with the Declaration of Helsinki and approved by the Ethics Commission of the Medical Faculty of the University Duisburg-Essen (study number 11-4898-BO). Written informed consent was obtained from each volunteer before the examination. After leaving the examination room all subjects were consulted about possible side effects.

Scanner and Coil System

Examinations were performed on a 7 Tesla whole-body MR system (Magnetom 7T, Siemens Healthcare Sector, Erlangen, Germany) in supine position. For image acquisition a custom-built eight channel body transmit/receive RF coil was utilized [20]. The body coil consisted of two arrays with four elements each placed ventral and dorsal on the upper abdomen. The field of view (FOV) was centered on the liver. In this region, manual adjustments, in particular B_0 shimming was performed utilizing a shim volume adapted to the region of interest. As MRI at higher field strength is known to be susceptible to transmit B_1 field inhomogeneities due to the reduced Larmor wavelength [21], static shimming of the eight individual transmit phases of the RF coil was performed to mitigate potential limitations and to achieve a more homogeneous excitation of the upper abdomen [22]. A phase increment of 90 degrees and equal amplitudes between neighboring elements (circularly polarized mode CP^{2+}) was found to be most compatible for this study in terms of image quality as it constrained the signal voids to a periaortal focus as shown in Figure 1. Here, flip angle maps obtained in transversal orientation with the Bloch-Siegert-Shift B1 mapping technique [23,24] demonstrate advantages of the CP^{2+} mode for the study objective in comparison to the CP^{+} mode. Furthermore, predefined phase settings allow an improved workflow as input power limits can be calculated prior to the study for the SAR supervision. For compliance with the International Electrotechnical Commission (IEC) guidelines [25], SAR calculations were performed in human adult male and female body models of the Virtual Family (CST Microwave Studio, Darmstadt, Germany) [26] prior to the study, resulting in a maximum permitted input power level of 24 W for which the localized 10 g-averaged SAR complies with the limit of 10 W/kg for both human body models used in the simulations. Given is the total RF power at the coil plug, which was equally split to all eight coil elements.

Sequence Protocol

With the increase of the magnetic field strength, sequence parameters need adjustments and modifications to provide best possible image quality while providing a good workflow for the whole imaging protocol and obeying RF power constraints. Therefore imaging parameters (e.g. repetition time (TR), echo time (TE), flip angle (α) and bandwidth) were adapted and modified to 7 Tesla in an exclusive group of three healthy volunteers prior to the start of the study. The examination protocol consisted of the following sequences:

1. T1w spoiled gradient-echo sequence (2D FLASH) in transversal orientation.
2. T1w spoiled gradient-echo sequence (3D FLASH) in transversal orientation.
3. T1w 2D FLASH Time-of-Flight (TOF) MRA in transversal orientation.

Aim of the optimization process was to achieve high contrast between vasculature and parenchyma at a high spatial resolution for the delineation of the vessels. However, nominal flip angles and transmit reference voltages in the sequences were set to allow continuous scanning without waiting times between individual scans to allow the subjects to cool down in case SAR limits would have been reached within the 6-minute averaging time-window requested by the safety guidelines. Achieving an acquisition time within breath-hold conditions for the rather high flip angle TOF sequence was found difficult. Best results regarding image quality and workflow were obtained by using a lower spatial resolution compared to FLASH acquisitions. However, to compensate for the reduced matrix the FOV of the TOF sequence was reduced to a minimum for whole-liver coverage. The above mentioned SAR limitations in the TOF sequence were also the rationale for including the other two gradient echo sequences in this study. Prior publications have demonstrated the feasibility of non-contrast enhanced MRA of those standard gradient echo sequences for intracranial or renal vessel imaging at 7 T [12,27]. Furthermore, it has to be mentioned, that 2D and 3D FLASH imaging were acquired at a higher spatial and temporal resolution which might be beneficial for a high quality vessel delineation and for clinical applicability providing a faster image acquisition. Imaging parameters of the above named sequences are summarized in Table 1. The total examination time was registered using a stop watch.

Data Analysis

All images were analyzed separately and blinded by two radiologists with 8 and 3 years experience in abdominal MRI on a standard Picture Archiving and Communication System (PACS) workstation (Centricity RIS 4.0i, GE Healthcare, USA). Qualitative image analysis was performed in the transversal source images for following vessel segments:

(1) *arterial*

a. proper hepatic artery (PHA)
b. 2nd order branch of the right hepatic artery in liver segment 5 (RHA)

(2) *portal venous*

a. main portal vein (PV)
b. 1st order branch of the right portal vein (RPV)

(3) *venous*

a. inferior vena cava (IVC)
b. middle hepatic vein (MHV).

Visual qualitative image analysis was carried out with regard to vessel delineation using a five-point scale (5 = excellent image quality with sharply defined vessels, 4 = good vessel delineation, 3 = moderate vessel delineation, 2 = poor vessel delineation, 1 = not visible or non-diagnostic) as well as overall image quality for each sequence. Additionally presence of artefacts was assessed

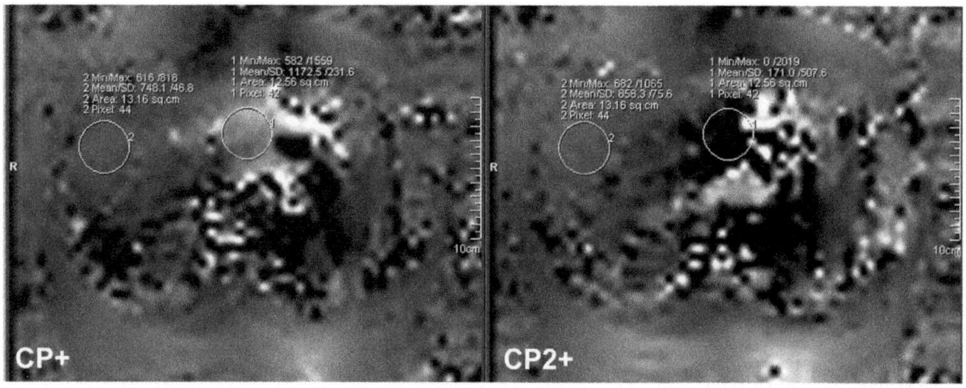

Figure 1. Flip angle maps obtained in two standard excitation modes in transversal orientation of the upper abdomen. Improved excitation of the liver is given with the CP^{2+} mode compared to the CP^{+} mode both in terms of general coverage, particularly of the right liver lobe as well as regarding mean reached flip angle. In the images, ROIs are displayed ventral of the aorta (ROI1) and within liver tissue of the right liver lobe (ROI2) yielding flip angle values encoded by a factor of 10.

for each sequence using five categories: 1 = massive impairment, non-diagnostic, 2 = strong impairment, 3 = moderate impairment, 4 = slight impairment or insignificant, 5 = no artifact present. The following artefacts were evaluated: (1) B_1 inhomogeneity, (2) inflow effects, (3) motion artefacts, (4) susceptibility artefact and (5) overall image impairment.

For quantitative image evaluation, contrast ratios ($CR = [S_{vessel} - S_{liver}] / [S_{vessel} + S_{liver}]$) of the above named vessel segments were assessed by placing ROIs (regions of interest) of identical size in the according vessel lumen and neighboring liver tissue.

Measurements of signal-to-noise and contrast-to-noise ratio (SNR, CNR) were performed for all vessel segments: [$SNR_{vessel} = Signal_{vessel}/noise$], [$SNR_{liver} = Signal_{liver}/noise$], [$CNR = SNR_{vessel} - SNR_{liver}$]. To accommodate for inhomogeneous noise due to the use of parallel imaging[28], it was measured by placing two maximum size ROIs out of the body and to use the mean value of the standard deviation of each noise value.

For statistical analysis, a Wilcoxon Rank Test was applied (Software: IBM SPSS Statistics 21). Score values for image quality and presence of artifacts were compared for each sequence. A p-value <0.05 was considered to establish statistically significant differences. In addition, interobserver reliability was calculated using the method of Landis et al. [29].

Results

All MR examinations at 7 T were successfully performed and well tolerated by the subjects without any side effects. The examination time amounted to 16 min (+/−2 min) including positioning, manual adjustments and data acquisition of the non-enhanced sequences.

Qualitative image analysis showed the superiority of TOF MRA, which provided best overall image quality (4.17 ± 0.38) as well as highest image quality values for all analyzed liver vessel segments and was least impaired by artifacts (overall artifacts 4.08 ± 0.28) (Fig. 2). 2D FLASH and 3D FLASH images revealed similar values, in terms of moderate to good overall image quality ratings (2D FLASH 3.42 ± 0.58, 3D FLASH 3.46 ± 0.51) and a low to moderate presence of artifacts (overall 2D FLASH 3.50 ± 0.51, 3D FLASH 3.46 ± 0.51). Nevertheless among the two sequences, 2D FLASH MRI yielded superior conspicuity of all assessed liver

Table 1. Sequence parameters.

	2D FLASH	3D FLASH	TOF
Repetition time TR [ms]	193	3.2	17
Echo time TE [ms]	3.57	1.36	4.7
Nominal Flip angle FA [°]	70	10	60
Bandwidth [Hz/pixel]	410	930	230
Slice orientation	transversal	transversal	transversal
Slices	42	104	20
Slice thickness [mm]	5	2	2.5
Field-of-view FOV [mm²]	350	350	230
Acquisition matrix [pixel]	448×448	448×448	256×128
Parallel imaging with GRAPPA	Yes (R = 2)	Yes (R = 2)	Yes (R = 2)
Reference lines	48	48	48
Acquisition time TA [min:s]	0:52 (breathhold with 2 concatenations)	0:24	0:33 (breathhold with 5 concatenations)

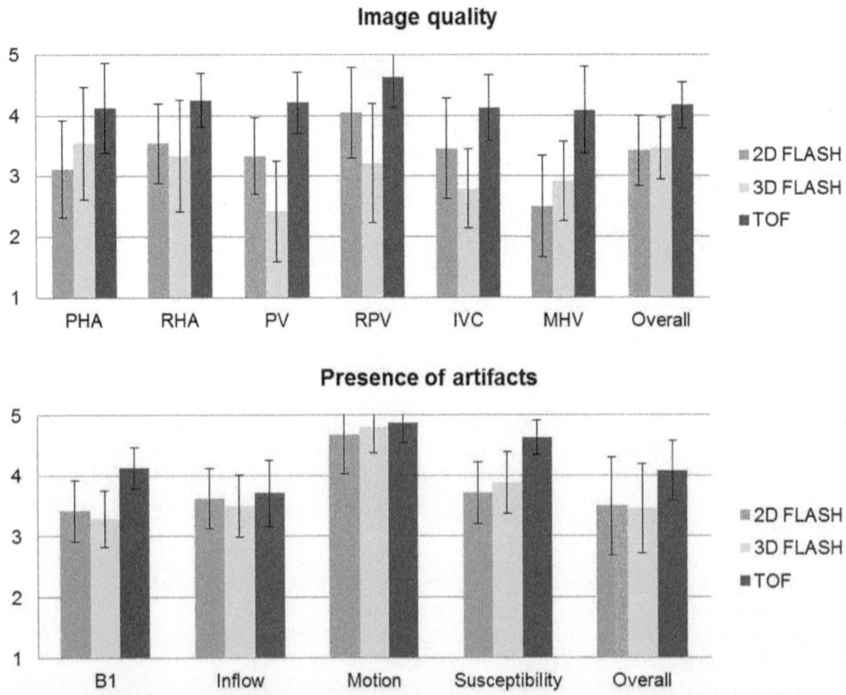

Figure 2. Qualitative analysis of image quality and presence of artifacts (5-point scales) for all analyzed liver vessel segments in all three sequences. (PHA = proper hepatic artery, RHA = 2nd order branch of right hepatic artery, PV = main portal vein, RPV = 1st order branch of right portal vein, IVC = inferior vena cava, MHV = middle hepatic vein).

vessels despite the common hepatic artery and the middle hepatic vein.

Quantitative image analysis confirmed the results of the qualitative image evaluation, in terms of superiority of the TOF sequence. TOF MRA showed highest CR values for the right portal vein (0.59±0.08), closely followed by the inferior vena cava and the middle hepatic vein (0.53±0.09, 0.50±0.08, respectively). In contrast, 2D and 3D FLASH imaging, achieved a considerably lower vessel contrast for all analyzed segments with values ranging from 0.07±0.05 (IVC at 3D FLASH) to 0.23±0.07 (RPV at 2D FLASH). TOF MRA provided comparable superiority for SNR and CNR measurements, yielding highest scores for SNR and CNR in all vessel segments (highest SNR and CNR for RPV: TOF SNR 129.73±33.98 and CNR 96.94±28.74, 2D FLASH SNR 97.75±23.33 and CNR 36.39±12.22, 3D FLASH SNR 60.44±16.88 and CNR 14.28±9.33). Mean scores for the qualitative analysis and the presence of artifacts are displayed in Figure 2. Figure 3 shows the mean CR, SNR and CNR values for all sequences. Detailed results for each sequence are described below.

T1w Spoiled Gradient-echo Sequence (2D FLASH)

Qualitative analysis of 2D FLASH imaging demonstrated a moderate delineation of the hepatic arteries (PHA 3.13±0.80, RHA 3.54±0.66) and veins (IVC 3.46±0.83, MHV 2.50±0.83). The sequence was moderately impaired by B_1 (3.42±0.50) and inflow (3.63±0.49) artifacts, mainly located in the periaortal region (Fig. 4). Signal loss due to susceptibility and motion artifacts caused only a slight disturbance of vessel delineation (mean values 3.71±0.81, 4.67±0.64, respectively).

Regarding quantitative evaluation, 2D FLASH imaging provided CR values ranging from 0.09 (RHA±0.07) to 0.23 (RPV±0.07), which were significantly lower compared to TOF imaging (RHA $p = 0.02$, RPV $p = 0.02$), yet marginally higher than for 3D FLASH MRI.

Assessment of interobserver reliability revealed a moderate agreement with a mean kappa value of 0.51 for qualitative analysis of all liver vessels. Regarding the presence of artifacts, a slightly higher strength of agreement was detected (mean 0.58).

T1w Spoiled Gradient-echo Sequence (3D FLASH)

Out of all three sequences, 3D FLASH MRI was the sequence to provide poorest vessel delineation, particularly for assessment of the main portal vein (2.42±0.83), inferior vena cava (2.79±0.66) and the middle hepatic vein (2.92±0.65) with statistically significant difference to TOF MRA (p-values ranging from to 0.00 to 0.012). Similar to 2D FLASH imaging, there was a moderate impairment caused by B_1 (3.29±0.46) and inflow artifacts (3.50±0.51) as well as a minor presence of susceptibility artifacts (3.88±0.74).

Quantitative analysis confirmed the predominantly moderate to poor vessel delineation at 3D FLASH imaging: CR values ranged from 0.07 (IVC±0.05) to 0.20 (MHV±0.10), being significantly lower compared to TOF imaging (IVC $p = 0.02$, MHV $p = 0.02$).

The interobserver agreement was rated moderate (mean 0.44) for vessel delineation and substantial (mean 0.63) for the presence of artifacts.

T1w Time-Of-Flight Sequence (TOF-MRA)

Analysis of all liver vessel segments demonstrated a significant superiority for TOF imaging, providing a homogeneous hyperintense delineation of all liver vessels (Fig. 5). Mean values of all assessed vessel segments were similar, ranging from 4.13±0.74 for assessment of the common hepatic artery to 4.13±0.54 for the inferior vena cava and 4.21±0.51 for the main portal vein. The right portal vein was the vessel segment to be best delineated with

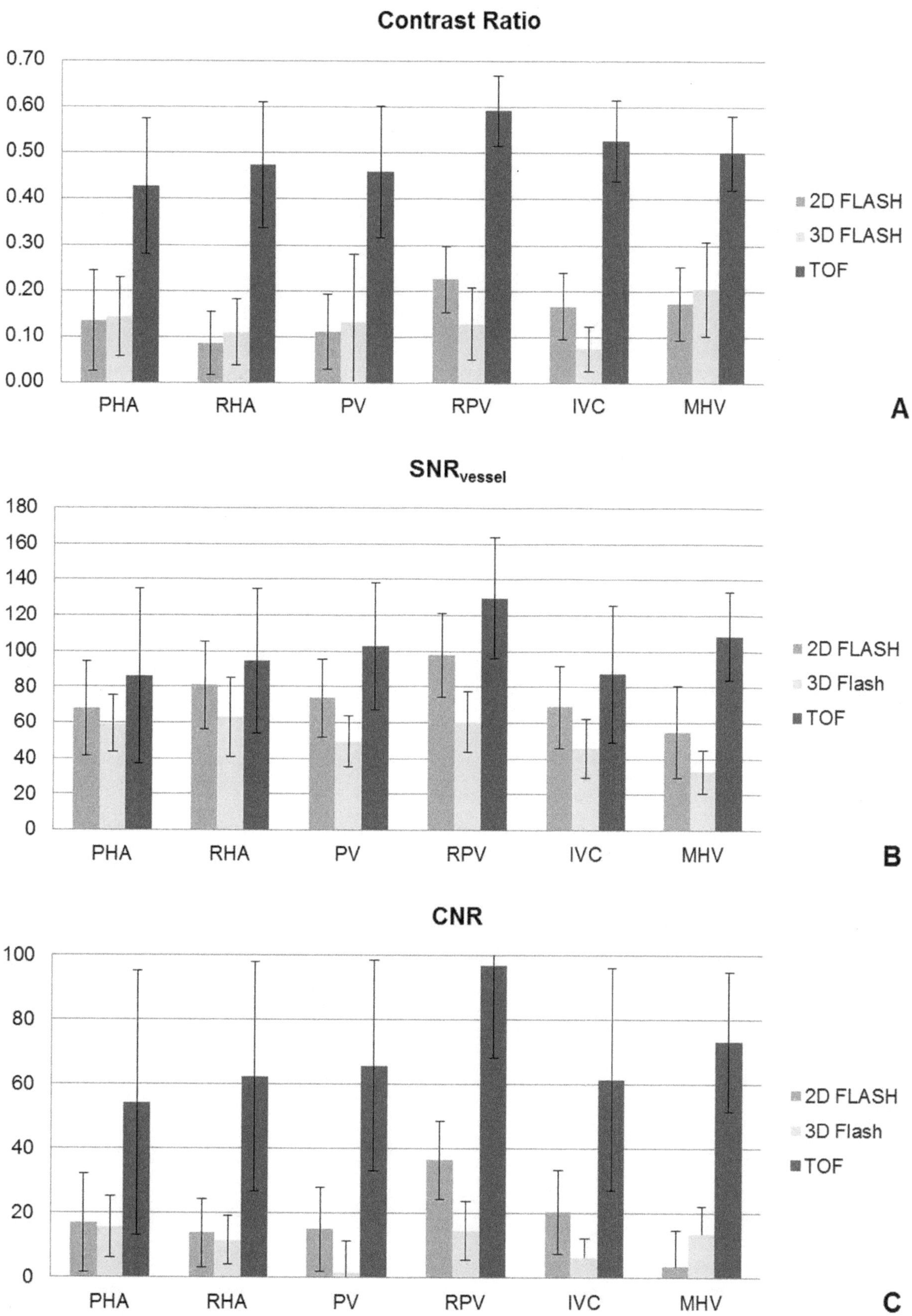

Figure 3. Quantitative analysis (A: Contrast ratios, B: SNR_{vessel}, C: CNR) for all analyzed liver vessel segments in all three sequences.

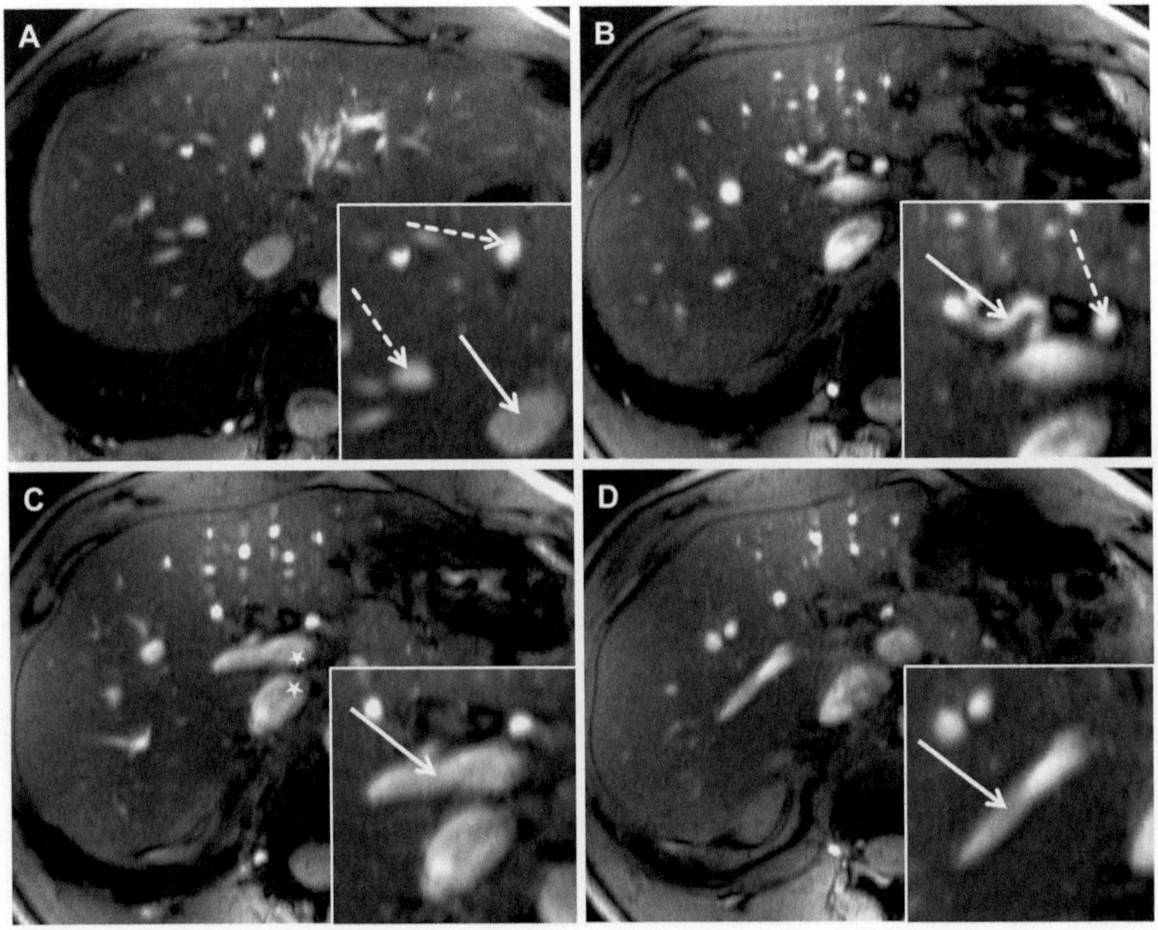

Figure 4. TOF MRA demonstrated high quality delineation of all analyzed liver vessel segments due to a hyperintensive vessel signal and an effective suppression of background signal. Figure A shows the inferior vena cava (arrow) as well as the right and middle hepatic veins (dashed arrow). A major part of the right hepatic artery (arrow) and a section of the common hepatic artery (dashed arrow) are visualized in Figure B. Figure C and D show the hyperintense delineation of the main portal vein (arrow) and the right portal vein (arrow). A slight intraluminal signal inhomogeneity could be depicted in the main portal vein and inferior vena cava (Figure C, star). Furthermore, signal drop outs due to susceptibility are visible in the stomach in the left ventral abdomen, but do not hamper vessel visualization (Figure B–D).

mean score values of 4.63±0.49. Furthermore, this sequence was least impaired by B_1 inhomogeneity (4.13±0.34) and susceptibility artifacts (4.63±0.49) out of all three sequences (p-value<0.01, respectively) (Fig. 6).

Quantitative analysis confirmed the high quality assessment of the arterial and venous liver vasculature with CR values ranging from 0.43±0.15 (PHA) to 0.59±0.08 (RPV). These CR values were considerably higher in TOF imaging compared to 2D and 3D FLASH imaging ($p = 0.02$) due to an effective background saturation of liver tissue signal.

Interobserver reliability was calculated moderate for the TOF sequence yielding mean values of 0.45 (image quality) and 0.40 (presence of artifacts).

Discussion

Noninvasive imaging techniques such as contrast-enhanced computed tomographic and magnetic resonance angiography have emerged to become excellent non-invasive alternatives to conventional catheter angiography for the evaluation of hepatic vasculature [30–35]. Gadolinium-based contrast agents for MRA were considered to be safe until first studies characterized Nephrogenic Systemic Fibrosis as a severe systemic side effect associated to the administration of gadolinium-based contrast agents in patients with acute or chronic renal insufficiency [36,37]. Owing to the onset of this severe side effect, the focus of research has shifted to non-contrast-enhanced MR angiographic techniques for the assessment of hepatic vasculature.

Recent studies at 1.5 Tesla have demonstrated the diagnostic potential of several strategies for liver vessel imaging without the need of contrast media [4,6,38]. The most common technique for non-enhanced MR angiography is based on the application of true steady-state free-precession sequences (SSFP).

Within the last few years ultra-high-field MR imaging at 7 Tesla has been introduced to in vivo human imaging. First approaches in neuro imaging revealed an interesting incidental finding, in terms of an inherently high signal intensity of the arterial vasculature in T1w imaging. This incidental finding has been shown beneficial and of high diagnostic value for non-enhanced intracranial MR angiographic applications [16,17,27,39]. With etiology remaining to be incompletely understood, a combination of steady-state and inflow effects as well as the utilization of local transmit/receive coils within a small excitation volume seem to be

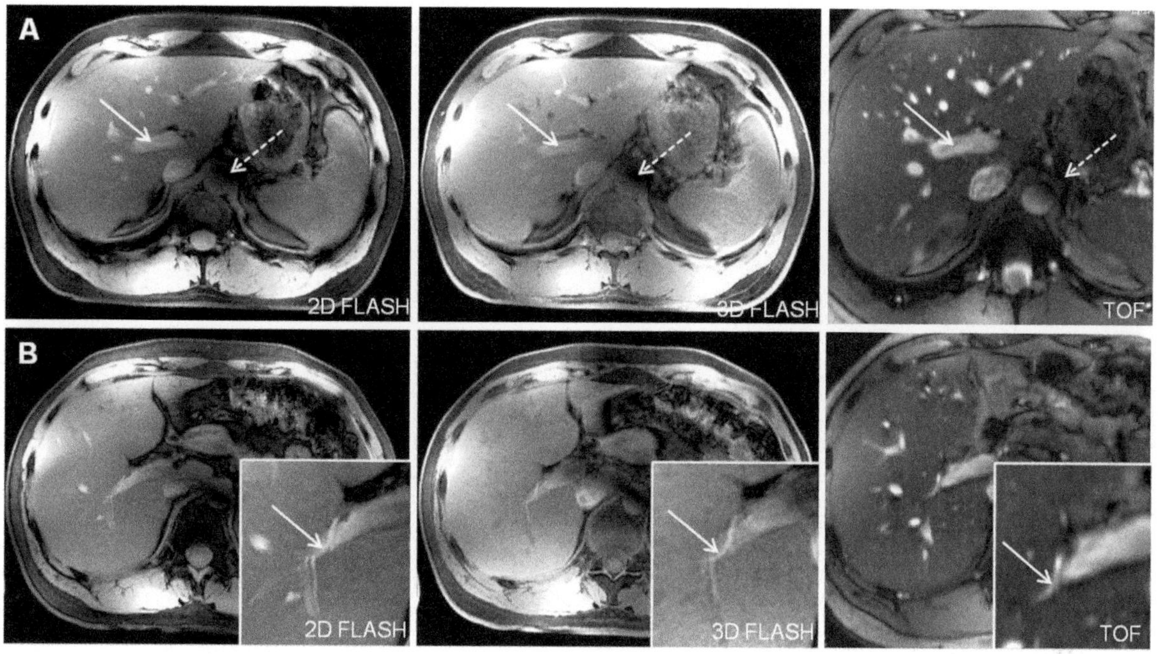

Figure 5. Depiction of the main portal vein (Figure A, arrows) and the right hepatic artery (Figure B, arrows) in all three sequences in one subject. 2D and 3D FLASH provided moderate to good image quality for both vessel segments with a slight advantage for 2D FLASH imaging due to a marginally higher contrast. TOF MRA was superior in the delineation of the liver arteries and veins from proximal to peripheral segments. Signal voids due to remaining B_1-inhomogeneity were shifted out of the liver to a periaortal focus, causing minor impairment of vessel delineation (dashed arrow in Fig. A).

accountable [40]. Thus, flowing spins are not pre-saturated by RF pulses when entering the imaging region [40].

Based on continuous development of multi-channel body coils and RF shimming technology at 7 T, the focus of research has expanded to whole-body applications, including abdominal imaging. Furthermore, the afore-mentioned hyperintense signal of the arterial vasculature could be confirmed for abdominal vessels [9,12,41,42]. Metzger et al. investigated the feasibility of non-enhanced renal MRA at 7 Tesla utilizing a respiratory triggered turbo-flash sequence [9,41]. In further 7 T studies, Umutlu et al. demonstrated the feasibility of non-enhanced as well as contrast-enhanced renal MRA. Their results showed promising results of non-enhanced renal arterial vessel imaging, utilizing T1w FLASH and TOF sequences with TOF MRA yielding best ratings in qualitative and quantitative analysis [12].

Our results go in line with previous publications on 7 T renal MRA in demonstrating the feasibility of high-quality T1w non contrast-enhanced imaging of abdominal vasculature at 7 Tesla. In accordance to a previous publication on non-enhanced renal MRA at 7 T by Umutlu et al. [12], our results also confirmed the considerable superiority of TOF MRA, regarding qualitative and quantitative evaluation due to sharply defined and homogeneously hyperintense vessel signal as well as an effective suppression of background signal. 2D and 3D FLASH imaging achieved a similar image quality and clearly lower contrast values with a slight advantage for the 2D FLASH sequence. Nevertheless, out of the three sequences, 3D FLASH imaging provided fastest acquisition (24 seconds) covering the entire liver during one breath-hold and offering high spatial resolution vessel imaging. Yet, in contrast to selective arterial vessel imaging, our results demonstrate the potential of T1w 7 T MRI not only for arterial vessels but for assessment of all three vessel types. TOF MRA revealed best delineation of the right portal vein and equivalently high quality delineation of the main portal vein as well as arterial and venous

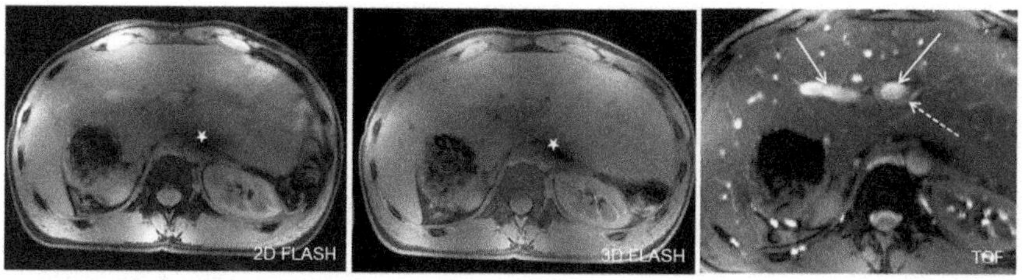

Figure 6. Figure 5 shows an anatomic variability of the upper abdomen in one healthy subject with a tall, centrally arranged liver and partially inverted situs, by means of mirrored location of spleen and stomach in the right upper abdomen. In this subject residual B_1-artifacts strongly impaired the conspicuity of central liver vessels in 2D and 3D FLASH imaging (stars in Figure A). Yet, being the sequence to be least impaired, TOF imaging allowed for a high-quality assessment of portal vein (arrow) and the left hepatic artery (dashed arrow). Figure B shows high quality delineation of the splenic artery and several small branches at the splenic hilus in all three sequences (arrows).

liver vasculature. Nevertheless, the comparatively long examination time for TOF-MRA has to be mentioned, as five imaging steps of 33 seconds each were necessary to cover the entire liver. Achieving an acquisition time within breath-hold conditions for the rather high flip angle TOF sequence was not possible. Best results regarding image quality and workflow were obtained by using a lower spatial resolution compared to FLASH acquisitions. However, to compensate for the reduced matrix the FOV of the TOF sequence was reduced to a minimum for whole-liver coverage. As an alternative, respiratory-gated imaging using a navigator is still restricted at 7 T due to an inhomogeneous excitation. At last, the breath-hold sequences acquired in the current study are advantageous regarding acquisition time compared to non-enhanced liver MRA studies at lower field strength based on SSFP imaging with acquisition times from 6–10 minutes [4,5].

Moreover, SSFP imaging is known to suffer from signal heterogeneity of the static magnetic field B_0 with increasing magnetic field strength, resulting in signal loss or dark banding artifacts [13]. An additional impairment of SSFP sequences can also be caused by SAR limitation, as SAR increases approximately with the square of the magnetic field and with the square of the flip angle. T2w Fast Spin Echo (FSE) imaging has also been proposed for non-enhanced MRA [43]. However, TSE performance at ultra-high field strength is strongly constrained by B_1 field signal alterations and by a lack of available RF power for generation of accurate refocusing pulses and high flip angles [13]. Hence, as described in previous trials on 7 T abdominal MRI, SSFP and T2w TSE imaging are strictly limited [10], leaving the exploitation of the inherently hyperintense vessel signal in T1 MRI to be a more promising method for non-contrast-enhanced liver vessel imaging at 7 Tesla.

Clearly, our initial study is not without some limitations. With increasing field strength, the Larmor wavelength is reduced to approximately 15 cm at 7 T, provoking significant B_1-field signal alterations and signal drop outs in large cross-sectional imaging [13]. These artifacts could be reduced in this trial with static RF shimming, pooling the majority of signal voids to a periaortal focus. Nevertheless, these residual B_1 artifacts caused a predominantly moderate impairment in 2D and 3D FLASH imaging, impeding the delineation of surrounding vessel structures as the main portal vein, the inferior vena cava and the common hepatic artery. Another limitation may be caused by the concomitant delineation of arterial, venous and portal venous vessels. Selective vessel delineation by dedicated vessel signal saturation would have been desirable. Yet, as stated in previous publications on 7 Tesla renal MRA [12], sufficient saturation of the inherently high vessel signal was not applicable, mainly based on B_1 inhomogeneities, SAR and peak RF power limitations associated with increasing field strength and limited coverage of the local transmit coil in contrast to a whole-body transmit coil used at clinical field strength. For body imaging at 7 T, hardware solutions in addition to improved pulse sequences are necessary. For example, Wu et al. have recently shown improved excitation homogeneity in liver MRI at 7 T with multi-spoke slice-selective parallel transmit RF pulse [44]. Additionally, further improvement of selective vessel signal suppression should be addressed in upcoming trials to improve dedicated vessel diagnostics. Finally, inflow effects depending on differences in slice thickness and TR between the three sequences, and in combination with aforementioned B1 inhomogeneities may have introduced a bias which might partially explain differences in the performance of the three sequences.

In conclusion, the initial results of our study demonstrate the feasibility of non-contrast-enhanced 7 Tesla liver vessel imaging and the challenges of this emerging technique. Non-enhanced T1w imaging in general and TOF MRA in particular, appear to be promising techniques for good quality liver vessel assessment at 7 T. Comparison trials to contrast-enhanced MRA in healthy subjects and patients with liver vessel pathologies should be addressed in future studies to assess the diagnostic competence of non-enhanced liver vessel MRI at 7 T.

Author Contributions

Conceived and designed the experiments: AF LU TCL OK. Performed the experiments: AF OK SM. Analyzed the data: AF KB. Contributed reagents/materials/analysis tools: MEL TCL MF. Wrote the paper: AF LU OK.

References

1. Saba L, Mallarini G (2008) Multidetector row CT angiography in the evaluation of the hepatic artery and its anatomical variants. Clin Radiol 63: 312–321.
2. Streitparth F, Pech M, Figolska S, Denecke T, Grieser C, et al. (2007) Living related liver transplantation: Preoperative magnetic resonance imaging for assessment of hepatic vasculature of donor candidates. Acta Radiol 48: 20–26.
3. Grobner T (2006) Gadolinium–a specific trigger for the development of nephrogenic fibrosing dermopathy and nephrogenic systemic fibrosis? Nephrol Dial Transplant 21: 1104–1108.
4. Shimada K, Isoda H, Okada T, Maetani Y, Arizono S, et al. (2009) Non-contrast-enhanced hepatic MR angiography with true steady-state free-precession and time spatial labeling inversion pulse: Optimization of the technique and preliminary results. Eur J Radiol 70: 111–117.
5. Shimada K, Isoda H, Okada T, Kamae T, Maetani Y, et al. (2009) Non-contrast-enhanced MR angiography for selective visualization of the hepatic vein and inferior vena cava with true steady-state free-precession sequence and time-spatial labeling inversion pulses: Preliminary results. J Magn Reson Imaging 29: 474–479.
6. Shimada K, Isoda H, Okada T, Kamae T, Arizono S, et al. (2009) Non-contrast-enhanced MR portography with time-spatial labeling inversion pulses: Comparison of imaging with three-dimensional half-fourier fast spin-echo and true steady-state free-precession sequences. J Magn Reson Imaging 29: 1140–1146.
7. Ramalho M, Altun E, Heredia V, Zapparoli M, Semelka R (2007) Liver MR imaging: 1.5T versus 3T. Magn Reson Imaging Clin N Am 15: 321–47, vi.
8. Vaughan JT, Snyder CJ, DelaBarre LJ, Bolan PJ, Tian J, et al. (2009) Whole-body imaging at 7T: Preliminary results. Magn Reson Med 61: 244–248.
9. Metzger GJ, Simonson J, Bi X, Weale P, Zuehlsdorff S, et al. (2010) Initial experience with non-contrast enhanced renal angiography at 7.0 tesla. ISMRM 403.
10. Umutlu L, Bitz AK, Maderwald S, Orzada S, Kinner S, et al. (2011) Contrast-enhanced ultra-high-field liver MRI: A feasibility trial. Eur J Radiol 82: 760–767.
11. Metzger GJ, Auerbach EJ, Akgun C, Simonson J, Bi X, et al. (2012) Dynamically applied B(1) (+) shimming solutions for non-contrast enhanced renal angiography at 7.0 tesla. Magn Reson Med 69: 114–126.
12. Umutlu L, Maderwald S, Kraff O, Kinner S, Schaefer LC, et al. (2012) A new look at renal vasculature: 7 tesla non-enhanced T1-weighted FLASH imaging. Investigative Radiology 36: 714–721.
13. Moser E, Stahlberg F, Ladd ME, Trattnig S (2012) 7-T MR-from research to clinical applications? NMR Biomed 25: 695–716.
14. Bernstein MA, Huston J 3rd, Ward HA (2006) Imaging artifacts at 3.0T. J Magn Reson Imaging 24: 735–746.
15. Ladd ME (2007) High-field-strength magnetic resonance: Potential and limits. Top Magn Reson Imaging 18: 139–152.
16. Umutlu L, Theysohn N, Maderwald S, Johst S, Lauenstein TC, et al. (2013) 7 tesla MPRAGE imaging of the intracranial arterial vasculature: Nonenhanced versus contrast-enhanced. Acad Radiol 20: 628–634.
17. Wrede KH, Dammann P, Monninghoff C, Johst S, Maderwald S, et al. (2014) Non-enhanced MR imaging of cerebral aneurysms: 7 tesla versus 1.5 tesla. PLoS One 9: e84562.
18. Fischer A, Maderwald S, Orzada S, Johst S, Schafer LC, et al. (2013) Nonenhanced magnetic resonance angiography of the lower extremity vessels at 7 tesla: Initial experience. Invest Radiol 48: 525–534.
19. Johst S, Orzada S, Fischer A, Schäfer L, Nassenstein K, et al. (2014) Sequence comparison for non-enhanced MRA of the lower extremity arteries at 7 tesla. PloS One 9: e86274.
20. Orzada S, Quick HH, Ladd ME (2009) A flexible 8-channel transmit/receive body coil for 7 T human imaging. ISMRM 2999.

21. Hoult DI, Phil D (2000) Sensitivity and power deposition in a high-field imaging experiment. J Magn Reson Imaging 12: 46–67.
22. Bitz AK, Brote I, Orzada S, Kraff O, Maderwald S, et al. (2009) An 8-channel add-on RF shimming system for whole-body 7 tesla MRI including real-time SAR monitoring. ISMRM 4767.
23. Sacolick LI, Wiesinger F, Hancu I, Vogel MW (2010) B1 mapping by bloch-siegert shift. Magn Reson Med 63: 1315–1322.
24. Duan Q, van Gelderen P, Duyn J (2013) Improved bloch-siegert based B1 mapping by reducing off-resonance shift. NMR Biomed 26: 1070–1078.
25. International Electrotechnical Commission (2002) Medical electrical equipment-part 2–33: Particular requirements for the safety of magnetic resonance diagnostic devices. IEC 60601-2-33.
26. Christ A, Kainz W, Hahn EG, Honegger K, Zefferer M, et al. (2010) The virtual family–development of surface-based anatomical models of two adults and two children for dosimetric simulations. Phys Med Biol 55: N23–38.
27. Maderwald S, Ladd SC, Gizewski ER, Kraff O, Theysohn JM, et al. (2008) To TOF or not to TOF: Strategies for non-contrast-enhanced intracranial MRA at 7 T. MAGMA 21: 159–167.
28. Dietrich O, Raya JG, Reeder SB, Ingrisch M, Reiser MF, et al. (2008) Influence of multichannel combination, parallel imaging and other reconstruction techniques on MRI noise characteristics. Magn Reson Imaging 26: 754–762.
29. Landis JR, Koch GG (1977) The measurement of observer agreement for categorical data. Biometrics 33: 159–174.
30. Carr JC, Nemcek AA Jr, Abecassis M, Blei A, Clarke L, et al. (2003) Preoperative evaluation of the entire hepatic vasculature in living liver donors with use of contrast-enhanced MR angiography and true fast imaging with steady-state precession. J Vasc Interv Radiol 14: 441–449.
31. Aslam R, Yeh BM, Yee J (2010) MR imaging evaluation of the hepatic vasculature. Magn Reson Imaging Clin N Am 18: 515–23, xi.
32. Lee MW, Lee JM, Lee JY, Kim SH, Park EA, et al. (2007) Preoperative evaluation of hepatic arterial and portal venous anatomy using the time resolved echo-shared MR angiographic technique in living liver donors. Eur Radiol 17: 1074–1080.
33. Lee MW, Lee JM, Lee JY, Kim SH, Park EA, et al. (2006) Preoperative evaluation of the hepatic vascular anatomy in living liver donors: Comparison of CT angiography and MR angiography. J Magn Reson Imaging 24: 1081–1087.
34. Sahani D, Mehta A, Blake M, Prasad S, Harris G, et al. (2004) Preoperative hepatic vascular evaluation with CT and MR angiography: Implications for surgery. Radiographics 24: 1367–1380.
35. Uchida K, Taniguchi M, Shimamura T, Suzuki T, Yamashita K, et al. (2010) Three-dimensional computed tomography scan analysis of hepatic vasculatures in the donor liver for living donor liver transplantation. Liver Transpl 16: 1062–1068.
36. Grobner T, Prischl FC (2007) Gadolinium and nephrogenic systemic fibrosis. Kidney Int 72: 260–264.
37. Lauenstein TC, Salman K, Morreira R, Tata S, Tudorascu D, et al. (2007) Nephrogenic systemic fibrosis: Center case review. J Magn Reson Imaging 26: 1198–1203.
38. Puippe GD, Alkadhi H, Hunziker R, Nanz D, Pfammatter T, et al. (2012) Performance of unenhanced respiratory-gated 3D SSFP MRA to depict hepatic and visceral artery anatomy and variants. Eur J Radiol 81: e823–9.
39. Monninghoff C, Maderwald S, Theysohn JM, Kraff O, Ladd SC, et al. (2009) Evaluation of intracranial aneurysms with 7 T versus 1.5 T time-of-flight MR angiography - initial experience. Rofo 181: 16–23.
40. Grinstead JW, Rooney W, Laub G (2010) The origins of bright blood MPRAGE at 7 tesla and a simultaneous method for T1 imaging and non-contrast MRA. ISMRM 1429.
41. Metzger GJ, Auerbach EJ, Akgun C, Simonson J, Bi X, et al. (2013) Dynamically applied B(1) (+) shimming solutions for non-contrast enhanced renal angiography at 7.0 tesla. Magn Reson Med 69: 114–26.
42. Umutlu L, Kraff O, Orzada S, Fischer A, Kinner S, et al. (2011) Dynamic contrast-enhanced renal MRI at 7 tesla: Preliminary results. Invest Radiol 46: 425–433.
43. Shimada K, Isoda H, Okada T, Kamae T, Arizono S, et al. (2009) Unenhanced MR portography with a half-fourier fast spin-echo sequence and time-space labeling inversion pulses: Preliminary results. AJR Am J Roentgenol 193: 106–112.
44. Wu X, Schmitter S, Auerbach EJ, Ugurbil K, Van de Moortele PF (2014) Mitigating transmit B 1 inhomogeneity in the liver at 7T using multi-spoke parallel transmit RF pulse design. Quant Imaging Med Surg 4: 4–10.

2

Non-Enhanced MR Imaging of Cerebral Aneurysms: 7 Tesla versus 1.5 Tesla

Karsten H. Wrede[1,2]*, Philipp Dammann[1,2], Christoph Mönninghoff[3], Sören Johst[1,3], Stefan Maderwald[1,3], I. Erol Sandalcioglu[2], Oliver Müller[2], Neriman Özkan[2], Mark E. Ladd[1,3], Michael Forsting[3], Marc U. Schlamann[3], Ulrich Sure[2], Lale Umutlu[1,3]

1 Erwin L. Hahn Institute for Magnetic Resonance Imaging, University Duisburg-Essen, Essen, Germany, **2** Department of Neurosurgery, University Hospital Essen, Essen, Germany, **3** Department of Diagnostic and Interventional Radiology and Neuroradiology, University Hospital Essen, Essen, Germany

Abstract

Purpose: To prospectively evaluate 7 Tesla time-of-flight (TOF) magnetic resonance angiography (MRA) in comparison to 1.5 Tesla TOF MRA and 7 Tesla non-contrast enhanced magnetization-prepared rapid acquisition gradient-echo (MPRAGE) for delineation of unruptured intracranial aneurysms (UIA).

Material and Methods: Sixteen neurosurgical patients (male n = 5, female n = 11) with single or multiple UIA were enrolled in this trial. All patients were accordingly examined at 7 Tesla and 1.5 Tesla MRI utilizing dedicated head coils. The following sequences were obtained: 7 Tesla TOF MRA, 1.5 Tesla TOF MRA and 7 Tesla non-contrast enhanced MPRAGE. Image analysis was performed by two radiologists with regard to delineation of aneurysm features (dome, neck, parent vessel), presence of artifacts, vessel-tissue-contrast and overall image quality. Interobserver accordance and intermethod comparisons were calculated by kappa coefficient and Lin's concordance correlation coefficient.

Results: A total of 20 intracranial aneurysms were detected in 16 patients, with two patients showing multiple aneurysms (n = 2, n = 4). Out of 20 intracranial aneurysms, 14 aneurysms were located in the anterior circulation and 6 aneurysms in the posterior circulation. 7 Tesla MPRAGE imaging was superior over 1.5 and 7 Tesla TOF MRA in the assessment of all considered aneurysm and image quality features (e.g. image quality: mean MPRAGE7T: 5.0; mean TOF7T: 4.3; mean TOF1.5T: 4.3). Ratings for 7 Tesla TOF MRA were equal or higher over 1.5 Tesla TOF MRA for all assessed features except for artifact delineation (mean TOF7T: 4.3; mean TOF1.5T 4.4). Interobserver accordance was good to excellent for most ratings.

Conclusion: 7 Tesla MPRAGE imaging demonstrated its superiority in the detection and assessment of UIA as well as overall imaging features, offering excellent interobserver accordance and highest scores for all ratings. Hence, it may bear the potential to serve as a high-quality diagnostic tool for pretherapeutic assessment and follow-up of untreated UIA.

Editor: Zhuoli Zhang, Northwestern University Feinberg School of Medicine, United States of America

Funding: An IFORES grant to KHW from the University Duisburg-Essen supported the research [http://www.uni-due.de/med/forschung/forschungsfoerderung/ifores.shtml]. The funders had no role in study design, data collection and analysis, decision to publish, or preparation of the manuscript.

Competing Interests: The authors have declared that no competing interests exist.

* E-mail: karsten.wrede@uk-essen.de

Introduction

Rupture of intracranial aneurysm is associated with high morbidity and mortality rates, as it is known to be accountable for 80% of all subarachnaoid hemorrhages (SAH), causing 25% of all cerebrovascular-related deaths, [1]. Size and shape of unruptured intracranial aneurysms (UIA) are known to be significantly affiliated with rupture rates, hence, high-quality assessment of UIA and its related features displays an important role on potential aneurysm treatment [2–4].

Digital subtraction angiography (DSA) is considered the gold standard for detection of UIA. Nevertheless, due to the application of ionizing radiation and iodinated contrast agent as well as the general risk affiliated to invasive interventional procedures, DSA is associated with a 0.2%–0.5% risk for severe permanent neurological complications [5,6].

Within the past 15 years, 1.5 Tesla magnetic resonance angiography (MRA) has evolved to become an excellent non-invasive diagnostic alternative to DSA, yielding sensitivity rates of 79–97% for the detection of small UIA [7–10]. With the successful introduction of (ultra-) highfield non-enhanced MRA of the intracranial vasculature, recent studies performed at 3 and 7 Tesla reported improved depiction of UIA with sensitivity rates comparable to the gold standard DSA [11–14]. The increase of the magnetic field strength from 1.5 to 3 Tesla, and respectively to 7 Tesla, allowed for a successful transition of the increased signal-to-noise (SNR) and contrast-to-noise ratio (CNR) to improvements in spatial resolution and vessel contrast.

The purpose of this prospective study was to evaluate the image quality and diagnostic ability in the assessment of UIA of 1.5 Tesla TOF MRA in comparison to ultra-high-field TOF MRA and non-enhanced MPRAGE imaging.

Table 1. Basic demographic data and aneurysm size and location.

aneurysm	subject	sex	age	location	side	7 Tesla TOF MRA Ø in mm*	1.5 Tesla TOF MRA Ø in mm*	7 Tesla MPRAGE Ø in mm*
1	1	female	52	ICA	left	8	7.5	7
2	2	female	56	giant ICA	right	36.5	34	35.5
3	3	female	69	ICA	left	16.5	17	18
4	4	female	56	MCA	left	8.5	8.5	9
5				BT		2.5	2.5	2.5
6	5	male	70	BT		6.5	6.5	6.5
7	6	male	45	PCA	left	18	13.5	16.5
8	7	female	66	ACA	right	1.5	1	1.5
9				PICA	right	4	3	4
10				MCA	left	5	5	5
11				MCA	right	10.5	10	10.5
12	8	female	54	MCA	right	4.5	4.5	6
13	9	female	60	ICA	right	17	17	16.5
14	10	female	44	ACA	right	2.5	2.5	2.5
15	11	female	53	MCA	right	8	8	8
16	12	male	45	MCA	left	5	5	4.5
17	13	female	49	MCA	left	6	5.5	5
18	14	male	38	PCA	left	4.5	4.5	3.5
19	15	male	55	PcomA	right	4.5	3.5	2.5
20	16	female	42	SC	right	3.5	2.5	2.5

internal carotid artery (ICA).
middle cerebral artery (MCA).
basilar tip (BT).
posterior cerebral artery (PCA).
anterior cerebral artery (ACA).
posterior inferior cerebellar artery (PICA).
posterior communicating artery (PcomA).
superior cerebellar artery (SC).
*mean diameter from both readers.

Materials and Methods

Ethics Statement

The study was conducted according to the principles expressed in the Declaration of Helsinki and was approved by the authorized ethical review board of the University Duisburg-Essen. Written informed consent was obtained before each examination.

Study Design and Population

This prospective study evaluates the diagnostic ability of 7 Tesla TOF MRA in comparison to 1.5 Tesla TOF MRA and 7 Tesla non-contrast enhanced MPRAGE for delineation of UIA. The study group comprised 16 neurosurgical patients (male n = 5, female n = 11, average age 53.38 years; range 38–70 years). Inclusion criteria were: 1) single or multiple UIA, 2) age 18–80 years, 3) ability to give informed consent and 4) legal

Table 2. Interobserver accordance (kappa-statistic).

	dome	neck	parent vessel	artifacts	vessel-tissue contrast	overall image quality
7 T TOF MRA	0.75	0.79	0.85	0.89	0.88	0.50
1.5 T TOF MRA	0.39	0.80	0.73	0.71	0.84	0.68
7 T MPRAGE	0.26	1.00	0.92	1.00	0.84	1.00

According to Landis the kappa coefficient (k) was rated as follows:
Poor (k<0.00), Slight (k = 0.00–0.20), Fair (k = 0.21–0.40), Moderate (k = 0.41–0.60).
Substantial (k = 0.61–0.80), Almost Perfect (k = 0.81–1.00).
Disagreements were weighted by 1– {(i–j)/(k–1)}2 where i and j index the rows and columns of the ratings by the two raters and k is the maximum number of possible ratings.

competence. Exclusion criteria were: 1) cardiac pacemakers or any other electronic implants, 2) metallic implants, 3) pregnancy or breast feeding period, 4) claustrophobia and 5) chronic or episodic vertigo. All patients were accordingly examined at a 7 Tesla (Magnetom 7T, Siemens) and a 1.5 Tesla MR scanner system (Espree, Siemens) utilizing dedicated head coils. The following sequences were obtained: (1) 7 Tesla TOF MRA, (2) 1.5 Tesla TOF MRA and (3) 7 Tesla non-contrast enhanced MPRAGE. A total of 20 intracranial aneurysms were detected, with two patients showing multiple aneurysms (2, respectively 4 aneurysms).

Scanners and Coil Systems

Ultra-high-field examinations were acquired on a 7 Tesla whole-body MRI system (Magnetom 7T, Siemens Healthcare, Erlangen, Germany) utilizing a 32-channel Tx/Rx head coil (Nova Medical, Wilmington, USA). The scanner is equipped with a gradient system of 45 mT/m maximum amplitude and a slew rate of 200 mT/m/ms.

Concomitant 1.5 Tesla examinations were acquired on a whole-body MRI system (Espree, Siemens Healthcare) equipped with a 12-channel Rx head coil (Siemens Healthcare, Erlangen, Germany). The scanner is equipped with a gradient system of 33 mT/m maximum amplitude and a slew rate of 200 mT/m/ms.

Examination at 7 Tesla

Prior to the acquisition of the diagnostic sequences B_0 shimming was performed using a vendor-provided gradient echo sequence and algorithm based on the work of Schar [15]. For B_1 field mapping and local flip angle optimization a vender provided spin-echo type sequence was used. After a slice selective excitation, two refocusing pulses generate a spin-echo and a stimulated echo, respectively. The algorithm is mainly based on the work of Hoult [16].

TOF MRA sequence at 7 Tesla

The TOF MRA sequence is based on a 3D FLASH sequence with flow compensation and tilt-optimized non-saturated excitation (TONE) across the slab [17]. Datasets were acquired with an excitation flip angle of $\alpha = 18°$, TE $= 4.34$ ms, TR $= 20$ ms, FOV 200 mm $\times$169 mm $\times$46 mm, 112 slices per slab (oversampling 14%), GRAPPA acceleration factor R = 4 (phase direction), partial Fourier 6/8 in both slice and phase directions, matrix of 896$\times$756 (non-interpolated), and a voxel size of $0.22\times0.22\times0.41$ mm^3 in a total acquisition time of 6 min 22 s. The variable-rate selective excitation (VERSE) algorithm {Conolly, 1988#1168} was used to reduce SAR contribution of excitation and venous saturation RF pulses {Schmitter, 2011#1484}. The flip angle of the saturation RF pulses was additionally reduced ($\alpha_{SAT} = 35°$ instead of 90° which is normally used) to further ameliorate SAR constraints [17].

MPRAGE sequence at 7 Tesla

MPRAGE imaging was obtained with the following sequence parameters: TR = 2500 ms, TE = 1.54 ms, TI = 1100 ms,

Table 3. Ratings for dome, neck and parent vessel delineation (mean ratings from both readers).

aneurysm	7 Tesla	1.5 Tesla	7 Tesla	7 Tesla	1.5 Tesla	7 Tesla	7 Tesla	1.5 Tesla	7 Tesla
	TOF MRA	TOF MRA	MPRAGE	TOF MRA	TOF MRA	MPRAGE	TOF MRA	TOF MRA	MPRAGE
	dome	dome	dome	neck	neck	neck	parent vessel	parent vessel	parent vessel
1	5	4	5	4	5	5	4	5	5
2	4.5	3	3.5	5	4	2	5	4	3.5
3	4	3	5	4.5	4	5	4	5	4
4	5	4	5	5	5	5	5	4.5	5
5	4.5	3.5	4.5	5	4	5	5	4.5	5
6	5	4	5	5	4	5	5	4	5
7	5	3.5	5	5	3	5	5	3	5
8	4	4	4.5	4.5	3.5	5	4	3	5
9	4	4.5	4	4	3.5	5	4	4	5
10	4.5	4.5	5	4.5	5	5	4.5	5	5
11	5	4	4.5	5	4.5	5	4.5	4	5
12	3	4	5	4	3	5	4	4	5
13	4	4	5	3	4	4	3	4	3
14	5	4	5	5	3.5	5	5	4	5
15	5	3.5	5	5	4	5	5	3.5	5
16	5	4.5	5	4	3	5	4	3	5
17	5	4.5	5	5	3	5	4	3	5
18	4	4	5	4	3	5	4	3.5	5
19	3.5	3	5	4	4	5	4	3.5	5
20	5	3.5	5	4	3	5	5	4	5
mean	**4.5**	**3.9**	**4.8**	**4.5**	**3.8**	**4.8**	**4.4**	**3.9**	**4.8**

5 = excellent. 4 = good. 3 = moderate. 2 = poor. and 1 = non-diagnostic vessel delineation.

Table 4. Combined readings of both raters for dome and neck diameter in mm and dome/neck ratio (DNR) for all aneurysms.

Subject	7 Tesla	7 Tesla	7 Tesla	7 Tesla	7 Tesla	7 Tesla	1.5 Tesla	1.5 Tesla	1.5 Tesla
	MPRAGE	MPRAGE	MPRAGE	TOF MRA	TOF MRA	TOF MRA	TOF MRA	TOF MRA	TOF MRA
	dome	neck	DNR	dome	neck	DNR	dome	neck	DNR
1	6.5	3	2.167	7	3	2.333	6	3	2
2	35	11	3.182	34	11	3.091	34	10.5	3.238
3	10	4	2.5	10	3	3.333	9.5	3	3.167
4	8	2	4	8	3	2.667	8.5	3	2.833
5	2.5	2	1.25	2.5	2	1.25	2.5	2	1.25
6	6.5	2	3.25	6.5	2.5	2.6	6.5	2	3.25
7	15	2	7.5	15	2	7.5	13.5	2	6.75
8	1.5	1	1.5	1.5	1	1.5	1	1	1
9	4	2	2	4	2	2	3	2.5	1.2
10	5	2	2.5	5	2	2.5	5	2	2.5
11	10.5	3	3.5	10	3	3.333	10	3	3.333
12	4	2	2	4	1	4	4	2	2
13	16.5	4.5	3.667	17	5	3.4	17	5.5	3.091
14	2.5	2	1.25	2.5	2	1.25	2.5	2	1.25
15	8	2	4	8	2	4	8	2	4
16	4.5	2	2.25	4	1.5	2.667	4	2	2
17	4	2	2	4	2	2	4	2	2
18	3	1	3	3	1	3	3	2	1.5
19	2.5	1	2.5	3	1	3	3	1	3
20	2.5	2	1.25	3	2	1.5	2.5	2	1.25
mean			*2.763*			**2.846**			***2.531***

*standard error = 0.318, 95% confidence interval [2.098–3.428].
**standard error = 0.307, 95% confidence interval [2.203–3.489].
***standard error = 0.299, 95% confidence interval [1.906–3.156].

TA = 6 min 13 s, GRAPPA acceleration factor R = 2, excitation flip angle $\alpha = 7°$, adiabatic WURST pulse for magnetization preparation [18], bandwidth = 570 Hz/px, 256 slices per slab (slice oversampling 75%), matrix 384×336 (non-interpolated), FOV = 270×236 mm^2, voxel size 0.7×0.7×0.7 mm^3.

TOF MRA sequence at 1.5 Tesla

The TOF MRA sequence was based on a clinically used standard 3D gradient echo sequence. Datasets were acquired with an excitation flip angle of $\alpha = 25°$, TE = 7 ms, TR = 26 ms, matrix 512×448 (interpolated), FOV 180 mm ×157 mm, 3 slabs with 44 slices per slab (oversampling 18.2%) and a voxel size of 0.35×0.35×0.7 mm^3 in a total acquisition time of 4 min 3 s.

Image Evaluation

Image evaluation was performed separately and independently by two experienced radiologists on standard post-processing Picture Archiving and Communcation system (PACS) workstations (Centricity RIS 4.0i, GE Healthcare, USA). Both radiologists were blinded to image acquisition methods and intracranial pathologies. Visual evaluation was performed using 3D image reconstructions; all measurements were performed on 2D multiplanar reconstructions of the 3D datasets. The total number of aneurysms, the maximal diameter as well as the diameter of neck and dome of each aneurysm were assessed. For qualitative analysis the following features were evaluated, utilizing a five-point scale (5 = excellent, 4 = good, 3 = moderate, 2 = poor, and 1 = non-diagnostic vessel delineation):

1. Delineation of aneurysm dome
2. Delineation of aneurysm neck
3. Delineation of parent vessel
4. Presence of artifacts
5. Vessel tissue contrast
6. Overall image quality.

Vessel-tissue contrast ratio $\left(VTCR = \frac{Signal_{MCA} - Signal_{GM}}{Signal_{MCA} + Signal_{GM}}\right)$ of the middle cerebral artery (MCA) was assessed in correlation to surrounding gray matter (GM) for 7 Tesla MPRAGE sequences, 7 Tesla TOF sequences and for 1.5 Tesla TOF sequences. Therefore, regions of interest (ROI) were placed in the largest diameter of the proximal left M1 segments ($Signal_{MCA}$) and adjacent gray matter ($Signal_{GM}$). The average diameter for the ROI of the vessel was 3–5 mm; the ROI for brain parenchyma amounted to approximately 10 mm.

Interobserver accordance for ordinal scale variables were rated using the kappa coefficient [19] (k) according to Landis [20] as follows: Poor (k<0.00), Slight (k = 0.00–0.20), Fair (k = 0.21–0.40), Moderate (k = 0.41–0.60), Substantial (k = 0.61–0.80), Almost Perfect (k = 0.81–1.00). Interobserver accordance for ratio scale variables were rated using Lin's [21,22] concordance correlation

Table 5. Ratings for artifacts. vessel-tissue contrast (VTC) and overall image quality (mean ratings from both readers).

aneurysm	7 Tesla	1.5 Tesla	7 Tesla	7 Tesla	1.5 Tesla	7 Tesla	7 Tesla	1.5 Tesla	7 Tesla
	TOF MRA	TOF MRA	MPRAGE	TOF MRA	TOF MRA	MPRAGE	TOF MRA	TOF MRA	MPRAGE
	artifacts	artifacts	artifacts	VTC	VTC	VTC	image quality	image quality	image quality
1	4.5	5	5	5	3.5	5	4	4.5	4.5
2	4	4.5	5	4.5	3	3.5	4	4	5
3	3.5	5	5	5	4	5	4.5	5	5
4	5	5	5	5	4.5	5	4.5	4.5	5
5	5	5	5	5	4	5	4.5	5	5
6	5	5	5	5	5	5	5	5	5
7	5	3.5	5	5	4	5	4.5	4.5	5
8	5	4	5	5	4	5	5	5	5
9	4	5	5	4.5	5	5	4.5	4.5	5
10	5	5	5	4	5	5	4	4	5
11	5	4.5	5	5	4	5	5	5	5
12	3	4	5	3	5	5	4	4	5
13	3	3.5	5	3	4	4	3	3	5
14	4	5	5	4	4	5	4	4	5
15	4	4	5	4	5	5	4.5	4	5
16	4	4	5	4	4	5	4	4	5
17	4	4	5	4	4	5	4	4	5
18	4	4	5	4	4	5	4	4	5
19	4	4	5	4	4	5	4	4	5
20	4	4	5	4	4	5	4	4	5
mean	**4.3**	**4.4**	**5.0**	**4.4**	**4.2**	**4.9**	**4.3**	**4.3**	**5.0**

5= excellent. 4= good. 3= moderate. 2= poor. and 1= non-diagnostic vessel delineation.

coefficient. For intermethod comparison the Wilcoxon signed rank test was applied. Differences of continuous scaled variables were tested by Student's t-test.

Statistical analysis was carried out with the STATA software package (Stata/SE 12.1 for Mac (64-bit Intel), StataCorp, 4905 Lakeway Drive, College Station, Texas 77845 USA).

Results

All 1.5 Tesla and 7 Tesla scans were performed successfully without any relevant side effects. Both readers identified twenty intracranial aneurysms in 1.5 Tesla and 7 Tesla TOF MRA and 7 Tesla MPRAGE imaging. Fourteen of the twenty intracranial aneurysms were located in the anterior circulation: middle cerebral artery (n = 7), anterior cerebral artery (n = 2), internal carotid artery (n = 4) and posterior communicating artery (n = 1). Six aneurysms were detected in the posterior circulation: basilar tip (n = 2), posterior cerebral artery (n = 2), posterior inferior cerebellar artery (n = 1) and superior cerebellar artery (n = 1). Two patients had multiple intracranial aneurysms (2, respectively 4 aneurysms). Ten of twenty identified aneurysms were defined as small (3–5 mm), five as medium-sized (6–10 mm), three as large (11–25 mm) and one was rated a giant cerebral aneurysm (>35 mm). The mean aneurysm size was 8.65 mm (Standard Error (SE) 1.823) for the 7 Tesla TOF MRA reading, 8.075 mm (SE 1.708) for the 1.5 Tesla TOF MRA reading and 8 mm (SE 1.826) for the 7 Tesla MPRAGE reading. Interobserver accordance measured by Lin's concordance correlation coefficient was substantial for 7 Tesla TOF MRA readings (ρc = 0.963) and 1.5 Tesla TOF MRA readings (ρc = 0.951) and moderate for 7 Tesla MPRAGE readings (pc = 0.922). Table 1 shows an overview on basic demographic data and aneurysm size and location.

Dome, neck and parent vessel

Mean score values of both readers' for delineation of the aneurysm dome were 4.5 (excellent) (SE 0.136) for 7 Tesla TOF MRA, 3.9 (good) (SE 0.109) for 1.5 Tesla TOF MRA and 4.8 (excellent) (SE 0.092) for 7 Tesla MPRAGE imaging. Wilcoxon matched-pairs two-sided signed-ranks test showed significant differences between 7 Tesla TOF MRA and 1.5 Tesla TOF MRA (p = 0.0042) ratings as well as between 7 Tesla MPRAGE and 1.5 Tesla TOF MRA (p = 0.0000) ratings. There were no significant differences between 7 Tesla TOF MRA and 7 Tesla MPRAGE (p = 0.1797) ratings.

The delineation of the aneurysm neck was rated 4.5 (excellent) (SE 0.128) in 7 Tesla TOF MRA, 3.8 (good) (SE 0.156) in 1.5 Tesla TOF MRA and 4.8 (excellent) (SE 0.156) in 7 Tesla MPRAGE MRI. Wilcoxon matched-pairs two-sided signed-ranks test showed significant differences between 7 Tesla TOF MRA and 1.5 Tesla TOF MRA (p = 0.0075) ratings, between 7 Tesla MPRAGE and 1.5 Tesla TOF MRA (p = 0.0005) ratings as well as between 7 Tesla TOF MRA and 7 Tesla MPRAGE (p = 0.0063) ratings.

Table 6. Combined readings of both raters for signal intensities of left middle cerebral artery, adjacent gray matter and calculated vessel-tissue contrast ratio for all subjects.

Subject	7T MPRAGE left MCA	7T MPRAGE GM	7T MPRAGE VTCR	7T TOF left MCA	7T TOF GM	7T TOF VTCR	1.5T TOF left MCA	1.5T TOF GM	1.5T TOF VTCR
1	1032	263	0.594	908	145	0.725	486	132	0.573
2	1071	282	0.583	1063	192	0.694	581	142	0.607
3	543	135	0.602	881	216	0.606	409	89	0.643
4	897	204	0.629	897	157	0.702	408	106	0.588
5	773	141	0.691	785	185	0.619	438	128	0.548
6	844	179	0.650	864	176	0.662	519	139	0.578
7	1014	205	0.664	951	193	0.663	532	143	0.576
8	913	188	0.658	1088	154	0.752	485	121	0.601
9	851	141	0.716	851	176	0.657	426	94	0.638
10	998	152	0.736	912	198	0.643	508	105	0.657
11	846	174	0.659	865	202	0.621	470	113	0.612
12	909	240	0.582	921	193	0.654	520	133	0.593
13	858	219	0.593	818	175	0.648	534	149	0.564
14	792	165	0.655	944	209	0.637	411	92	0.634
15	831	141	0.710	902	196	0.643	540	127	0.619
16	926	186	0.665	843	184	0.642	494	108	0.641
mean			*0.649*			**0.660**			***0.604***

Vessel-tissue contrast ratio $\left(VTCR = \frac{Signal_{MCA} - Signal_{GM}}{Signal_{MCA} + Signal_{GM}}\right)$ of the middle cerebral artery (MCA) were assessed in correlation to surrounding gray matter (GM) for 7 Tesla (T) magnetization prepared rapid acquisition gradient echo (MPRAGE) sequences, 7T time-of-flight (TOF) sequences and for 1.5T TOF sequences. Therefore, regions of interest (ROI) were defined in the largest diameter of the proximal left M1 segments ($Signal_{MCA}$) and adjacent gray matter ($Signal_{GM}$). The average diameter for the ROI of the vessel was 3–5 mm; the ROI for brain parenchyma amounted to approximately 1 cm.
*standard error = 0.012, 95% confidence interval [0.623 - 0.675].
**standard error = 0.010, 95% confidence interval [0.639 - 0.681].
***standard error = 0.008, 95% confidence interval [0.587 - 0.622].

Quantitative measurements for dome and neck diameter showed larger dome/neck ratio for 7 Tesla MPRAGE ($p = 0.0597$) and 7 Tesla TOF MRA ($p = 0.0305$) compared to 1.5 Tesla TOF MRA. There was no significant difference between dome/neck ratio in 7 Tesla MPRAGE and 7 Tesla TOF MRA ($p = 0.5586$).

In accordance with the delineation of the aneurysm dome and neck, 7 Tesla MPRAGE also offered best assessment of the parent vessel 4.8 (excellent) (SE 0.128). TOF MRA yielded good assessment of the parent vessel at both field strengths (1.5 Tesla TOF MRA mean: 4.4 (SE 0.129); 7 Tesla TOF MRA mean: 3.9 (SE 0.146).

Wilcoxon matched-pairs two-sided signed-ranks test showed significant differences between 7 Tesla TOF MRA and 1.5 Tesla TOF MRA ($p = 0.0309$) ratings, between 7 Tesla MPRAGE and 1.5 Tesla TOF MRA ($p = 0.0075$) ratings as well as between 7 Tesla TOF MRA and 7 Tesla MPRAGE ($p = 0.0117$) ratings.

Interobserver accordance was substantial to almost perfect for most readings, with slightly lower accordance (fair) for delineation of the dome for 1.5 Tesla TOF MRA and 7 Tesla TOF MRA. Details are shown in Table 2.

Table 3 shows mean ratings for delineation of dome, neck and parent vessel of both readers. Table 4 lists the combined readings of both raters for dome and neck diameter in mm and calculated dome/neck ratio for all aneurysms.

Examples for aneurysm dome, neck and parent vessel delineation in all three MRI sequences are shown in Figures 1 and 2.

Artifacts, vessel-tissue contrast and overall image quality

Seven Tesla MPRAGE imaging was the sequence to be least impaired by artifacts (excellent) with mean value of 4.9 (SE 0.000). 7 Tesla and 1.5 Tesla TOF MRA showed equivalent artifact impairment (good) with mean values of 4.3 (SE 0.147) for 7 Tesla and mean 4.4 (SE 0.124) for 1.5 Tesla imaging.

Wilcoxon matched-pairs two-sided signed-ranks test showed significant differences between 7 Tesla MPRAGE and 7 Tesla TOF MRA ($p = 0.0002$) ratings and between 7 Tesla MPRAGE and 1.5 Tesla TOF MRA ($p = 0.0005$) ratings. No significant differences were detected between 7 Tesla TOF MRA and 1.5 Tesla TOF MRA ($p = 0.3438$) ratings. Figure 3 shows examples of pulsation artifacts for 1.5 Tesla and 7 Tesla TOF MRA sequences.

Vessel-tissue contrast was rated equally good for TOF MRA at both field strengths, with mean values of 4.4 (good) (SE 0.146) for 7 Tesla and 4.2 (good) (SE 0.122) for 1.5 Tesla MRI. MPAGE imaging provided highest vessel-tissue contrast with excellent mean values of 4.9 (SE 0.088). Wilcoxon matched-pairs two-sided signed-ranks test showed significant differences between 7 Tesla MPRAGE and 7 Tesla TOF MRA ($p = 0.0063$) ratings and between 7 Tesla MPRAGE and 1.5 Tesla TOF MRA ($p = 0.0001$) ratings. There were no significant differences detected between 7 Tesla TOF MRA and 1.5 Tesla TOF MRA ($p = 0.5811$) ratings. Quantitative measurements of signal intensities showed significantly higher vessel-tissue contrast for 7 Tesla MPRAGE ($p = 0.0018$) and 7 Tesla TOF MRA ($p = 0.0014$) compared to 1.5 Tesla TOF MRA. No difference between vessel-tissue contrast

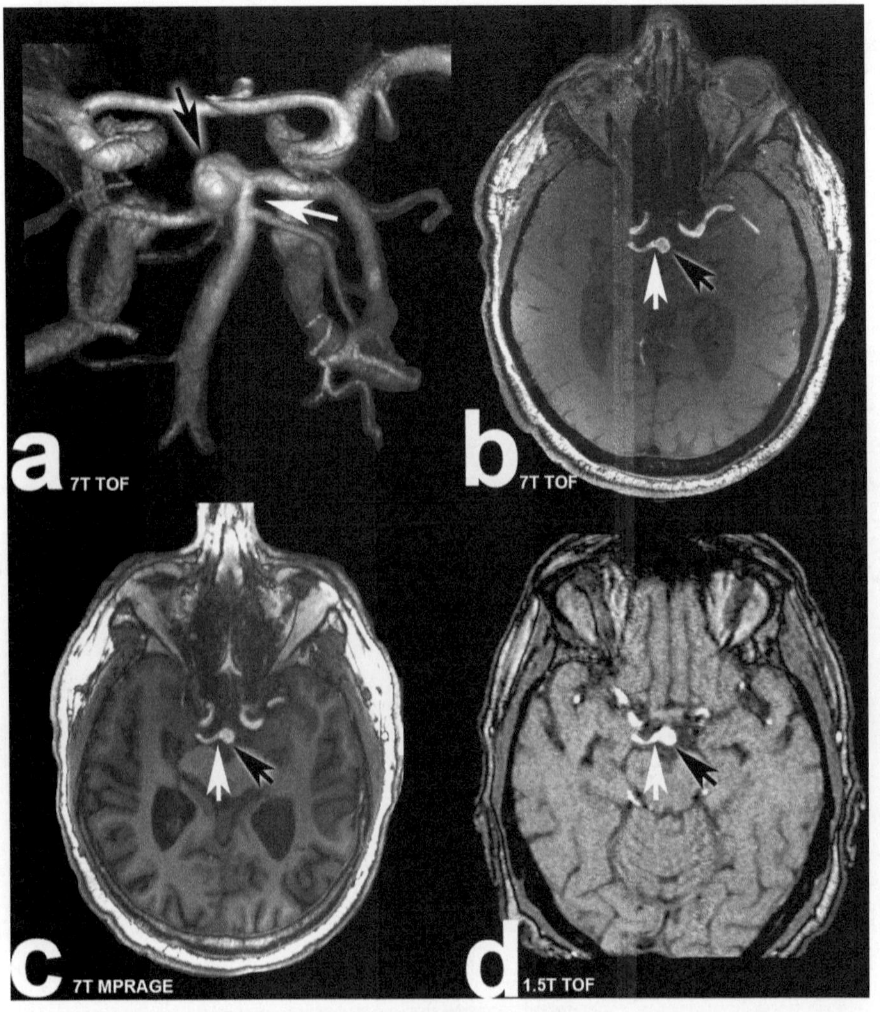

Figure 1. Seventy years old male patient (subject 5) suffering from basilar tip aneurysm. White arrows are marking the aneurysm neck, black arrows are marking the aneurysm dome. **a:** Volume rendering of the 7 Tesla TOF MRA demonstrating the three dimensional structure of the aneurysm; **b:** transverse plane of the 7 Tesla TOF MRA clearly depicting the aneurysm dome, neck and parent vessel; **c:** 7 Tesla MPRAGE sequence with excellent delineation of the aneurysm; **d:** 1.5 Tesla TOF MRA scan with minor irregularities of the parent vessel and aneurysm dome.

could be detected in 7 Tesla MPRAGE and 7 Tesla TOF MRA ($p = 0.5337$).

Overall image quality was rated equivalently good (4.3) for 7 Tesla (SE 0.105) and 1.5 Tesla (SE 0.117) TOF MRA and excellent (5.0) (SE 0.025) for 7 Tesla MPRAGE imaging. Wilcoxon matched-pairs two-sided signed-ranks test showed significant differences between 7 Tesla MPRAGE and 7 Tesla TOF MRA ($p = 0.0000$) ratings and between 7 Tesla MPRAGE and 1.5 Tesla TOF MRA ($p = 0.0001$) ratings. There were no significant differences detected between 7 Tesla TOF MRA and 1.5 Tesla TOF MRA ($p = 0.6250$) ratings.

Interobserver accordance was almost perfect (kappa coefficient) for most readings with slightly lower accordance (substantial) for artifact and overall image quality assessment in 1.5 Tesla TOF MRA Details are shown in Table 2.

Table 5 shows mean ratings for artifact delineation, vessel-tissue contrast and overall image quality. Table 6 lists the combined readings of both raters for signal intensities of left middle cerebral artery, adjacent gray matter and calculated vessel-tissue contrast ratio for all subjects.

Discussion

With DSA remaining to be the gold standard, 1.5 Tesla TOF MRA has evolved to become a reliable and equivalent non-invasive technique for detection and follow-up of UIA larger than 3 mm [1,23–27]. The increase in SNR and CNR affiliated to the increase in magnetic field strength has been shown to result in superior vessel (disease) assessment at 3 Tesla compared to 1.5 Tesla [26]. With further increase of the field strength to 7 Tesla, the combination of the associated increase in SNR (up to 4–5 fold higher than at 1.5 Tesla) and longer T1 relaxation times [28] are known to offer an improved vessel-tissue contrast based on more efficient background tissue suppression [29]. Studies in healthy volunteers at 7 Tesla have shown superior vessel delineation compared to 1.5 Tesla [30,31]. Furthermore, patient studies demonstrated the high diagnostic ability and superiority of 7 Tesla non-enhanced TOF MRA for evaluation of intracranial vasculature and aneurysm detection compared to DSA and/or 1.5 Tesla TOF MRA [13,32].

Initial studies of 7 Tesla non-enhanced T1w brain imaging revealed an incidental finding, by means of a homogeneously

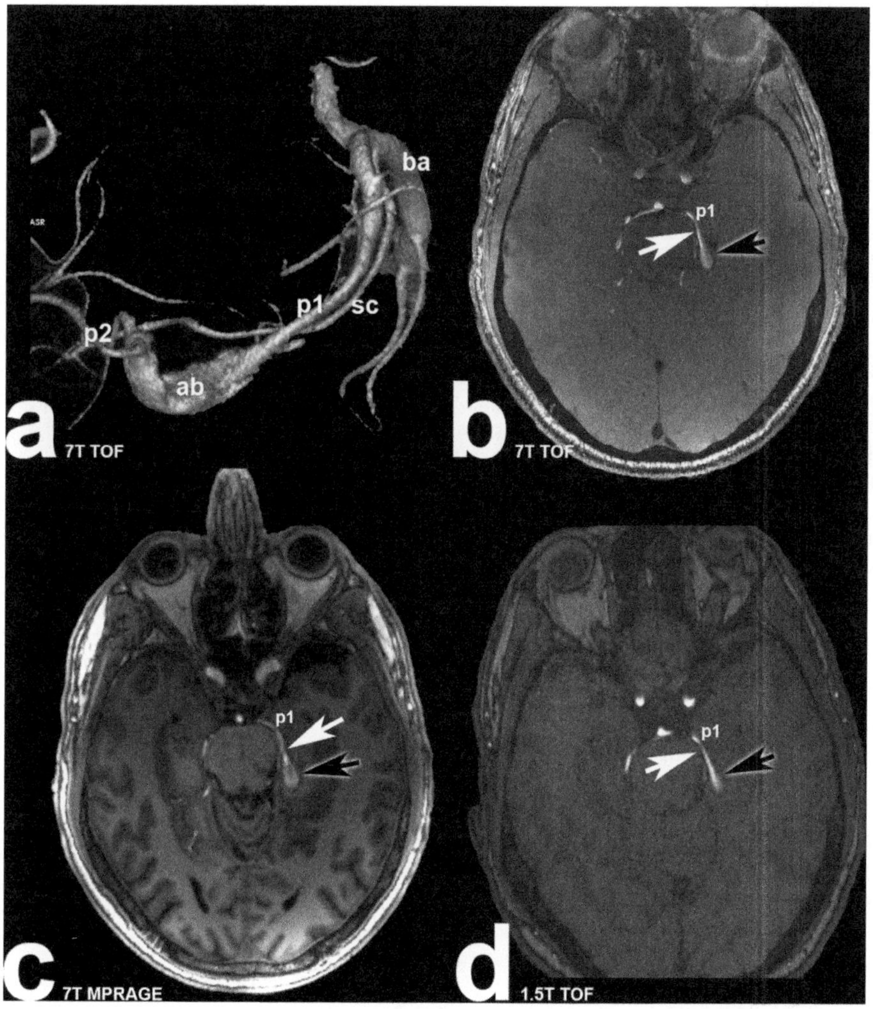

Figure 2. Forty-five years old male patient (subject 6) with partially thrombosed left sided fusiform posterior cerebral artery aneurysm. White arrows are marking the aneurysm neck, black arrows are marking the aneurysm dome. p1: posterior cerebral artery (p1 segment) **a:** Volume rendering of the 7 Tesla TOF MRA illustrating the three dimensional structure of the aneurysm (ba: basilar artery; sc: superior cerebellar artery; p2: posterior cerebral artery (p2 segment); ab: aneurysm body); **b:** transverse plane of the 7 Tesla TOF MRA depicting the parent vessel and part of the aneurysm body; **c:** Excellent delineation of parent vessel and part of the aneurysm body in 7 Tesla MPRAGE scan; **d:** Moderate depiction of parent vessel and aneurysm body in 1.5 Tesla TOF MRA.

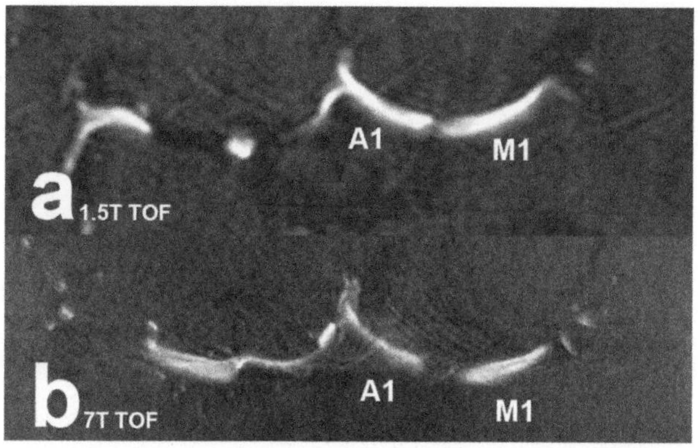

Figure 3. Pulsation artifacts near the carotid bifurcation in TOF MRA scans. The artifacts in 1.5 Tesla (**a**) and 7 Tesla (**b**) TOF MRA scans make vessel depiction more difficult (M1: middle cerebral artery (M1 segment); A1: anterior cerebral artery (A1 segment)).

hyperintense signal of arterial vasculature. This incidental finding bears a strong diagnostic potential for non-enhanced high-quality vessel imaging at 7 Tesla, as demonstrated in numerous studies [18,32–36]. In a study presented at the ISMRM 2010, Grinstead et al. analyzed the primary source of the hyperintense vessel signal. Their investigations showed an association of the high vessel signal to the lack of body RF transmit coils at 7 Tesla, resulting in the utilization of head coils for transmit and receive. Hence, non-selective infrared pulses effectively become slab-selective infrared-pulses. Furthermore a combination of steady state and inflow effects seems to be accountable.

To investigate the diagnostic ability of T1w non-enhanced 7 Tesla MRI, Maderwald et al. [32] published an intra-individual comparison trial of 7 Tesla TOF MRA, VIBE imaging (three-dimensional volume interpolated breath hold examination) and MPRAGE imaging of the intracranial vasculature in 25 subjects. Their results demonstrated the superiority of MPRAGE imaging in the assessment of non-enhanced vasculature, providing high-quality delineation of all vessel segments and least impairment due to intraluminal signal variations. Furthermore, MPRAGE and VIBE imaging offered full brain coverage in contrast to TOF MRA. Zwanenburg et al. [37] confirmed the high diagnostic potential of non-enhanced MPRAGE MRI at 7 Tesla, yielding excellent assessment of cerebral perforating arteries and related anatomical parenchymatous structures. In another recent study, the potential diagnostic benefit of the application of contrast agent to 7 Tesla MPRAGE MRI was investigated. The study results revealed only minor non-significant improvement based on the administration of contrast agent, underlining the high-diagnostic potential of non-enhanced 7 Tesla MPRAGE MRI [36].

Based on these previous study results, we decided to include non-enhanced MPRAGE imaging to our 7 Tesla protocol and compare its diagnostic ability to 7 Tesla and 1.5 Tesla TOF MRA regarding the assessment of intracranial aneurysms and their related features. Our study results go in line with previous publications regarding the superiority of 7 Tesla TOF MRA over 1.5 Tesla TOF MRA as well as 7 Tesla MPRAGE over 7 Tesla and 1.5 Tesla TOF MRA. However, while previous studies mainly focused on the evaluation of the overall image quality and overall delineation of the aneurysms, our study results deepen the assessment of the diagnostic ability based on a dedicated analysis of numerous aneurysm features and image quality parameters. Due to its high spatial resolution and excellent vessel-to-tissue contrast MPRAGE MRI offered best delineation of all assessed aneurysm features. It also yielded highest scores in overall image quality and least artifact impairment with significant difference to TOF MRA at 7 Tesla and 1.5 Tesla. Furthermore, aside from excellent vessel delineation, it also offers the potential for simultaneous high quality assessment of related anatomical parenchymatous structures and full brain coverage. While 7 Tesla TOF MRA yielded superior diagnostics of the aneurysm dome and neck over 1.5 Tesla, it was slightly inferior in the assessment of the parent vessel. This inferiority was mainly due to amplified intraluminal signal variations at 7 Tesla, resulting in impaired parent vessel delineation.

Clearly, our study is not free of limitations. The study group comprised a rather small population of 16 patients with a total of 20 untreated IA. Nevertheless, to our knowledge this is one of the largest neurosurgical patients cohorts suffering from UIA scanned at 7 Tesla and 1.5 Tesla MRI, published in literature. Further investigations with larger patient cohorts, also including patients with clipped or coiled intracranial aneurysms should be the focus of future studies. Ultrahighfield imaging in patients with treated aneurysms has been a restricted so far, as neither Guglielmi detachable coils nor aneurysm clips are certified for 7 Tesla MR imaging. Nevertheless, first promising preliminary results on implant safety in cerebral 7 Tesla MRI have been recently demonstrated {Kraff, 2013#1639}{Noureddine, 2012#1640}{Noureddine, 2013#1641}. Future studies on the diagnostic potential of 7 Tesla MRI for follow-up of coiled aneurysms would be of high scientific and clinical interest with special focus on aneurysm recanalization and its precise detection, comparing MRA at different magnetic field strengths to DSA.

Furthermore, another limitation is posed by the lack of a comparison to the diagnostic gold standard, in terms of digital subtraction angiography. However, with MRA offering equivalent non-invasive vessel diagnostics to DSA, particularly applied for aneurysm monitoring (as in our patient cohort), the main focus of this trial was set on a direct comparison of the diagnostic ability of different magnetic field strengths. Finally, as known from previous studies, 3 Tesla MRA is considered to provide improved vessel delineation over 1.5 Tesla. Hence, a comparison of 7 Tesla MRA to 3 Tesla MRA instead of 1.5 Tesla imaging would have been desirable. Unfortunately, this was not applicable due to availability reasons in this clinical setting. Nevertheless, 1.5 Tesla MRI is still considered the worldwide clinical standard. Hence, in order to investigate the diagnostic ability of 7 Tesla MRA, a comparison to the clinical worldwide standard (1.5 Tesla) may be a fair comparison after all.

In conclusion, we believe our study demonstrates the superiority of 7 Tesla MRA over 1.5 Tesla MRA and underlines the high diagnostic potential of 7 Tesla non-enhanced MPRAGE imaging for assessment, screening and follow-up of UIA.

Acknowledgments

The authors would like to thank Lena C. Schäfer (RT) for performing all 7 Tesla examinations.

Author Contributions

Conceived and designed the experiments: KHW PD CM SJ SM IES OM NÖ MEL MF MUS US LU. Performed the experiments: KHW PD CM SJ SM IES OM NÖ MEL MF MUS US LU. Analyzed the data: KHW PD CM SJ SM IES OM NÖ MEL MF MUS US LU. Contributed reagents/materials/analysis tools: KHW PD CM LU. Wrote the paper: KHW PD CM SJ SM IES OM NÖ MEL MF MUS US LU.

References

1. Fogelholm R, Hernesniemi J, Vapalahti M (1993) Impact of early surgery on outcome after aneurysmal subarachnoid hemorrhage. A population-based study. Stroke 24: 1649–1654.
2. Kashiwazaki D, Kuroda S, on behalf of the Sapporo SAHSG (2013) Size Ratio Can Highly Predict Rupture Risk in Intracranial Small (<5 mm) Aneurysms. Stroke.
3. Lawson MF, Neal DW, Mocco J, Hoh BL (2013) Rationale for Treating Unruptured Intracranial Aneurysms: Actuarial Analysis of Natural History Risk versus Treatment Risk for Coiling or Clipping Based on 14,050 Patients in the Nationwide Inpatient Sample Database. World Neurosurgery 79: 472–478.
4. Steinberg GK (2013) Controversy: Clipping of Asymptomatic Intracranial Aneurysm That is <7 mm: Yes. Stroke 44: S97–99.
5. Kaufmann TJ, Huston J III, Mandrekar JN, Schleck CD, Thielen KR, et al. (2007) Complications of diagnostic cerebral angiography: evaluation of 19,826 consecutive patients. Radiology 243: 812–819.
6. Willinsky RA, Taylor SM, TerBrugge K, Farb RI, Tomlinson G, et al. (2003) Neurologic complications of cerebral angiography: prospective analysis of 2,899 procedures and review of the literature. Radiology 227: 522–528.
7. Chung TS, Joo JY, Lee SK, Chien D, Laub G (1999) Evaluation of cerebral aneurysms with high-resolution MR angiography using a section-interpolation technique: correlation with digital subtraction angiography. AJNR Am J Neuroradiol 20: 229–235.
8. Okahara M (2002) Diagnostic Accuracy of Magnetic Resonance Angiography for Cerebral Aneurysms in Correlation With 3D-Digital Subtraction Angiographic Images: A Study of 133 Aneurysms. Stroke 33: 1803–1808.
9. White PM, Teadsale E, Wardlaw JM, Easton V (2001) What is the most sensitive non-invasive imaging strategy for the diagnosis of intracranial aneurysms? Journal of Neurology Neurosurgery and Psychiatry 71: 322–328.
10. White PM, Teasdale EM, Wardlaw JM, Easton V (2001) Intracranial aneurysms: CT angiography and MR angiography for detection prospective blinded comparison in a large patient cohort. Radiology 219: 739–749.
11. Shahzad R, Younas F (2011) Detection and characterization of intracranial aneurysms: Magnetic resonance angiography versus digital subtraction angiography. Journal of the College of Physicians and Surgeons Pakistan 21: 325–329.
12. Nakiri GS, Santos AC, Abud TG, Aragon DC, Colli BO, et al. (2011) A comparison between magnetic resonance angiography at 3 teslas (time-of-flight and contrastenhanced) and flat-panel digital subtraction angiography in the assessment of embolized brain aneurysms. Clinics 66: 641–648.
13. Monninghoff C, Maderwald S, Theysohn JM, Kraff O, Ladd SC, et al. (2009) Evaluation of intracranial aneurysms with 7 T versus 1.5 T time-of-flight MR angiography – initial experience. RoFo: Fortschritte auf dem Gebiete der Rontgenstrahlen und der Nuklearmedizin 181: 16–23.
14. Ferré JC, Carsin-Nicol B, Morandi X, Carsin M, de Kersaint-Gilly A, et al. (2009) Time-of-flight MR angiography at 3 T versus digital subtraction

angiography in the imaging follow-up of 51 intracranial aneurysms treated with coils. European Journal of Radiology 72: 365–369.
15. Schar M, Kozerke S, Fischer SE, Boesiger P (2004) Cardiac SSFP imaging at 3 Tesla. Magnetic resonance in medicine 51: 799–806.
16. Hoult DI (2000) The Principle of Reciprocity in Signal Strength Calculations – A Mathematical Guide. Concepts in Magnetic Resonance 12: 173–187.
17. Johst S, Wrede KH, Ladd ME, Maderwald S (2012) Time-of-Flight Magnetic Resonance Angiography at 7 T Using Venous Saturation Pulses With Reduced Flip Angles. Invest Radiol 47: 445–450.
18. Wrede KH, Johst S, Dammann P, Umutlu L, Schlamann MU, et al. (2012) Caudal Image Contrast Inversion in MPRAGE at 7 Tesla Problem and Solution. Acad Radiol 19: 172–178.
19. Cohen J (1960) A Coefficient of Agreement for Nominal Scales. Educational and Psychological Measurement 20: 37–46.
20. Landis JR, Koch GG (1977) The measurement of observer agreement for categorical data. Biometrics 33: 159–174.
21. Lin LI-K (1989) A concordance correlation coefficient to evaluate reproducibility. Biometrics 45: 255–268.
22. Lin LIK (2000) Erratum: A note on the concordance correlation coefficient (Biometrics (1989) (214)). Biometrics 56: 324–325.
23. Adams WM, Laitt RD, Jackson A (2000) The role of MR angiography in the pretreatment assessment of intracranial aneurysms: A comparative study. American Journal of Neuroradiology 21: 1618–1628.
24. Chung TS, Joo J, Lee SK, Chien D, Laub G (1999) Evaluation of cerebral aneurysms with high-resolution MR angiography using a section-interpolation technique: Correlation with digital subtraction angiography. American Journal of Neuroradiology 20: 229–235.
25. Gaa J, Weidauer S, Requardt M, Kiefer B, Lanfermann H, et al. (2004) Comparison of intracranial 3D-ToF-MRA with and without parallel acquisition techniques at 1.5T and 3.0T: Preliminary results. Acta radiologica 45: 327–332.
26. Gibbs GF, Huston J III, Bernstein MA, Riederer SJ, Brown RD Jr (2004) Improved image quality of intracranial aneurysms: 3.0-T versus 1.5-T time-of-flight MR angiography. AJNR Am J Neuroradiol 25: 84–87.
27. Willinek WA, Born M, Simon B, Tschampa HJ, Krautmacher C, et al. (2003) Time-of-Flight MR Angiography: Comparison of 3.0-T Imaging and 1.5-T Imaging-Initial Experience. Radiology 229: 913–920.
28. Edelstein WA, Glover GH, Hardy CJ, Redington RW (1986) The intrinsic signal-to-noise ratio in NMR imaging. Magn Reson Med 3: 604–618.
29. Majoie CBLM, Sprengers ME, Van Rooij WJJ, Lavini C, Sluzewski M, et al. (2005) MR angiography at 3T versus digital subtraction angiography in the follow-up of intracranial aneurysms treated with detachable coils. American Journal of Neuroradiology 26: 1349–1356.
30. Heverhagen JT, Bourekas E, Sammet S, Knopp MV, Schmalbrock P (2008) Time-of-flight magnetic resonance angiography at 7 tesla. Investigative Radiology 43: 568–573.
31. Nowinski WL, Puspitasaari F, Volkau I, Marchenko Y, Knopp MV (2011) Comparison of Magnetic Resonance Angiography Scans on 1.5, 3, and 7 Tesla Units: A Quantitative Study of 3-Dimensional Cerebrovasculature. Journal of Neuroimaging: Epub DOI: 10.1111/j.1552-6569.2011.00597.x.
32. Maderwald S, Ladd SC, Gizewski ER, Kraff O, Theysohn JM, et al. (2008) To TOF or not to TOF: strategies for non-contrast-enhanced intracranial MRA at 7 T. MAGMA 21: 159–167.
33. Fischer A, Maderwald S, Orzada S, Johst S, Schafer LC, et al. (2013) Nonenhanced magnetic resonance angiography of the lower extremity vessels at 7 tesla: initial experience. Invest Radiol 48: 525–534.
34. Umutlu L, Kraff O, Fischer A, Kinner S, Maderwald S, et al. (2013) Seven-Tesla MRI of the female pelvis. Eur Radiol.
35. Umutlu L, Maderwald S, Kraff O, Kinner S, Schaefer LC, et al. (2012) New look at renal vasculature: 7 tesla nonenhanced T1-weighted FLASH imaging. J Magn Reson Imaging.
36. Umutlu L, Theysohn N, Maderwald S, Johst S, Lauenstein TC, et al. (2013) 7 Tesla MPRAGE Imaging of the Intracranial Arterial Vasculature: Nonenhanced\ versus Contrast-Enhanced. Acad Radiol.
37. Zwanenburg JJ, Hendrikse J, Takahara T, Visser F, Luijten PR (2008) MR angiography of the cerebral perforating arteries with magnetization prepared anatomical reference at 7 T: comparison with time-of-flight. Journal of magnetic resonance imaging: JMRI 28: 1519–1526.

3

Enhancement Characteristics and Impact on Image Quality of Two Gadolinium Chelates at Equimolar Doses for Time-Resolved 3-Tesla MR-Angiography of the Calf Station

Jan Hansmann[1], Henrik J. Michaely[1], John N. Morelli[2], André Luckscheiter[1], Stefan O. Schoenberg[1], Ulrike I. Attenberger[1]*

1 Institute of Clinical Radiology and Nuclear Medicine, University Medical Center Mannheim, Medical Faculty Mannheim – Heidelberg University, Mannheim, Germany, 2 The Russel H. Morgan Department of Radiology and Radiological Science, The Johns Hopkins Hospital, Baltimore, Maryland, United States of America

Abstract

Purpose: To compare enhancement characteristics and image quality of two macrocyclic gadolinium chelates, gadoterate meglumine and gadobutrol, in low-dose, time-resolved MRA of the calf station.

Materials and Methods: 100 consecutive patients with peripheral arterial disease (stages II-IV) were retrospectively analysed. Fifty patients were included in each group - 32 men and 18 women for gadobutrol (mean age 67 years) and 34 men, 16 women for gadoterate meglumine (mean age 64 years). 0.03 mmol/kg bw of either gadobutrol or gadoterate meglumine was injected. Gadobutrol was diluted 1:1 with normal saline (0.9% NaCl) to provide similar injection volume and bolus geometry compared to the undiluted 0.5 M dose of gadoterate meglumine. Signal-to-noise-ratio (SNR), contrast-to-noise-ratio (CNR) and image quality were analysed and compared between the two groups.

Results: Mean SNR ranged from 83.0±46.7 (peroneal artery) to 96.4±64.5 (anterior tibial artery) for gadobutrol, and from 37.6±13.8 (peroneal artery) to 45.3±16.4 (anterior tibial artery) for the gadoterate meglumine group ($p<0.0001$). CNR values ranged from 30.1±20.1 (peroneal artery) to 37.6±26.0 (anterior tibial artery) for gadobutrol and from 14.9±8.0 (peroneal artery) to 18.6±16.4 (anterior tibial artery) for gadoterate meglumine ($p<0.0001$). No significant difference in image quality was found except for the peroneal arteries ($p=0.006$ and $p=0.04$). Interreader agreement was excellent (kappa 0.87–0.93)

Conclusion: The significantly better enhancement as assessed by SNR and CNR provided by gadobutrol compared to gadoterate meglumine does not translate into substantial differences in image quality in an equimolar, low-dose, time-resolved MRA protocol of the calves.

Editor: Andreas-Claudius Hoffmann, West German Cancer Center, Germany

Funding: We acknowledge financial support by the Deutsche Forschungsgemeinschaft and the Ruprecht-Karls-Universitaet Heidelberg within the funding program Open Access Publishing. The funders had no role in study design, data collection and analysis, decision to publish, or preparation of the manuscript.

Competing Interests: Ulrike I. Attenberger is a consultant for Bayer Healthcare, Berlin, Germany. Bayer Healthcare had no role in study design, data collection and analysis, decision to publish, or preparation of the manuscript. All other authors have declared that no competing interests exist. Please also note that Ulrike I. Attenberger is a consultant for Bayer Healthcare, Berlin, Germany.

* E-mail: ulrike.attenberger@umm.de

Introduction

The diagnostic value of contrast-enhanced MR-angiography (CE MRA) for the evaluation of the lower extremity vasculature at 3 Tesla (3 T) is well-established in the literature [1,2]. Increasingly available high field MR systems operating at 3 T allow markedly shortened acquisition times without a corresponding loss in spatial resolution [1]. This is in part due to intrinsically higher SNR at these field strengths combined with the development of other innovations such as parallel imaging and multi-element coils [3,4]. In particular, CE MRA enables accurate gradation of disease stage in patients suffering from peripheral artery disease (PAD): comparisons with conventional angiography, the clinical gold standard, have demonstrated a high degree of overall diagnostic accuracy with CE MRA, with values of 80% for stenosis detection and 93.5% for the detection of high grade vessel stenosis [5].

Evaluation of the relatively small caliber vasculature of the calf station is often impaired by venous overlay due to altered patient hemodynamics. This may result from soft tissue inflammation—a common finding in patients with advanced stages of PAD. Such limitations can be successfully avoided through implementation of time-resolved MRA sequences such as time-resolved imaging of contrast kinetics (TRICKS) [6] and time-resolved angiography with interleaved stochastic trajectories (TWIST). These sequences eliminate the need for a test-bolus and have been shown to provide arterial-phase imaging free of venous contamination in different vascular territories [7]. In peripheral MR-angiography applications, time-resolved MRA sequences have been proven to allow for an accurate assessment even in patients whose CE MRA images had been non-diagnostic due to venous contamination [8,9].

Patients suffering from PAD also often present with multiple comorbidities including impaired renal function and are thus at an increased risk of developing nephrogenic systemic fibrosis (NSF). The incidence of NSF is not only related to the molecular structure of the administered gadolinium chelate, with macrocyclic chelates being more stable than linear compounds, but also to the injected dose. Therefore, low-dose injection protocols or nonenhanced MRA [10,11] are preferred to minimize the risk of NSF in this particular patient group [4,5]. The implementation of low-dose protocols together with the increased use of macrocyclic MR contrast agents has led to a significantly reduced risk for NSF in high-risk patients [12,13]. Among the macrocyclic chelates available, gadobutrol is unique in its availability at an 1.0 M formulation and its higher r^1 relaxivity when compared to other contrast agents. We hypothesized that the latter factor should thus lead to improvements in signal to noise ratio (SNR), contrast to noise ratio (CNR) and image quality [14,15].

The aim of the current investigation was therefore to compare equimolar doses of gadobutrol and gadoterate meglumine with respect to SNR, CNR and image quality in a time-resolved, low-dose MRA protocol of the calf region.

Materials and Methods

Patients

Institutional review board approval was obtained for this study. The institutional review board (IRB name: Medizinische Ethikkommission II der Medizinischen Fakultaet Mannheim, Heidelberg University, Germany) waived the requirement for informed patient consent for this retrospective study. The information gathered on this retrospective patient population was performed in compliance with HIPAA guidelines. 100 consecutive patients with PAD (Fontaine stages II-IV) who underwent routine MRA of the peripheral vasculature at our institution between October 2008 and March 2011 were included for retrospective data analysis (32 men and 18 women; mean age 67 years in gadubutrol group and 34 men, 16 women for gadoterate meglumine, mean age 64 years in the gadoterate meglumine group). Either gadobutrol or gadoterate meglumine was utilized as the contrast agent, based upon the clinical necessities of the examination day (i.e. patient renal function, contrast agent utilized for previous examinations).

MR-Protocol

All MRA examinations were performed on a 3 T, 32-channel whole-body MR system (MAGNETOM Tim Trio [102×32], Siemens AG, Healthcare Sector, Erlangen, Germany). To cover the entire field of view (FoV) from the diaphragm to the calves, a dedicated 36-element peripheral angiography matrix coil, as well as 2 body 6-element matrix coils and 2 clusters of the inbuilt spine matrix coil were utilized. Patients were positioned supine feet-first in the MR bore. A 20 G cannula in the left or right antecubital vein was used for contrast agent administration, which was performed with an automated power injector (Medrad Spectris Solaris EP, Medrad Indianola, PA). Detailed scan parameters are summarized in Table 1.

Contrast agents

Two macrocyclic gadolinium based contrast agents were utilized for this study: gadobutrol (Gadovist, Bayer Healthcare AG, Berlin, Germany) formulated at 1.0 molar (M) and gadoterate meglumine (Dotarem, Guerbet, France) formulated at 0.5 M. The r^1 relaxivity of gadobutrol versus gadoterate meglumine is 5.0±0.3 vs. 3.5±0.2 L*mmol^{-1}s^{-1} (in plasma, at 3 T and 37°C) [15]. To allow for a more equal comparison between the two different contrast agents in terms of bolus geometry the 1 M gadobutrol was diluted 1:1 with normal saline (0.9% NaCl). Thus, contrast agents administered to the patients were equimolar on a per bodyweight basis (0.03 mmol/kg BW) and were administered in equivalent concentrations (0.5 M).

MR imaging

2D gradient echo sequence localizers were obtained in coronal and axial planes to allow for planning of the examination. After acquisition of continuous table movement-MRA (CTM-MRA) images, an additional 0.03 mmol/kg body weight of the respective contrast agent was administered at a rate of 1.5 ml/s followed by a 30 ml normal saline (0.9% NaCl) chaser at the same injection rate for time-resolved MRA with interleaved stochastic trajectories (TWIST) of the calf station.

SNR/CNR evaluation

Image evaluation was performed offline utilizing a standard DICOM-viewer (OsiriX, The OsiriX Foundation, Geneva, Switzerland). Region-of-Interest (ROI) measurements were performed by a single reader for SNR and CNR measurements. The reader was blinded to the contrast agent administered. ROIs were placed in vessel segments in the anterior and posterior tibial as well as peroneal arteries on the pre-contrast scans. Noise calculations were performed by placing a ROI in an artifact-free background area of the subtracted coronal maximum intensity projection images. A ROI was placed in the corresponding vessel at consecutive time points and signal intensity then was measured at the time point of maximum vessel enhancement. The above ROIs were carefully placed in vessel segments displaying homogenous contrast enhancement while avoiding the vessel borders. SNR and CNR were calculated according to the following formulas [16]:

$$SNR = SI\ vessel / SD_{noise} \quad (1)$$

$$CNR = (SI\ vessel_{post} - SI\ vessel_{pre}) / SD_{noise} \quad (2)$$

Qualitative assessment

For the qualitative assessment, two blinded readers assessed image quality on a scale of 1 to 4 (1 = poor image quality and blurring of the arterial segment; 2 = fair image quality, inadequate arterial enhancement for confident diagnosis; 3 = good image quality and arterial enhancement, adequate for confident diagnosis; 4 = excellent image quality and arterial enhancement, for highly confident diagnosis) within 4 arterial segments in the bilateral lower extremities (tibioperoneal trunk, anterior tibial, posterior tibial, and the peroneal arteries). Data from both limbs in the patients was pooled, resulting in possible evaluation of 96 (2×48) data points for each territory. Territories in a given patient were excluded if arterial occlusions within a segment led to no significant vascular enhancement, one of the limbs was amputated, or vascular evaluation was not possible secondary to patient motion.

Table 1. Sequence parameters for TWIST MR Angiography.

Parameter	TWIST MRA
Parallel Imaging	Grappa 2
Acquisition time (sec)	96
Spatial resolution (mm^3)	1.1×1.1×1.1
Temporal resolution (sec)	5.49
Field of view (mm)	500×375
Repetition time (msec)	3.75
Echo time (msec)	1.12
Flip angle (degrees)	20
Matrix	448×336
Bandwidth (Hertz per pixel)	660

Statistical analysis

Statistical analysis was performed using JMP 9.0 (SAS Institute, Cary, North Carolina, USA). Continuous variables are expressed as mean, standard deviation (± SD), and range (min–max). Continuous variables for SNR and CNR are expressed as mean and standard deviation. SNR and CNR values between the two groups were compared using a Student t-test after normally distribution of data was confirmed using the Shapiro–Wilk test. A 2-tailed p-value of <0.05 was considered statistically significant. To assess qualitative differences in quality between scans performed with gadobutrol and gadoterate meglumine, median image quality for each reader in 4 arterial segments was computed. Image quality ratings for each reader were compared between images obtained with gadobutrol and gadoterate meglumine utilizing a Mann-Whitney U Test. Inter-reader variability was assessed via Cohen's Kappa statistics. Kappa values greater than 0.75 were taken to represent excellent agreement, values between 0.4-0.75 to represent good agreement, and values below 0.4 as poor agreement.

Results

SNR/CNR evaluation

All measurements were completed successfully, and no examinations were excluded due to inadequate image quality. SNR measurements for gadobutrol demonstrated a mean signal intensity of 83.0±46.7 for the peroneal artery, 92.9±58.9 for the posterior tibial artery, and 96.4±64.5 for the anterior tibial artery. Gadoterate meglumine SNR was 37.6±13.8 for the peroneal artery, 41.2±13.8 for the posterior tibial artery, and 45.3±16.4 for the anterior tibial artery. SNR measurements were statistically significantly different for all three vessel segments evaluated (peroneal artery p<0.0001; posterior tibial artery p< 0.0001, anterior tibial artery p<0.0001) (Table 2).

CNR measurements for gadobutrol in the peroneal artery demonstrated a mean signal intensity of 30.1±20.1 for the peroneal artery, 37.1±26.8 for the posterior tibial artery, and 37.6±26.0 for the anterior tibial artery. Gadoterate meglumine exhibited CNR of 14.9±8.0 for the peroneal artery, 16.9±9.2 for the posterior tibial artery and 18.6±16.4 for the anterior tibial artery. CNR measurements were statistically significantly different for all three vessel segments evaluated (peroneal artery p<0.0001; posterior tibial artery p<0.0001, anterior tibial artery p<0.0001) (Table 2).

Qualitative assessment

For reader 1, qualitative assessments were possible for the gadobutrol scans in 91% (87/96) of cases for the anterior tibial artery, 81% (78/96) of cases for the posterior tibial artery, and 90% (86/96) of cases for the peroneal artery. For the gadoterate meglumine scans, these respective assessments were possible in 89% (85/96), (89%) 85/96, and 93% (89/96) of cases. For reader 2, qualitative assessments were possible for the gadobutrol scans in 91% (87/96) of cases for the anterior tibial artery, 80% (77/96) of cases for the posterior tibial artery, and 90% (86/96) of cases for the peroneal artery. For the gadoterate meglumine scans these respective assessments were possible in 90% (85/96), 90% (85/96), and 92% (88/96) of cases. Image quality ratings ranged from values of 1–4 for each reader. Median ratings of image quality are provided in Table 3. Statistically significant differences in image quality were observed between gadobutrol and gadoterate meglumine in the peroneal arteries for both readers. Kappa values demonstrated excellent interobserver agreement for all qualitative assessments (Table 3). An example of individual SNR and CNR values as well as the pertinent image quality ratings by both readers is provided in figure 1.

Discussion

The results of the present study demonstrate superior SNR and CNR for equimolar doses of gadobutrol versus gadoterate meglumine for time-resolved MRA of the calves at 3 T. Our results demonstrate a significant difference in SNR and CNR measurements in all three vessel segments evaluated, with gadobutrol achieving SNR and CNR values up to 100% higher than gadoterate meglumine. However, this did not translate into the expected degree of improved subjective image quality as gadobutrol scans were only rated to have statistically significantly better image quality in one of three assessed vascular segments.

A previous study by Voth et al. showed equimolar doses of gadobutrol, also diluted to 0.5 M with saline, provided greater image quality for peripheral MRA in all vessel segments from the diaphragm to the calves versus gadoterate meglumine utilizing CTM-MRA. Both contrast agents were injected at a dose of 0.07 mmol/kg bw in this instance and at a constant injection rate of 1.5 ml/sec [17]. A recent study performed by Haneder et al. compared SNR, CNR, and image quality on an intraindividual basis in 14 patients who underwent static, CTM-MRA using either gadobutrol or gadoterate meglumine [18]. Haneder et al. found that while SNR and CNR were statistically significantly greater for

Table 2. SNR/CNR.

Contrast agent		Anterior tibial artery	Posterior tibial artery	Peroneal artery
Gadobutrol	*Mean SNR*	96.4±64.5	92.9±58.9	83.0±46.7
Gadoterate meglumine	*Mean SNR*	45.3±16.4	41.2±13.8	37.6±13.8
	p-value	*<0.0001*	*<0.0001*	*<0.0001*
Gadobutrol	*Mean CNR*	37.6±26.0	37.1±26.8	30.1±20.1
Gadoterate meglumine	*Mean CNR*	18.6±16.4	16.9±9.2	14.9±8.0
	p-value	*<0.0001*	*<0.0001*	*<0.0001*

Note – SNR = Signal to noise ratio; CNR = Contrast to noise ratio.

gadobutrol, gadoterate meglumine images were rated as superior in terms of image quality and diagnostic confidence. In distinction to that work, our study included a larger number of patients and focused solely on time-resolved imaging of the calves. The value of TWIST-MRA relative to static MRA is primarily due to its stability in conditions of altered flow, conditions often present in higher stages of PAD [4]. Contrast agent comparisons for MR angiography applications often lead to controversial discussions focusing on study design and the fairness of comparisons between agents. Crucial considerations include injection dose, volume, and rate. The complexity of comparisons increases when comprehensive evaluations of contrast agents at non-equimolar formulations are performed. Considering these factors, the mixed conclusions of prior studies in this field are not surprising. Achenbach et al. found no significant differences in terms of image quality, diagnostic accuracy, signal intensity, SNR, and CNR between 0.5 M gadobenate dimeglumine and 1.0 M gadobutrol in 74 Patients at 1.5 T [19]. Gadobenate dimeglumine is known to bind temporarily to serum proteins such as albumin, which in consequence leads to an increased r^1-relaxation rate relative to non-protein binding agents like gadobutrol [20].

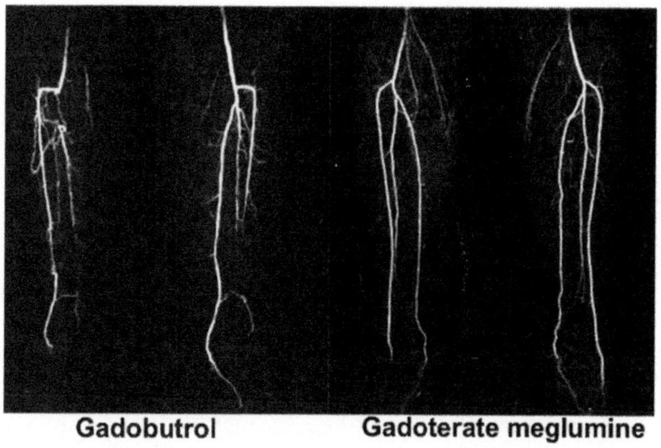

Figure 1. Higher SNR and CNR in time resolved MR-Angiography does not translate into improved image quality. Gadobutrol was utilized as the contrast agent in a 80 year old female with SNR/CNR values of 93/65 for the anterior tibial artery, 125/101 for the posterior tibial artery and 90/62 for the peroneal artery. Gadoterate meglumine administered in a 61 year old female resulted in SNR/CNR values of 60/21 for the anterior tibial artery, 55/21 for the posterior tibial artery and 52/19 for the peroneal artery. Image quality was rated good to excellent by both readers in both cases.

Szucs-Farkas et al. concluded that gadobutrol did not show significant differences in regards to SNR, CNR or image quality in CE-MRA performed at 1.5 Tesla compared to gadoterate meglumine. Szucs-Farkas et al. did not dilute gadoterate meglumine, but did inject the agents at equimolar doses per bodyweight. The major drawback of that study was the slow injection rates of 0.4 and 0.8 ml/sec for gadobutrol and gadoterate meglumine, respectively. This may have resulted in insufficient bolus definition, particularly in the peripheral vasculature of the calves. The authors concluded that further investigation was warranted to determine whether a higher injection rate would translate into better image quality [21]. Comparison of results obtained at 3 and 1.5 Tesla is even more difficult due to differences in relaxivity of contrast agents at different field strengths [15] and different T1 relaxation times of the background tissue.

Our study utilized an equimolar dose of the contrast agents, with dilution of the 1 M gadobutrol 1:1 with normal saline (NaCl), thus allowing for an equivalent concentration and similar bolus geometry compared to the 0.5 M gadoterate meglumine. Dilution allowed for injection of the same volume of contrast material for both injection protocols, minimizing the potential for technologist error. Thus, using the same technical parameters, gadobutrol performed significantly better than gadoterate meglumine in terms of objective image quality. However, our initital hypothesis that the higher relaxivity of gadoterate would translate into improved diagnostic image quality did not hold true. This is in agreement with prior work by Fink et al. and Haneder et al. [18,22], who suggested that measurable differences in SNR and CNR are irrelevant for subjectively rated image quality.

Several limitations of our study warrant further discussion. Neither age, gender, nor PAD stage was matched; however, both groups contain similar numbers of male and female patients of similar mean ages. Contrast agent was already present in the vessel segments evaluated on pre-contrast scans due to the prior CTM-MRA, however this possible confounder was equivalently present in both groups. In addition, intra-individual comparisons could not be performed due to the retrospective study design. By definition, retrospective studies are limited, and therefore larger scale prospective studies are required to validate our results.

In conclusion, the significantly better enhancement as assessed by SNR and CNR provided by gadobutrol does not translate into improved image quality in an equimolar, low-dose, time-resolved MRA protocol.

Table 3. Image Quality.

Distribution	Reader	Median Rating (Gadobutrol, Gd-DOTA)	P-values	Kappa**
Anterior Tibial Artery	Reader 1	4, 4	0.29	0.88
	Reader 2	4, 4	0.42	
Posterior Tibial Artery	Reader 1	4, 4	0.56	0.93
	Reader 2	4, 4	0.68	
Peroneal Artery	Reader 1	4, 4	0.006*	0.87
	Reader 2	4, 4	0.04*	

*Statistically significantly better image quality with gadobutrol.
**All Kappa values are statistically significant.
Gd-DOTA = gadoterate meglumine.

Author Contributions

Conceived and designed the experiments: JH HJM SOS UIA. Performed the experiments: JH HJM AL SOS UIA. Analyzed the data: JH JNM AL HJM UIA. Wrote the paper: JH HJM JNM AL SOS UIA.

References

1. Kramer H, Michaely HJ, Matschl V, Schmitt P, Reiser MF, et al. (2007) High-resolution magnetic resonance angiography of the lower extremities with a dedicated 36-element matrix coil at 3 Tesla. Invest Radiol 42: 477–483.
2. Menke J, Larsen J (2010) Meta-analysis: Accuracy of contrast-enhanced magnetic resonance angiography for assessing steno-occlusions in peripheral arterial disease. Ann Intern Med 153: 325–334.
3. Kramer H, Zenge M, Schmitt P, Glaser C, Reiser MF, et al. (2008) Peripheral magnetic resonance angiography (MRA) with continuous table movement at 3.0 T: initial experience compared with step-by-step MRA. Invest Radiol 43: 627–634.
4. Voth M, Haneder S, Huck K, Gutfleisch A, Schonberg SO, et al. (2009) Peripheral magnetic resonance angiography with continuous table movement in combination with high spatial and temporal resolution time-resolved MRA With a total single dose (0.1 mmol/kg) of gadobutrol at 3.0 T. Invest Radiol 44: 627–633.
5. Attenberger UI, Haneder S, Morelli JN, Diehl SJ, Schoenberg SO, et al. (2010) Peripheral arterial occlusive disease: evaluation of a high spatial and temporal resolution 3-T MR protocol with a low total dose of gadolinium versus conventional angiography. Radiology 257: 879–887.
6. Korosec FR, Frayne R, Grist TM, Mistretta CA (1996) Time-resolved contrast-enhanced 3D MR angiography. Magn Reson Med 36: 345–351.
7. Blackham KA, Passalacqua MA, Sandhu GS, Gilkeson RC, Griswold MA, et al. (2011) Applications of time-resolved MR angiography. AJR American journal of roentgenology 196: W613–620.
8. Andreisek G, Pfammatter T, Goepfert K, Nanz D, Hervo P, et al. (2007) Peripheral arteries in diabetic patients: standard bolus-chase and time-resolved MR angiography. Radiology 242: 610–620.
9. Hansmann J, Michaely HJ, Morelli JN, Diehl SJ, Meyer M, et al. (2013) Impact of Time-Resolved MRA on Diagnostic Accuracy in Patients With Symptomatic Peripheral Artery Disease of the Calf Station. AJR American journal of roentgenology 201: 1368–1375.
10. Lanzman RS, Schmitt P, Kropil P, Blondin D (2011) [Nonenhanced MR angiography techniques]. Rofo 183: 913–924.
11. Miyazaki M, Lee VS (2008) Nonenhanced MR angiography. Radiology 248: 20–43.
12. Abujudeh HH, Rolls H, Kaewlai R, Agarwal S, Gebreananya ZA, et al. (2009) Retrospective assessment of prevalence of nephrogenic systemic fibrosis (NSF) after implementation of a new guideline for the use of gadobenate dimeglumine as a sole contrast agent for magnetic resonance examination in renally impaired patients. J Magn Reson Imaging 30: 1335–1340.
13. Wang Y, Alkasab TK, Narin O, Nazarian RM, Kaewlai R, et al. (2011) Incidence of Nephrogenic Systemic Fibrosis after Adoption of Restrictive Gadolinium-based Contrast Agent Guidelines. Radiology.
14. Anzalone N, Scarabino T, Venturi C, Cristaudo C, Tartaro A, et al. (2011) Cerebral neoplastic enhancing lesions: Multicenter, randomized, crossover intraindividual comparison between gadobutrol (1.0 M) and gadoterate meglumine (0.5 M) at 0.1 mmolGd/kg body weight in a clinical setting. Eur J Radiol.
15. Rohrer M, Bauer H, Mintorovitch J, Requardt M, Weinmann HJ (2005) Comparison of magnetic properties of MRI contrast media solutions at different magnetic field strengths. Invest Radiol 40: 715–724.
16. Reeder SB, Wintersperger BJ, Dietrich O, Lanz T, Greiser A, et al. (2005) Practical approaches to the evaluation of signal-to-noise ratio performance with parallel imaging: application with cardiac imaging and a 32-channel cardiac coil. Magn Reson Med 54: 748–754.
17. Voth M, Attenberger UI, Luckscheiter A, Haneder S, Henzler T, et al. (2011) "Number needed to read"—how to facilitate clinical trials in MR-angiography. Eur Radiol 21: 1034–1042.
18. Haneder S, Attenberger UI, Schoenberg SO, Loewe C, Arnaiz J, et al. (2012) Comparison of 0.5 M gadoterate and 1.0 M gadobutrol in peripheral MRA: a prospective, single-center, randomized, crossover, double-blind study. J Magn Reson Imaging 36: 1213–1221.
19. Achenbach M, Figiel JH, Burbelko M, Heverhagen JT (2010) Prospective comparison of image quality and diagnostic accuracy of 0.5 molar gadobenate dimeglumine and 1.0 molar gadobutrol in contrast-enhanced run-off magnetic resonance angiography of the lower extremities. J Magn Reson Imaging 32: 1166–1171.
20. Giesel FL, von Tengg-Kobligk H, Wilkinson ID, Siegler P, von der Lieth CW, et al. (2006) Influence of human serum albumin on longitudinal and transverse relaxation rates (r1 and r2) of magnetic resonance contrast agents. Invest Radiol 41: 222–228.
21. Szucs-Farkas Z, Froehlich JM, Ulrich M, Wuersten HU, Guignard D, et al. (2008) 1.0-M gadobutrol versus 0.5-M gadoterate for peripheral magnetic resonance angiography: a prospective randomized controlled clinical trial. J Magn Reson Imaging 27: 1399–1405.
22. Fink C, Bock M, Kiessling F, Lichy MP, Krissak R, et al. (2004) Time-resolved contrast-enhanced three-dimensional pulmonary MR-angiography: 1.0 M gadobutrol vs. 0.5 M gadopentetate dimeglumine. J Magn Reson Imaging 19: 202–208.

4

Low-Dose High-Pitch CT Angiography of the Supraaortic Arteries Using Sinogram-Affirmed Iterative Reconstruction

Dietrich Beitzke[1]*, Richard Nolz[1], Sylvia Unterhumer[1], Christina Plank[1], Michael Weber[1], Rüdiger Schernthaner[1], Veronika Schöpf[2], Florian Wolf[1], Christian Loewe[1]

1 Department of Biomedical Imaging and Image-guided Therapy, Division of Cardiovascular and Interventional Radiology, Medical University Vienna, Vienna, Austria, **2** Department of Biomedical Imaging and Image-guided Therapy, Division of Neuroradiology and Musculoskeletal Radiology, Medical University Vienna, Vienna, Austria

Abstract

Objective: To prospectively evaluate image quality and radiation dose using a low-dose computed tomography angiography protocol and iterative image reconstruction for high-pitch dual-source CT-angiography (DSCTA) of the supraaortic arteries.

Material and Methods: DSCTA was performed in 42 patients, using either 120 kVp tube voltage, 120 mAS tube current, 2.4 pitch and filtered back projection, or 100 kVp tube voltage, 100 mAs tube current, 3.2 pitch, and sinogram affirmed iterative reconstruction. Measurements of vessel attenuation, of the contrast-to-noise ratio (CNR) and the signal-to-noise ratio (SNR) were performed to objectively evaluate image quality. Two readers evaluated subjective image quality and image noise, using a four-point scale. Effective dose was used to compare the differences in radiation dose.

Results: Low-dose protocol application showed significantly higher vessel opacification ($p = 0.013$), and non-significantly higher CNR and SNR values. There was no difference in the subjective image quality and image noise reading between the protocols. Effective dose was significantly lower using the low-dose protocol (1.29 ± 0.21 mSv vs. 2.92 ± 0.72 mSv; $p < 0.001$).

Conclusion: The combined use of reduced tube voltage, reduced tube current, and iterative reconstruction reduces radiation dose by 55.4% in high-pitch DSCTA of the supraaortic arteries without impairment of image quality.

Editor: Rozemarijn Vliegenthart, University of Groningen, Netherlands

Funding: The authors have no support or funding to report.

Competing Interests: The authors have declared that no competing interests exist.

* E-mail: dietrich.beitzke@meduniwien.ac.at

Introduction

Computed tomography angiography (CTA) of the supraaortic arteries has become a standard imaging technique for arteriosclerotic disease, acute stroke imaging, and for imaging traumatic arterial dissection [1,2]. Advantages of this technique include the high spatial resolution, the short acquisition times that reduce motion artifacts and venous overlay, and the high accuracy for the detection of stenosis [3]. The ability to image the entire supraaortic vasculature and to combine CTA of the supraaortic arteries with a computed tomography (CT) of the cerebrum and/ or a CT perfusion protocol leads to broad clinical use of this method during the last several years [4]. In 2006 computed tomography was accountable for about 25% of the annual per-capita effective radiation dose in the US [5]. Although until now there is no clear evidence about cancer induction through cumulative radiation doses of below 100 mSv, radiation exposure from medical imaging has drawn widespread attention within the last years [6]. Recent advances in computed tomography have introduced new possibilities for significant radiation dose reduction, including iterative reconstruction algorithms and the introduction of high-pitch scanning. The efficacy and usefulness of radiation dose reduction by using reduced tube voltage and reduced tube current settings have already been reported, but this technique leads to increased image noise, which may alter diagnostic image quality if using filtered back projection (FBP) for image reconstruction [7]. Therefore, the use of FBP in low dose CT scanning is limited, as increased image noise is associated with and reduced image quality [8]. To overcome this limitation and to provide diagnostic image quality even at low dose, iterative reconstruction algorithms for image noise correction may be used [9,10]. These reconstruction algorithms allow for image noise reduction during postprocessing, as loop-wise comparison and noise correction to the raw data images are performed [11].

Sinogram-affirmed iterative reconstruction (SAFIRE) is a raw data-based iterative reconstruction algorithm that is based on a noise modelling technique. SAFIRE tries to discover picture building and non-picture building pixels during image postprocessing. Therefore SAFIRE utilizes the known propagation of signal and noise in projection data to separate information from noise. With each iterative step, the noise content is determined and subtracted from the image data-set. After each reconstruction loop (also called iteration) the resulting image is then compared to the initial raw data for image validation. The resulting CT data may be considered as a "noise free" base and additive statistical noise. The number of iterations determines the level of noise reduction and image smoothing [9,11,12].

In addition, the latest generation of dual-source scanners, can be used high-pitch scanning with a maximum pitch of 3.2. In single-source CT the maximum pitch is usually limited to <1.5. Single source scanning with a pitch above 1.5 will result in sampling gaps. In high-pitch scanning two separated 128-slice detectors are operated with similar energy at a rotation time of 0.28 sec and a table feed up to 46 cm/sec. This allows for gapless scanning at higher pitch values as the second detector is used to fill up the gaps [13]. In various studies that focused on the coronary arteries and other scan regions, this scanning technique confirmed the possibility of significant dose reduction without the loss of diagnostic imaging quality [14,15]. Recent literature also showed lowered radiation dose values by using the high-pitch mode at CTA of the supraaortic arteries [16].

The purpose of this study was to evaluate image quality and radiation dose of a low-dose, dual source, single energy CTA protocol of the supraaortic arteries using a reduced tube voltage, a reduced tube current, and iterative reconstruction algorithms in high pitch scanning, and to compare this protocol to the standard institutional DSCTA protocol using FBP in order to prove the possibility of significant dose reduction while maintaining image quality [10].

Materials and Methods

Patient Population

The study has been approved by the local ethics committee at the Medical University of Vienna, Austria (Local IRB NR: 127/2011). All subjects gave written and informed consent prior to study inclusion. Forty-two consecutive patients with suspected or previously diagnosed vascular disease of the supraaortic arteries and referred for CTA of the supraaortic arteries were enrolled in this prospective, randomized study and assigned to one of the studies groups using a computer-generated randomization list (Table 1). Indications for CTA included stenosis of the subclavian artery (n = 5), stenosis of the brachiocephalic trunk (n = 2), stenosis of the common carotid artery (n = 1), suspected stenosis of the internal carotid artery (n = 24), suspected occlusion of the internal carotid artery (n = 2), suspected aneurysm of the common carotid artery (n = 1), suspected aneurysm of the vertebral artery (n = 1), evaluation of the supraaortic vessels prior to axillo-femoral bypass operation (n = 1), assessment of suspected in-stent restenosis (n = 4),and suspected arteriovenous fistula (n = 1).

Exclusion criteria included renal insufficiency, known allergic reaction to iodinated contrast media, age <18, hyperthyroidism, pregnancy and breast feeding.

Computed Tomography Angiography Image Acquisition

All examinations were performed using a 128–row, dual-source, multi-slice CT scanner (Siemens Somatom Definition Flash, Siemens Medical Systems, Erlangen, Germany). CTA was performed in a caudocranial direction from the level of the aortic arch to the calvarium. Acquisition parameters were 2×64×0.6 mm collimation and 280 ms gantry rotation time in both groups. Scanner settings for the standard protocol were as follows: 120 kVp tube voltage for both tubes; 120 mAs per rotation tube current time product with tube current modulation turned on (CAREDose 4D); and pitch 2.4. In contrast to the standard protocol, the scanner settings for the low-dose protocol were as follows: 100 kVp tube voltage for both tubes; 100 mAs per rotation tube current time product with tube current modulation turned on; and pitch 3.2 (Table 1). Scanner settings for the low dose protocol were based on previous reports in the literature and adopted to the second generation dual source scanner used in our study [7,16,17]. For the low dose groups 100 kVp tube voltage was chosen as previous reports using 80 kVp without SAFIRE were associated with increased image noise at the level of the shoulder belt [7]. To achieve further radiation dose reduction in the low dose group, reference tube current settings were lowered to 100 mAs per rotation.

Contrast agent injections were performed using a programmable power injector (OptiVantage, Digital Injection System, Liebel-Flarsheim Company, Cincinnati OH, USA). Optiray, a non-ionic iodinated contrast medium, was used at a concentration of 350 mg iodine/mL for all CTA studies in both groups (Optriray 350, Covidien, Dublin, Ireland).

An eighteen- (40 Patients) or 20-gauge (2 Patients) intravenous catheter was placed, wherever applicable, into the right antecubital vein for the injection of contrast agent. In three patients, the catheter had to be placed into the left antecubital vein because adequate venous access could not be provided on the right side. Bolus tracking technique was used for scan timing, with the reference image at the level of the descending thoracic aortic artery and a threshold for aortic enhancement of 150 HU. Despite using the high pitch mode, the post-threshold delay was set to 5 s in all examinations in order to avoid venous contrast agent remnants and venous contrast agent reflux at the upper thoracic outlet. Seventy mL of contrast material was injected at a constant injection rate of 5 mL/s in patients with an 18 gauge catheter and 4 ml/sec in the two patients with a 20 gauge catheter. All injections were followed by a saline flush of 40 ml.

Image Reconstruction

All images were reconstructed at 1 mm and 3 mm slice thicknesses. For image reconstruction in the standard group, FBP with a standard medium soft kernel (B31F) was used. SAFIRE with a noise reduction level 3 and the corresponding medium soft kernel for iterative reconstruction I31F was used in the low-dose group.

In addition, standardized curved planar reformats (CPR), as well as maximum intensity projections (MIP), were reconstructed in the coronal and sagittal planes, respectively.

Objective Image Analysis

A segment based analysis was chosen for the evaluation of objective image quality. Intravascular attenuation values (Hounsfield Units; HU) for the calculation of the contrast-to-noise ratio (CNR) and signal-to-noise ratio (SNR) were obtained at the level of the aorta, and bilaterally at three different anatomical levels in the course of the carotid arteries, using 3 mm thick axial reconstructed images. Measurements of vessel attenuation were performed within the aortic arch, the common carotid artery 2 cm distal to its origin, at the level of the carotid bifurcation, within the extracranial course of internal carotid artery, in the carotid sinus, and within the M1 segment of the medial cerebral artery. Care was taken to avoid measurements directly next to vessel wall calcifications.

To quantify venous enhancement vessel and reflux of contrast agent into cervical veins, attenuation measurements within the sagittal sinus, the transverse sinus and the jugular veins at the level of the bifurcation were performed.

CT attenuation values for the cervical CNR calculation were obtained from the sternocleidomastoid muscle (at the same level of

Table 1. CT study protocols and patient characteristics. Scan Range/Patients data presented as means±standard deviations (range).

	Standard	Low-dose	p-value
CT Protocol:			
CT scanner	Somatom Definition Flash		
Slice collimation	2×64×0.625 mm		
Kilovoltage (kV)	120	100	
Tube current (mAs) ref.	120	100	
Tube current modulation	CareDose4D		
Pitch	2.4	3.2	
Contrast/flow	70 ml Optiray 350 at 5 ml/sec		
Image reconstruction	FBP	SAFIRE (Level 3)	
Scan Range (cm)	42±3.5 (35.8–48.5)	42.1±2.9 (37.4–48.6)	0.83 (n.s.)
Patients:			
Sex (female/male)	9/12	7/14	
Age (years)	66.5±12 (43–86)	64.1±11.8 (39–90)	0.69 (n.s.)
Body Mass Index	27.3±4.1 (20,7–36,2)	27.1±2.8(22.1–33.5)	0.49 (n.s.)

the vessel measurements), and background noise (BN) was obtained from three areas of the surrounding air (right, left, anterior). As the field of view did not allow BN measurements in all patients at the level of the aorta, the level of the common carotid artery was used for CNR and SNR calculation at the aortic level. The area of the region of interest for HU measurements was kept constant (0.11–0.13 cm^2) during all measurements. CNR and SNR data were also calculated from the source data of axial 3 mm thick slices and was derived using the following formulas:

$$CNR = \frac{HUVes - HUSterno}{SDBN}$$

$$SNR = \frac{HUVes}{SDBN}$$

(*HUVes* = attenuation value within the vessel, *HUSterno* = attenuation value within the sternocleidomastoid muscle, *SDBN* = average standard deviation of the surrounding air at right, left, and anterior positions). All data was read in three sessions.

Subjective Image Quality Analysis

Two readers, not involved in the objective image quality reading and blinded to the protocol, performed the image quality reading independently, using a four-point scale:

Grade 0 (non-diagnostic): vascular segments cannot be assessed because of streak artifacts, vascular contrast, or graininess of the images.

Grade 1 (poor-diagnostic): patency or occlusion of the vascular segment can be assessed, but image quality is unsatisfactory.

Grade 2 (good quality): good image quality providing all details necessary for an adequate diagnosis.

Grade 3 (excellent): excellent image quality enabling sufficient differentiation of even small structures.

Readers were also asked to rate image noise on a four-point scale (0–3).

Grade 0: no noise.

Grade 1: little noise, natural graininess of the images.

Grade 2: noise above average but no impairment of the diagnostic image quality.

Grade 3: strong image noise with impairment of the diagnostic image quality.

Image quality and image noise scoring was obtained from the following segments: Aortic arch, common carotid artery, carotid bifurcation, internal carotid artery (extracranial course), carotid sinus, medial cerebral artery (M1), origin of the vertebral artery (V1), extracranial course of the vertebral artery (V2–V3) and the intradural course of the vertebral artery (V4). With the exception of the aortic arch, image quality and noise ratings were obtained from the left and right side separately.

Radiation Dose

For the estimation of radiation dose, the Dose Length Product (DLP) was calculated automatically by the CT scanner system, based on the multiplication of the Computed Tomography Dose Index (CTDI) according to the imaging range. Effective dose (ED) was subsequently calculated by using a standard conversion factor of 0.0051 mSv mGy^{-1} cm^{-1}, and as the DLP values provided by the scanner system were based on a 32-cm body phantom, the values were then multiplied by a correction factor of 2.4 to correct for a 16 cm phantom as proposed by Lell et al [18,19].

Statistical Analysis

Patient characteristics, imaging range, signal parameters, DLP, and the ED of both groups were analysed using the SPSS statistical package (SPSS Windows, version 20.0; SPSS, Chicago, IL, USA). Metric data, such as age, BMI, or scan length were expressed using means ± standard deviations. Nominal data are presented using percentages. Unpaired t-tests were performed for metric data to assess differences between the study protocols. In order to compare results of 100 and 120 kVp for all arterial and venous segments, two-way mixed model ANOVAs using unstructured covariance matrices were assessed separately, taking multiple measures per patient into account.

Agreement about subjective image quality between the two raters was tested using Cohen's kappa statistics. Image quality and noise ratings between the two study groups were compared using a

Mann-Whitney Test. The alpha level for all tests was set at $p = 0.05$.

Results

All CT scans were performed without complications according to the study protocol.

Patient Population

19 female patients and 23 male patients were included in this study. The mean age was 64.3 years (range, 22 to 85 years), and mean body mass index (BMI) was 27.6 (range 19.5 to 36.5). Patient characteristics, including height, weight, and body mass index, were equally distributed within the two groups, with no significant differences between the groups (Table 1).

Image Quality

Objective image quality. Evaluation of arterial intravascular attenuation values showed significantly higher intravascular HU values at low-dose CTA ($p = 0.013$) (Fig. 1, 2). Measured HU values within the sternocleidomastoid muscle were significantly higher at low-dose CTA ($p = 0.006$). BN was non-significantly lower ($p = 0.059$) at the low dose. Calculated CNR and SNR values showed non-significantly higher values at the low dose (CNR: $p = 0.197$; SNR: $p = 0.152$) (Table 2; Fig. 1, 2).

Mean venous opacification values did not differ between the study groups ($p = 0.121$). Venous overlay at the level of the sagittal sinus and the transverse sinus was higher at low dose, but at the same time higher attenuation differences between the arterial (M1) and the venous territory (sagittal sinus) were measured at low dose (Table 2). HU values within the jugular veins showed mean attenuation values between 100 and 126.

Subjective image quality. Of the 1428 vascular segments in both study groups, 4.1% ($n = 58$) were occluded, and thus, were excluded from further analysis. Overall image quality ratings and noise ratings did not differ between the protocols ($p = 0.4$; noise: $p = 0.91$). The majority of the segments in both protocols were rated to be of excellent image quality (Grade 3), with 86.4% in the standard dose and 86.1% at the low dose group (Fig. 2). There were 10.6% of the segments at the standard protocol and 9.1% of the segments at the low dose that were rated to be of good image quality (Grade 2), and 0.3% ($n = 2$) of the segments in both protocols were rated to be of poor image quality (Grade 1). Insufficient image quality in these two patients was based on low cardiac output resulting in reduced vessel attenuation at the level of the carotid sinus. The interrater agreement was moderate for image quality ratings ($\kappa = 0.532$; CI [0.43; 0.63]) (Table 3).

The evaluation of subjective image noise ratings showed 77.6% rated as having no noise in the standard protocol (Grade 0) and 75.9% of the segments rated as such in the low dose protocol. Moderate noise (Grade 1) was evident in 19.5% of the segments in the standard group and in 19.3% of the segments at low dose. Again, 0.3% of the segments in each group ($n = 2$) were classified having noise above the average (Grade 2). The two patients with noise ratings above the average presented with BMI values >30 and image noise was located at the level of the thoracic aperture.

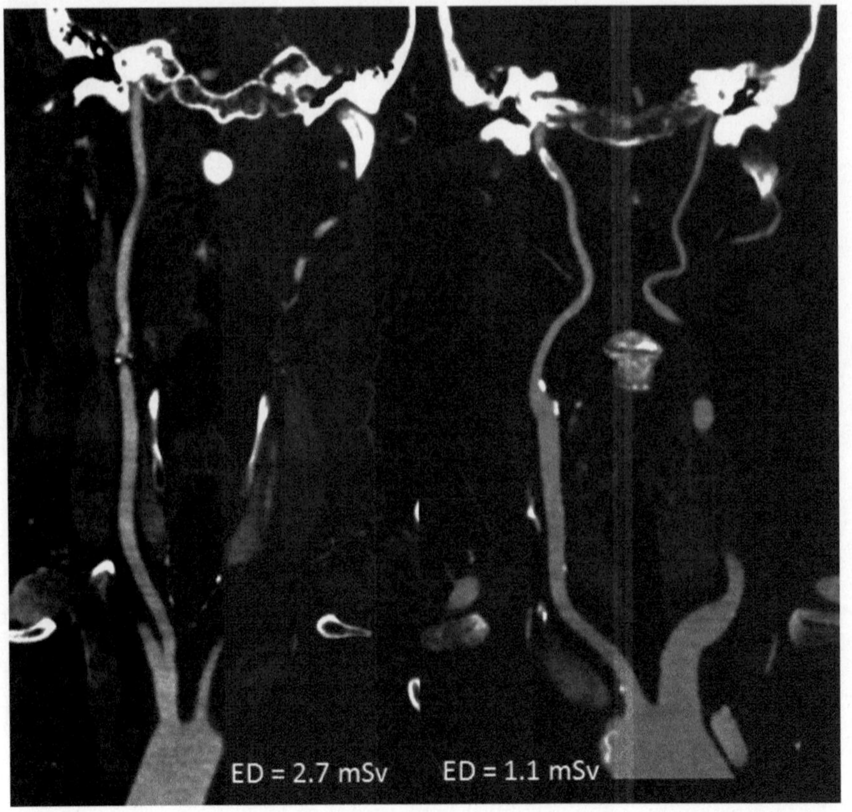

Figure 1. Comparison of image quality in two patients with suspected stenosis of the internal carotid artery. Curved planar reconstructions of (A) the standard protocol and (B) the low-dose protocol demonstrate similar diagnostic image quality in both protocols with a more smoothed appearance and reduced image noise at the level of the common carotid arteries using SAFIRE. Significantly lower radiation dose at B.

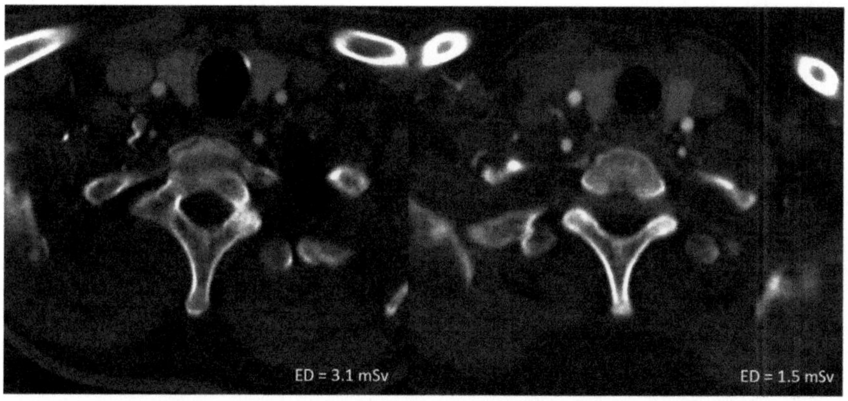

Figure 2. Comparison of image quality at the thoracic outlet. Axial images with similar window setting (W900/L250) using the standard protocol and FBP (A) and at low-dose, using SAFIRE for image reconstruction (B). Both studies were rated having excellent diagnostic image quality. Higher vessel attenuation and reduced image noise is evident at low-dose and SAFIRE (B).

The interrater agreement was good for the noise ratings ($\kappa = 0.724$; 95% CI [0.64; 0.79]) (Table 3).

Radiation Exposure

There was no significant difference in the imaging range between the groups (41.8±2.7 cm vs. 42.6±4.7 cm; $p = 0.57$; Table 1), enabling a comparison of the DLP between the two groups. Mean CTDI was 5.3±1.1 mGy for the standard protocol and 2.4±0.8 mGy at low dose ($p<0.001$). Mean DLP was 225.4±55.315 mGy*cm in the standard protocol, and 99.2±15.2 mGy*cm at low-dose ($p<0.001$). Estimated mean ED was 1.21±0.19 mSv for the low dose protocol and 2.76±0.68 mSv for the standard protocol ($p<0.001$; Table 4; Fig. 3). The latter equals an average reduction in the ED of 55.4%.

Discussion

In imaging of carotid artery disease invasive angiography as the gold standard has nowadays been replaced by non-invasive imaging modalities like ultrasound (US) magnetic resonance angiography (MRA) and CTA. CTA has a high sensitivity, specificity and accuracy in detection and characterization arteriosclerotic disease of the carotid artery and proofed to be a valuable tool, especially in the acute setting, if there is discordance between US and MRA, or if MRA is contraindicated [3]. With the introduction of new scanner techniques, enormous improvements in CT technique could be observed, including mainly advances in spatial and temporal resolution, making CT applicable for many different indications all through the body. As a consequence, the total number of CT scans performed has increased, and the exposure to radiation doses through CT imaging has become a cause for concern, particularly regarding the potential for cancer induction by CT-associated radiation dose exposure [5,20].

Different ways to reduce the radiation dose in CT, including scanning at low kV and reduced mAs settings, use of high pitch scanning, and dose modulation techniques, have been evaluated in clinical trials [7,21,22]. Using FBP for image reconstruction, most of these techniques are associated with increased image noise, impairing diagnostic image quality at low dose. Recently published studies using iterative reconstruction algorithms on so-called 'half-dose' images showed the possibility of an up to 50% dose reduction in CTA, compared to FBP in an intraindividual comparison [23]. Our study evaluated a low-dose protocol for CTA of the supraaortic arteries by combining three different, already established techniques for radiation dose reduction, including low kV settings, reduced mAs settings, and an elevated pitch. To overcome the limitation of increased image noise at low dose, SAFIRE for image reconstruction was applied to the low-dose study group. Our study underlined the possibility of a significant radiation dose reduction of more than 50% at CTA of the supraaortic arteries an unselected patient collective.

Using a lower tube voltage in CTA has two major advantages. First, it is the most effective way to reduce radiation dose. Lowering the tube voltage from 120 to 100 kVp has the potential to reduce the radiation dose applied during scanning by up to 40% [24]. In a recent study 70% dose reduction using 80 kV tube voltage at CTA of the supraaortic arteries using a 64-slice scanner and FBP was reported [7]. However the authors were confronted with streak artefacts and increased image noise at the level of the shoulder belt. Therefore, 100 kVp tube voltage was chosen for our study, as a further dose reduction was achieved by using reduced tube current settings and a high pitch. The second advantage of low kVp settings in CTA is the increase in intravascular contrast due to an increase in intravascular iodine attenuation at low kVp, as the mean photon energy of the x-rays approaches the k-edge of iodine (33.2 keV) [8]. Consequently in our study, significantly higher intravascular attenuation was evident in our low-dose group at 100 kVp (Fig. 1, 2). This effect can positively be used in CTA to either increase the vessel-to-background contrast, and thus, the image quality, or to reduce the total amount of iodinated contrast agents, as shown in previous studies [25,26]. However, to maintain full comparability of the low-dose protocol to the standard protocol, the total amount of iodinated contrast agent was not changed for the low kVp group in our study.

Since the kVp settings were not lowered to the maximum of 80 kVp to avoid severe artifacts at the level of the thoracic aperture, the tube current time product was lowered by 20% as an additional radiation dose reduction strategy in our study. SAFIRE was successfully used in the low-dose group to eliminate potentially upcoming image noise at low dose. Several published studies using lowered kVp settings in abdominal, pulmonal and supraaortic CTA showed significant higher BN or image noise in their results [7,27,28]. Contrary to these reports, the application of SAFIRE in the low-dose group resulted in a tendency toward lower background noise and non-significantly higher CNR und SNR values in the study group. This shows that the expected increase in image noise at low dose was completely compensated by the application of iterative reconstructions providing similar image

Table 2. Group comparison of objective image quality (mean vessel attenuation, muscle attenuation, background noise, CNR, SNR).

	Standard Protocol mean±SD		Low-dose protocol mean±SD		p-value
Arterial Vesselattenuation (HU)					
Aorta	362.3±91.48		420.2±75.97		
	Right	Left	Right	Left	
Common carotid artery	358.1±93.3	370.4±115.1	419.1±79.5	423.5±81.1	
Bifurcation	405.3±93.9	417.3±114.2	477.8±91.7	480.7±95.7	
Internal carotid artery	354.2±87.1	370.4±104.9	433.8±78.4	436.3±81.2	
Carotid sinus	362,6±81,5	378,3±103,6	475,4±87,6	462,3±84,8	
Medial cerebral artery	345,5±75,3	349,0±93,8	428,9±81,0	444,9±89,3	
Overall p					*0.013†*
Backgroundnoise*					
Common carotid artery	6.32±1.9		6.08±1.7		
Bifurcation	5.53±1.5		5.34±0.7		
Internal carotid artery	6.13±1.4		6.12±1.2		
Overall p					*0.59*
Muscle (HU)					
Aorta	46.7±12.71		50±13.33		
	Right	Left	Right	Left	
Common carotid artery	58.3±14.7	56.3±17.3	70.8±17.8	67.7±21.9	
Bifurcation	58.4±10.1	59.6±11.7	64.8±7.9	61±9.1	
Internal carotid artery	49.5±13.9	50.2±10.7	54.3±16.2	53.3±11.8	
Overall p					*0.006†*
CNR					
Aorta	55.78±28.40		65.81±23.10		
	Right	Left	Right	Left	
Common carotid artery	53.4±29.6	55.5±36.7	62.2±23.1	63.6±24.3	
Bifurcation	68.1±27.9	70.6±32.7	77.7±19.9	80.5±23.8	
Internal carotid artery	52.6±21.5	58.6±31.9	64.5±19.8	63.6±18.2	
Overall p					*0.2*
SNR					
Aorta	58.41±27.9		73.11±26.9		
	Right	Left	Right	Left	
Common carotid artery	63.4±32.1	66.1±38.1	74.5±24.9	75.3±26	
Bifurcation	79.3±30.3	82.2±35.2	89.8±20.9	91.9±23.9	
Internal carotid artery	61.1±22.7	67.5±33.6	73.4±20	72.9±20.3	
Overall p					*0.15*
Venous Vesselattenuation (HU)					
Sagital Sinus	238.5±74.76		256.1±60.2		
Δ to M1 (mean)	108.7		224		
	Right	Left	Right	Left	
Transverse Sinus	194.0±44.15	192.2±47.5	230.8±60.5	221±44.1	
Jugular Vein	126.5±129.7	106.4±34.4	108.2±23.9	102.2±22	
Δto Bifurcation (mean)	278.8	310.9	369.6	378.5	
Overall p					*0.121*

Mixed model ANOVA was used for group comparison of objective image quality. Data are means±standard deviations.
HU = Houndsfield units, CNR = contrast-to-noise ratio, SNR = signal-to-noise ratio. BN = Standard deviation HU.
*BN at the level of the aorta = BN ACC.
† = Significance level <0.05.

Table 3. Image reading parameters including interrater agreement measures for both protocols.

Image Quality	Standard Protocol		Low-dose Protocol	
0	0.0%	n = 0	0.0%	n = 0
1	0.3%	n = 2	0.3%	n = 2
2	10.6%	n = 76	9.1%	n = 65
3	86.4%	n = 617	86.1%	n = 615
Occluded Segments	2.7%	n = 23	4.5%	n = 36
	p		*p = 0.21*	
	95% CI		*0.43; 0.63*	
	Interrater agreement		*κ = 0.52*	
Image Noise	**Standard Protocol**		**Low-dose Protocol**	
0	77.6%	n = 554	75.9%	n = 542
1	19.5%	n = 139	19.3%	n = 138
2	0.3%	n = 2	0.3%	n = 2
3	0.0%	n = 0	0.0%	n = 0
Occluded Segments	2.6%	n = 23	4.5%	n = 36
	p		*p = 0.5*	
	95% CI		*0.66; 0.79*	
	Interrater agreement		*κ = 0.72*	

CI indicates confidence interval.

quality while saving half of the radiation dose. Especially at the origin of the vertebral artery and within the carotid sinus, representing difficult to image areas in CTA of the supraaortic arteries, no differences were observed between the study groups. The results of our prospective study go along with reports in the literature describing the effectiveness of iterative reconstruction on so called "half dose images" in abdominal CT or in CTA of the thoracic aorta [9,23].

Results from the subjective image quality reading are probably even more important for the evaluation of low-dose protocols and

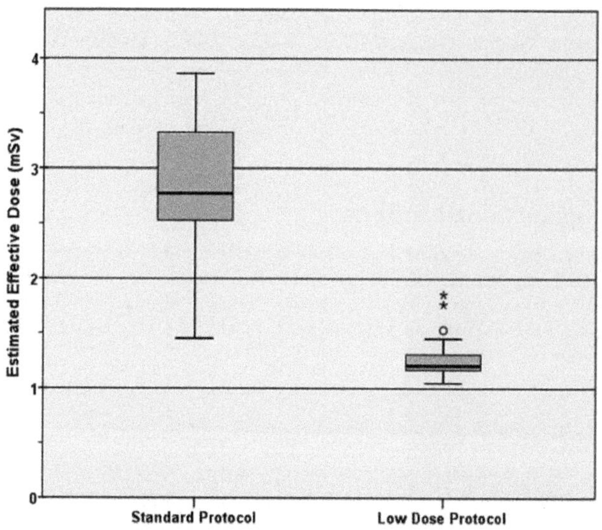

Figure 3. Box-Whisker plots of the estimated mean effective dose (mSv) for the study protocols.

to test their practicality in the clinical practice, as vessel attenuation is not the only important factor in preserving diagnostic image quality at low-dose. The scan range for CTA of the supraaortic arteries includes the bony structures of the upper thoracic aperture and the skull base, two anatomic areas that can potentially interfere with low-dose scanning [29]. Despite this, results from the subjective image quality rating in our study completely concur with results from objective image quality calculations. Both readers rated 86% of all vascular segments in both study groups as having excellent image quality. The interrater agreement concerning image quality was moderate, which may be explained by the more smooth appearance of the CT images reconstructed with SAFIRE. These images may appear "unnatural" to radiologists trained in FBP. There was also no difference in the rating of noise between the readers, and interrater agreement in noise ratings was good. These findings are different to previous work, reporting on increased image noise at low kVp without the use of SAFIRE [7]. Our results could be achieved in a clinical representative patient collective including obese patients and/or patients presenting with vascular pathologies, mainly stenosis. In our study Level 3 of SAFIRE was used in order to avoid an exaggeratedly smooth appearance of the low-dose CT images. If the noise reduction level is set too high or images at standard dose are postprocessed with iterative reconstruction algorithms the images will become blurred. If the noise reduction is set too low on the other hand, image noise remains and may result in impaired diagnostic image quality at low-dose.

Streak artifacts due to dense contrast agent remnants within the veins at the upper thoracic outlet may also alter diagnostic image quality in CTA of the supraaortic arteries, as neighbouring arteries become obscured [30]. These artifacts may be prevented by the application of the contrast agent into a right-sided cubital vein. However, if this is not possible, or in case of insufficient contrast

Table 4. Results from group comparison of radiation dose (unpaired t-test).

	Standard protocol mean±SD	Low-dose protocol mean±SD	p-value
Radiation Dose			
CTDI (mGy)	5.3±1.1	2.4±0.8	<0.01
DLP (mGy*cm)	225.4±55.3	99.2±15.9	<0.01
ED (mSv)	2.8±0.7	1.2±0.2	<0.01

Data are means±standard deviations.
CDTI = Computed Tomography Dose Index (mGy); DLP = Dose Length Product (mGy*cm); ED = estimated effective dose (mSv).

agent mobilisation (e.g. heart failure), iterative reconstruction may also be useful in the reduction of these artifacts.

Beside the above described advantages of iterative reconstruction in CTA there may also be some pitfalls. Based on the functionality of SAFIRE by small hypodens structures adjacent to very hyperdens structures may be interpreted as non-picture building pixels during image reconstruction and may be filtered during iterations. In question of in-stent restenosis or intimal hyperplasia this may theoretically false negative results if dealing with small vessel and stent diameters or in case of severe beam hardening artifacts from the stent material [11]. On the other hand there are first reports about an improved instent visibility in cardiac CTA by using raw data based iterative reconstruction in cardiac CTA [31,32].

The last adaption of the image acquisition protocol for dose-saving attempts was the use of a pitch factor of 3.2 in the study group, compared to 2.4 in the reference group examined with the standard protocol. Application of the high-pitch mode reduces acquisition of overlapping slices, as two radiation sources allow for gap free scanning at a high table feed. Additionally short scanning times also reduce radiation exposure to the patient [33]. In an evaluation of various pulmonary CTA protocols including 100 kVp settings at high pitch De Zordo et al. showed significant lower DLP values using the high pitch mode in DSCTA in comparison to single source CTA at 100 kVp at comparable tube current settings [34]. Lowest dose was found at 100 kVp and high pitch in this study. In a recent published study by Korn et al. high-pitch DSCTA showed 35% lower radiation dose values compared to single source low-pitch CTA of the supraaortic arteries [35]. In both study groups 120 kV tube voltage was used. In our study, a high pitch was used with both groups (2.4 vs. 3.2), and, from our data, we are not able to clearly estimate the contribution of the difference in pitch to the overall scan dose-saving. But, as a 2.4 pitch represents our approved standard institutional CTA protocol, it was not changed for study purposes in order to avoid higher radiation doses for the reference group by reducing the pitch factor in the study. An additional benefit of using the high pitch mode is the fast scanning time reducing the likelihood of motion artifacts during the scanning in restless and pediatric patients [36].

Venous overlay is another important aspect in CTA of the supraaortic arteries [30]. While using the high pitch moderate venous enhancement of 200 to 250 HU was evident at the intracranial sinuses in both groups but no essential enhancement was measured within the internal jugular veins in both groups. Therefore high pitch scanning with bolus tracking enables to capture the bolus mainly within the arterial system and the intracranial sinuses and disturbing venous overlay within the cervical veins can be avoided.

Some limitations of our study have to be addressed. An intra-individual comparison to exclude hemodynamic factors of vessel attenuation was not performed due to ethical considerations. No direct comparison to a single source CT scanner was performed, as all scans in our institution are performed at dual source. However, from the literature ED values ranging from approximately 4 to 6 mSv are described for standard single source CT, showing even much lower dose in our standard group compared to single source low pitch CT [4,7]. No comparison to the gold standard invasive angiography was performed. Finally, although more than 1400 vascular segments were analysed in this study, a larger sample size may have detected differences in subjective and objective image reading between the study groups.

In conclusion, iterative reconstruction algorithms enable a significant radiation dose reduction by deleting the increased image background noise at lowered tube voltage and tube current settings during image postprocessing. Image quality did not differ between our study protocols, with an even greater intravascular attenuation at low dose. Therefore, the use of 100 kVp tube voltage, reduced tube current, a high pitch, and the use of sinogram-affirmed iterative reconstruction algorithms in CTA of the surpaaortic arteries enables a radiation dose reduction of more than 50% in an unselected patient collective without the loss of diagnostic image quality.

Author Contributions

Conceived and designed the experiments: DB CL SU RN FW. Performed the experiments: SU CP FW RS DB CL RN. Analyzed the data: MW VS DB CP FW CL. Contributed reagents/materials/analysis tools: SU VS RS RN FW MW. Wrote the paper: DB CL RN FW RS VS MW SU CP.

References

1. Tholen AT, de Monye C, Genders TS, Buskens E, Dippel DW, et al. (2010) Suspected carotid artery stenosis: cost-effectiveness of CT angiography in work-up of patients with recent TIA or minor ischemic stroke. Radiology 256: 585–597.
2. Gonzalez RG, Lev MH, Goldmacher GV, Smith WS, Payabvash S, et al. (2012) Improved outcome prediction using CT angiography in addition to standard ischemic stroke assessment: results from the STOPStroke study. PloS one 7: e30352.
3. Anderson GB, Ashforth R, Steinke DE, Ferdinandy R, Findlay JM (2000) CT angiography for the detection and characterization of carotid artery bifurcation disease. Stroke; a journal of cerebral circulation 31: 2168–2174.
4. Mnyusiwalla A, Aviv RI, Symons SP (2009) Radiation dose from multidetector row CT imaging for acute stroke. Neuroradiology 51: 635–640.
5. Mettler FA, Jr., Bhargavan M, Faulkner K, Gilley DB, Gray JE, et al. (2009) Radiologic and nuclear medicine studies in the United States and worldwide: frequency, radiation dose, and comparison with other radiation sources–1950–2007. Radiology 253: 520–531.

6. Hendee WR, O'Connor MK (2012) Radiation risks of medical imaging: separating fact from fantasy. Radiology 264: 312–321.
7. Beitzke D, Wolf F, Edelhauser G, Plank C, Schernthaner R, et al. (2011) Computed tomography angiography of the carotid arteries at low kV settings: a prospective randomised trial assessing radiation dose and diagnostic confidence. European radiology 21: 2434–2444.
8. Huda W, Lieberman KA, Chang J, Roskopf ML (2004) Patient size and x-ray technique factors in head computed tomography examinations. I. Radiation doses. Med Phys 31: 588–594.
9. Winklehner A, Karlo C, Puippe G, Schmidt B, Flohr T, et al. (2011) Raw data-based iterative reconstruction in body CTA: evaluation of radiation dose saving potential. European radiology 21: 2521–2526.
10. Noel PB, Renger B, Fiebich M, Munzel D, Fingerle AA, et al. (2013) Does iterative reconstruction lower CT radiation dose: evaluation of 15,000 examinations. PloS one 8: e81141.
11. Beister M, Kolditz D, Kalender WA (2012) Iterative reconstruction methods in X-ray CT. Physica medica: PM: an international journal devoted to the applications of physics to medicine and biology: official journal of the Italian Association of Biomedical Physics 28: 94–108.
12. von Falck C, Bratanova V, Rodt T, Meyer B, Waldeck S, et al. (2013) Influence of sinogram affirmed iterative reconstruction of CT data on image noise characteristics and low-contrast detectability: an objective approach. PloS one 8: e56875.
13. Flohr TG, Leng S, Yu L, Aiimendinger T, Bruder H, et al. (2009) Dual-source spiral CT with pitch up to 3.2 and 75 ms temporal resolution: image reconstruction and assessment of image quality. Medical physics 36: 5641–5653.
14. Achenbach S, Goroll T, Seltmann M, Pflederer T, Anders K, et al. (2011) Detection of coronary artery stenoses by low-dose, prospectively ECG-triggered, high-pitch spiral coronary CT angiography. JACC Cardiovascular imaging 4: 328–337.
15. Amacker NA, Mader C, Alkadhi H, Leschka S, Frauenfelder T (2012) Routine chest and abdominal high-pitch CT: an alternative low dose protocol with preserved image quality. European journal of radiology 81: e392–397.
16. Korn A, Fenchel M, Bender B, Danz S, Thomas C, et al. (2013) High-pitch dual-source CT angiography of supra-aortic arteries: assessment of image quality and radiation dose. Neuroradiology 55: 423–430.
17. Waaijer A, Prokop M, Velthuis BK, Bakker CJ, de Kort GA, et al. (2007) Circle of Willis at CT angiography: dose reduction and image quality–reducing tube voltage and increasing tube current settings. Radiology 242: 832–839.
18. Lell MM, May M, Deak P, Alibek S, Kuefner M, et al. (2011) High-pitch spiral computed tomography: effect on image quality and radiation dose in pediatric chest computed tomography. Investigative radiology 46: 116–123.
19. Deak PD, Smal Y, Kalender WA (2010) Multisection CT protocols: sex- and age-specific conversion factors used to determine effective dose from dose-length product. Radiology 257: 158–166.
20. Carpeggiani C, Landi P, Michelassi C, Marraccini P, Picano E (2012) Trends of increasing medical radiation exposure in a population hospitalized for cardiovascular disease (1970–2009). PloS one 7: e50168.
21. Thai WE, Wai B, Lin K, Cheng T, Heist EK, et al. (2012) Pulmonary venous anatomy imaging with low-dose, prospectively ECG-triggered, high-pitch 128-slice dual-source computed tomography. Circulation Arrhythmia and electrophysiology 5: 521–530.
22. Kulkarni NM, Uppot RN, Eisner BH, Sahani DV (2012) Radiation dose reduction at multidetector CT with adaptive statistical iterative reconstruction for evaluation of urolithiasis: how low can we go? Radiology 265: 158–166.
23. May MS, Wust W, Brand M, Stahl C, Allmendinger T, et al. (2011) Dose reduction in abdominal computed tomography: intraindividual comparison of image quality of full-dose standard and half-dose iterative reconstructions with dual-source computed tomography. Investigative radiology 46: 465–470.
24. Wintersperger B, Jakobs T, Herzog P, Schaller S, Nikolaou K, et al. (2005) Aorto-iliac multidetector-row CT angiography with low kV settings: improved vessel enhancement and simultaneous reduction of radiation dose. Eur Radiol 15: 334–341.
25. Cho ES, Chung TS, Oh DK, Choi HS, Suh SH, et al. (2012) Cerebral computed tomography angiography using a low tube voltage (80 kVp) and a moderate concentration of iodine contrast material: a quantitative and qualitative comparison with conventional computed tomography angiography. Investigative radiology 47: 142–147.
26. Fujikawa A, Tsuchiya K, Imai M, Nitatori T CT angiography covering both cervical and cerebral arteries using high iodine concentration contrast material with dose reduction on a 16 multidetector-row system. Neuroradiology 52: 291–295.
27. Marin D, Nelson RC, Schindera ST, Richard S, Youngblood RS, et al. Low-tube-voltage, high-tube-current multidetector abdominal CT: improved image quality and decreased radiation dose with adaptive statistical iterative reconstruction algorithm–initial clinical experience. Radiology 254: 145–153.
28. Wintermark M, Arora S, Tong E, Vittinghoff E, Lau BC, et al. (2008) Carotid plaque computed tomography imaging in stroke and nonstroke patients. Ann Neurol 64: 149–157.
29. Ertl-Wagner BB, Hoffmann RT, Bruning R, Herrmann K, Snyder B, et al. (2004) Multi-detector row CT angiography of the brain at various kilovoltage settings. Radiology 231: 528–535.
30. Kim JJ, Dillon WP, Glastonbury CM, Provenzale JM, Wintermark M (2010) Sixty-four-section multidetector CT angiography of carotid arteries: a systematic analysis of image quality and artifacts. AJNR American journal of neuroradiology 31: 91–99.
31. Ebersberger U, Tricarico F, Schoepf UJ, Blanke P, Spears JR, et al. (2013) CT evaluation of coronary artery stents with iterative image reconstruction: improvements in image quality and potential for radiation dose reduction. European radiology 23: 125–132.
32. Oda S, Utsunomiya D, Funama Y, Takaoka H, Katahira K, et al. (2013) Improved coronary in-stent visualization using a combined high-resolution kernel and a hybrid iterative reconstruction technique at 256-slice cardiac CT-Pilot study. European journal of radiology 82: 288–295.
33. Achenbach S, Marwan M, Ropers D, Schepis T, Pflederer T, et al. (2010) Coronary computed tomography angiography with a consistent dose below 1 mSv using prospectively electrocardiogram-triggered high-pitch spiral acquisition. European heart journal 31: 340–346.
34. De Zordo T, von Lutterotti K, Dejaco C, Soegner PF, Frank R, et al. (2012) Comparison of image quality and radiation dose of different pulmonary CTA protocols on a 128-slice CT: high-pitch dual source CT, dual energy CT and conventional spiral CT. European radiology 22: 279–286.
35. Korn A, Fenchel M, Bender B, Danz S, Thomas C, et al. (2012) High-pitch dual-source CT angiography of supra-aortic arteries: assessment of image quality and radiation dose. Neuroradiology.
36. Schulz B, Jacobi V, Beeres M, Bodelle B, Gruber T, et al. (2012) Quantitative Analysis of Motion Artifacts in High-pitch Dual-source Computed Tomography of the Thorax. Journal of thoracic imaging 27: 382–386.

5

Development and Validation of Intracranial Thrombus Segmentation on CT Angiography in Patients with Acute Ischemic Stroke

Emilie M. M. Santos[1,2,3,4]*, Henk A. Marquering[3,4], Olvert A. Berkhemer[3], Wim H. van Zwam[5], Aad van der Lugt[1], Charles B. Majoie[3], Wiro J. Niessen[1,2,6] on behalf of the MR CLEAN investigators¶

1 Dept. of Radiology, Erasmus MC, Rotterdam, the Netherlands, 2 Dept. of Medical Informatics, Erasmus MC, Rotterdam, the Netherlands, 3 Dept. of Radiology, AMC, Amsterdam, the Netherlands, 4 Dept. of Biomedical Engineering and Physics, AMC, Amsterdam, the Netherlands, 5 Dept. of Radiology, Maastricht University Medical Centre, Maastricht, the Netherlands, 6 Faculty of Applied Sciences, Delft University of Technology, Delft, the Netherlands

Abstract

Background and Purpose: Thrombus characterization is increasingly considered important in predicting treatment success for patients with acute ischemic stroke. The lack of intensity contrast between thrombus and surrounding tissue in CT images makes manual delineation a difficult and time consuming task. Our aim was to develop an automated method for thrombus measurement on CT angiography and validate it against manual delineation.

Materials and Methods: Automated thrombus segmentation was achieved using image intensity and a vascular shape prior derived from the segmentation of the contralateral artery. In 53 patients with acute ischemic stroke due to proximal intracranial arterial occlusion, automated length and volume measurements were performed. Accuracy was assessed by comparison with inter-observer variation of manual delineations using intraclass correlation coefficients and Bland–Altman analyses.

Results: The automated method successfully segmented the thrombus for all 53 patients. The intraclass correlation of automated and manual length and volume measurements were 0.89 and 0.84. Bland-Altman analyses yielded a bias (limits of agreement) of −0.4 (−8.8, 7.7) mm and 8 (−126, 141) mm^3 for length and volume, respectively. This was comparable to the best interobserver agreement, with an intraclass correlation coefficients of 0.90 and 0.85 and a bias (limits of agreement) of −0.1 (−11.2, 10.9) mm and −17 (−216, 185) mm^3.

Conclusions: The method facilitates automated thrombus segmentation for accurate length and volume measurements, is relatively fast and requires minimal user input, while being insensitive to high hematocrit levels and vascular calcifications. Furthermore, it has the potential to assess thrombus characteristics of low-density thrombi.

Editor: Jean-Claude Baron, INSERM U894, Centre de Psychiatrie et Neurosciences, Hopital Sainte-Anne and Université Paris 5, France

Funding: Technology Foundation STW under Grant 11632, MRCLEAN (Dutch Heart Foundation). http://www.carisma-airspace.nl. ITEA3 project MEDUSA under grant number 10004. https://itea3.org/project/medusa.html. The funders had no role in study design, data collection and analysis, decision to publish, or preparation of the manuscript.

Competing Interests: The authors have declared that no competing interests exist.

* Email: e.santos@erasmusmc.nl

¶ MR CLEAN investigators are provided in the Acknowledgments.

Introduction

Treatment of acute ischemic stroke aims to reopen the cerebral arteries and restore cerebral perfusion. Numerous studies have related image characteristics of thrombus (size, location, and density) measured on CT, with treatment success [1–5]. Although in various studies, positive associations have been reported, their predictive value for treatment success is still under debate. The methods that were used to assess thrombus characteristics vary widely. Therefore, thrombus characteristics and outcome reported in different studies cannot be compared. An automated, objective, and reliable measurement tool would be of great value in investigating the association between thrombus characteristics and treatment outcome, and in facilitating an objective comparison tool between studies.

The composition of thrombus may vary. White clots consist of platelets and fibrin, whereas red clots are erythrocyte-rich [6]. Clots dominantly composed of red blood cells can be detected on non-contrast CT (NCCT), where it is expressed as a hyperdense artery sign. Using an automated method, Riedel & al [7] measured hyperdense middle cerebral artery thrombus length on NCCT with mean deviations from the reference values and limits of agreement of 0.1 mm±0.7 mm using <2.5 mm slice images, demonstrating that hyperdense thrombi can be measured accurately. The reported prevalence of hyperdense thrombi in patients with ischemic stroke ranges from 2% to 58% depending on thrombus location [8–10]. A challenge for hyperdense thrombus segmentation techniques on NCCT data is the possible presence of hyperdensities in intracranial vessels due to calcified arterial walls or high hematocrit [11] that mimics hyperdense thrombus. Because of the lack of contrast between low-density thrombi and surrounding tissue on NCCT, low-density thrombi can only be visualized and quantified in CTA images using the absence of contrast-enhanced lumen. However, this approach requires sufficient retrograde filling of the occluded vessel via collateral arteries, which occurs in 51% to 87% of the cases [5,12] and is related to the scan protocol [13]. The Clot Burden Score has been proposed as an alternative approach for the assessment of thrombus extent. It is a semi-quantitative measurement that assesses the volume and location of the thrombus on CTA [1]. However, the Clot Burden Score is a rather crude measure since it does not include the actual length and volume of the thrombus, which may be predictors of treatment outcome.

Our aim was to develop and validate an automated method to detect and quantify thrombus on CTA, requiring minimal user input. The method exploits the absence of contrast at the site of thrombus by using anatomical information from the contralateral arteries. The method was validated for high density thrombus by comparison with manual delineation of thrombus visible on NCCT.

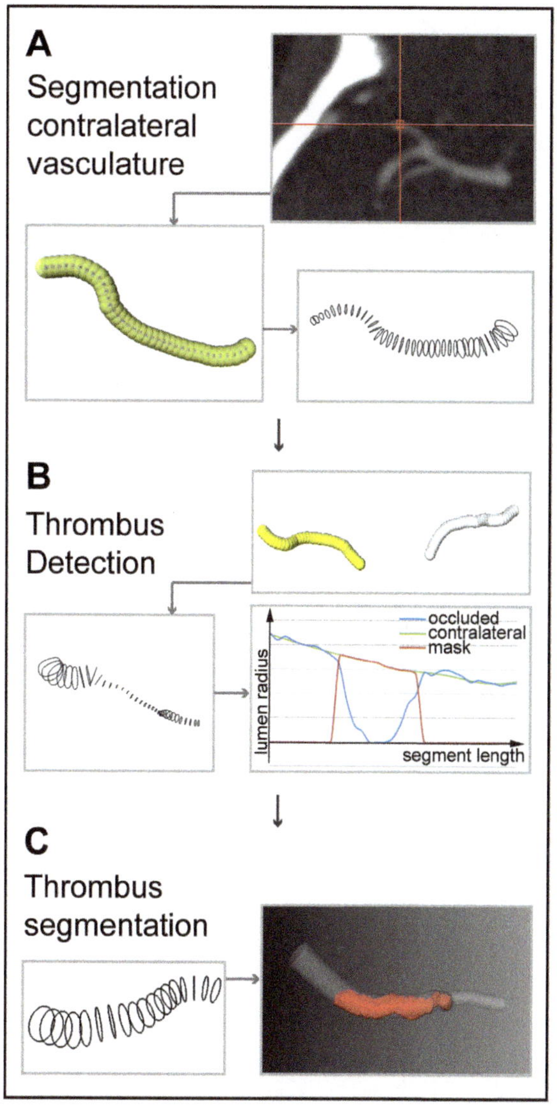

Figure 1. Illustration of the pipeline of the automated method. (A) The segmentation of the contralateral vasculature is started after manual seeds point placement. The lumen is segmented using a graph cut segmentation.(B) The thrombus is detected by mirroring the centerline and a Bspline registration followed by the segmentation of the occluded segment. Distal and proximal thrombus position is detected using the lumen radii.(C) Thrombus is segmented using tubular masking and region growing.

Materials and Methods

Patients

We retrospectively collected baseline thin slice (<2.5 mm) NCCT and CTA image data from the Dutch multi-center image database of the MR CLEAN clinical trial (Registries: NTR1804/ ISRCTN10888758; protocol available at www.mrclean-trial.org). CTA was used for the automated thrombus segmentation method. Thin slice NCCT was used in this study for the manual delineation of thrombus to validate the automated method. Therefore both baseline thin slice NCCT and CTA was required for a patient to be included. All patients had a clinical diagnosis of acute ischemic stroke due to proximal intracranial arterial occlusion with a deficit on NIHSS of 2 points or more; occlusion of the distal internal, middle, or anterior cerebral arteries, the possibility to start treatment within 6 hours from onset, and age 18 or over. Exclusion criteria for this study were low quality scans, and incomplete volume of interest.

Ethic statement

This retrospective study has been approved by the Medical and Ethical Review Committee (Medisch Ethische Toetsings Commissie; http://www.erasmusmc.nl/commissies/metc/) from Erasmus MC, Rotterdam, The Netherlands. Moreover, all participating centers providing image data received approval from their local medical ethical committee. All patient records, informations and images were anonymized and de-identified prior to analysis. All patients or legal representatives signed informed consent.

Automated Thrombus Segmentation Method

The proposed automated thrombus segmentation consists of three steps: (1) segmentation of the contralateral vasculature; (2) creation of a mask in the occluded arterial segment by mapping the contralateral segmentation using mirror symmetry; (3) segmentation of the thrombus using intensity based region growing. The image processing pipeline was implemented in MeVisLab [14] (www.mevislab.de), the different steps are visualized in Figure 1 and the main parameters used are presented in the Table 1.

The contralateral vasculature was segmented in two steps. First, proximal and distal seed points were placed manually ensuring that they covered the contralateral thrombus. Next, a curve was created through the contralateral vasculature using an optimal path calculation on a cost image generated with a vesselness filter [15,16]. Using this curve as an initial estimation of the centerline, cross-sectional lumen boundary contours were obtained using a graph-cut technique with kernel regression [17]. A refined centerline was generated by connecting all centers of mass of the lumen boundary contours. Subsequently, the vessel radius along

Table 1. Image segmentation parameters and their corresponding values.

Parameters	Values (unit)
Vesselness filter (σ_{low}, σ_{up})	1.0, 3.5
Graph cut (σi_{nside}, $\sigma_{outside}$)	20, 20 (Hounsfield unit)
Radial Reg. ($fraction_{outside}$, $P_{outside}$, $blur\sigma_{distance}$)	0.75, 0.5, 2 (mm)
Weighed Gaussian Reg. (Iteration, σ_{radius})	2, 0.5 (mm)
3D-BSpline registration (Grid spacing, grey level)	2 (mm), 32 (bit)
Mathematical morphology (opening, dilatation (3D kernel (2n+1)))	n = 1(voxel), n = 1(voxel)

the centerline was defined as the average distance from each center of mass to their respective lumen boundary contour. To correct for large variations in radii along the center line, which may be the result of blooming artifacts caused by calcifications, the radius along the centerline was smoothed with a weighted Gaussian kernel [18].

An initial estimate of the centerline of the occluded arterial segment was obtained by mirroring the contralateral centerline. This estimation was improved by performing a 3D-Bspline registration using Elastix [19] (www.elastix.isi.uu.nl), of the mirrored region of interest of the contralateral side with the region of interest of the occluded arterial segment. The mirrored centerline was used as an initialization for graph-cut segmentation with kernel regression. As it was done for the contralateral vasculature, the lumen radii along the centerline were estimated. Because the intensity of thrombi (<80 Hounsfield unit) was much lower than contrast enhanced lumen (~150 to 300 Hounsfield unit), this segmentation never includes the thrombus. As a result, the estimated lumen radius at the position of the thrombus was much smaller than the radius at the contralateral artery. The start and end positions where the estimated radius was smaller than 0.05 times the radius of the contralateral site were used as an initial estimation of the proximal and distal location of the occlusion. In some cases, due to expected insufficient contrast flow from collaterals, the method used the end part of the vasculature as distal reference for the masking step.

In the next step the thrombus was segmented. First, a mask was generated to exclude the surrounding tissues and the contrast enhanced lumen that should not be considered in the intensity based region growing segmentation. The mask was defined as a tube around the centerline of the occluded arterial segment with the radius of the contralateral arterial segment. The mask ranges from the estimated proximal and distal location of the occlusion. Intensity based region growing for thrombus segmentation was initialized at the centerline approximately 0.5 mm distal to the estimated proximal location of the occlusion. The region growing method requires two thresholds. The maximum threshold was defined as the average intensity along the contralateral centerline subtracted with the standard deviation of the intensity values along the same centerline. The minimum threshold was defined as the minimal intensity along the occluded arterial centerline in the estimated thrombus added with the standard deviation of the intensity values. A mathematical morphological opening was performed to smooth the contours of the thrombus. Length and volume are automatically measured from the resulting segmentation. The volume was determined by computing the number of segmented voxels multiplied by the size of a voxel and the length was measured from the extremities of the segmented volume along the centerline.

Manual delineations

Manual delineations of the thrombi were used to assess the accuracy of the automated method. Three neuroradiologists (CBM, WHvZ and AvdL), each with more than 10 years of experience, performed the manual delineations. The observers only had access to baseline NCCT and CTA images of the patient during thrombus delineation and were blinded from all clinical information apart from the symptom side. To assist manual delineation, a custom made tool was developed in MeVisLab. With this tool, a manual centerline was first obtained by interpolating a polynomial curve through manually placed points in the thrombus on the baseline NCCT scan. Next, the thrombus contours were delineated on a stretched-vessel view through the occluded arterial segment. Thrombus volume and length were subsequently determined from these contours. The different steps of the manual delineation pipeline are visualized in Figure 2. Because low-density thrombi were not visible on the NCCT image data, only high-density thrombi were selected for validation. The

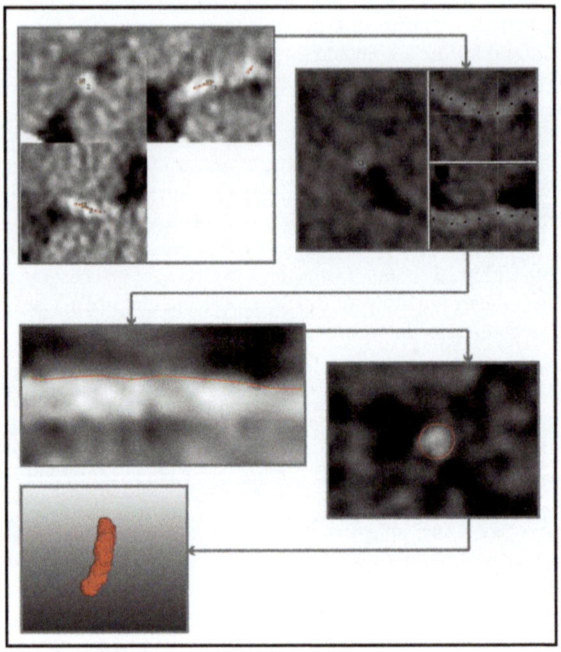

Figure 2. Illustration of the manual segmentation process. A centerline is drawn in orthogonal views and subsequently corrected using MPR viewing. The contours of the thrombus are drawn first in a longitudinal view and subsequently corrected using on a transversal view.

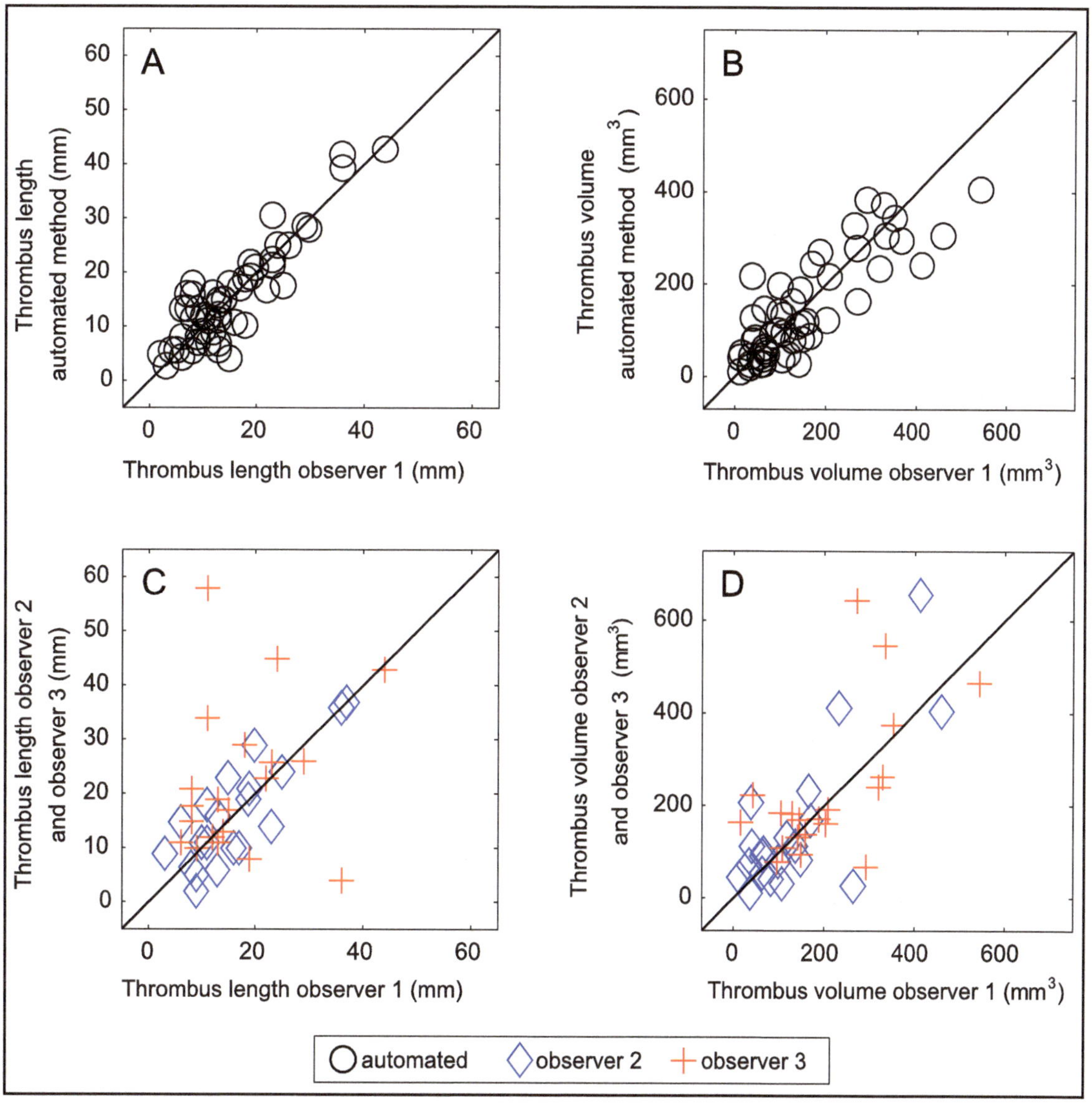

Figure 3. Scatter plot of thrombus length and volume of observer 1 and automated method (A, B). Scatter plot of thrombus length and volume of observer1 and observer 2 and 3 (C, D). The solid line represents the identity line.

time needed for automated segmentation and manual delineation was recorded.

Statistical analysis

To assess the accuracy, automated length and volume measurements were compared with the manual delineations performed by observer 1. Because of the lack of a reference standard, we compared variation between the automated method and observer 1 with the interobserver variation of the manual delineation. To assess the interobserver agreement, 20 datasets were delineated by both observer 1 and 2, and 20 other datasets were delineated by both observer 1 and 3. SPSS (SPSS version 20.0) was used to calculate the intraclass correlation coefficient (ICC) and to perform a Bland & Altman analyses.

Results

We included 78 consecutive patients with thin slice CTA and NCCT. In two patients the NCCT and/or CTA scans were incomplete. Fifty-seven (77%) of the remaining 74 patients had a visible hyperdense thrombus on NCCT. Four patients were randomly included in the training set, the remaining 53 constituted the test set. Forty-one percent of the patients were female and the mean age was 63.4 (±11.8) years. The method successfully segmented the thrombus for all patients. Figure 3 shows a scatter plot of thrombus length and volume measurements of observer1 versus observers 2, 3, and the automated method. Table 2 shows the results of the statistical analysis of the volume and length measurements. There was a high agreement between observer1 and the automated method with ICC of 0.89 and 0.84 for length and volume respectively. These values were similar to the agreement between observer 1 and 2 with ICC of 0.90 and 0.85 respectively and exceeded the agreement between observer 1 and 3. For brevity, we omitted the comparison of the automated method with observer 2 and 3, which were somewhat lower but comparable to the agreement with observer 1. Figure 4 shows the results of the Bland-Altman analysis, the agreement between

Table 2. Comparison of volume and length measurements for the automated method and observers.

	Average ± SD	(min, max)	N	Average paired difference ± SD	Limits of agreement, upper/lower limit	ICC
Length (mm)						
Observer 1	15.1±9.0	(2.0, 43.8)	53	−0.4±4.3	−8.8/7.7	0.89*
Automated	15.4±9.3	(2.7, 42.8)				
Observer 1	15.9±9.0	(3.0, 36.9)	20	−0.1±5.7	−11.2/10.9	0.90*
Observer 2	16.1±9.8	(2.0, 36.9)				
Observer 1	17.1±10.0	(6.0, 43.8)	20	−5.0±15.1	−34.7/24.6	0.31
Observer 3	22.1±13.9	(4.0, 57.9)				
Volume (mm^3)						
Observer 1	152±125	(12, 542)	53	7.5±67	−126/141	0.84*
Automated	145±110	(11, 406)				
1Observer 1	137±122	(13, 460)	20	−17±103	−218/185	0.85*
Observer 2	154±163	(12, 656)				
Observer 1	205±127	(15, 542)	20	−25±127	−340/224	0.61†
Observer 3	230±157	(68, 644)				

*p-value <0.001
†p-value <0.005.

observer 1 and the automated method was similar to the interobserver agreement. This figure also shows that there are couples of strong outliers in the comparison of observer 1 and 3. The automated segmentation required 5–7 minutes, while the manual delineations took in average 20 minutes per patient.

Discussion

In this study, a method for automated thrombus segmentation on CTA using information from the contralateral arterial segment was proposed. The method is relatively fast and requires minimal user input. The validation showed a high accuracy in automated length and volume measurement, comparable with the best interobserver agreement.

Current methods to measure thrombus characteristics are either based on manual or semi-automated measurement of hyperdense thrombus on non-contrast CT or on quantification of absence of contrast-enhanced lumen in CT angiography.

Most of these methods are based on direct measurement using a straightforward ruler tool available on a diagnostic workstation or visual scoring. More advanced length measurements have been performed on hyperdense middle cerebral thrombus on NCCT [6]. The interobserver agreement found in our study is somewhat smaller than the values reported in a previous study with a mean deviation from the reference values and limits of agreement of 0.1 mm ±0.7 mm for length [7]. This may be explained by the smaller thrombi that were present in their patient population; all thrombi were smaller than <20.0 mm and <150 mm^3. In contrast to their approach, our method does not rely on intensities of high-density thrombus and therefore is suitable for segmentation and measurement of hypodense thrombus. However, we could not validate the accuracy of automated measurement of low density thrombus owing to the difficulty of manual segmentation. Fifty seven (77%) patients had a visible thrombus on NCCT. This finding is rather high compared to the literature, which suggests that high-density thrombi are more often observed in thin slice reconstructions [20].

This study has some limitations. Because the trial was still ongoing, for many patients not all image data was available in the image database at the time of this study. Only for 74 out of 230 patients, thin slice (<=2.5 mm) NCCT and CTA data were available. As a result, further studies on larger cohorts are necessary to confirm our results in other populations. Moreover, this study does not determine predictive value of the different parameters of the thrombus (length, volume or density) as the patient outcome was not available at the current stage of the trial. The accuracy of the method could be limited by the large variety of scanner manufacturers in this study. As a result, imaging parameters such as reconstruction parameters and slice thickness varied considerably. However, since our method successfully segmented the thrombi for all used scans, it appears to be robust to these variations. Additionally, in our population we did not observe large variations in the protocols.

Another limitation is the lack of a gold standard for the thrombus characteristics. Theoretically, measurements of the surgically removed thrombus could serve as gold standard. However endovascular techniques disrupt the integrity of the thrombus. Therefore, we used the current reference standard (manual delineation) for assessing the accuracy of the automated method. This comparison indicated that the difference between the method and the manual delineation is within the range of interobserver disagreement. Because of the large effort required for manual assessment, the number of measurements of observer 2 and 3 was rather limited.

Because manual segmentation of low-density thrombus on NCCT was difficult even for very experienced neuroradiologists, accuracy of automated measurement could not be validated for these thrombi. For segmentation of low density thrombi, good collateral retrograde filling may be required. Current literature suggests that good collateral retrograde filling of an occluded artery is common but not always the case [5,12]. Poor retrograde filling may result in overestimation of the thrombus on CTA. However, due to the intensity based region growing segmentation used in our pipeline, our method is not sensitive for poor

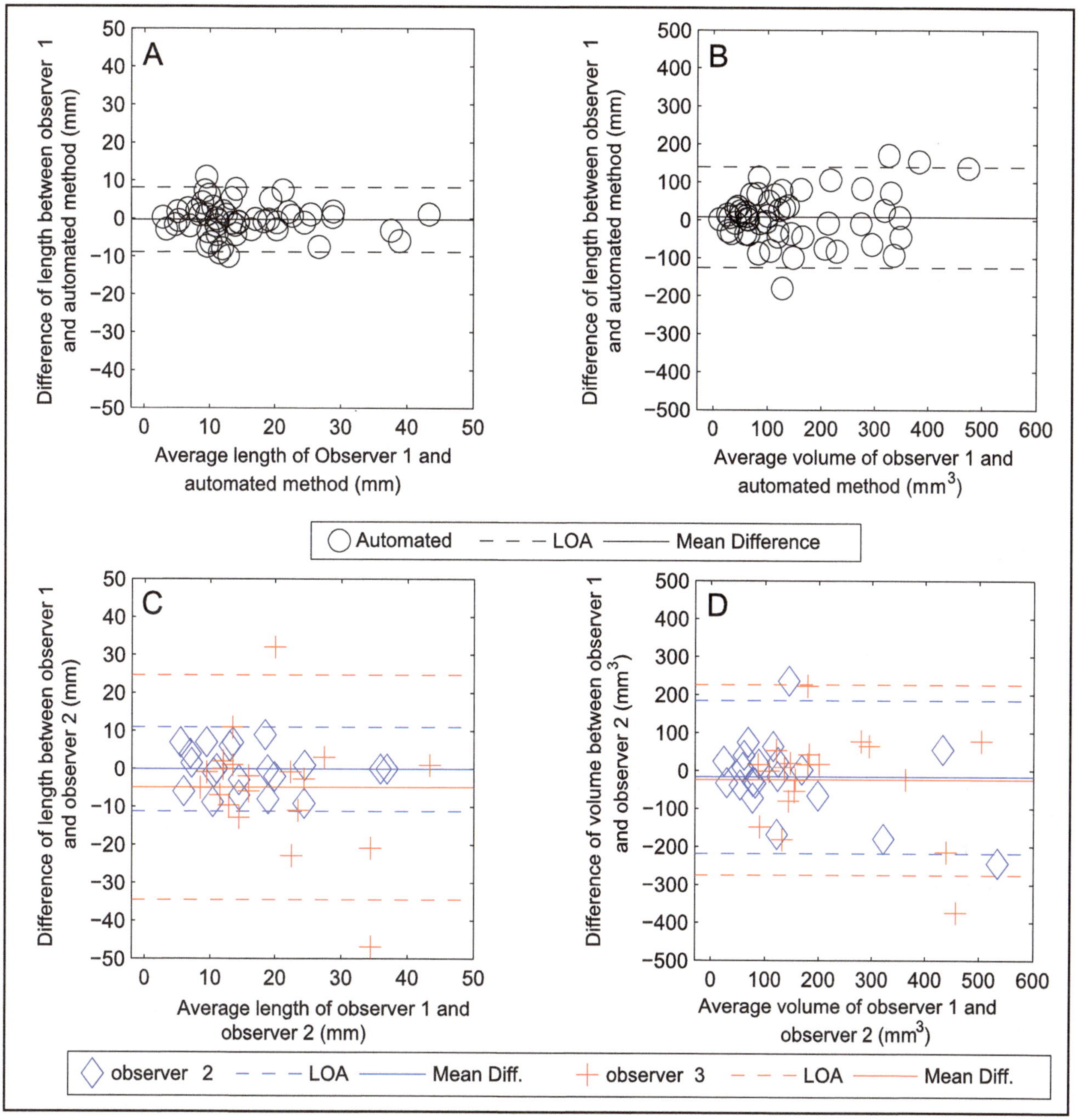

Figure 4. Bland-Altman plot comparing thrombus volume and length as measured by observer 1 and the automated method (A, B), and for all observers (D, C).

retrograde filling. Actually the large agreement between the automated method using CTA and the manual delineation on NCCT indicates that the method indeed is robust for delayed retrograde filling. In future studies, low-density thrombus segmentation could be validated by comparison with other measurements such as clot-burden score.

In our method, we assumed symmetry in order to retrieve the radius of the occluded segment for background masking. However, the occluded vascular tree and the contralateral vascular tree are not perfectly symmetric. To deal with this asymmetry, we used an elastic, non-rigid registration, which allows for differences in length, shape, and location of bifurcation. Because the accuracy of the method in 53 cases is in the range of the interobserver variability, we believe that the non-rigid registration accurately corrects for these contralateral differences. Yet, little is known about the degree of symmetry of radii of the proximal intracranial arteries. Violation of this assumption may result in errors. This could explain the larger limit of agreement for volume measurements compared to length measurement.

In three cases, we observed a strong disagreement between observer 1 and observer 3. Retrospective analysis of these three outliers revealed that this could be explained by high hematocrit level and vascular calcifications. Arteries in image datasets of patients with elevated hematocrit are known to mimic high density thrombi in CT images because of the higher attenuation on CT [20]. It is not uncommon to exclude patients with high hematocrit in thrombus analysis [4]. We believe that the observers disagreed on the interpretation of these hyperdense arteries. By excluding patients with high-hematocrit levels, as was done in previous studies, the interobserver agreement significantly improved to ICC of 0.85 and 0.78 for length and volume respectively. These values are in the range of the ICC of observer 1 and observer 2.

Image-supported treatment decision for patients with acute ischemic stroke was recently, recommended before treatment initialization by the American Society of Neuroradiology as well as number of current studies aim to it [4,12,21,22]. Predictors of successful recanalization are likely to differ for mechanical thrombectomy and intra-arterial fibrinolysis. Thrombus characteristics have been suggested to be a determinant for inclusion for IV treatment. Indeed, the thrombus length might particularly be useful as a parameter to better identify patients who are unlikely to benefit from IVT [21]. In an ongoing randomized controlled trial, it is currently uses as an inclusion criterion [http://clinicaltrials.gov/show/NCT01429350]. Whereas thrombus burden was an important predictor for the success of IV treatment, mechanical thrombectomy may be more influenced by other target characteristics like thrombus branching and vessel curvature [23].

The presented method has the potential to support current clinical research and to be introduced in clinical practice to support treatment decisions for patients with acute ischemic stroke. With this method, multivariate analysis of many thrombus characteristics (length, volume, density, curvature, etc.) could be performed to relate these to stroke subtype, response to treatment, and patient outcome measures. This way, thrombus characteristics with the most prognostic value could be determined. However, further prospective studies will have to demonstrate the feasibility of this method in acute clinical setting and determine the predictive value of imaging features of thrombus on CTA.

Conclusions

We developed and validated an automated tool performing thrombus length and volume measurements. We have shown that for high-density thrombi, this method is highly accurate, with accuracies comparable to interobserver agreements. Furthermore, this method was shown to be able to segment thrombi even for cases with high hematocrit level or calcifications, and thus could facilitate segmentation of hypodense thrombi. However, further studies on larger cohorts are necessary to confirm our results in larger and different populations.

Acknowledgments

The MR CLEAN investigators: *Local principal investigators*: Diederik W. Dippel, Patrick A. Brouwer, (Erasmus Medical Center, [ErasmusMC] Rotterdam, the Netherlands); Yvo B. Roos, Charles B. Majoie, (Academic Medical Center [AMC], Amsterdam, the Netherlands); Robert J. van Oostenbrugge, Wim H. van Zwam, (University Medical Center Maastricht [MUMC], Maastricht, the Netherlands); Jelis Boiten, Geert J. Lycklama à Nijeholt, (Medical Center Haaglanden, Den Haag, the Netherlands); Marieke J. Wermer, Marianne A. van Walderveen, (Leiden University Medical Center [LUMC], Leiden, the Netherlands); L. Jaap Kappelle, Rob T. Lo, (University Medical Center Utrecht [UMCU], Utrecht, the Netherlands); Ewoud J. van Dijk, Joost de Vries, (University Medical Center St. Radboud, Nijmegen, the Netherlands); Wouter J. Schonewille, Jan Albert Vos, (St. Antonius Ziekenhuis, Nieuwegein, the Netherlands); Jeannette Hofmeijer, Jacques A.van Oostayen, (Rijnstate Ziekenhuis, Arnhem, the Netherlands); Patrick C. Vroomen, Omid Eshghi, (University Medical Center, Groningen, the Netherlands); Paul L. de Kort, Willem Jan van Rooij, (St. Elisabeth Ziekenhuis, Tilburg, the Netherlands); Koos Keizer, Xander Tielbeek,(Catharina Ziekenhuis Eindhoven, the Netherlands); Bas F. de Bruijn, Lukas C. van Dijk, (Haga Ziekenhuis, Den Haag, the Netherlands); J.S. Peter van den Bergh, Boudewijn A. van Hasselt, (Isala Klinieken, Zwolle, the Netherlands); Leo A. Aerden, René J Dallinga, (Reinier de Graaf Gasthuis, Delft, the Netherlands); Heleen M. den Hertog, Dick G. Gerrits, (Ziekenhuis Medisch Spectrum Twente, Enschede, the Netherlands); Marieke C. Visser, Joost C. Bot, (VU University Medical Center [VUmc], Amsterdam, the Netherlands). *Executive committee*: Diederik W.J. Dippel, Aad van der Lugt (ErasmusMC); Charles B. Majoie, Yvo B.W.E.M. Roos, (AMC); Robert J. van Oostenbrugge, Wim H. van Zwam, (MUMC). *Imaging assessment committee*: Charles B. Majoie; Wim H. van Zwam; Geert J. Lycklama à Nijeholt; Marianne A. van Walderveen; Joost C. Bot; Henk A. Marquering, Ludo F. Beenen; Marieke E. Sprengers; René van den Berg, *Independent DSA reader*: Albert J. Yoo, (Massacussets General Hospital, Boston, USA). *Outcome assessment committee*: Yvo B. Roos; Peter J. Koudstaal; Jelis Boiten; Ewoud J. van Dijk. *Adverse event committee*: Robert J. van Oostenbrugge, Marieke J. Wermer, Zwenneke H. Flach. *PhD-students and study coordinators*: Puck S.S. Fransen, (ErasmusMC); Debbie Beumer, (MUMC); Olvert A. Berkhemer, Lucie van den Berg, (AMC). *Trial statisticians*: Ewout W. Steyerberg, Hester F. Lingsma, (Dept. of Public Health, Center for Clinical Decision Sciences, ErasmusMC). *Data Monitoring Committee*: Martin M Brown, (UC London,UK). Thomas Liebig, Uniklinik Köln, Theo Stijnen, (LUMC). *Trial managers*: Esther S. van der Heijden (ErasmusMC), Nadine M. Fleitour, (AMC). Consortium contact: Charles B. Majoie; c.b.majoie@amc.uva.nl

Author Contributions

Conceived and designed the experiments: ES HM WN. Performed the experiments: WZ AL CM. Analyzed the data: ES HM WN. Contributed reagents/materials/analysis tools: ES OB. Contributed to the writing of the manuscript: ES HM OB WZ AL CM WN.

References

1. Volker P, Dzialowski I, Hill MD, Subramaniam S, Sylaja PN, et al. (2008) Intracranial thrombus extent predicts clinical outcome, final infarct size and hemorrhagic transformation in ischemic stroke: the clot burden score. Neuroradiology 3: 230–236.
2. Marder VJ, Chute DJ, Starkman S, Abolian AM, Kidwell C, et al. (2006) Analysis of thrombi retrieved from cerebral arteries of patients with acute ischemic stroke. Stroke 37: 2086–2093.
3. Molina CA (2005) Imaging the clot: does clot appearance predict the efficacy of thrombolysis? Stroke 36: 2333–2334.
4. Spiotta AM, Vargas J, Hawk H, Turner R, Chaudry MI, et al. (2013) Hounsfield unit value and clot length in the acutely occluded vessel and time required to achieve thrombectomy, complications and outcome. J Neurointerv Surg: in press.
5. Puig J, Pedraza S, Demchuk A, Blasco G, Soria G, et al. (2012) Quantification of Thrombus Hounsfield Units on Noncontrast CT Predicts Stroke Subtype and Early Recanalization after Intravenous Recombinant Tissue Plasminogen Activator. AJNR Am J Neuroradiol. 33: 90–96.
6. Liebeskind DS, Sanossian N, Yong WH, Starkman S, Tsang MP, et al. (2011) CT and MRI early vessel signs reflect clot composition in acute stroke. Stroke 42: 1237–1243.
7. Riedel CH, Jensen U, Rohr A, Tietke M, Alfke K, et al. (2010) Assessment of thrombus in acute middle cerebral artery occlusion using thin-slice nonenhanced Computed Tomography reconstructions. Stroke 41: 1659–1664.
8. Leys D, Pruvo JP, Godefroy O, Rondepierre P, Leclerc X (1992) Prevalence and significance of hyperdense middle cerebral artery in acute stroke. Stroke 23: 317–324.
9. Fitzsimmons PR, Biswas S, Hill AM, Kumar R, Cullen C, et al. (2011) The hyperdense internal carotid artery sign: prevalence and prognostic relevance in stroke thrombolysis. Stroke Res Treat: in press.
10. Krings T, Noelchen D, Mull M, Willmes K, Meister IG, et al. (2006) The hyperdense posterior cerebral artery sign: a computed tomography marker of acute ischemia in the posterior cerebral artery territory. Stroke 37: 399–403.
11. New P, Saul A (1976) Attenuation Measurements of Whole Blood and Blood Fractions in Computed Tomography. Radiology.121: 635–640.
12. Christoforidis G, Mohammad Y, Kehagias D, Avutu B, Slivka AP (2005) Angiographic assessment of pial collaterals as a prognostic indicator following intra-arterial thrombolysis for acute ischemic stroke. AJNR Am J Neuroradiol 26: 1789–1797.
13. Yoo AJ, Pulli B, Gonzalez RG (2012) arterial stroke therapies: a comprehensive review. Expert Rev Cardiovasc Ther 9: 857–876.

14. Heckel F, Schwier M, Peitgen H (n.d.) Object-oriented application development with MeVisLab and Python. Lecture Notes in Informatics (Informatik 2009: Im Focus das Leben). 154: 1338–1351.
15. Frangi AF, Niessen WJ, Vincken KL, Viergever MA (1998) Multiscale vessel enhancement filtering. Medical Image Computing and Computer-Assisted Intervention–MICCAI 1998, 130–137.
16. Metz CT, Schaap M, Walsum T Van, Niessen WJ (2008) Two Point Minimum Cost Path Approach for CTA Coronary Centerline Extraction: 3D segmentation in the clinic: a grand challenge II. MICCAI 2008 workshop proceedings.
17. Schaap M, van Walsum T, Neefjes L, Metz C, Capuano E, et al. (2011) Robust shape regression for supervised vessel segmentation and its application to coronary segmentation in CTA. IEEE Trans Med Imaging 30: 1974–1986.
18. Shahzad R, Walsum T Van, Kirisli H, Tang H (2012) Automatic Stenoses Detection, Quantification and Lumen Segmentation of the Coronary Arteries using a Two Point Centerline Extraction Scheme, 3D Cardiovascular Imaging: A MICCAI segmentation challenge. MICCAI 2012 workshop proceedings.
19. Klein S, Staring M, Murphy K, Viergever MA, Pluim JPW (2010) Elastix: a Toolbox for Intensity-Based Medical Image Registration. IEEE Trans Med Imaging 29: 196–205.
20. Riedel CH, Zoubie J, Ulmer S, Gierthmuehlen J, Jansen O (2012) Thin-Slice Reconstructions of Nonenhanced CT Images Allow for Detection of Thrombus in Acute Stroke. Stroke: 2319–2323.
21. Riedel CH, Zimmermann P, Jensen-Kondering U, Stingele R, Deuschl G, et al. (2011) The importance of size: successful recanalization by intravenous thrombolysis in acute anterior stroke depends on thrombus length. Stroke 42: 1775–1777.
22. Wintermark M, Sanelli PC, Albers GW, Bello JA, Derdeyn CP, et al. (2013) Imaging recommendations for acute stroke and transient ischemic attack patients: a joint statement by the American Society of Neuroradiology, the American College of Radiology and the Society of NeuroInterventional Surgery. J Am Coll Radiol 10: 828–832.
23. Zhu L, Liebeskind DS, Jahan R, Starkman S, Salamon N, et al. (2012) Thrombus branching and vessel curvature are important determinants of middle cerebral artery trunk recanalization with Merci thrombectomy devices. Stroke 43: 787–792.

6

Clinical Significance of A Single Multi-Slice CT Assessment in Patients with Coronary Chronic Total Occlusion Lesions Prior to Revascularization

Xinkai Qu[1], Weiyi Fang[1]*, Kaizheng Gong[2], Jianding Ye[3], Shaofeng Guan[1], Ruogu Li[1], Yingjia Xu[1], Yan Shen[3], Min Zhang[1], Hua Liu[1], Wenhui Xie[4]

1 Department of Cardiology, Shanghai Chest Hospital, Shanghai Jiao Tong University, Shanghai, China, **2** Department of Cardiology, The Second Clinical Medical School of Yangzhou University, Jiangsu Province, China, **3** Department of Radiology, Shanghai Chest Hospital, Shanghai Jiao Tong University, Shanghai, China, **4** Department of Nuclear medicine, Shanghai Chest Hospital, Shanghai Jiao Tong University, Shanghai, China

Abstract

Accurate assessment of coronary chronic total occlusion (CTO) lesion is essential to design an appropriate procedural strategy before revascularization. The present study aims to evaluate the significance of a single multislice computed tomography (MSCT) examination in patients with CTO lesion. We retrospectively analyzed the clinical data of 23 CTO lesions in twenty patients underwent computed tomography coronary angiography (CTCA) and SPECT. The CTCA was more powerful and sensitive to determine the CTO lesion length (100% v.s 47.8%) and to identify the length and location of calcification in occluded vessels compared with the coronary angiography (CAG). The LVEF measured by MSCT was comparable to that from the gated SPECT. Myocardial perfusion imaging showed that the location of the early defect region identified by MSCT was corresponded to the nuclide filling defect on the stressed ^{201}thallium-SPECT imaging. The late hyperenhancement on MSCT was presented as incomplete nuclide filling on the ^{99m}Tc-MIBI imaging. The results suggested that a single MSCT examination in previous myocardial infarction without revascularization facilitates to provide some valuable information on the nature of the occluded lesion, myocardial perfusion and globe cardiac function, which would be helpful to design appropriate revascularization strategy in these subjects.

Editor: Rozemarijn Vliegenthart, University of Groningen, Netherlands

Funding: This study was partly supported Scientific Research Program of Shanghai Municipal Health Bureau (No. 2010091). The grant was 5000 dollars. And the funder's website is http://www.smhb.gov.cn/wsj/. The funders had no role in study design, data colloction and analysis, decision to publish, or preparation of the manuscript.

Competing Interests: The authors have declared that no competing interests exist.

* E-mail: fwychest@163.com

Introduction

Chronic total occlusion (CTO) of a coronary artery was documented in nearly 15% patients undergoing coronary angiography (CAG), and represents of 10% lesions treated by percutaneous coronary intervention (PCI)[1]. Successful recanalization of CTO lesions in patients with viable myocardium not only facilitates to reduce angina symptoms, avoid bypass surgery and decrease incidence of myocardial infarction, but also may improve long-term survival[2,3]. An analysis of 25 years of experience in the Mayo Clinic showed that the procedural success rate for CTO remained around 70%[4]. However, with the remarkable advancements in the instruments and the techniques of PCI for CTO lesions, the success rate of PCI for CTO in the few international cardiovascular interventional centers have raised up to 80% to 90%[5]. It is noted that the application of new instruments and the techniques of PCI often are limited due to various reasons. Therefore, the recanalization of CTO lesion still remains as one of major challenges for the most interventional cardiologists in current clinical practice. Using the traditional antegrade wire approach, the lesion characteristics including long lesion length and occlusion duration, no stump, presence of a large side branch with a takeoff adjacent to the occlusion, serious calcification and bad collateral circulation, often became the unfavorable factors for successful recanalization for CTO lesion[6,7]. Therefore, a detailed comprehensive assessment for CTO arteries has become very important before PCI revascularization.

Recently, noninvasive imaging techniques, including computed tomography coronary angiography (CTCA), magnetic resonance imaging and single-photon emission computed tomography (SPECT), on the assessment of coronary artery disease have been developed and well documented in many studies[8–10]. For example, based on its high spatial and temporal resolution, multislice computed tomography (MSCT) can not only non-invasively assess the coronary arteries and detect coronary stenosis (≥50%) with high sensitivity and specificity compared with quantitative CAG, but also provides excellent information concerning cardiac function and myocardial perfusion[11,12]. More recently, Schuleri *et al*[13] demonstrated that a delayed enhancement (DE)-MSCT had ability to provide a more detailed assessment of the peri-infarct zone in a model of pig with chronic myocardial infarction compared with magnetic resonance imaging. However, few data are available on the value of MSCT in patients with CTO[14]. Also, it is noted that the diagnosis of CTO by MSCT sometimes may be underestimated or missed because the vessel distal to the CTO is often visualized or opacified with contrast because of retrograde collateral flow[15,16]. Therefore, we hypothesized that combination of multiple non-invasive modalities can provide more accurate information in the assessment of CTO lesion compared with the traditional CAG. The aim of this study was to evaluate the diagnostic value of a single MSCT examination on patients with CTO lesion by retrospectively comparing the data from MSCT, SPECT imaging and CAG.

Methods

The research was approved by Shanghai Chest Hospital ethics committee. Written consent was given by the patients for their information to be stored in the hospital database and used for research.

Patients

During Jan 2010 to Dec 2010, a total of 600 patients with coronary heart disease were diagnosed in the Shanghai Chest Hospital Affiliated to Shanghai Jiaotong University. Patients with atrial fibrillation, renal insufficiency (serum creatinine > 120 mmol/L), known allergy to iodine contrast media, unstable clinical conditions, and other routine contraindications for MSCT or SPECT were excluded. After exclusion, 20 patients with a total of 23 CTO lesions identified by invasive CAG and MSCT were entered in this retrospective study.

MSCT Data Acquisition

MSCT imaging was performed using a 64-detector single-source CT scanner (Philips Medical Systems Corporation). Beta-blockade was used if the heart rate was >65 beats/min. Scanning parameters were as follows: tube voltage 80 to 100 kV, tube current 650–800 mA, depending on body mass index, slice thickness = 0.6 mm, increment = 0.3 mm. An 80 ml bolus of Ultravist 370 was injected intravenously at a rate of 4 ml/s, followed by 25 ml saline flush at same flow rate was used. To time the scan, automated detection of peak enhancement in the aortic root was used. All images were acquired during an inspiratory breath hold, while an electrocardiogram (ECG) was used simultaneously for retrospective analysis of the data. MSCT images were acquired at 45 seconds and 5 minutes after bolus injection, and raw data were stored for subsequent reconstruction. Source images were analyzed by software, at 60–75% of the RR interval with a retrospective multi-cycle ECG gating algorithm, slice thickness = 3 mm, reconstruction increment = 0.3 mm to assure image quality. Axial slices were reconstructed for assessment of necrotic myocardium, various myocardial signal intensities, left ventricular ejection fraction (LVEF) and coronary artery stenosis. Radiation dose was determined based on the dose-length product documented in the CT scan protocol, separately for the 'test bolus' acquisition and the coronary CTA acquisition. Effective dose was estimated based on the dose-length product, using a conversion factor of 0.014 for chest CT in adults.

MSCT Data Analysis

Images were analyzed by two experienced cardiovascular radiologists, using a dedicated workstation with multiplanar reconstruction images, and volume rendering (VR). The VR allowed reconstruction of three-dimensional (3D) images (Tree, Heart, Outline). For each slice, endocardial and epicardial contours of the left ventricle in both end-systolic and end-diastolic periods were drawn manually and independently by a radiologist, and global function parameters, including end-systolic volume, end-diastolic volume and LVEF were calculated. To assess myocardial viability, the signal intensity in a separate myocardial area was measured.

Thallium-201 Chloride (^{201}TICI) Perfusion imaging After Dobutamine Stress

Dobutamine was injected intravenously at a rate of 5 μg/kg/min initially, then increased by 5 μg/kg/min every 3 minutes to 20 μg/kg/min. Injection of 111–148 MBq (3–4 mCi) ^{201}TICI was performed when stress was induced, as indicated by any of the following: heart rate 85% of the expected highest heart rate or ≥ 130 bpm; severe angina symptoms; serious arrhythmia; systolic blood pressure ≥28 KPa or blood pressure decreased by >3 KPa; ST segment decreased by ≥2 mm. Myocardium perfusion imaging was performed 10 minutes later, and nuclide myocardial perfusion was observed.

Delayed ^{201}TICI Resting Perfusion imaging

Delayed ^{201}TICI resting perfusion imaging was performed 4 hours after the first examination, and ^{201}TI distribution was observed. ^{201}TI redistribution was defined as an ischemic myocardial region; no redistribution was defined as an infarcted region; and reverse redistribution was defined as a damaged region.

Technetium-99m Hexakis-2-methoxy-2-isobutylisonitrile (^{99m}Tc-MIBI) Perfusion Imaging

Nitroglycerin (0.5 mg) was given immediately after delayed ^{201}TICI resting perfusion imaging. ^{99m}Tc-MIBI 1110 MBq (30 mCi) was injected after 5 minutes, followed by ^{99m}Tc-MIBI perfusion imaging 1 hour later. The region with residual nuclide filling defect was defined as necrotic myocardium.

All above SPECT data were collected at three examination time-points. Parameter settings were as follows: low energy high resolution parallel-hole collimators, 64×64 matrix, 1.00 zoom, peak energy 70–80 keV, window width 20%, and dual-detector with an angle of 60°. Original data were collected for reconstruction. Horizontal long-axis, vertical long-axis and short-axis images were acquired to define early perfusion defect (ED) regions and LVEF, and to compare qualitatively between MSCT-derived zones.

Invasive CAG Examination

After the above noninvasive imaging examination, a conventional CAG was performed in all 20 patients according to the standard technique. An experienced operator blinded to the MSCT data visually evaluated the coronary angiograms.

Statistical Analysis

Continuous variables were expressed as mean ± standard deviation. Agreement between MSCT- and SPECT-derived LVEF was assessed with the Pearson's correlation coefficient and by Bland-Altman analysis.25 Statistical analysis was performed with SPSS 13.0 software. For Bland-Altman analysis, MedCalc® software was used. Statistical significance was defined as two-sided P value <0.05.

Results

Clinical characteristics

The study population consisted of seventeen men and three women, mean age was 66±10 years. Mean heart rate was 61±3

Table 1. Clinical characteristics of the study population ($n = 20$).

Mean age (yrs)	66±10
Male, n (%)	17 (85.0%)
Smoker	4 (20.0%)
Diabetes mellitus	4 (20.0%)
Hypertension	12 (60.0%)
Previous infarction	5 (25.0%)

beats/min, duration of breath hold was 15s. Clinical characteristics of the study population are summarized in Table 1. All patients underwent coronary artery MSCT and invasive CAG examination. Effective radiation dose for dual-stage MSCT scanning was 31.60±1.92 mGy. Among, 10 patients also performed successfully myocardial perfusion SPECT imaging. Measurement of serum creatinine remained similar level before and after there invasive examines. Subsequently, successful revascularization procedure were performed in 17/23 CTO lesions according the information from MSCT examination.

Comparative of CTO lesion features: CTCA vs. CAG

A total of twenty-three CTO lesions were assessed by CTCA and CAG in 20 patients, including eight CTOs in the left anterior descending coronary artery, seven in the left circumflex coronary artery and eight in the right coronary artery. The length of the occluded segment was determined by CTCA examination in all 23 CTOs. In contrast, only 11 CTOs was measured by CAG because of missing collateral angiography. In eleven patients with data acquired both by MSCT and CAG, the length of the CTOs showed no significant difference between two methods (23±12 mm vs. 22±11 mm, P>0.05). However, CTCA had higher sensitivity in the rate of detection of calcification lesion compared with CAG (69.6% vs. 43.4%, P<0.05). Also, the length of calcification lesion could be successfully measured by CTCA (10.1±5.5 mm), but not by CAG. It is noted that CTCA could detect the detailed location (proximal, middle and distal segment) of calcification in occlusive vessels, and facilitated to visualize the tract of the occluded segment by using 3D reconstruction (Fig. 1).

Comparison of LV function: MSCT vs. SPECT

The assessment of global LV function has important diagnostic and prognostic values in patients with CAD, especially for CTO. The average LVEF (58%±11%) obtained by gated SPECT was comparable to that measured with MSCT (57%±15%). The measurement of LVEF by using MSCT and SPECT methods are highly correlated with a r Pearson coefficient value of 0.79 (P< 0.01). Bland-Altman plot analysis indicated a good agreement between the two methods (Fig. 2).

Comparison of Myocardium Perfusion: MSCT vs. SPECT

Quantitative analysis from MSCT biphasic imaging in all CTO patients showed a statistically significant difference in attenuation values between the normal and the perfusion defect regions in early scanning images (92±13 HU vs. 42±12 HU, P<0.001). Three patients had residual perfusion defect regions in late scanning images and the attenuation values were lower than those in the normal regions (57±16 HU vs. 86±18 HU, P<0.01). Late hyperenhancement (LH) regions were detected in eight patients

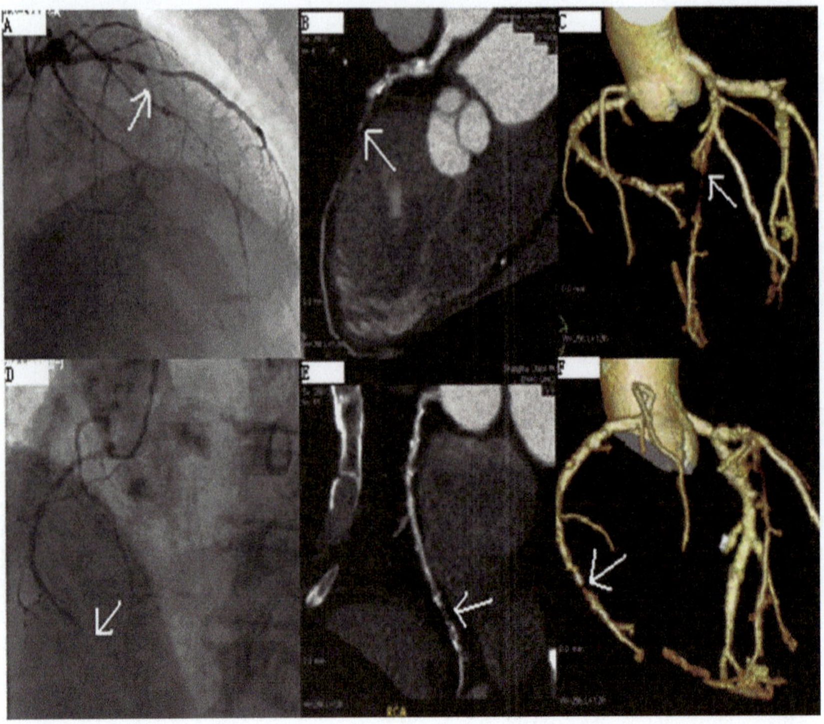

Figure 1. Representative Reconstructed Images of CTO Lesions at the Left Anterior Descending Coronary Artery (LAD) and Right Coronary Artery (RCA). 1A, 1D: Coronary angiography (CAG) image; 1B, 1E: Multiplanar reconstruction images; 1C, 1F: Three-dimensional volume rendering (Tree) image.

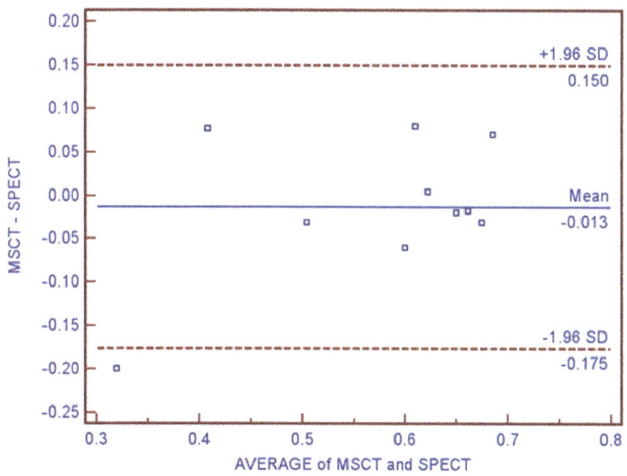

Figure 2. Bland-Altman Plots of Left Ventricular Ejection Fraction using Multislice Computed Tomography (MSCT) and Single-photon Emission Computed Tomography (SPECT).

and had higher attenuation values compared with the normal regions (135±29 HU vs. 86±18 HU, P<0.001).

In addition, table 2 showed that a total of 10 patients with CTO finished myocardial perfusion imaging using both MSCT and SPECT. The location of the early perfusion defect region identified by MSCT was corresponded to the nuclide filling defect detected by stressed ^{201}TI-SPECT perfusion imaging. In patients with late hyperenhancement in MSCT, ^{99m}Tc-MIBI imaging showed incomplete nuclide filling. By contrast, the complete nuclide filling was shown on ^{99m}Tc-MIBI imaging in patients without late hyperenhancement on MSCT scan. Figure 3 shows an example of a large perfusion defect on MSCT and SPECT.

Discussion

Accurate assessment of CTO lesion is essential to design the strategy of revascularization before PCI procedure. Accumulating evidence demonstrated that combination of multiple coronary artery imaging techniques provides a comprehensive assessment on coronary artery lesions[17,18]. In the present study, we evaluate the diagnosis value of a single MSCT examination on CTO lesion by comparative analysis of the data from traditional invasive CAG and myocardial perfusion SPECT imaging.

Many studies have demonstrated that the success rates of PCI for CTO are influenced by marked lesion calcification at the stump, severe tortuosity of the proximal vessel, the orientation and long length of the occluded segment as well as the location of the vessel distal to the occlusion[5,7]. Our results demonstrated that all above-mentioned unfavorable features of PCI treatment can be easily identified by CTCA. By contrast, the lesion features can not be often well detected by traditional CAG. As a result of the relatively long time that transpires between intravenous injection of contrast and the time required for scan acquisition, the distal site of the occlusion could be identified by retrograde collateral flow of contrast.

Serious calcification was shown to have strong association with the success rate of CTO recanalization[7,19]. Although sometimes it is difficult to identify calcification using CAG, but CTCA has been confirmed to be a useful tool for the identification of calcification[20]. The present study showed that the location, extent and length of calcification could be accurately evaluated by CTCA.

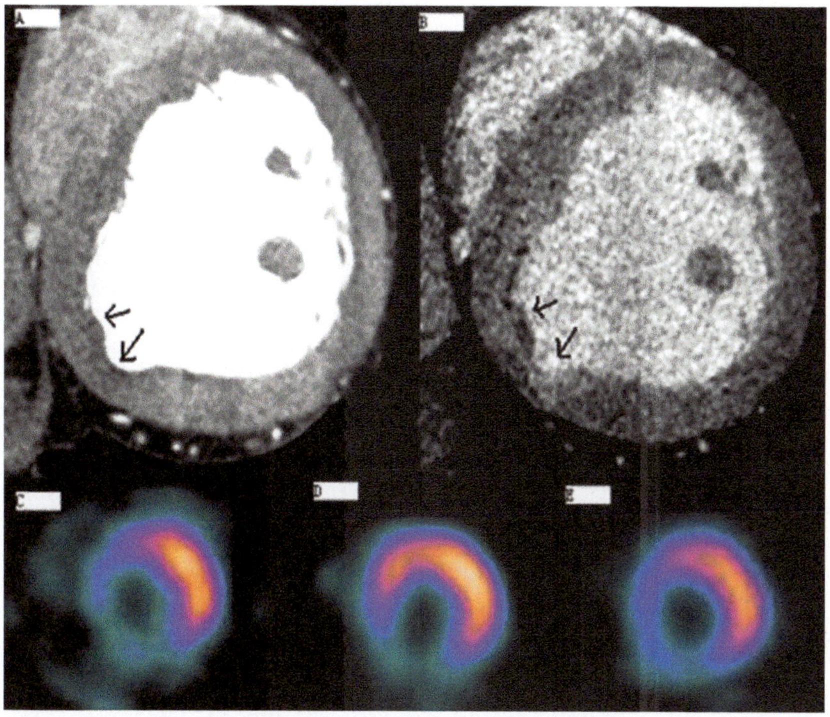

Figure 3. Representative Myocardial Perfusion Images of the Left Anterior Descending Coronary Artery (LAD) and Right Coronary Artery (RCA) using both MSCT and SPECT Examination. 3A: MSCT early scanning; 3B: MSCT late scanning; 3C: Stressed thallium-201 (^{201}TI)-SPECT imaging; 3D: ^{99m}Tc-MIBI imaging; 3E: ^{201}TI-SPECT late resting image.

Table 2. Myocardial perfusion comparison between MSCT and SPECT.

Patient	CTO location	MSCT			SPECT		
		ED	RD	LH	Stressed image	Delayed resting image	^{99m}Tc-MIBI image
1	LAD LCX	Anteroseptal	Anteroseptal	Anteroseptal	Anteroseptal, Inferior	INF	INF
2	RCA	Inferior	N	Inferior	Inferior	INF	INF
3	LAD	Anteroseptal	N	Anteroseptal	Anteroseptal	INF	INF
4	RCA	Inferior	N	Inferior	Inferolateral	INF	INF
5	LAD, RCA	Anteroseptal	N	Anteroseptal	Apicalinferior	INF	CNF at apical wall INF at inferior wall
6	LCX	Anterolateral	N	N	Lateral	INF	CNF
7	LAD	Anteroseptal	N	Anteroseptal	Anteroseptal	INF	INF
8	LAD	Anterior	N	N	Anteroseptal	INF	CNF
9	RCA	Inferior	N	N	Inferior	INF	CNF
10	LAD	Anteroseptal	N	Anteroseptal	Anteroseptal	INF	INF

CTO, chronic total occlusion; ED, early perfusion defect; RD, residual perfusion defect; LH, late hyperenhancement; INF, incomplete nuclide filling; CNF, complete nuclide filling; LCX, left circumflex coronary artery; ^{99m}Tc-MIBI, technetium-99m hexakis-2-methoxy-2-isobutylisonitrile.

The most common reasons for procedural failure of PCI for CTOs include the inability to cross the lesion into the true lumen of the distal vessel with a guidewire (>60%), intimal dissection with creation of a false lumen, contrast extravasation, failure to cross the lesion with a balloon, or failure to dilate adequately. In fact, the absence of morphological information of occluded artery including tortuosity or bending, exact occlusion length or vessel diameter, localization of soft or calcified plaque with traditional CAG, significantly increase the difficulty of CTO recanalization by PCI[21]. Therefore, if the features of CTO could be well identified prior to PCI, adequate pre-procedural planning and scheduling could be undertaken. Our results have demonstrated that the features of CTO, including length of occluded segment, location and extent of calcification, orientation and path of the CTO, could be identified by CTCA, suggesting a role of CTCA in assessing CTO features. Also, 3-D vascular reconstruction images for CTO lesion can be used to map and determinate the optimal working view angle that best demonstrates the target lesion with least foreshortening. The information will be helpful to predict the success rate of CTO recanalization and to design optional procedural strategies and guide the operation of PCI[16,22].

Previous studies have shown that LVEF measured by MSCT had an excellent correlation with that by SPECT or transthoracic echocardiography[12,23]. Similar with these results, we also showed a good correlation between the data from MSCT and SPECT.

In addition, with its high spatial and temporal resolution achievable, MSCT recently was used to assess cardiac function and myocardial perfusion[11,12]. Francone et al[24] reported that MSCT could detect 25 of 30 myocardial infarction, showing an overall sensitivity of 83% and specificity of 91%. Henneman et al[25] has demonstrated that MSCT not only was used to detect healed myocardial infarction, evaluate LV function and myocardial perfusion in patients with previous MI, but also showed a good correlation with the results from SPECT examination. However, since the results were from post-myocardial infarction patients, it remains unclear whether the findings can be extended to all patients with a CTO lesion. Delayed hyperenhancement in a chronic collagenous myocardial scar results from an accumulation of contrast media in the interstitial space between collagen fibers, resulting in an increased volume of contrast distribution in the scar tissue compared with that of tightly packed myocytes[26]. The present study showed that the location of the early perfusion defect region identified by MSCT was corresponded to the nuclide filling defect on stressed ^{201}TI-SPECT perfusion imaging. The late hyperenhancement on MSCT examination was shown to be incomplete nuclide filling on ^{99m}Tc-MIBI imaging. The results suggested that during a single examination, MSCT can provide a comprehensive cardiac assessment of lesion morphological, myocardial perfusion and cardiac function, indicating the feasibility of MSCT in assessment of CTO lesion.

For patients with CTO, comprehensive cardiac assessment, including the occluded segment, cardiac function and the viable myocardium should be performed prior to decision-making. The present study confirmed the ability of MSCT to provide comprehensive cardiac information of CTO lesions. However, there are still some limitations. For example, because of exposure of patients to X-rays and potentially toxic contrast agents, MSCT perfusion imaging is presently unlikely to become a first-line test to assess myocardial viability in all patients. Until now, this modality has only been recommended for use in patients with definite CTO or previous myocardial infarction. Also, it is still difficult and time-consuming to analyze the myocardial perfusion images. With the development of dedicated software, the problem of the heavy workload could be diminished in the future.

Conclusions

In conclusion, in this study, we have demonstrated that except for screening diagnostic purpose on coronary heart disease, a single MSCT examination in previous myocardial infarction without revascularization might provide some valuable information on the nature of CTO lesion, myocardial perfusion and globe cardiac function, which would be helpful for subsequently designing appropriate revascularization strategy in these subjects.

Author Contributions

Conceived and designed the experiments: XKQ WYF. Performed the experiments: XKQ SFG RGL YJX MZ HL. Analyzed the data: KZG SFG JDY YS WHX. Contributed reagents/materials/analysis tools: KZG SFG JDY YS WHX. Wrote the paper: XKQ KZG WYF.

References

1. Park HJ, Kim HY, Lee JM, Choi YS, Park CS, et al (2012) Randomized comparison of the efficacy and safety of zotarolimus-eluting stents vs. sirolimus-eluting stents for percutaneous coronary intervention in chronic total occlusion. Circ J 76: 868–875.
2. Claessen BE, van der Schaaf RJ, Verouden NJ, Stegenga NK, Engstrom AE, et al (2009) Evaluation of the effect of a concurrent chronic total occlusion on long-term mortality and left ventricular function in patients after primary percutaneous coronary intervention. JACC Cardiovasc Interv 2: 1128–1134.
3. Grantham JA, Jones PG, Cannon L, Spertus JA (2010) Quantifying the early health status benefits of successful chronic total occlusion recanalization: Results from the FlowCardia's Approach to Chronic Total Occlusion Recanalization (FACTOR) Trial. Circ Cardiovasc Qual Outcomes 3: 284–290.
4. Prasad A, Rihal CS, Lennon RJ, Wiste HJ, Singh M, et al (2007) Trends in outcomes after percutaneous coronary intervention for chronic total occlusion. J Am Coll Cardiol 49: 1611–1618.
5. Galassi AR, Tomasello SD, Reifart N, Werner GS, Sianos G, et al (2011) In-hospital outcomes of percutaneous coronary intervention in patients with chronic total occlusion: insights from the ERCTO (European Registry of Chronic Total Occlusion) registry. EuroIntervention 7: 472–479.
6. Yamane M (2012) Current percutaneous recanalization of coronary chronic total occlusion. Rev Esp Cardiol 65: 265–277.
7. Hsu JT, Kyo E, Chu CM, Tsuji T, Watanabe S (2011) Impact of calcification length ratio on the intervention for chronic total occlusions. Int J Cardiol 150: 135–141.
8. Gaemperli O, Bengel FM, Kaufmann PA (2011) Cardiac hybrid imaging. Eur Heart J 32: 2100–2108.
9. Takimura H, Muramatsu T, Tsukahara R (2012) CT coronary angiography-guided percutaneous coronary intervention for chronic total occlusion combined with retrograde approach. J Invasive Cardiol 24: E5–9.
10. de Graaf FR, Schuijf JD, Delgado V, van Velzen JE, Kroft LJ, et al (2010) Clinical application of CT coronary angiography: state of the art. Heart Lung Circ 19: 107–116.
11. Lardo AC, Cordeiro MA, Silva C, Amado LC, George RT, et al (2006) Contrast-enhanced multidetector computed tomography viability imaging after myocardial infarction: characterization of myocyte death, microvascular obstruction, and chronic scar. Circulation 113: 394–404.
12. Yamaguchi K, Nomura M, Tsujikawa T, Koshiba K, Ito S (2007) Accurate estimation of regional and global cardiac function in old myocardial infarction patients by multidetector-row computed tomography. J Med Invest 54: 72–82.
13. Schuleri KH, Centola M, George RT, Amado LC, Evers KS, et al (2009) Characterization of peri-infarct zone heterogeneity by contrast-enhanced multidetector computed tomography. J Am Coll Cardiol 53: 1699–1707.
14. Choi JH, Song YB, Hahn JY, Choi SH, Gwon HC, et al (2011) Three-dimensional quantitative volumetry of chronic total occlusion plaque using coronary multidetector computed tomography. Circ J 75: 366–375.
15. Kirschbaum SW, Nieman K, Springeling T, Weustink AC, Ramcharitar S, et al (2011) Non-invasive diagnostic workup of patients with suspected stable angina by combined computed tomography coronary angiography and magnetic resonance perfusion imaging. Circ J 75: 1678–1684.
16. Soon KH, Cox N, Wong A, Chaitowitz I, Macgregor L, et al (2007) CT coronary angiography predicts the outcome of percutaneous coronary intervention of chronic total occlusion. J Interv Cardiol 20: 359–366.
17. Liew GY, Feneley M, Worthley SG (2011) Noninvasive coronary artery imaging: current clinical applications: Cardiac Society of Australia and New Zealand guidelines. Heart Lung Circ 20: 425–437.
18. Toriyama T, Takase H, Goto T, Sugiura T, Nakazawa A, et al (2007) Coronary artery disease investigated using 99mTc-tetrofosmin myocardial SPECT. Eur J Clin Invest 37: 478–482.
19. van der Hoeven BL, Schalij MJ, Delgado V (2012) Multimodality imaging in interventional cardiology. Nat Rev Cardiol 14: 333–346.
20. Maffei E, Seitun S, Nieman K, Martini C, Guaricci AI, et al (2011) Assessment of coronary artery disease and calcified coronary plaque burden by computed tomography in patients with and without diabetes mellitus. Eur Radiol 21: 944–953.
21. Ehara M, Terashima M, Kawai M, Matsushita S, Tsuchikane E, et al (2009) Impact of multislice computed tomography to estimate difficulty in wire crossing in percutaneous coronary intervention for chronic total occlusion. J Invasive Cardiol 21: 575–582.
22. Cury RC, Nieman K, Shapiro MD, Butler J, Nomura CH, et al (2008) Comprehensive assessment of myocardial perfusion defects, regional wall motion, and left ventricular function by using 64-section multidetector CT. Radiology 248: 466–475.
23. Henneman MM, Schuijf JD, Jukema JW, Lamb HJ, de Roos A, et al (2006) Comprehensive cardiac assessment with multislice computed tomography: evaluation of left ventricular function and perfusion in addition to coronary anatomy in patients with previous myocardial infarction. Heart 92: 1779–1783.
24. Francone M, Carbone I, Danti M, Lanciotti K, Cavacece M, Mirabelli F, et al (2006) ECG-gated multi-detector row spiral CT in the assessment of myocardial infarction: correlation with non-invasive angiographic findings. Eur Radiol 16: 15–24.
25. Henneman MM, Schuijf JD, Petra DS, Stokkel MP, van der Geest RJ, et al (2008) Comparison of multislice computed tomography to gated single-photon emission computed tomography for imaging of healed myocardial infarcts. Am J Cardiol 101: 144–148.
26. Wu KC, Lima JA (2003) Noninvasive imaging of myocardial viability: current techniques and future developments. Circ Res 93: 1146–1158.

Initial Imaging Analysis of Budd-Chiari Syndrome in Henan Province of China: Most Cases Have Combined Inferior Vena Cava and Hepatic Veins Involvement

Pengli Zhou[❖]**, Jianzhuang Ren**[❖]**, Xinwei Han*, Gang Wu, Wenguang Zhang, Pengxu Ding, Yonghua Bi**

Department of Interventional Radiology, The First Affiliated Hospital, Zhengzhou University, Zhengzhou, Henan Province, China

Abstract

Aim: To evaluate the type of venous involvement in Chinese Budd-Chiari syndrome (BCS) patients and the relative diagnostic accuracy of the different imaging modalities.

Methods: Using digital subtraction angiography (DSA) as a reference standard, color Doppler ultrasound (CDUS), computed tomography angiography (CTA), and magnetic resonance angiography (MRA) were performed on 338 patients with BCS. We analyzed the course of the main and any accessory hepatic veins (HVs) and the inferior vena cava (IVC) to assess the etiology of obstructed segments and diagnostic accuracy of CDUS, CTA and MRA.

Results: Among the 338 cases, there were 8 cases (2.4%) of isolated IVC membranous obstruction, 45 cases (13.3%) of isolated HV occlusion, and 285 cases (84.3%) with both IVC membranous obstruction and HV occlusion. Comparing with DSA, CDUS, CTA had a diagnostic accuracy of 89.3% and 80.2% in detecting BCS, and 83.4% of cases correctly correlated by MRA.

Conclusion: In Henan Province, most patients with BCS have complex lesions combining IVC and HV involvement. The combination of CDUS and CTA or MRI is useful for diagnosis of BCS and guiding therapy.

Editor: Sang Hoon Ahn, Yonsei University College of Medicine, Republic of Korea

Funding: The authors have no support or funding to report.

Competing Interests: The authors have declared that no competing interests exist.

* E-mail: hanxinwei2006@163.com

❖ These authors contributed equally to this work.

Introduction

Budd-Chiari syndrome (BCS) is a rare disease in Western countries. The prevalence is approximately 1:100,000, [1] and thrombotic obstruction of hepatic veins (HVs) is the most important cause. [2,3,4] One predisposing thrombophilic factor, such as Myeloproliferative neoplasms (MPNs), JAK2 V617F mutation and factor V G1691A mutation (FLVM), can be found in at least 90% of BCS patients, of which, MPNs are the most common cause and account for about 41% of cases. [5,6,7] However, the prevalence of BCS is higher in less developed countries, such as China, South Africa, India and Nepal. For example, BCS is more common in areas along the Yellow River and Huaihe River Basin, especially in Henan and Shandong Provinces of China. Unlike the Western countries, it is reported that membranous obstruction of inferior vena cava (IVC) represents the most common etiological factor, and only a few cases have an underlying thrombotic factor. [5,8,9] These differences excite wildly interest and need further investigation.

The Henan Province has a population of 130 million, accounting for one-thirteenth of the total population of China, which is also the region with considerably high BCS incidence rate. Unfortunately, there is a lack of knowledge about BCS etiology and its imaging features. Nowadays, research on BCS has been growing, especially with the availability of Doppler ultrasound (US), CT angiography (CTA), magnetic resonance angiography (MRA), and digital subtraction angiography (DSA). [10,11,12] This study aims to evaluate the type of venous involvement in Chinese Budd-Chiari syndrome (BCS) patients and the relative diagnostic accuracy of the different imaging modalities.

Materials and Methods

Ethics

This study has been approved by The First Affiliated Hospital of Zhengzhou University Ethics Review Committee and the National Ethics Review Committee. Written informed consents were obtained from all patients and the guardians, caretakers, or the next of kin on the behalf of the participants involved in this study.

Patients

All patients came from the regions along the Yellow and Huaihe Rivers, and most of them lived in rural areas under adverse socioeconomic and public health conditions. From August 2006 to

October 2010, 338 BCS patients were admitted to the interventional wards of No.1 Affiliated Hospital of Zhengzhou University.

Procedures of Doppler US, MRI, CT and DSA

Doppler US was performed on a seven-color apparatus (General Electric, USA), examining the HV and IVC using acoustic windows under the xiphoid and costal margin. A 6-slice spiral CT (Brilliance, Philips, Holland), a 16-slice CT (Lightspeed, General Electric, USA), and 64 rows of CT machines (Lightspeed, General Electric, USA) were used. After acquisition of baseline unenhanced images, a bolus of iodinated contrast material was administered and images of the liver were acquired in the arterial phase (25–30 s after injection), portal venous phase (60 s after injection), and IVC phase (180 s after injection). The IVC phase was timed in order to enable a stenotic IVC to fill with contrast medium. [13] Images were formatted in the axial, sagittal, and coronal planes. MRI with a dynamic enhanced angiography sequence was performed on a 1.5 Tesla or 3.0 Tesla Signa (HDxt 3.0T, General Electronic, USA). Enhanced scanning was commenced 15 s after injecting of contrast agent (0.2–0.4 ml/kg body weight) to obtain dynamic 3D images. By using Shimadzu Digitex (Shimadzu, Tokyo, Japan) equipment, DSA was performed to opacify the IVC via femoral vein injection. Hepatic venous opacification was achieved by retrograde injection or, if necessary, percutaneous transhepatic catheterization. [14].

Image Evaluation

Doppler US examinations were evaluated by two experienced operators (Ren JZ and Wu G) together, with a third physician (Han XW) required in case of different opinions. Diagnosis was not made until two physicians agreed. All the scanning images were viewed separately by two experienced associate chief physicians (Ren JZ and Wu G), with a third physician (Han XW) required in case of different opinions. All the radiologists diagnosed randomly and respectively, they were blinded to patient information and did not know the results of the DSA images when they are reading the ultrasound, CTA or MRA images.

Statistical Analysis

All qualitative data were expressed as proportions. The chi-square test was for study the categorical variables (SPSS Inc., Chicago, IL, USA). Differences were considered statistically significant when P was less than 0.05.

Results

There were 209 males and 129 females, ranging from 12 to 72 years old, with an average age of 41.7±10.1 years. The imaging examinations were completed within one week for patients suspected by clinical symptoms. All patients were firstly scanned by CDUS, CTA and/or MRA were further performed if necessary. All BCS cases underwent DSA to confirm the diagnosis of BCS during radiological intervention. Fifty-five cases were confirmed by CDUS, 126 cases by CDUS and CTA, and 157 cases by CDUS and MRA.

Evaluation of CDUS, MRI, CT and DSA

Comparing with DSA, CDUS had a diagnostic accuracy of 89.3% (302/338) in detecting BCS, with a 3.6% (12/338) of false-positive diagnoses of BCS and 7.1% (14/338) of false-negative. Among 126 cases confirmed by Doppler US and CTA, CTA has an overall accuracy of 80.2% (101/126), with a 6.3% (8/126) of false-positive and 13.5% (17/126) of cases indeterminate when compared with DSA findings. Among 157 patients studied by MRA, 83.4% (131/157) of cases correctly correlated with DSA findings. The false-positive and false-negative were 11.5% (18/157) and 5.1% (8/157), respectively.

CDUS is sensitive for membranous obstruction of IVC. HVs and IVC were devoid of flow signal once completely obstructed. HV may compensatory enlarge (Figure 1). Turbulent, reversed or stagnant flow in HVs can be easily depicted by CDUS. Heterogeneous patchy enhancement, nonvisualization of HVs, intrahepatic collaterals and obstruction of the IVC are important findings of CT or MRI. MRI allows good anatomic orientation of HVs or IVC due to its multiplanar capacity, and IVC can be better visualized on coronal images (Figure 2). DSA are useful for showing the level and extent of obstruction (Figure 3). The CT examination results were consistent with those of DSA (Figure 4).

Focal Liver Abnormality

68.6% (232/338) of cases were of hepatic cirrhosis, and ascites were often found during image assessment. Intrahepatic collateral circulation and collateral circulation in the body were identified in 62.1% (210/338) and 65.1% (220/338) of cases due to portal hypertension. 48.2% (163/338) of those patients had wider accessory HVs or large HV collaterals. About half of cases showed caudate lobe enlargement, the caudate lobe hypertrophied and reached a mean diameter of 33.1±3.2 mm. Benign regenerative nodules were found in 23.4% (79/338) of cases, which were typically small and multiple, with hypervascularity during the arterial and portal venous phases. Hepatocellular carcinoma was found in 7.7% (26/338) of patients. For identifying parenchymal abnormalities, CT and MRI had a higher sensitive modality than CDUS (90.5%, 91.3% versus 76.8%, $P<0.05$).

Type Analysis of BCS

Out of 338 patients with BCS, 293 cases (86.7%) showed IVC involvement, in which, 285 cases had an associated HV obstruction (84.3%), and 8 cases had isolated IVC involvement (2.4%). Of 330 cases with HV involvement (97.6%), 45 cases (13.3%) had isolated HV obstruction with a normal IVC. Among 285 patients with venous lesions involving both the IVC and HV, there were 186 cases (55.0%) with obstruction of the left, middle and right HV branches and 82 cases (24.3%) with obstruction of two branches (77 cases were obstructed in the left and middle branches; 2 cases in the left and right branches; and 3 cases in the middle and right branches), the remaining 17 cases (5.0%) displayed obstruction of one HV branch, of which 11 cases had obstruction of the right HV, 3 cases of the middle HV, and 3 cases of the left HV. IVC lesions included 200 cases (59.2%) of complete occlusion and 93 cases (27.5%) of stenosis (Table 1). Of the 200 occlusive cases, there were 163 cases (48.2%) of membranous obstruction and 37 cases (10.9%) of thrombotic obstruction of the IVC. 209 cases (61.8%) were membranous obstruction if adds the stenotic cases caused by membrane in IVC.

Among 45 patients with isolated HV obstructive lesions (Table 1), there were 44 cases of involving the left, middle, and right HVs, and one case with the obstruction of only the right HV. Among 8 patients with isolated IVC obstructive lesions, 6 cases were occlusive and 2 cases were stenotic. All of 8 cases were of the membranous type. There was no significant difference among the findings of CDUS, CTA, MRA, or DSA according to the chi-square test ($P>0.05$).

Discussion

Thrombotic obstruction of HVs is considered as the most important cause of BCS in European regions. [2,3,4] The

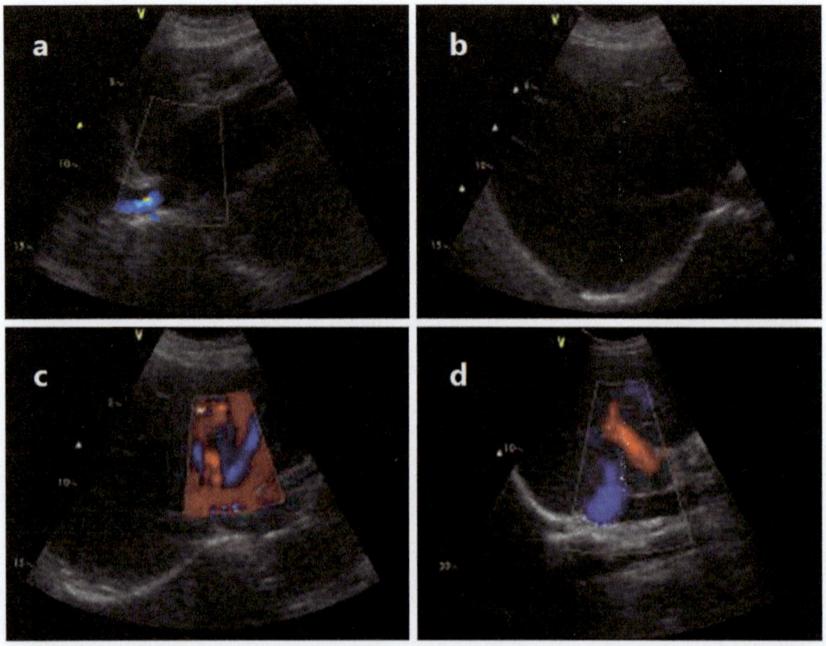

Figure 1. The preoperative color Doppler flow imaging. CDUS shows a membranous obstruction of IVC wiht thin beam-like flow (Figure 1 a), and the right HV is completely obstructed (Figure 1 b); There is a obliteration after the confluence of left HVs without blood flows (Figure 1 c), the right HV has compensatory enlargement, with blood flow draining into IVC (Figure 1 d).

predisposing thrombophilic factors, particularly thrombosis due to the hypercoagulable state, or thrombophlebitis resulted from long-term oral contraceptives, cause the secondary onset of thrombus in HV and obstruction of HV. [15] In the Eastern countries, Africa and other less developed countries, BCS was considered to be due to IVC membranous obstruction in the rear segment of the liver, rarely due to thrombosis, and there was no intravasculitis, hypercoagulability or thrombosis, [16] which was once called IVC diaphragm obstructive syndrome. In 1962, Kimura initially conducted the IVC diaphragm intervention through the heart. [17] More cases were then reported in Japan, India, Asia, and Africa. China is one of the areas suffering from a high incidence of BCS, and Chinese BCS is generally considered as one of the subtypes. The type of BCS in the West is quite different from that of less developed regions in the East. Among 338 cases of BCS confirmed by various imaging modalities, the most common type had involved both the IVC and HV, accounting for 84.3% of all cases. This result suggests that IVC and HV involvement is the predominant pattern of Chinese BCS, or at least in Henan Province, which is consistent with the relevant reports in recent years. Similarly, Cheng D et al. reported that 61% of cases are membranous obstruction, only 5% of cases have MPNs with a JAK2 V617F mutation, and most of BCS patients (63%) suffered from both HVs and IVC obstruction. [9].

As for the reason, inherited predisposition and acquired thrombogenic stimulus may converge in the pathogenesis of BCS. [18,19] FLVM is quite common in Caucasian populationsbe and is found in at least 90% of BCS patient, interestingly, this

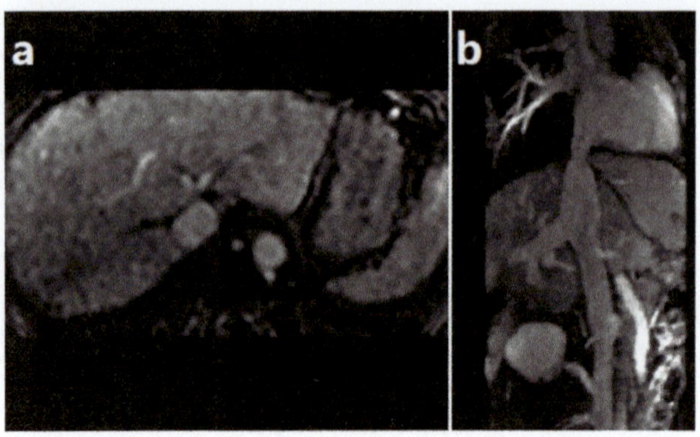

Figure 2. MRI axial and 3D reconstruction images for showing HVs and IVC. The right HV is completely obstructed and the middle and left HVs are obstructed after their confluence (Figure 2 a). The IVC shows a membranous stenosis, and the right HV is compensatory enlarged (Figure 2 b).

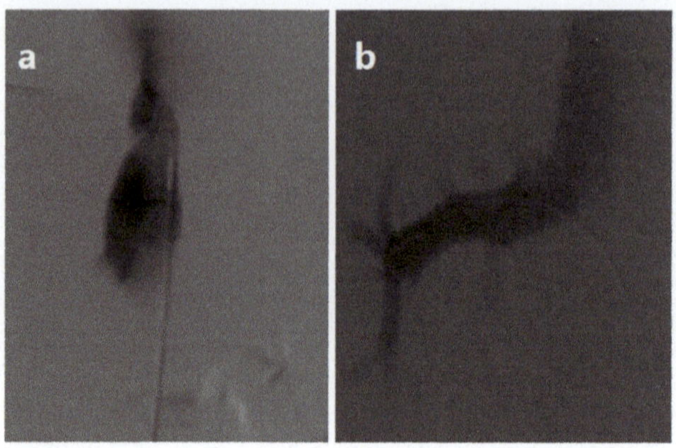

Figure 3. The inferior venocavography through the femoral access. The IVC is obstructed at the secondary porta of liver, and the adopted contrast agent is thin and beam-like (Figure 3 a), the right and rear HVs are remarkably dilated (Figure 3 b).

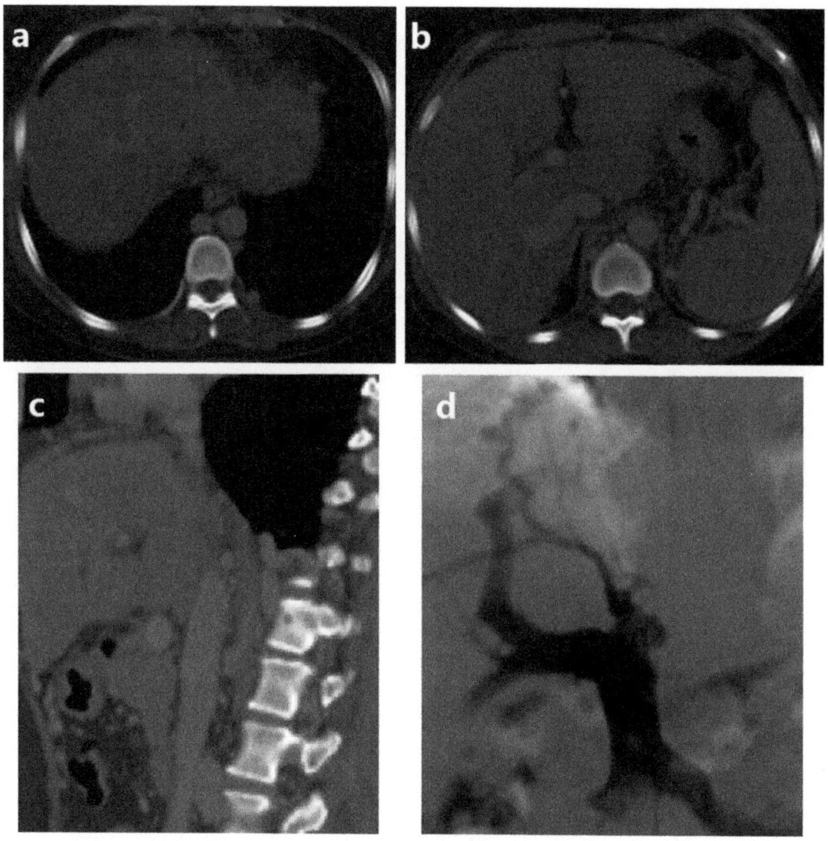

Figure 4. The CTA images of portal venous phase and DSA image during intervention. The middle HV is obstructed, the right and left HVs are completely obstructed (Figure 4 a); The right, rear and inferior HVs are expanded (Figure 4 b), and the segmental IVC is obstructed (Figure 4 c); DSA image shows a segmental obstruction of the inferior caval vein, and intrahepatic collateral circulation for drainage of HV flows (Figure 4 d).

mutated allele is not determined in Eastern populations, which indicates that genetics differences between Western and Eastern populations should account for the discordance of BCS. [20] The most patients are chornic BCS and the course of disease is quite long in China and Japan. [9,21] The situation in the East is different from that in the West where most patients are acute BCS, and the type of lesion may vary according to geography. [9].

Table 1. Types distribution of venous lesions in patients with BCS.

Lesion types	Cases	Proportion (%)
IVC and HV involvement	285	84.3
Obstruction of three main HVs	186	55.0
Obstruction of two main HVs	82	24.3
Obstruction of one HV	17	5.0
Isolated HV involvement	45	13.3
Obstruction of three main HVs	44	13.0
Obstruction of two main HVs	0	0.3
Obstruction of one HV	1	2.2
Isolated IVC involvement	8	2.4
Occlusive IVC	6	1.8
Stenotic IVC	2	0.6

IVC: inferior vena cava; HV: hepatic vein.

BCS is distributed regionally in China, and there is the highest prevalence in the Huanghuai region. [22] The most prevalent etiological factor of BCS is also membranous obstruction in China. Females of childbearing age are more likely to develop BCS in Western countries, however, males with the median age of 46 years account for the majority of cases, and most of cases are chronic BCS. [9] The HVs obstruction is lower, but the IVC obstruction rate in Chinese patients is far higher when compared with those in Western countries, indicating that BCS may vary from region to region. In Henan Province, more than 80% of BCS cases are peasant, and people in countryside are more likely to develop BCS than oppidan in city. These indicate that BCS is related to environmental conditions, diet and economic factors to some extent in Henan Province, or even in China.

Various imaging modalities are available for dignosing BCS in the clinical setting, including CDUS, CT, MRI and conventional venography. The CDUS should be performed as the first imaging method of choice in BCS due to its high diagnostic sensitivity, inexpensiveness and convince, without contrast material. [23,24] The CDUS has a diagnostic sensitivity of 75.0% to 90%. [23,24,25] HVs and IVC devoid of flow signal and collateral hepatic venous circulation can be indicative of BCS. [26] Echogenic membrane can be easily depicted by sonography. However, sonography is operator-dependent and interfered with intestinal gas and excessive ascites. [27].

The second line of investigation should be CT or MRI. Heterogeneous patchy enhancement, nonvisualization of hepatic veins, intrahepatic collaterals and obstruction of the IVC are their important findings. For identifying the status of hepatic venous thrombosis, CT has an overall accuracy of 50%. [28,29] CT has a higher sensitive modality than sonography (90.0% versus 70.0%) in showing parenchymal abnormalities. [28] Our results confirmed those findings. Moreover, CTA is useful in investigating the patency of TIPS shunt and vascular involvement. [27] The limitations of CT are the possible allergic reaction and nephrotoxicity due to the use of contrast material, and CT is often unable to show web in IVC.

MRI allows good anatomic orientation of HVs or IVC due to its multiplanar capacity. The status of 80.0% of cases correctly correlated with pathology when using MRI. [28] The advantages of MRA over CDUS include better anatomic orientation, short examination time without operator-dependency or restriction from intestinal gas. [27] MRI is also advantageous over CT imaging in some aspects. [27] The combination of CDUS and CT or MRI is useful for guiding therapy due to the optimal delineation of HV and IVC obstruction. [26].

Hepatic venography and inferior venocavography are conventional diagnostic method for BCS, which currently serve as a third line of investigation. Venography combined with venous pressure measurements should be performed when radiological intervention or surgical shunting is considered. [25,26] However, venography often requires cannulation of HVs and large amounts of contrast medium. [26].

Most of Chinese patients are chronic, ascites, caudate lobe enlargement and abnormal hepatic configuration are present in vast majority of the BCS cases. [27] Half of patients have wider accessory HVs or large HV collaterals, which can help to drain off the blocked HVs blood to relieve portal hypertension. [9] Caudate lobe may hypertrophy due to its separate drainage into the IVC. [30] Contrast-enhanced CT reveals inhomogeneous enhancement of liver, such as peripheral regions with low attenuation due to portal hypoperfusion and focal enhancing area owning to arterio-portal shunting. [30] Benign regenerative nodules, intrahepatic collateral circulation, body collateral circulation and hepatic cirrhosis can be seen in chronic BCS cases. [31] Hepatocellular carcinoma often develops in chronic end-stage liver disease, [27,31] sometimes it will be shown in BCS cases.

Knowledge of the morphologic type of BCS is useful for guiding the therapeutic approach and assessing operation risk. Shunt surgery is no longer the standard care for BCS, with advances in radiological interventions and a good midterm outcome. [32] Interventional techniques can aid in treating and stabilising the patient for possible orthotopic liver transplantation when liver dysfunction progressive. [33].

Percutaneous transluminal angioplasty (PTA) can be used for patients with post-hepatic IVC membranous-type obstruction, balloon dilatation and percutaneous stent placement have been found to be the techniques for those with segmental IVC obstruction [34] or IVC web [35]. PTA is seldom adopted in Western countries, however, and stenting are effective and safe for treating BCS, with a good long-term outcome, [36] because most chronic BCS are caused by membranous obstruction. According to our experiences, large balloon dilation with a diameter of 25–30 mm ballon catheter is safe and effective for most IVC obstruction cases, and only few cases need further stenting after large balloon dilation. The blood backflow of HV and liver function can be basically compensated, as long as there was a widely patent HV, regardless of which branch of the main HVs was or whether it was the accessory HV. PTA, mainly balloon dilation, is suitable for this kind of BCS. TIPS and orthotopic liver transplantation are usually adopted in Western countries, although the survival rate is poor. [37].

In case of short segment occlusion or stenosis of HV and/or IVC, the obstruction between remnant HV and IVC should be reopened by means of balloon angioplasty with or without stent placement. [38] TIPS and surgical options are reserved for patients with failure of interventions due to complete occlusion of HV. [32] Patients with both the and segmental IVC occlusion require opening of both occlusive segments, these may be difficult and challenging and the several multiple approaches should be required. [32] The IVC occlusion should be reopened as long as they have unobstructed HV blood flow. [34] Besides, additional therapies with anticoagulation, pharmacological or endoscopic treatment for variceal bleeding and diuretics for ascites should be considered. [26].

Author Contributions

Conceived and designed the experiments: PZ XH JR. Performed the experiments: PZ JR GW WZ PD. Analyzed the data: GW WZ PD. Contributed reagents/materials/analysis tools: PZ XH JR. Wrote the paper: PZ JR YB. Revised the manuscript: YB.

References

1. Darwish Murad S, Valla DC, de Groen PC, Zeitoun G, Hopmans JA, et al. (2004) Determinants of survival and the effect of portosystemic shunting in patients with Budd-Chiari syndrome. Hepatology 39: 500–508.
2. Rav-Acha M, Gur C, Ilan Y, Verstandig A, Eid A (2004) [Budd-Chiari syndrome: updated treatment modalities]. Harefuah 143: 372–376, 389.
3. Okuda K (2002) Obliterative hepatocavopathy-inferior vena cava thrombosis at its hepatic portion. Hepatobiliary Pancreat Dis Int 1: 499–509.
4. Valla D, Hadengue A, el Younsi M, Azar N, Zeitoun G, et al. (1997) Hepatic venous outflow block caused by short-length hepatic vein stenoses. Hepatology 25: 814–819.
5. Plessier A, Rautou PE, Valla DC (2012) Management of hepatic vascular diseases. J Hepatol 56 Suppl 1: S25–38.
6. Smalberg JH, Arends LR, Valla DC, Kiladjian JJ, Janssen HL, et al. (2012) Myeloproliferative neoplasms in Budd-Chiari syndrome and portal vein thrombosis: a meta-analysis. Blood 120: 4921–4928.
7. Pemmaraju N, Hamilton JP, Cameron AM, Sisson S, Moliterno AR (2012) Abdominal venous thrombosis presenting in myeloproliferative neoplasm with JAK2 V617F mutation: a case report. J Med Case Rep 6: 102.
8. Singh V, Sinha SK, Nain CK, Bambery P, Kaur U, et al. (2000) Budd-Chiari syndrome: our experience of 71 patients. J Gastroenterol Hepatol 15: 550–554.
9. Cheng D, Xu H, Lu ZJ, Hua R, Qiu H, et al. (2013) Clinical features and etiology of Budd-Chiari syndrome in Chinese patients: a single-center study. J Gastroenterol Hepatol 28: 1061–1067.
10. Yanaga K, Matsumata T, Hayashi H, Shimada M, Urata K, et al. (1994) Isolated hepatic caudate lobectomy. Surgery 115: 757–761.
11. Sato TJ, Hirai I, Murakami G, Kanamura T, Hata F, et al. (2002) An anatomical study of short hepatic veins, with special reference to delineation of the caudate lobe for hanging maneuver of the liver without the usual mobilization. J Hepatobiliary Pancreat Surg 9: 55–60.
12. Goldsmith NA, Woodburne RT (1957) The surgical anatomy pertaining to liver resection. Surg Gynecol Obstet 105: 310–318.
13. Meng WC, Shao CX, Mak KL, Lau PY, Yeung YP, et al. (2003) Anatomical justification of Belghiti's 'liver hanging manoeuvre' in right hepatectomy with anterior approach. ANZ J Surg 73: 407–409.
14. Elias H, Petty D (1952) Gross anatomy of the blood vessels and ducts within the human liver. Am J Anat 90: 59–111.
15. Deltenre P, Denninger MH, Hillaire S, Guillin MC, Casadevall N, et al. (2001) Factor V Leiden related Budd-Chiari syndrome. Gut 48: 264–268.
16. Nakamura S, Tsuzuki T (1981) Surgical anatomy of the hepatic veins and the inferior vena cava. Surg Gynecol Obstet 152: 43–50.
17. Kimura C (1964) Surgical Treatment of Portal Hypertension of Post-Hepatic Origin, with Special Reference to Trans-Cardiac Membranotomy for Membranous Obstruction of the Hepatic Portion of the Inferior Vena Cava. Jpn Circ J 28: 181–183.
18. Janssen HL, Meinardi JR, Vleggaar FP, van Uum SH, Haagsma EB, et al. (2000) Factor V Leiden mutation, prothrombin gene mutation, and deficiencies

in coagulation inhibitors associated with Budd-Chiari syndrome and portal vein thrombosis: results of a case-control study. Blood 96: 2364–2368.
19. Mahmoud AE, Mendoza A, Meshikhes AN, Olliff S, West R, et al. (1996) Clinical spectrum, investigations and treatment of Budd-Chiari syndrome. QJM 89: 37–43.
20. Rees DC, Cox M, Clegg JB (1995) World distribution of factor V Leiden. Lancet 346: 1133–1134.
21. Okuda H, Yamagata H, Obata H, Iwata H, Sasaki R, et al. (1995) Epidemiological and clinical features of Budd-Chiari syndrome in Japan. J Hepatol 22: 1–9.
22. Wang ZG, Zhang FJ, Yi MQ, Qiang LX (2005) Evolution of management for Budd-Chiari syndrome: a team's view from 2564 patients. ANZ J Surg 75: 55–63.
23. Bolondi L, Gaiani S, Li Bassi S, Zironi G, Bonino F, et al. (1991) Diagnosis of Budd-Chiari syndrome by pulsed Doppler ultrasound. Gastroenterology 100: 1324–1331.
24. Chawla Y, Kumar S, Dhiman RK, Suri S, Dilawari JB (1999) Duplex Doppler sonography in patients with Budd-Chiari syndrome. J Gastroenterol Hepatol 14: 904–907.
25. Kamath PS (2006) Budd-Chiari syndrome: Radiologic findings. Liver Transpl 12: S21–22.
26. Janssen HL, Garcia-Pagan JC, Elias E, Mentha G, Hadengue A, et al. (2003) Budd-Chiari syndrome: a review by an expert panel. J Hepatol 38: 364–371.
27. Erden A (2007) Budd-Chiari syndrome: a review of imaging findings. Eur J Radiol 61: 44–56.
28. Miller WJ, Federle MP, Straub WH, Davis PL (1993) Budd-Chiari syndrome: imaging with pathologic correlation. Abdom Imaging 18: 329–335.
29. Noone TC, Semelka RC, Siegelman ES, Balci NC, Hussain SM, et al. (2000) Budd-Chiari syndrome: spectrum of appearances of acute, subacute, and chronic disease with magnetic resonance imaging. J Magn Reson Imaging 11: 44–50.
30. Bargallo X, Gilabert R, Nicolau C, Garcia-Pagan JC, Bosch J, et al. (2003) Sonography of the caudate vein: value in diagnosing Budd-Chiari syndrome. AJR Am J Roentgenol 181: 1641–1645.
31. Maetani Y, Itoh K, Egawa H, Haga H, Sakurai T, et al. (2002) Benign hepatic nodules in Budd-Chiari syndrome: radiologic-pathologic correlation with emphasis on the central scar. AJR Am J Roentgenol 178: 869–875.
32. Mukund A, Gamanagatti S (2011) Imaging and interventions in Budd-Chiari syndrome. World J Radiol 3: 169–177.
33. Buckley O, O'Brien J, Snow A, Stunell H, Lyburn I, et al. (2007) Imaging of Budd-Chiari syndrome. Eur Radiol 17: 2071–2078.
34. Xue H, Li YC, Shakya P, Palikhe M, Jha RK (2010) The role of intravascular intervention in the management of Budd-Chiari syndrome. Dig Dis Sci 55: 2659–2663.
35. Khuroo MS, Al-Suhabani H, Al-Sebayel M, Al Ashgar H, Dahab S, et al. (2005) Budd-Chiari syndrome: long-term effect on outcome with transjugular intrahepatic portosystemic shunt. J Gastroenterol Hepatol 20: 1494–1502.
36. Qiao T, Liu CJ, Liu C, Chen K, Zhang XB, et al. (2005) Interventional endovascular treatment for Budd-Chiari syndrome with long-term follow-up. Swiss Med Wkly 135: 318–326.
37. Plessier A, Valla DC (2008) Budd-Chiari syndrome. Semin Liver Dis 28: 259–269.
38. Eapen CE, Velissaris D, Heydtmann M, Gunson B, Olliff S, et al. (2006) Favourable medium term outcome following hepatic vein recanalisation and/or transjugular intrahepatic portosystemic shunt for Budd Chiari syndrome. Gut 55: 878–884.

8

Transcatheter Pulmonary Valve Replacement by Hybrid Approach Using a Novel Polymeric Prosthetic Heart Valve: Proof of Concept in Sheep

Ben Zhang[1,2]⁹, Xiang Chen[3]⁹, Tong-yi Xu[1], Zhi-gang Zhang[3], Xin Li[1], Lin Han[1], Zhi-yun Xu[1]*

1 Department of Cardiothoracic Surgery, Changhai Hospital, Second Military Medical University, Shanghai, China, **2** Centre of Cardiovascular Surgery, Guangzhou General Hospital of Guangzhou Military Region, Guangzhou, China, **3** Department of Cardiology, Changhai Hospital, Second Military Medical University, Shanghai, China

Abstract

Background: Since 2000, transcatheter pulmonary valve replacement has steadily advanced. However, the available prosthetic valves are restricted to bioprosthesis which have defects like poor durability. Polymeric heart valve is thought as a promising alternative to bioprosthesis. In this study, we introduced a novel polymeric transcatheter pulmonary valve and evaluated its feasibility and safety in sheep by a hybrid approach.

Methods: We designed a novel polymeric trileaflet transcatheter pulmonary valve with a balloon-expandable stent, and the valve leaflets were made of 0.1-mm expanded polytetrafluoroethylene (ePTFE) coated with phosphorylcholine. We chose glutaraldehyde-treated bovine pericardium valves as control. Pulmonary valve stents were implanted in situ by a hybrid transapical approach in 10 healthy sheep (8 for polymeric valve and 2 for bovine pericardium valve), weighing an average of 22.5±2.0 kg. Angiography and cardiac catheter examination were performed after implantation to assess immediate valvular functionality. After 4-week follow-up, angiography, echocardiography, computed tomography, and cardiac catheter examination were used to assess early valvular function. One randomly selected sheep with polymeric valve was euthanized and the explanted valved stent was analyzed macroscopically and microscopically.

Findings: Implantation was successful in 9 sheep. Angiography at implantation showed all 9 prosthetic valves demonstrated orthotopic position and normal functionality. All 9 sheep survived at 4-week follow-up. Four-week follow-up revealed no evidence of valve stent dislocation or deformation and normal valvular and cardiac functionality. The cardiac catheter examination showed the peak-peak transvalvular pressure gradient of the polymeric valves was 11.9±5.0 mmHg, while that of two bovine pericardium valves were 11 and 17 mmHg. Gross morphology demonstrated good opening and closure characteristics. No thrombus or calcification was seen macroscopically.

Conclusions: This design of the novel ePTFE transcatheter pulmonary valve is safe and effective to deploy in sheep by hybrid approach, and the early valvular functionality is good.

Editor: Giacomo Frati, Sapienza University of Rome, Italy

Funding: The authors have no support or funding to report.

Competing Interests: The authors have declared that no competing interests exist.

* E-mail: zhiyunxu168@gmail.com

⁹ These authors contributed equally to this work.

Introduction

Since the first sucessful clinical application of transcatheter pulmonary valve replacement (TPVR) was reported by Bonhoeffer and colleagues in 2000 [1], TPVR has steadily advanced and become readily adopted for the patients with stenotic or regurgitant pulmonary valve diseases, especially for patients with congenital heart disease (CHD) who had surgical pulmonary valvectomy or transannular pulmonary patches [2,3].

However, the available prosthetic pulmonary valves are restricted to bioprosthesis which currently have various problems. First, most of the prospective patients for TPVR are young, the deterioration of bioprosthesis will lead to reoperation which means more agony for the young patients. Second, the sizes of currently available bioprosthetic valves are not suitable for use in all concerned patients due to anatomic variability [4]. Moreover, valved stent deployment during TPVR has been proved to be responsible for traumatic injury to bioprosthetic valve leaflets [5,6], which concievably impact on the durability of bioprosthetic valves.

Polymeric prosthetic heart valve (PPHV) is a so-called "biomechanical valve" which is thought as a combination of the advantages of mechanical and bioprosthetic valves: long-term durability and no necessity for permanent anticoagulation [7], and as a promising alternative to bioprosthetic valves for TPVR [8]. Recently, Metzner et al [9] have demonstrated an excellent outcome of polyurethane valves with a self-expanding stent in the pulmonary position of sheep in a period of 4 weeks.

Currently, clinically used transcatheter pulmonary valve stents are disigned for percutaneous therapy. With currently available stents, it is not possible to treat all concerned patients. So far, patients with small or distorted peripheral vessels and patients with wide or severely calcified and kinked RVOTs are not suitable for percutaneous therapy. New stent designs and hybrid approaches are desired to overcome these problems.

In this study, we designed a novel trileaflet polymeric transcatheter pulmonary valve (PTPV) with a balloon-expandable stent, and the valve leaflets were made of 0.1-mm expanded polytetrafluoroethylene (ePTFE) coated with phosphorylcholine. The aim of this study was to evaluate the feasibility and safety of this novel valve for TPVR in sheep by a hybrid approach and assess the function of this valve during a 4-week period using angiographic, hemodynamic, echocardiographic, and macroscopic analyses and histologic assessment.

Materials and Methods

Ethics Statement

All the animal experimental protocols were approved by the ethics committee of Changhai Hospital, Shanghai. All animals received care in compliance with the Guide for the Care and Use of Laboratory Animals.

Phosphorylcholine (PC) Coating of ePTFE Membranes

The 0.1-mm ultramicroporous ePTFE membranes (Gore-Tex, WL Gore and Associates, Inc., Flagstaff, AZ) were coated with a derivative of PC as previously described [10,11]. Briefly, 2-methacryloxyethyl phosphorylcholine (MPC, 1 mol eq) and N-butyl methacrylate (BMA, 2 mol eq) were polymerized by a solution free radical process using azobisisobutyronitrile (0.2 mol eq) as initiator. Polymer (MPC–BMA) was dispersed in ethanol to give a 1% (w/v) mixture. The 0.1-mm ePTFE membranes were coated by a dip coating process, whereby the membranes were immersed in the solution and withdrawn at a rate of 30 cm/min. The coated membranes were dried at room temperature for 1 h and sterilized by autoclave.

Valved Stent Construction

The balloon-expandable stent was made of cobalt-chromium alloy. Bare stents were 24.6 mm in length and 20 or 23 mm in diameter when fully expanded. The valve leaflets of PPHV were made of the PC-coated ePTFE membrane, which was trimmed into 3 identically shaped valve leaflets according to the valve model profile and sutured onto the stent using 7–0 polypropylene threads (Johnson & Johnson, New Brunswick City, NJ). The bottom one-third of the stent is covered with the PC-coated ePTFE sealing cuff designed to reduce the potential for paravalvular leaks (Fig. 1).

Reference Valve

Bovine pericardium was used for the leaflets of reference valves. The bovine pericardium was processed by removal of surface fat tissue, agitated digestion with 0.01% trypsin for 8 hours, subsequent cross-linking with 0.6% glutaraldehyde for 36 hours, and, finally, repeated washing with 2%L-glutamine (to eliminate glutaraldehyde toxicity)[12]. The bovine pericardium was mounted on the stents by the similar method as PTPV.

Animals

Ten healthy male sheep, 5 to 8 months old and weighing an average of 22.5±2.0 kg, were used. No cardiac murmurs were detected. Preoperative electrocardiogram, chest film, and echocardiogram revealed no abnormalities.

Preoperative Preparation and Anesthetization

Animals were fasted for 12 hours and water deprived for 8 hours before surgery. Hair was removed from the right side of the chest wall. After intramuscular injection of ketamine (10–15 mg/kg, IM), diazepam (0.2 mg/kg, IM) and atropine (0.05 mg/kg, IM), a venous transfusion access on the foreleg was established and a 6-French leak-proof sheath was introduced percutaneously via the left femoral vein. Anesthesia was induced with fentanyl (2–4 ug/kg, IV), midazolam (0.05 mg/kg, IV), and vecuronium bromide (0.05 mg/kg, IV) and maintained with infusions of fentanyl (1–4 ug/kg·h) and propolfol (0.3 mg/kg·h). Ventilation was supported by use of a volume-limited ventilator with inspiratory volume of 10–15 ml/kg, respiratory rate of 18–24/min, and pressure support of 8–12cm H_2O. Electrocardiogram, SpO2, and non-invasive blood pressure were routinely monitored throughout the whole procedure.

Hybrid Approach and Implantation Procedure

The sheep were positioned in the left lateral decubitus. The thoracic cavity was opened via the right anterolateral thoracotomy at the fourth intercostal space. Then the right ventricular apex was exposed, and two felt strip-buttressed purse-string sutures using 5–0 polypropylene threads (Johnson & Johnson, New Brunswick City, NJ) were made at the right ventricular apex, almost 10 mm far away from the left anterior descending coronary artery (Fig. 2).

Heparin (1.5 mg/kg) was introduced via the sheath in the left femoral vein. A 6-French pigtail catheter (Cordis, Johnson and Johnson, New Brunswick City, NJ) was introduced through the femoral vein sheath, and imaging of the right ventricle and pulmonary valve were performed using digital subtraction angiography (DSA) (Siemens, Munich, Germany) (Fig. 3A). The pulmonary valve was identified, and its position was marked according to imaging results, and the radius of the pulmonary valve annulus was measured. A valved stent, size larger than the measured annulus, was selected to avoid paravalvular leaks and in consideration of the growth of the young sheep. Then the valved stent was crimped symmetrically using a specialized crimping device onto the inflatable portion of a 20 or 23 mm×3 cm high-pressure balloon catheter (volume driven) (Fig. 4). The balloon catheter loaded with valved stent was subsequently inserted into the auxiliary short sheath (Fig. 4). After that, the prepared right ventricular apex was punctured in the direction of the right ventricular outflow tract (RVOT), and an over-the-needle 7F introducer system (Arrows, Reading, Pa) was inserted. Under fluoroscopic guidance, a soft-tip 0.035-inch guide wire was first advanced into the right pulmonary artery and then transcatheter exchanged for an ultrastiff Back-up Meier wire (0.038 inches, 185 cm; Boston Scientific, Medi-tech, Watertown, Mass). After that, the 7F introducer was removed, and the 22F introducer sheath set (Fig. 4) was inserted over the guide wire during fluoroscopy. Then the 22F sheath and the guide wire were fixed, and the introducer was removed. The auxiliary short sheath and the prepared balloon catheter loaded with valved stent was inserted into the 22F sheath. Thereafter, the valved stent was advanced to the previously marked position of the pulmonary valve (Fig. 3B). After it was confirmed that the valved stent had been delivered to the optimal position, the valved stent was then balloon-expanded (Fig. 3C). The balloon was subsequently deflated, and the catheter and the 22F sheath were removed. Imaging of the artificial pulmonary valve and the right ventricle was performed by deploying a pigtail catheter via the left femoral

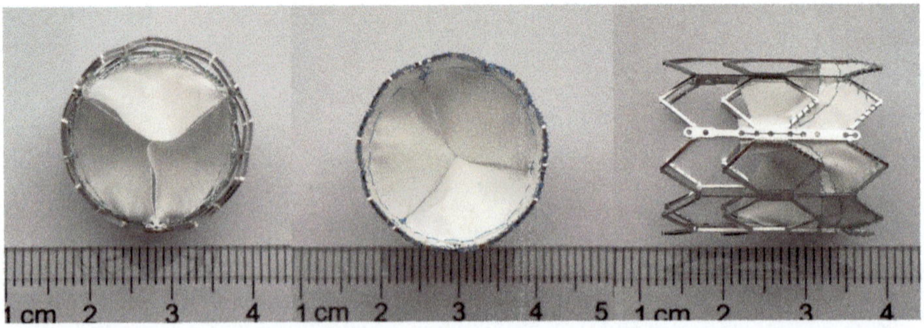

Figure 1. Views of the polymeric prosthetic pulmonary valve. Top view, bottom view, and side view of the balloon-expandable cobalt-chromium alloystent (length, 24.6 mm; diameter, 20 mm) containing a 3-leaflet ePTFE valve.

vein (pressure 800 psi, total amount of contrast 20 ml, speed 20 ml/s) (Fig. 3D). A chest tube was placed and the chest was closed.

Postoperative Treatment

All sheep received postoperative intramuscular injections of cefradine (25 mg/kg, 1/12 h) for 3 days and subcutaneous injections of low molecular heparin (60–80 IU/kg, 1/12 h) for 7 days. Oral aspirin (3 mg/kg·d) was given for the entire study period. One week after surgery, the sheep returned to the animal facility, where their general health was checked daily.

Angiography

Angiography was performed before the procedure to locate the precise position of the native pulmonary valve, after the procedure, and at 4-week follow-up to confirm the appropriate position and verify the function of the implanted valve. (Fig. 3).

Echocardiographic and Hemodynamic Measurements

Transthoracic echocardiography (TTE) was performed at 4-week follow-up. Right ventricular pressure, pulmonary artery pressure, and peak-peak transvalvular pressure gradient (PTPG) were collected before and after the implantation and at 4-week follow-up by cardiac catheterization.

Computed Tomography

The 64-row computed tomography was performed at 4-week follow-up to confirm the appropriate position and intact configuration of the stent.

Laboratory Blood Chemistry Measurements

Erythrocyte and white blood cell counts, hematocrit, free hemoglobin, platelet count, coagulation parameters, and levels of aspartate aminotransferase, alanine aminotransferase, lactate dehydrogenase, bilirubin, creatinine, serum calcium and phosphorus were checked 4 weeks after implantation and compared with preoperative values.

Valved Stent Retrieval

One randomly selected sheep with polymeric valve was euthanized and the valved stent was explanted 4 weeks after implantation. Before harvesting, heparin (100 IU/kg IV) was administered. Autopsy with macroscopic and histologic examination of heart, lungs, liver, kidneys, and spleen was performed. The valved stent was rinsed with a saline solution to remove excess blood, and then was examined macroscopically, histologically, and by electron microscopic analysis. The histology stains included standard hematoxylin and eosin (H&E) to detect tissue deposition, and von Kossa staining to detect calcium deposition on the leaflets.

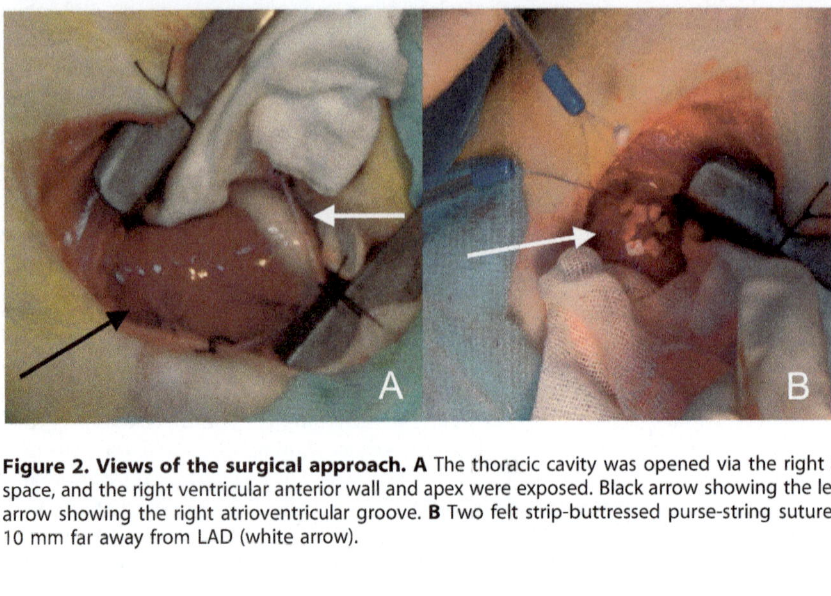

Figure 2. Views of the surgical approach. A The thoracic cavity was opened via the right anterolateral thoracotomy at the fourth intercostal space, and the right ventricular anterior wall and apex were exposed. Black arrow showing the left anterior descending coronary artery (LAD). White arrow showing the right atrioventricular groove. **B** Two felt strip-buttressed purse-string sutures were placed at the right ventricular apex almost 10 mm far away from LAD (white arrow).

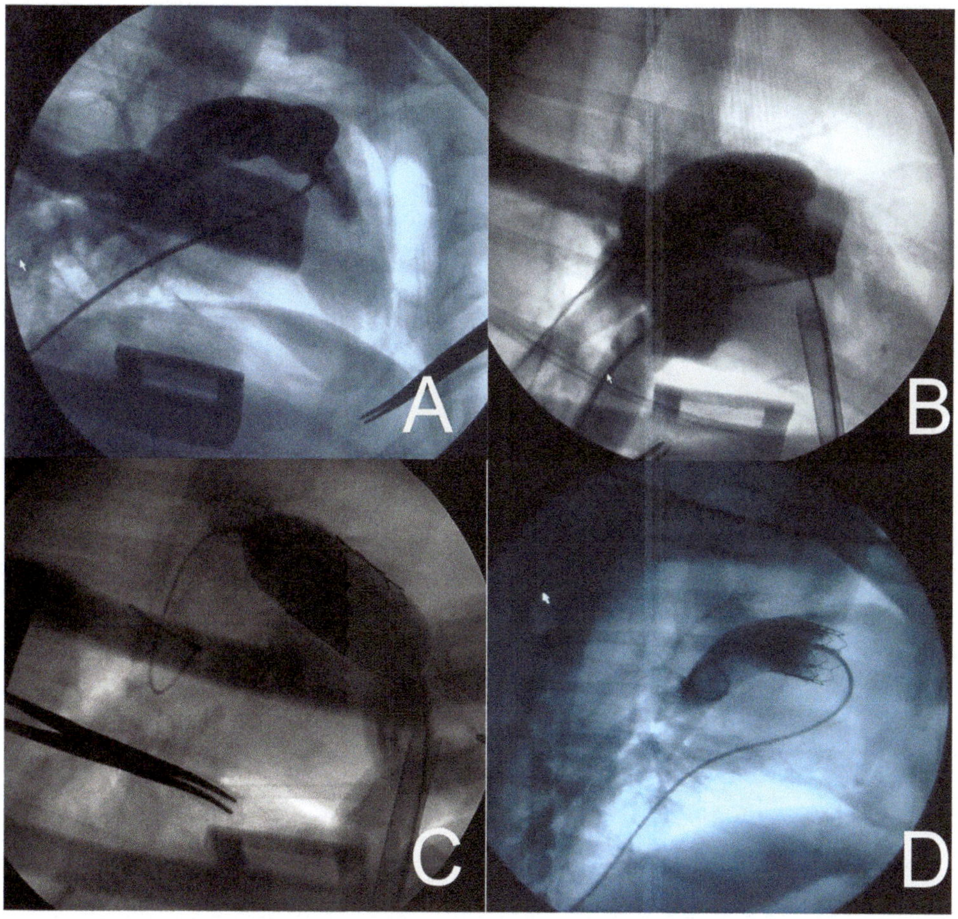

Figure 3. Valved stent implantation process (representative images). **A** Imaging of the pulmonary valve was performed to measure the pulmonary valve radius and location. **B** After the valved stent was advanced to the pulmonary valve via the 22F sheath, a right ventricular angiography was performed to confirm that the valved stent was at the optimal position. **C** The valved stent was fully balloon-expanded. **D** A pulmonary angiography showing correct position of the valved stent in the pulmonary position in an sheep model. No regurgitation was assessed.

Electron Microscopic Analysis

Samples for electron microscopy analysis were taken from the explanted valve leaflets and were rinsed in a solution of paraformaldehyde. For scanning electron microscopy (SEM), the tissue samples were dehydrated in a graded acetone series, and critical-point dried. Specimens were then glued to metal stubs, coated with gold, and examined in a Hitachi S-520 scanning electron microscope (Hitachi, Ltd., Chiyoda, Tokyo). For transmission electron microscope (TEM), the tissue samples were postfixed in osmium tetroxide and embedded in araldite. Ultrathin sections were stained with uranylacetate and lead citrate and observed with a Hitachi H-7650 transmission electron microscope (Hitachi, Ltd., Chiyoda, Tokyo).

Statistics

Values are presented as means±standard deviations. Changes in right ventricular pressure, pulmonary artery pressure, and transvalvular gradients (before, right after, and 4 weeks after implantation) were compared using repeated measurements or Friedman test. Statistical analyses were performed by using SPSS 16.0 software (SPSS, Inc, Chicago, Ill). P values of less than 0.05 were considered statistically significant.

Results

Implantation was successful in 9 sheep. Angiography at implantation showed one 20 mm PTPV failed to be located at orthotopic position and the stent was in RVOT. All the other prosthetic valves demonstrated orthotopic position and exhibited normal open and close functionality and no stenosis or insufficiency. Six sheep were implanted with 20 mm PTPV, and two sheep with 23 mm PTPV. The other 2 sheep were implanted with reference valve (20 mm and 23 mm valve, respectively).

The mean diameter of the pulmonary annulus was 16.8±1.4 mm and 17.5±1.1 mm as revealed by TTE and angiography, respectively. Mean surgery duration was 82±10.6 minutes. The mean x-ray exposure time was 7.5±1.6 minutes. The mean stent diameter (except the unsuccessful one) measured by angiography after the procedure was 20.5±1.6 mm (range: 18–23 mm).

In one sheep, postoperative chest drainage was above normal. The bloody chest drainage was 80 ml 3 h after surgery, and 160 ml 24 h after surgery. The chest tube was extracted 48 h after surgery. One sheep developed pneumothorax postoperatively, which was self-healing 48 h after surgery. Vomit and aspiration happened to one sheep before extubation during the surgery. The sheep developed cough and pneumonia postoperatively, and was successfully cured by antibiotic, expectorant, and chest physio-

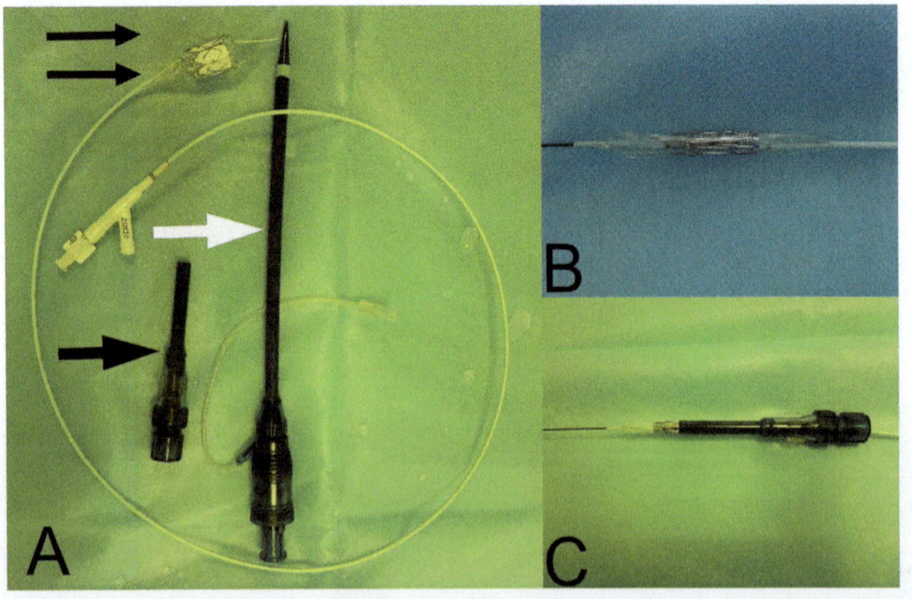

Figure 4. Views of the delivery system. A. Views of the 22F introducer sheath set (white arrow), the auxiliary short sheath (black arrow), and the 20 mm×3 cm high-pressure balloon catheter (double black arrows). **B** The valved stent was crimped symmetrically onto the inflatable portion of a balloon catheter. **C** Placement of valved stent into the auxiliary short sheath.

therapy for one week. The other sheep were uneventful postoperatively. All 10 sheep including the unsuccessful one survived and did well in the 4-week follow-up. The 4-week follow-up data excluded the unsuccessful one.

Echocardiography 4 weeks after implantation (Fig. 5) showed all the prosthetic valves exhibited normal functionality and no significant insufficiency, paravalvular leakage, or valve excrescence. Left ventricular and right ventricular function and dimensions appeared normal. PTPG of the polymeric valves was 14.1±6.6 mmHg, while that of two reference valves were 9 and 16 mmHg.

Four-week angiography demonstrated good opening and closure characteristics in all 9 sheep after 4 weeks. Paravalvular leakages were not observed. The mean stent diameter measured by 4-week angiography was 20.1±1.5 mm (range: 18.5–22 mm).

The results of cardiac catheterization revealed that PTPG of the polymeric valves was 3.9±1.1 mmHg before implantation, 5.9±1.3 mmHg right after implantation and 11.9±5.0 mmHg at follow-up ($P<0.01$). While, PTPG of the two reference valves were 2 and 4 mmHg before implantation, 4 and 7 mmHg right after implantation, and 11 and 17 mmHg at follow-up. Right ventricular pressure, pulmonary artery pressure, and PTPG of the polymeric valves before and after the implantation and at 4-week follow-up are shown in Figure 6.

CT 4 weeks after implantation demonstrated orthotopic position and no evidence of stent fracture or deformation of all 9 stents (Fig. 7).

Blood parameters of all sheep did not show any significant changes from preoperative values.

Postmortem examination of the randomly selected sheep confirmed the correct position of the valved stent and that the native pulmonary valve was stuck between the pulmonary wall and the stent. No paravalvular defects were visible. The valve leaflets were thin, pliable, and competent, without thrombus or calcification. No significant tissue deposits were noted in the outflow side of the ePTFE valved stent, while the inflow side of the ePTFE valved stent showed slight fibrous overgrowth at the bottom of the leaflet, in the commissural areas and on the sealing cuff. Cardiac structures were unscathed (Fig. 8).

On microscopic evaluation (Fig. 9), there was no cellular infiltration or structural deterioration of the ePTFE membrane noted. Slight fibrous overgrowth was observed on the sealing cuff and at the bottom of the leaflets. The fibrous overgrowth attached loosely to the ePTFE membrane which itself had no obvious cell or tissue infiltration. No evidence of calcification of the stented valve including the valve leaflets and sealing cuff was found after von Kossa staining. The surrounding tissue of the pulmonary artery showed normal H&E staining and von Kossa staining.

No cell or tissue attachment/infiltration was found in the SEM or TEM images (Fig. 10). Pathological findings showed no abnormality in the organs of the sheep.

Discussion

Since 2000, TPVR technology has steadily advanced [2,13,14]. Clinically, TPVR appears to offer significant benefits over standard surgical procedures for patients following surgery for CHD, including tetralogy of Fallot, pulmonary atresia and other surgical procedures requiring reconstruction of RVOT [2]. Not only is the process superior in smaller incisions, less postoperative pain, shorter hospital stay, and lower costs, but the short and medium follow-up data show satisfactory clinical effectiveness and good freedom from reoperation, and demonstrate that TPVR can potentially reduce the lifetime number of open heart operations [2,14,15]. Bonhoeffer et al [2] successfully performed 155 procedures with no early deaths, only 4 procedural complications, and a good survival rate of 96.9% after 83 month.

However, clincally available stented valves for TPVR are restricted to transcatheter bioprosthetic valves (TBVs), which have some significant defects. Firstly, the target population for TPVR are almost the young. The unsatisfactory durability of bioprosthesis certainly will increase the pain of the young patients. Secondly, the leaflets of TBVs, especially with balloon expandable valved stents, are proved to be injured after crimped and uncrimped

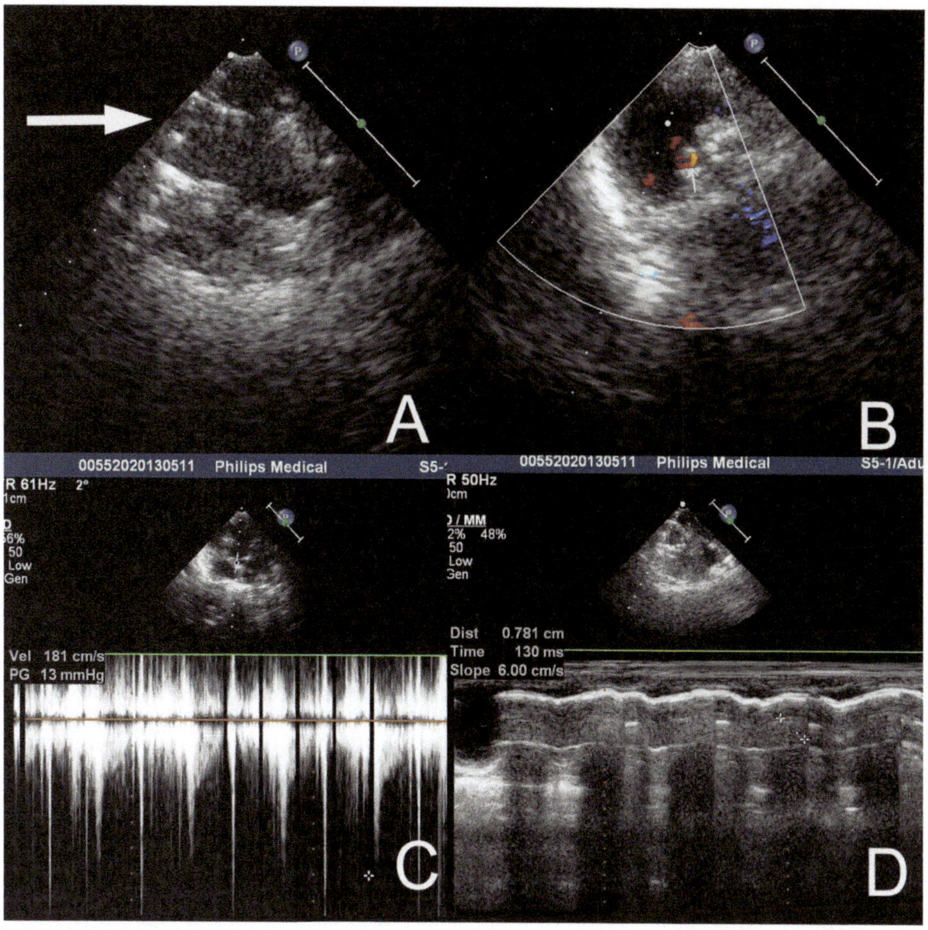

Figure 5. Echocardiography 4 weeks after implantation from a representative. sheep with a 20 mm PTPV. A The two parallel lines of echo enhancement showed appropriate position and open shape of the stent (white arrow). **B** Color Doppler ultrasonography revealed no regurgitation or paravalvular leakage. **C** Doppler ultrasonography revealed the peak-peak transvalvular pressure gradient of the stented valve was 13 mmHg. **D** The motion distance of the valve cusp was 0.781 cm measured by Doppler ultrasonography, meaning normal function of the valve leaflet.

during implantation. Zegdi et al [5] report the microscopic analysis of 4 Sapien-Edwards TBVs, which have been crimped and deployed in humans or ex vivo. Collagen fibers fragmentation and disruption in the valve leaflets could be found in all of them. The thickness of the leaflets was involved and areas of plasmatic insudation was found. These findings were also proved by animal experiment [6], in which the TBVs leaflets were implanted subcutaneously in rats for 12 weeks after crimped and uncrimped, and microscopic analysis revealed intense fragmentations of the collagen and elastic fibers and moderate invasion of macrophages, giant cells and signs of phagocytosis. These changes will conceivably impact on the long-term durability of TBVs. Thirdly, the resulting anatomic spectrum from pulmonary regurgitation after surgical intervention for CHD is broad. With currently

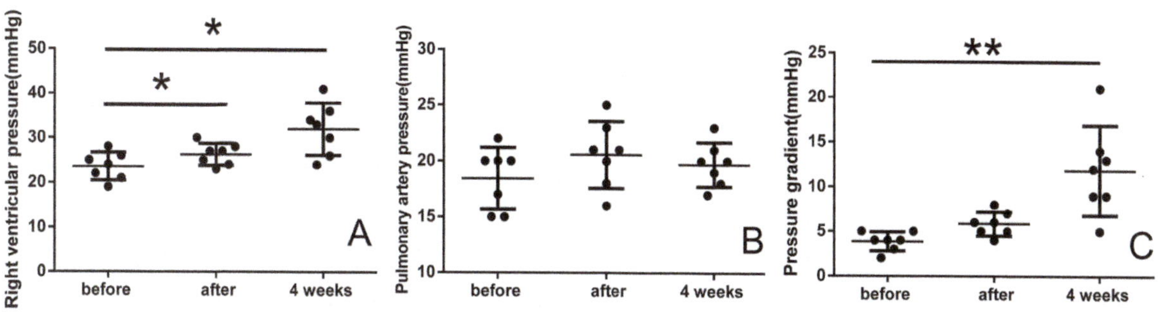

Figure 6. Hemodynamic data before, immediately after, and 4 weeks after implantation. Right ventricular systolic pressure (A), pulmonary artery systolic pressure (B), and peak-peak transvalvular pressure gradient (C) were assessed. vs. before group, *P<0.05, **P<0.01.

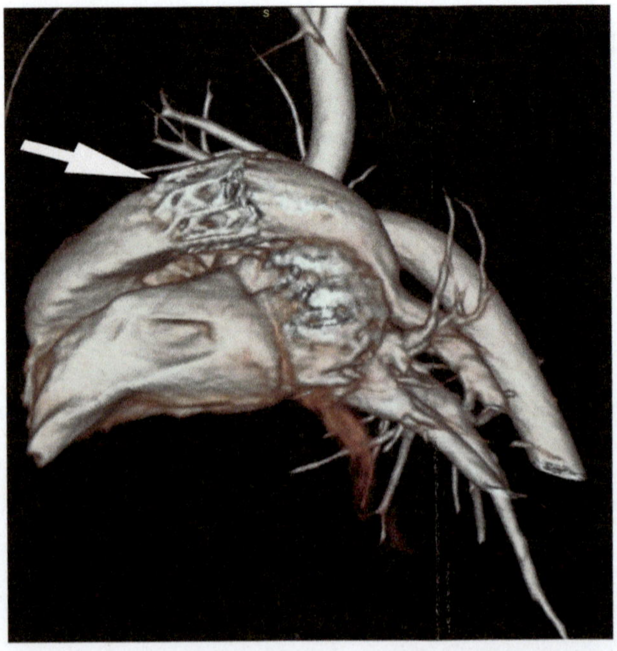

Figure 7. The 3D reconstruction CT image 4 weeks after implantation from a representative sheep with a 20 mm PTPV. The image demonstrated orthotopic position and no deformation of the stent (white arrow).

available TBVs, it is not possible to treat all concerned patients. Moreover, with younger patients, especially children, the overall size of the currently available TBVs are too large. So, the indications for TPVR includes the conduit RVOT diameter should be between 16 mm and 22 mm and the weight should be more than 20 kg [16].

The advancement in the study of PPHV has brought emerging hope to these patients by remedying those weaknesses of TBVs. Over the past 20 years, significant advances in material science has resulted in new materials with improved properties, which have the advantages of good durability and antithrombotic performance and being easily engineered and designed to reproduce the geometry and haemodynamic characteristics of natural valves, making them potential materials of choice in the development of valve substitutes [17]. Moreover, the application of low-profile PPHV could be an advantage for TPVR because it is easy for PPHV to be folded and introduced into delivery catheters [17].

Recently, several transcatheter PPHVs [18,19] have been designed and the results of in vitro test were good. Moreover, Metzner et al [9] have demonstrated an excellent valve function of polyurethane valves with a self-expanding stent in the pulmonary position of 7 sheep in a period of 4 weeks. Gross morphology demonstrated good opening and closure characteristics and the valve leaflets were thin and pliable without indurations or calcification.

ePTFE is a hydrophobic and polyporous polymer, with chemically inert, low friction, and low tissue affinity. The main advantages of ePTFE is its electronegative surface charge, which mimics the normal endothelium and would supposedly decrease its thrombogenicity [20]. This low tendency to **produce thrombotic events**, together with suitable mechanical properties and fatigue resistance, made this material a good choice for PPHV. In 1990s, Nistal et al [20] designed a PPHV in which the cuspal material was made of ePTFE with low porosity and the material covering the valve frame was made of ePTFE with high porosity, and sucessfully implanted ten PPHVs in the tricuspid position in sheep for 3 to 42 weeks with no postoperative anticoagulation. They found that the PPHVs had a moderate calcification rate and that calcium deposits appeared to be always related to the presence of ePTFE with high porosity. No evidence of valve thrombosis was found in 9 animals. Microscopy disclosed a complete lack of infiltrating cells within the cuspal material made of ePTFE with low porosity, however, those parts made of ePTFE with high porosity did show infiltration by host cells and calcium. These results presented that PPHV made of ePTFE had excellent anti-thrombotic function and the substitution of the ePTFE with high porosity might eventually eliminate these aforementioned problems.

In this century, a novel ultramicroporous ePTFE (UEPTFE) became a popular material for PPHV, especially in the pulmonary valve position. This extremely low porosity (distance of fiber nodes <1 um) of UEPTFE makes cellular or fibrinous adherence more difficult and is theoretically resistant to pannus formation or calcification. The monocusp valve [21], bicuspid valve [22], and

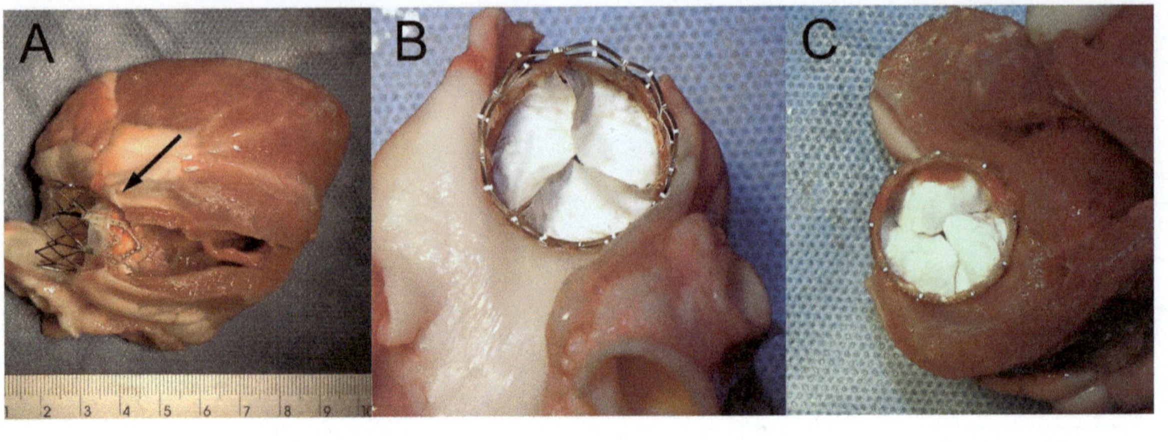

Figure 8. Gross morphology of the ePTFE valved stent explanted from a sheep 4 weeks after surgery. A The native pulmonary valve can be seen (arrow), confirming the correct position of the valved stent. **B** The outflow side of ePTFE valved stent showed the leaflets were thin without significant tissue deposits. **C** The inflow side of ePTFE valved stent showed slight fibrous overgrowth at the bottom of the leaflets, in the commissural areas and on the sealing cuff.

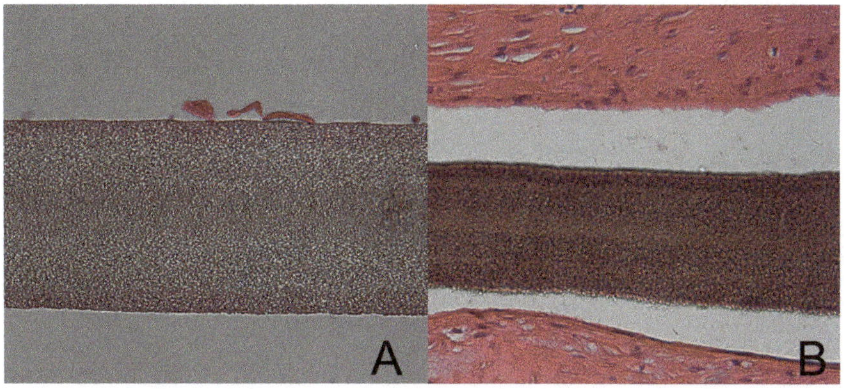

Figure 9. Histologic images of the ePTFE valve leaflets explanted from a sheep 4 weeks after surgery. A The surface of ePTFE leaflet was smooth, without obvious cell or tissue infiltration. The ePTFE membrane showed multilayered structure.(HE×400). **B** The surface of ePTFE on the sealing cuff revealed fibrous overgrowth, which attached loosely to the ePTFE membrane which itself had no obvious cell or tissue infiltration.(HE×200).

trileaflet valve [23] made of UEPTFE have successfully been implanted in men with CHD for pulmonary reconstruction, and have demonstrated satisfactory clinical effects. Ando et al [23] reported their ten-year experience with handmade trileaflet UEPTFE valved conduit used for pulmonary reconstruction in 139 patients with no postoperative anticoagulation. Estimated freedom from conduit explantation was 88.0%, and pulmonary insufficiency was less than or equal to mild in 75.0% at 10 years. All valves maintained their motion, and no evidence of valve thrombus was noted.

These achivement of UEPTFE valve in the pulmonary reconstruction has brought hope for further developing a transcatheter UEPTFE pulmonary valve.

However, some problems with UEPTFE valves remain to be resolved. Concerns have been raised about leaflet thickening and decreased mobility caused by neointimal and fibrous overgrowth after valve repair with UEPTFE membrane [24,25]. Given this, in this study, we used the PC-coating technique to provide a more biocompatible and nonthrombogenic surface for UEPTFE membrane. PC is a zwitterionic head group with no overall charge found in cell membrane lipid bilayers, which is nonthrombogenic. A coating of PC derivatives onto polymetric materials has shown decreased platelet adhesion and neointimal hyperplasia to the polymer surface in many studies [10,11,26,27]. The advantage of such an approach is that the blood that comes into contact with PC-coated surfaces maintains its homeostatic potential. After 4-week follow-up, we found the PPHVs with PC-coated UEPTFE showed good antithrombotic property and resistance to tissue affinity. However, mild fibrosis developed on the sealing cuff of this UEPTFE valve, and it spread to the commissural areas and the bottom of the leaflets. The stagnant flow in these areas might facilitate the apposition of fibrin and blood cell elements, and lead to fibrosis. The mild fibrosis didn't influenced the valve function in period of 4-week follow-up, while further results remained to be observed.

There are two available surgical approaches for TPVR: transvascular or transventricular approach. Currently, clinically used surgical approach for TPVR is confined to transvascular approach. For patients with small or distorted peripheral vessels and patients with wide or severely calcified and kinked RVOTs, hybrid operation and transventricular approach will be the only option. So, developing a safe and minimally invasive hybrid

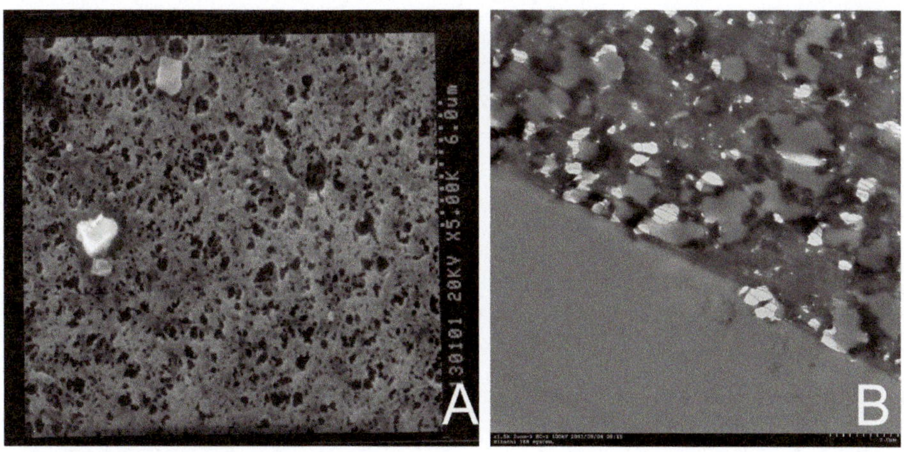

Figure 10. Electron microscopic images of the ePTFE leaflets explanted from a sheep 4 weeks after surgery. A Scanning electron microscopic appearance of the outflow side of a ePTFE valve cusp showing polyporous structure of ePTFE and no obvious cell or tissue attachment (×5000). **B** Transmission electron microscopic appearance of the outflow side of a ePTFE valve cusp showing polyporous structure of ePTFE and no obvious cell or tissue infiltration. (×1500).

approach is meaningful. Moreover, although less trauma, transvascular approach can bring two problems in sheep model: first, the diameter of peripheral vein in sheep is often small, which restricts the choice of valved stent size; second, the position and direction of heart and main artery are different between tetrapod sheep and bipedal human. The angles from inferior vena cava to right ventricle and from right ventricle to pulmonary artery in sheep are more sharp than those in human. So, it is difficult to deliver the sheath from femoral vein to pulmonary valve in sheep model [28], and it is easy to induce arrhythmia during this procedure [9]. In Metzner's study [9], rhythm disturbances occurred in all animals. Likewise, in our preliminary test, we had tried transfemoral approach in sheep with a 14F sheath, but we failed to deliver the sheath to pulmonary valve because of the sharp turning from tricuspid valve to pulmonary valve in sheep, and the repeated procedure led to ventricular fibrillation and death. After autopsy, we found endocardium scathed in the anterior wall of right ventricle. So, in this study, we chose the hybrid method and transapical approach for all sheep. We found TPVR by the hybrid method and transapical approach with this novel ePTFE stented valve was safe and effective. No serious arrhythmia occurred, and cardiac structures were intact.

To avoid stent migration, a right choice of valved stent size and a good coaxality between valved stent and pulmonary artery root when expanding balloon are important. We suggest a ratio of 1.2~1.3:1 between the diameter of the valved stent and the pulmonary valve ring, and a projection position of RAO 20/CRA 20 (sheep in left lateral decubitus), in which the angle from right ventricular long axis to main pulmonary artery would be as straight as possible. In one sheep, the valved stent was located below the right position. We thought a bad coaxality was the reason.

In conclusion, TPVR with the novel PC-coated UEPTFE stented valves by the hybrid method and right ventricular apical approach in an ovine model is feasible and safe. The early valvular functionality of the novel UEPTFE stented valves are as good as bovine pericardium valves. The PC-coated UEPTFE valves have demonstrated good antithrombotic performance and low cell or tissue affinity. The medium-term results remain to be observed.

Acknowledgments

The authors would like to acknowledge Lepu Medical Technology Co., Ltd. (Beijing, China) for manufacturing the balloon-expandable stents and the delivery system, and Yu-hao Zhou for his suppprt on statistic analysis.

Author Contributions

Conceived and designed the experiments: LH ZX. Performed the experiments: BZ XC TX ZZ XL LH. Analyzed the data: BZ XC. Contributed reagents/materials/analysis tools: ZX. Wrote the paper: BZ XC.

References

1. Bonhoeffer P, Boudjemline Y, Saliba Z, Merckx J, Aggoun Y, et al. (2000) Percutaneous replacement of pulmonary valve in a right-ventricle to pulmonary-artery prosthetic conduit with valve dysfunction. Lancet 356: 1403–1405.
2. Lurz P, Coats L, Khambadkone S, Nordmeyer J, Boudjemline Y, et al. (2008) Percutaneous pulmonary valve implantation: impact of evolving technology and learning curve on clinical outcome. Circulation 117: 1964–1972.
3. Kenny D, Hijazi ZM, Kar S, Rhodes J, Mullen M, et al. (2011) Percutaneous implantation of the Edwards SAPIEN transcatheter heart valve for conduit failure in the pulmonary position: early phase 1 results from an international multicenter clinical trial. J Am Coll Cardiol 58: 2248–2256.
4. Attmann T, Quaden R, Jahnke T, Muller-Hulsbeck S, Boening A, et al. (2006) Percutaneous pulmonary valve replacement: 3-month evaluation of self-expanding valved stents. Ann Thorac Surg 82: 708–713.
5. Zegdi R, Bruneval P, Blanchard D, Fabiani JN (2011) Evidence of leaflet injury during percutaneous aortic valve deployment. Eur J Cardiothorac Surg 40: 257–259.
6. Kiefer P, Gruenwald F, Kempfert J, Aupperle H, Seeburger J, et al. (2011) Crimping May Affect the Durability of Transcatheter Valves: An Experimental Analysis. The Annals of Thoracic Surgery 92: 155–160.
7. Sachweh JS, Daebritz SH (2006) Novel "biomechanical" polymeric valve prostheses with special design for aortic and mitral position: a future option for pediatric patients? ASAIO J 52: 575–580.
8. Claiborne TE, Slepian MJ, Hossainy S, Bluestein D (2012) Polymeric trileaflet prosthetic heart valves: evolution and path to clinical reality. Expert Rev Med Devices 9: 577–594.
9. Metzner A, Iino K, Steinseifer U, Uebing A, de Buhr W, et al. (2010) Percutaneous pulmonary polyurethane valved stent implantation. J Thorac Cardiovasc Surg 139: 748–752.
10. Chen C, Ofenloch JC, Yianni YP, Hanson SR, Lumsden AB (1998) Phosphorylcholine coating of ePTFE reduces platelet deposition and neointimal hyperplasia in arteriovenous grafts. J Surg Res 77: 119–125.
11. Campbell EJ, O'Byrne V, Stratford PW, Quirk I, Vick TA, et al. (1994) Biocompatible surfaces using methacryloylphosphorylcholine laurylmethacrylate copolymer. ASAIO J 40: M853–857.
12. Zong GJ, Bai Y, Jiang HB, Li WP, Wu H, et al. (2009) Use of a novel valve stent for transcatheter pulmonary valve replacement: an animal study. J Thorac Cardiovasc Surg 137: 1363–1369.
13. Coats L, Bonhoeffer P (2007) New percutaneous treatments for valve disease. Heart 93: 639–644.
14. McElhinney DB, Hellenbrand WE, Zahn EM, Jones TK, Cheatham JP, et al. (2010) Short- and medium-term outcomes after transcatheter pulmonary valve placement in the expanded multicenter US melody valve trial. Circulation 122: 507–516.
15. Lurz P, Nordmeyer J, Giardini A, Khambadkone S, Muthurangu V, et al. (2011) Early versus late functional outcome after successful percutaneous pulmonary valve implantation: are the acute effects of altered right ventricular loading all we can expect? J Am Coll Cardiol 57: 724–731.
16. Lee YS, Lee HD (2012) Percutaneous pulmonary valve implantation. Korean Circ J 42: 652–656.
17. Ghanbari H, Viatge H, Kidane AG, Burriesci G, Tavakoli M, et al. (2009) Polymeric heart valves: new materials, emerging hopes. Trends Biotechnol 27: 359–367.
18. Claiborne TE, Bluestein D, Schoephoerster RT (2009) Development and evaluation of a novel artificial catheter-deliverable prosthetic heart valve and method for in vitro testing. Int J Artif Organs 32: 262–271.
19. Tzamtzis S, Ghanbari H, Seifalian A, Burriesci G (2010) A new generation aortic valve device for transcatheter implantation. Cardiology 115: 292.
20. Nistal F, Garcia-Martinez V, Arbe E, Fernandez D, Artinano E, et al. (1990) In vivo experimental assessment of polytetrafluoroethylene trileaflet heart valve prosthesis. J Thorac Cardiovasc Surg 99: 1074–1081.
21. Gil-Jaurena J, Ferreiros M, Castillo R, Conejo L, Cuenca V, et al. (2010) Use of a pulmonary neovalve with a transannular patch for repair of tetralogy of fallot. Rev Esp Cardiol 63: 1438–1443.
22. Lee C, Lee CH, Kwak JG, Song JY, Shim WS, et al. (2012) Bicuspid pulmonary valve implantation using polytetrafluoroethylene membrane: early results and assessment of the valve function by magnetic resonance imaging. Eur J Cardiothorac Surg 43: 468–472.
23. Ando M, Takahashi Y (2009) Ten-year experience with handmade trileaflet polytetrafluoroethylene valved conduit used for pulmonary reconstruction. J Thorac Cardiovasc Surg 137: 124–131.
24. Quintessenza JA, Jacobs JP, Chai PJ, Morell VO, Lindberg H (2010) Polytetrafluoroethylene bicuspid pulmonary valve implantation: experience with 126 patients. World J Pediatr Congenit Heart Surg 1: 20–27.
25. Ito T, Maekawa A, Yamana K, Yoshizumi T, Sunada M (2010) Use of an expanded polytetrafluoroethylene patch as an artificial leaflet in mitral valve plasty: an early experience. Ann Thorac Surg 89: 1620–1624.
26. Duraiswamy N, Choksi TD, Pinchuk L, Schoephoerster RT (2009) A phospholipid-modified polystyrene-polyisobutylene-polystyrene (SIBS) triblock polymer for enhanced hemocompatibility and potential use in artificial heart valves. J Biomater Appl 23: 367–379.
27. Dahe GJ, Kadam SS, Sabale SS, Kadam DP, Sarkate LB, et al. (2011) In vivo evaluation of the biocompatibility of surface modified hemodialysis polysulfone hollow fibers in rat. PLoS One 6: e25236.
28. Bonhoeffer P, Boudjemline Y, Saliba Z, Hausse AO, Aggoun Y, et al. (2000) Transcatheter implantation of a bovine valve in pulmonary position: a lamb study. Circulation 102: 813–816.

9

Myocardial Defect Detection Using PET-CT: Phantom Studies

Eugene S. Mananga[1,2], Georges El Fakhri[1,2], Joshua Schaefferkoetter[3], Ali A. Bonab[1,2], Jinsong Ouyang[1,2]*

1 Center for Advanced Medical Imaging Sciences, Division of Nuclear Medicine and Molecular Imaging, Massachusetts General Hospital, Boston, Massachusetts, United States of America, **2** Department of Radiology, Harvard Medical School, Boston, Massachusetts, United States of America, **3** A*STAR-NUS Clinical Imaging and Research Centre (CIRC), Singapore, Singapore

Abstract

It is expected that both noise and activity distribution can have impact on the detectability of a myocardial defect in a cardiac PET study. In this work, we performed phantom studies to investigate the detectability of a defect in the myocardium for different noise levels and activity distributions. We evaluated the performance of three reconstruction schemes: Filtered Back-Projection (FBP), Ordinary Poisson Ordered Subset Expectation Maximization (OP–OSEM), and Point Spread Function corrected OSEM (PSF–OSEM). We used the Channelized Hotelling Observer (CHO) for the task of myocardial defect detection. We found that the detectability of a myocardial defect is almost entirely dependent on the noise level and the contrast between the defect and its surroundings.

Editor: Xiaoyuan Chen, NIH, United States of America

Funding: This research was supported in part by the National Institutes of Health (NIH) Grants R01-HL110241 and T32-EB013180. The funders had no role in study design, data collection and analysis, decision to publish, or preparation of the manuscript.

Competing Interests: The authors have declared that no competing interests exist.

* E-mail: ouyang.jinsong@mgh.harvard.edu

Introduction

The utility of ^{13}N-ammonia, ^{15}O-water, and ^{82}Rb as PET perfusion tracers has been well documented in the cardiac PET community [*1,2*]. Furthermore, ^{18}F-BMS-747158 [*2–5*] has the potential to replace SPECT for perfusion studies. In addition, ^{18}F-fluorodeoxyglucose (FDG) uptake in the myocardium has been well validated as an indicator of myocardial viability [*6*]. In the clinical setting, diagnosis of cardiac disease is often strongly correlated with the detectability of a defect, which can be affected by noise level as well as activity distribution. Therefore, it is important to investigate defect detectability under different injection doses/imaging times and activity distributions. Myocardial defect detectability can be impacted by the activity distribution in both the heart and other organs or tissues surrounding the heart. It would be very difficult to use clinical data to study such impact.

Lesion detection is an important clinical task for medical imaging. In oncology, lesion detectability is critically important for early diagnosis and staging of patients. Typically, lesion detectability pertains to hot lesions (e.g., tumors, inflammation), where the uptake is higher within the lesions as compared to their surrounding background [*7,8*]. Previous research on myocardial defect detection using PET is limited. Tang *et al.* [*9*] studied defect detection using ^{82}Rb-PET Monte Carlo simulation. Other myocardial defect detection results are reported on SPECT imaging by Chen *et al.* [*10*], Wollenweber *et al.* [*11*], and Matsunari *et al.* [*12*].

In this paper, we propose a methodology to study myocardial defect detectability using phantom studies on a PET–CT scanner. We performed cardiac phantom studies to characterize myocardial defect detectability as a function of total number of counts, which is related to noise level, and variable activity distributions. We modeled defect-present and defect-absent studies and used the Channelized Hotelling Observer (CHO) [*13–15*] as a surrogate of human observer performance. Observer SNR was evaluated in the task of defect detection in a signal–known–exactly/background–known–exactly (SKE-BKE) paradigm with three types of image reconstruction: Filtered Back-Projection (FBP), Ordinary Poisson–Ordered Subsets Expectation Maximization (OP–OSEM), and Point Spread Function corrected OSEM (PSF–OSEM).

Materials and Methods

1. Data acquisitions

An anthropomorphic torso phantom (Data Spectrum, Hillsborough, NC) with a cardiac insert was used for all the acquisitions (See Fig. 1). The phantom simulates upper torso of average to large male/female subjects (38×26 cm). This phantom included heart (myocardium wall, defect, and myocardium cavity), left and right lungs, liver, spine, and a soft tissue compartment. The fillable defect placed within the myocardium cavity has 45°×2 cm with 3.8 mL volume. All the phantom experiments were performed on a Siemens Biograph PET–CT at Massachusetts General Hospital (MGH). Virtually noise-free ^{18}F data were acquired for the following five data sets:

1) *Myocardium*: The myocardium wall was filled with radioactive water while the defect, the liver, the lung, and the soft tissue background compartments were filled with "cold" water.

2) *Defect*: The defect compartment was filled with radioactive water and all other compartments were filled with "cold" water.
3) *Liver*: The liver compartment was filled with radioactive water and all other compartments were filled with "cold" water.
4) *Lung*: The lung compartments were filled with radioactive water and all other compartments were filled with "cold" water.
5) *Background*: The soft tissue background compartment was filled with radioactive water while the liver, the lung, the defect, and the myocardium wall compartments were filled with cold water.

For all the acquisitions, the phantom was always placed at the same position on the bed of the scanner.

2. Data set combinations

Fig. 2 shows the flow chart of data set combinations, image reconstruction, and the analysis of defect detection. From *myocardium, defect, liver, lung, and background* data sets, we generated various activity combinations. For each activity combination, we created two virtually "noise-free" sinogram data sets: defect-absent and defect-present. Each original data set was scaled before mixing to account for the radioactive decay, scan time, and injected activity (measured by a dose calibrator). The synthesized sinogram data sets were then scaled again to yield total 20 million counts in the soft-tissue background. We then added Poisson noise to the "noise-free" sinogram data sets to generate 64 noise realizations. The acquired CT images of the phantom were used for accurate modeling of attenuation and scatter media during the image reconstruction.

In order to combine *myocardium, defect, liver, lung, and background* data sets to generate a realistic activity distribution, we first investigated a cardiac PET patient study with ^{18}F-BMS747158 flow agent (see Fig. 3). The patient study was approved by Partners Institutional Review Board (IRB). The patient study showed that the myocardium-to-background, liver-to-background, lung-to-background, and defect-to-myocardium concentration ratios were 11.14, 6.02, 0.63, and 0.825, respectively. The total number of detected coincidence events from the soft-tissue background was around 20 million. These concentration ratios and total number of counts were used as the default for our phantom studies except the parameter under investigation.

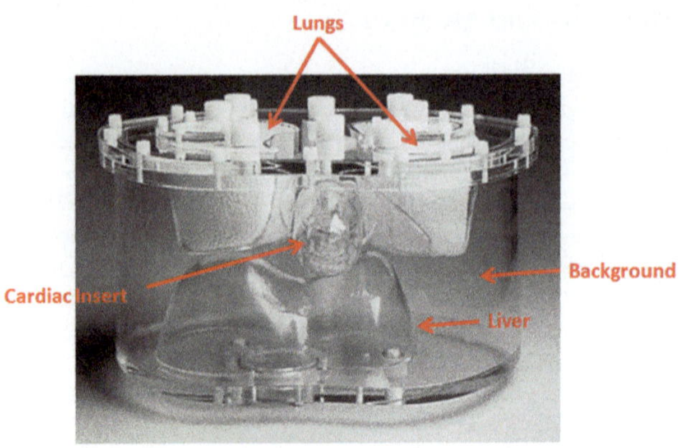

Figure 1. The anthropomorphic torso phantom used for the study.

3. Reconstructions

Three reconstruction schemes were considered: FBP, OP-OSEM, and PSF-OSEM. The image reconstruction was performed using Siemens e7-tools, which incorporated attenuation and scatter corrections using the acquired CT map of the phantom. For both OP-OSEM and PSF-OSEM, we used 2 iterations and 8 subsets unless stated otherwise. No post-reconstruction filtering was applied. All the image reconstruction was performed using $168\times168\times81$ matrix size and $4.07\times4.07\times2.02$ mm voxel size.

4. Observer Model

The acquisition and processing schemes were assessed on the basis of performance of a model observer in detecting the presence of a defect of known position. The CHO, which has been shown to have a good agreement with human performance [*16*], is the numerical observer used in this work. The model used a 3-channel Hotelling observer, in which the $168\times168\times81$ image volume data were processed through the frequency channels that are believed to exist in the human visual system. Sixty four defect-present and 64 defect-absent noise realizations were used to compute the 3–dimensional CHO SNR for myocardial defect detection. The CHO–SNR is given by:

$$SNR=\left[\frac{[\bar{\lambda}_1-\bar{\lambda}_0]^2}{0.5\mathrm{var}(\lambda)_1+0.5\mathrm{var}(\lambda)_0}\right]^{1/2},$$

where $\bar{\lambda}_i$ and $\mathrm{var}(\lambda)_i$ are the mean and variance ($i=1$ for defect-present; $i=0$ for defect-absent), respectively. We used the CHO with sparse difference–of–Gaussian (S–DOG) channel configuration (three radially symmetric channel profiles). The DOG channels are defined by:

$$C_j(\rho)=e^{-\frac{1}{2}\left(\frac{\rho}{Q\sigma_j}\right)^2}-e^{-\frac{1}{2}\left(\frac{\rho}{\sigma_j}\right)^2},$$

where ρ is the radial frequency, $j=1,2,3$ is the channel index, and σ_j is defined by:

$$\sigma_j=\sigma_0\alpha^j,$$

where σ_j is the variance of the two Gaussian curves in frequency domain. The channel parameters used were $\sigma_0=0.015$, $Q=2$, and $\alpha=2$.

Theoretically, a channel model is used to reduce the dimensionality of the data. In our study, we chose the above system of radially symmetric channels for simplification. This type of CHO reduces the dimensionality of the covariance matrix to the number of channels by the number of channels. For instance, in our case, for the image volume $168\times168\times81$, the covariance matrix size is of 2.3 M×2.3 M. Using the three channel model, the covariance matrix reduces to $3\times3\times3$. This massive reduction in dimensionality of the covariance matrix allows for the estimation problem to be tractable with a reasonable sized data set of images.

Overall, Fig. 2 shows the flow chart used to combine data, scale data, create noise realizations, reconstruct data for both lesion-absent and lesion-present cases, and perform CHO analysis.

Results and Discussion

Fig. 4 shows one reconstructed slice through the myocardial defect for the default case described in Sec. 2, Materials and

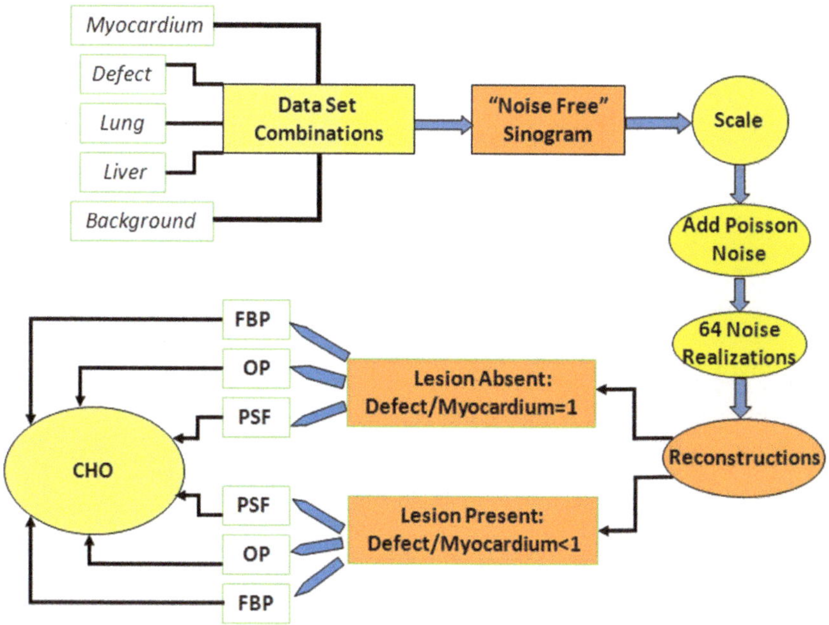

Figure 2. Flow chart of the data set combination, reconstruction, and CHO analysis.

Methods. As expected, the image reconstructed by FBP appears noisier and has lower contrast than images reconstructed by iterative algorithms. PSF-OSEM yields almost the same contrast as compared to OP-OSEM.

Fig. 5(A) shows CHO SNR versus total number of background counts ranging from 5 to 60 million for each reconstruction algorithm. As expected, the SNR increases as the total number of background counts increases. The SNR value was found to be approximately proportional to the square root of the number of total counts. For each total number of counts, PSF-OSEM reconstruction was performed twice; one with 2 iterations and 8 subsets (denoted PSF-OSEM) and the other with 8 iterations and 8 subsets (denoted PSF^+-OSEM). The CHO SNRs for both OP-OSEM and PSF^+-OSEM are almost the same. PSF^+-OSEM was found to yield almost the same noise level in the background region as OP-OSEM. This implies that PSF^+-OSEM yields almost the same defect contrast as OP-OSEM. Although PSF modeling is expected to correct partial volume effect (PVE) and improve defect contrast, the improvement is negligible for the defect we used, which has relatively large size. The reason that PSF-OSEM yields higher SNR as compared to OP-OSEM is mostly due to the fact the noise level produced by PSF-OSEM is lower than OP-OSEM at the same iteration number because PSF-OSEM converges more slowly than OP-OSEM. Fig. 5(B) shows that SNRs decreases as the number of iterations increases for the default case using eight subsets. As the number of iterations increases, SNR decreases due to increased noise level.

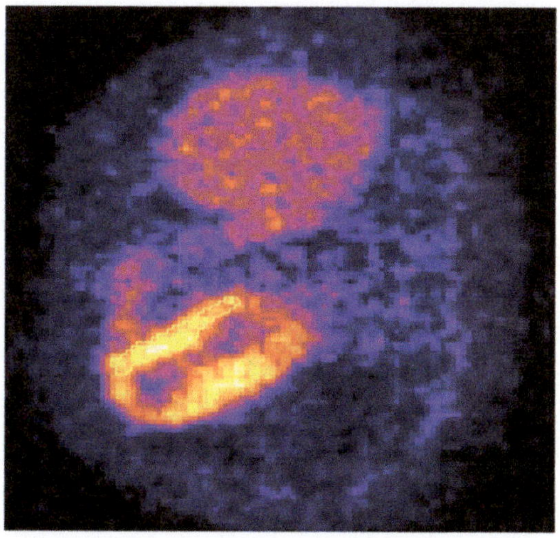

Figure 3. A reconstructed image slice through the myocardium for an ^{18}F-BMS747158 patient study.

Fig. 6(A) shows CHO SNR versus defect/myocardium activity concentration ratio ranging from 0.15 to 0.9. The coefficients of determination (R^2) for the least squares linear regression lines are: 0.978, 0.976, and 0.989 for FBP, OP-OSEM, and PSF-OSEM, respectively. The defect detectability increases as the defect/myocardium decreases. The SNR value vanishes as defect/myocardium approaches 1, i.e., defect-absent myocardium. Fig. 6(B) illustrates the defect detectability as a function of myocardium/background concentration ratio. The R^2 coefficients are: 0.926, 0.939, and 0.969 for FBP, OP-OSEM, and PSF-OSEM, respectively. Because we fixed defect/myocardium ratio to be 0.825 for this study, defect/background ratio increases as myocardium/background increases. That results in increased SNRs, which is partially determined by the contrast of the defect relative to its surrounding region, as myocardium/background increases.

Fig. 7(A) shows CHO SNR versus the activity concentration ratio of liver/background ranging from 1.5 to 8. This figure shows that the SNR is relatively insensitive to the liver/background concentration ratios. SNR decreases slightly as the concentration ratio liver/background increases from 1.5 to 8. On the other hand, Fig. 7(B) shows CHO SNR versus the activity concentration ratio of lung/background ranging from 0.2 to 0.8. This figure also

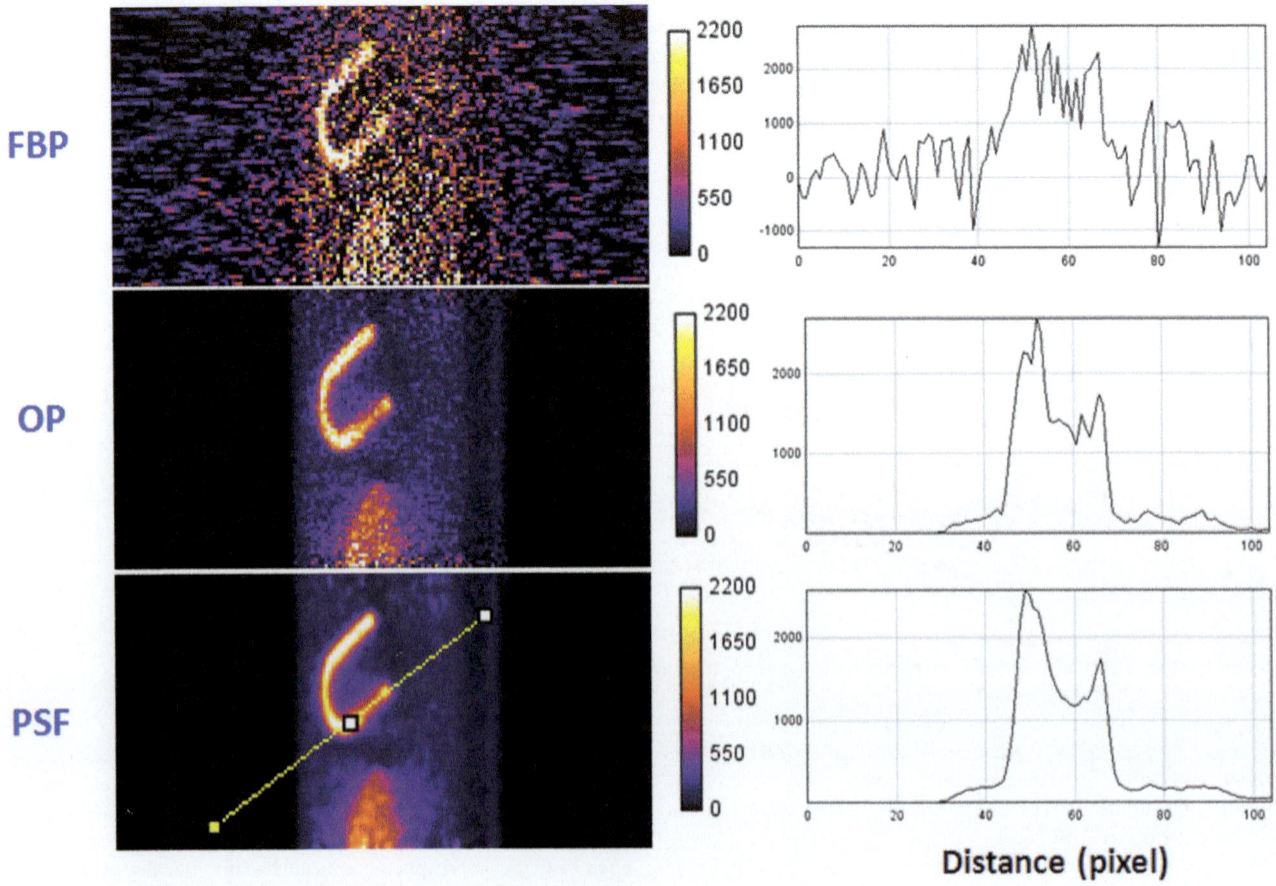

Figure 4. Reconstructed image slices and line profiles through the myocardial defect.

illustrates that the SNR is insensitive to the lung/background activity concentration ratios for all the data points.

For all the studies, FBP always yields the lowest CHO SNRs. For the same iteration number and the same number of subsets, PSF-OSEM always yields the higher CHO SNR than OP-OSEM.

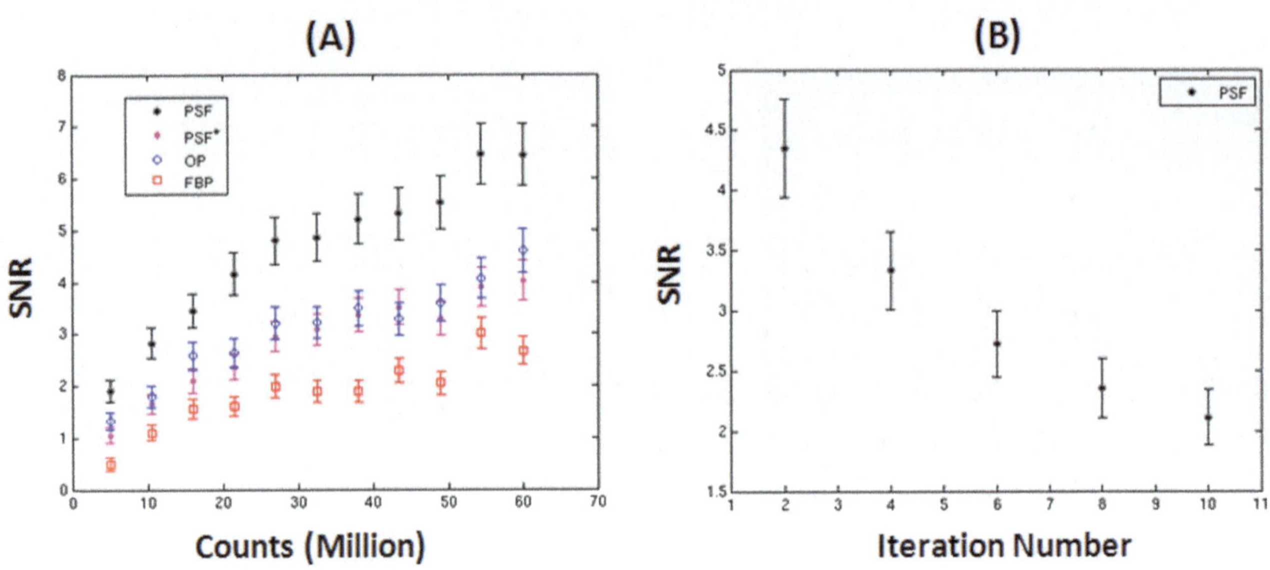

Figure 5. CHO SNR versus total number of counts in the background (A) and iteration number using PSF-OSEM for the default case described in Sec. 2, Materials and Methods.

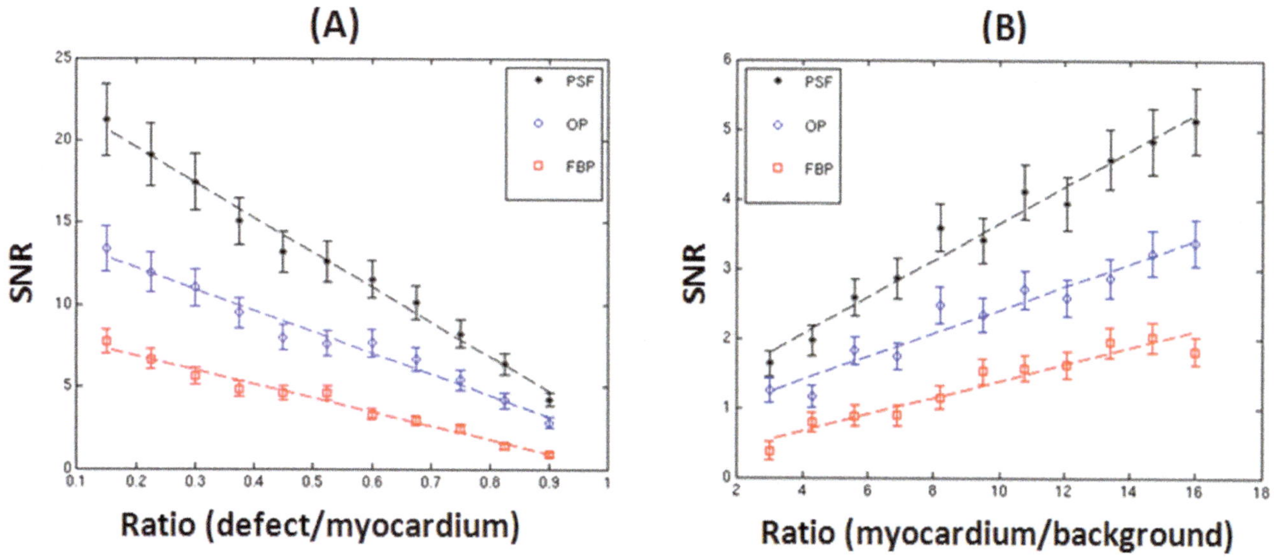

Figure 6. CHO SNR versus defect/myocardium (A) and myocardium/background (B) concentration ratios. The dashed lines were obtained using weighted least squares linear regression.

Conclusions

Defect detectability was assessed as a function of total number of background counts (noise level), defect/myocardium, myocardium/background, liver/background, and lung/background concentration ratios. As expected, the SNR increases as the noise level decreases. The SNR also increases as the defect/myocardium concentration ratio decreases. The results show that the SNR is relatively insensitive to the liver/background and lung/background concentration ratios. FBP yields the lowest CHO SNRs as compared to iterative reconstruction algorithms. Also, PSF-OSEM yields higher CHO SNRs than OP-OSEM for the same iteration number and same number of subsets. However, PSF-OSEM and OP-OSEM yield almost the same CHO SNR if noise levels are the same. This is mainly due to the fact that the defect size we used was relatively big.

Our phantom study shows that the detection SNR is dominated by the contrast of defect to its surrounding background and the noise level. The study of defect detection SNR as function of total number of coincidence counts can be useful to optimize injection dose and/or imaging time. The studies of defect detection versus various activity distributions in the lungs and liver prove that activity uptake in the liver and lungs will not have a major impact on the detection of a myocardial defect. In summary, this phantom study shows that the detectability of a myocardial defect is dominated by the noise level and the contrast between the defect and its surroundings. Therefore, accurate identification of a myocardial defect can be achieved using PET regardless of activity distribution.

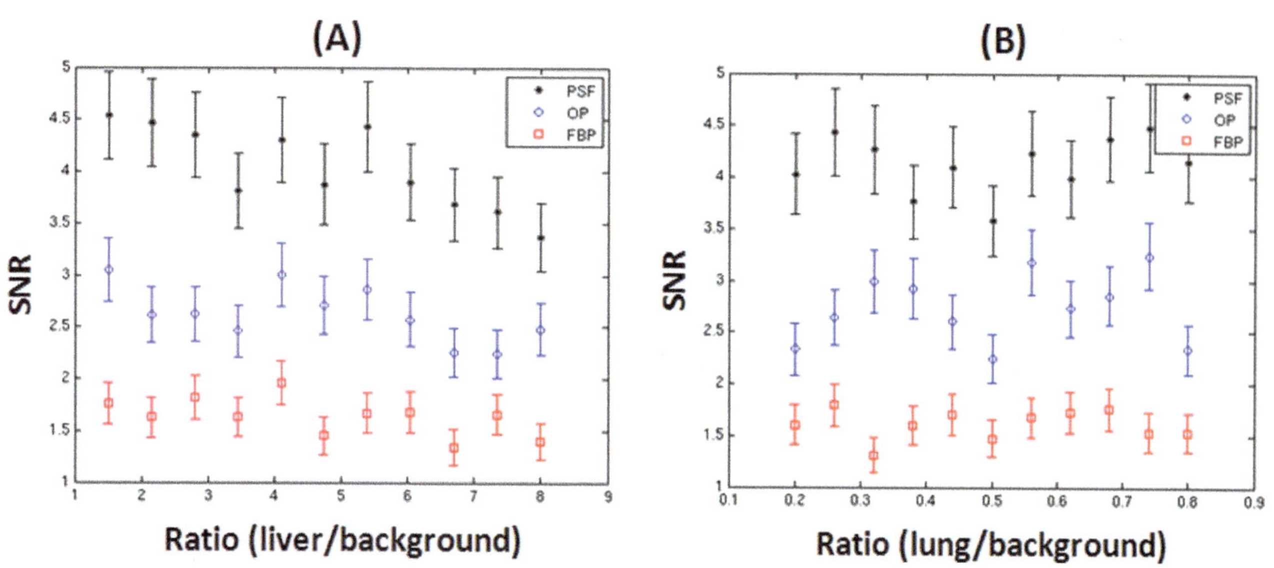

Figure 7. CHO SNR versus liver/background (A) and lung/background (B) concentration ratios.

Acknowledgments

We want to thank Zak Levin at Massachusetts General Hospital for his help with some of MATLAB programs used in the data analysis.

Author Contributions

Conceived and designed the experiments: GEF JO. Performed the experiments: AB JO. Analyzed the data: ESM JO. Contributed reagents/materials/analysis tools: JS JO. Wrote the paper: ESM JO. Edited the manuscript: JS.

References

1. Lin JW, Sciacca RR, Chou RL, Laine FA, Bergmann SR (2001) Quantification of myocardial perfusion in human subjects using 82Rb and wavelet-based noise reduction. J Nucl Med 42:201–208.
2. Vallabhajosula S, Solnes L, Vallabhajosula B (2011) A broad overview of Positron Emission Tomography Radiopharmaceuticals and clinical applications: what is new? Semin Nucl Med 41:246–264.
3. Fukumoto D, Nishiyama S, Harada N, Yamamoto S, Tsukada H (2012) Detection of ischemic neuronal damage with [18F]BMS-747158-02, a mitochondrial complex-1 positron emission tomography ligand: small animal PET study in rat brain. Synapse 66:909–917.
4. Maddahi J, Czernin J, Lazewatsky J, Huang SC, Dahlbom, et al. (2011) Phase I, first-in-human study of BMS747158, a novel 18F-labeled tracer for myocardial perfusion PET: dosimetry, biodistribution, safety, and imaging characteristics after a single injection at rest. J Nucl Med 52(9):1490–8.
5. Nekolla SG, Reder S, Saraste A, Higuchi T, Dzewas G, et al. (2009) Evaluation of the Novel Myocardial Perfusion Positron-Emission Tomography Tracer 18F-BMS-747158-02. Circulation 119:2333–2342.
6. Schelbert H (2002) F-18-deoxyglucose and the assessment of myocardial viability. Semin Nucl Med. 32:60–69.
7. Kadrmas D, Casey M, Conti M, Jakoby B, Lois C, Townsend D (2009) Impact of time-of-flight on PET tumor detection. J Nucl Med 50(8):1315–1323.
8. Surti S, Karp J (2009) Experimental evaluation of a simple lesion detection task with time-of-flight PET. Phys Med Biol. 54(2):373–384.
9. Tang J, Rahmin A, Lautamaki R, Lodge M, Bengel F, Tsui B (2009) Optimization of Rb-82 PET acquisition and reconstruction protocols for myocardial perfusion defect detection. Phys Med Biol. 54:3161–3171.
10. Chen M, Jaszczak R, Bowsher J, Gilland D (2001) An evaluation of cardiac uniformity, contrast and SNR with dual-head 180 degree and triple-head 360 degree SPECT scans. IEEE Trans Nucl Sci. 48(4):1428–1434.
11. Wollenweber S, Tsui B, Lalush D, Frey E, LaCroix K, Gullberg G (1999) Comparision of Hotelling Observer Models and Human Observers in Defect Detection from Myocardial SPECT Imaging. IEEE Trans Nucl Sci. 46:2098.
12. Matsunari I, Yoneyama T, Kanayama S, Matsudaira M, Nakajima K, et al. (2001) Phantom studies for estimation of defect size on cardiac 18F SPECT and PET: implications for myocardial viability assessment. J Nucl Med. 42:1579–1585.
13. Gifford H, King M, de Vries D, Soares E (2000) Channelized Hotelling and human observer correlation for lesion detection in hepatic SPECT imaging. J Nucl Med. 41:514–521.
14. Barrett HH, Yao J, Rolland JP, Myers KJ (1993) Model observers for the assessment of image quality. Proc Natl Acad Sci USA. 90:9758–9765.
15. Yao J, Barrett HH (1992) Predicting human performance by a channelized Hotelling observer model. Proc SPIE 1768:161–168.
16. Abbey CK, Barrett HH (2001) Human- and model-observer performance in ramp-spectrum noise; effects of regularization and object variability. J Opt Soc Am A. 18(3):473–488.

10

Abnormal T2-STIR Magnetic Resonance in Hypertrophic Cardiomyopathy: A Marker of Advanced Disease and Electrical Myocardial Instability

Giancarlo Todiere[1*⊙], Lorena Pisciella[2], Andrea Barison[1], Annamaria Del Franco[1], Elisabetta Zachara[2], Paolo Piaggi[3], Federica Re[2], Alessandro Pingitore[4], Michele Emdin[1], Massimo Lombardi[5], Giovanni Donato Aquaro[1⊙]

1 Fondazione G. Monasterio Regione Toscana-National Research Council, Pisa, Italy, **2** Cardiologia 2 Azienda Ospedaliera San Camillo-Forlanini, Rome, Italy, **3** Endocrinology Unit, University Hospital, Pisa, Italy, **4** Institute of Clinical Physiology, National Research Council, Pisa, Italy, **5** Multimodality Imaging Section, San Donato, Milano, Italy

Abstract

Background: Myocardial hyperintensity on T2-weighted short-tau inversion recovery (STIR) (HyT2) cardiac magnetic resonance (CMR) images has been demonstrated in patients with hypertrophic cardiomyopathy (HCM) and is considered a sign of acute damage. The aim of the current study was to evaluate the relationship between HyT2 and both a) markers of ventricular electrical instability and b) clinical and CMR parameters.

Methods: Sixty-five patients underwent a thorough clinical examination, consisting of 24-h ECG recording and CMR examination including functional evaluation, T2-STIR images and late gadolinium enhancement (LGE).

Results: HyT2 was detected in 27 patients (42%), and subjects with HyT2 showed a greater left ventricle (LV) mass index ($p < 0.001$), lower LV ejection fraction ($p = 0.05$) and greater extent of LGE ($p < 0.001$) compared to those without HyT2. Twenty-two subjects (34%) presented non-sustained ventricular tachycardia (NSVT) on the 24-h ECG recording, 21 (95%) of whom exhibited HyT2. Based on the logistic regression analysis, HyT2 (odds ratio [OR]: 165, 95% CI 11–2455, $p < 0.001$) and LGE extent (1.1, 1.0–1.3, $p < 0.001$) served as independent predictors of NSVT, while the presence of LGE was not associated with NSVT occurrence ($p = 0.49$). The presence of HyT2 was associated with lower heart rate variability ($p = 0.006$) and a higher number of arrhythmic risk factors ($p < 0.001$).

Conclusions: In HCM patients, HyT2 upon CMR examination is associated with more advanced disease and increased arrhythmic burden.

Editor: Alena Talkachova, University of Minnesota, United States of America

Funding: The authors received no specific funding for this work.

Competing Interests: The authors have declared that no competing interests exist.

* Email: todiere@alice.it

⊙ These authors contributed equally to this work.

Introduction

The prevention of sudden cardiac death is the most relevant challenge in patients with hypertrophic cardiomyopathy (HCM) [1–4]. The presence of myocardial fibrosis, as evaluated by cardiac magnetic resonance (CMR) imaging with the late gadolinium enhancement (LGE) technique, is associated with the occurrence of non-sustained ventricular tachycardia (NSVT), as observed via 24-h Holter electrocardiography (ECG) recording [5–7], and a worse clinical outcome [8–10]. However, the vast majority of HCM patients (60–85% prevalence at the first CMR evaluation, increasing up to >95% during follow-up) show LGE [11], which may be considered a nonspecific marker of this disease.

Myocardial hyperintensity upon CMR T2-weighted short-tau inversion recovery (STIR) imaging (HyT2) is a sign of edema that is secondary to acute ischemic or inflammatory damage [12–13] and is present in a subset of patients with HCM, where it is likely caused by myocardial ischemia [14]. Myocardial ischemia seems to be associated with microvascular impairment in HCM, where it is considered a trigger for arrhythmic events and has been associated with worse prognoses [15–16]. Although the relationship between HyT2 and NSVT was initially reported in patients with HCM [17,18], it has never been prospectively evaluated. Therefore, the aims of the current study were as follows: a) to assess the relationship between HyT2 and signs of ventricular electrical instability (premature ventricular contractions, PVC, and NSVT), autonomic impairment according to heart rate variability on 24 h-Holter ECG recordings, and the arrhythmic risk score [16] and b) to compare HyT2 to other CMR parameters, such as

Table 1. Clinical characteristics of the population.

		Whole population	Hy-T2	No-HyT2	p value
Population characteristics:	n(%)	65	27(42)	38(58)	
Age (years)	mean±SD	49±17	52±14	46±17	0.59
Male	n(%)	51 (78)	22(81)	29(76)	0.84
LVOT obstruction	n(%)	15(23)	6(22)	9(24)	0.98
History of paroxysmal atrial fibrillation	n(%)	16(25)	8(30)	8(21)	0.59
Reduced ejection fraction (<50%)	n(%)	6(9)	5(19)	1(3)	0.08
Hypertension	n(%)	32(49)	9(33)	23(61)	0.07
Diabetes Mellitus	n(%)	6(9)	0	6	0.08
Hospitalized	n(%)	11(17)	5(19)	6(16)	0.97
Increased HS-Troponine	n(%)	33(51)	20(74)	13(34)	0.39
Arrhyhtmic Risk Factors:					
Family history of SCD	n(%)	11(17)	5(19)	6(16)	0.97
VT at 24 h Holter monitoring	n(%)	22(34)	21(78)	1(3)	<0.001
Resuscitated SCD	n(%)	0	0	0	ns
Maximal wall thickness≥30	n(%)	8(12)	7(26)	1(3)	0.02
Unexplained Syncope	n(%)	6(9)	4(15)	2(5)	0.31
Outflow gradient >30 mmHg	n(%)	11(17)	4(15)	7 (18)	0.86
Abnormal pressure response during effort	n(%)	0	0	0	ns
Patients with 0 risk factors	n(%)	36(55)	3(11)	33(87)	<0.001
Patients with 1 risk factors	n(%)	18(28)	14(52)	4(11)	<0.001
Patients with≥2 risk factors	n(%)	11(17)	10(37)	1(3)	<0.001
Symptoms:					
Angina	n(%)	13(20)	7(26)	6(16)	0.42
Syncope	n(%)	6(9)	4(15)	2(5)	0.31
Palpitation	n(%)	26(40)	17(63)	9(24)	0.002
Dyspnea	n(%)	34(52)	11(41)	23(61)	0.18
NYHA class II	n(%)	26(40)	14(52)	12(32)	0.17
NYHA class III-IV	n(%)	5(8)	3(11)	2(5)	0.69
24 h Holter ECG monitoring:					
PVC	median(IQR)	37 (9–505)	33(14–1253)	41 (8–474)	0.74
NSVT	n(%)	22	21	1	<0.001
SDNN (ms)	mean±SD	130±51	110±38	154±64	<0.01
SDANN (ms)	mean±SD	95±25	86±25	102±21	0.02
pNN50(%)	mean±SD	8±5	9±6	7±5	0.15
RMSSD(ms)	mean±SD	49±24	48±17	50±30	0.75
Therapy:					
Beta-blockers	n(%)	35(54)	17(63)	18(47)	0.29
Calcium antagonists	n(%)	5(8)	4(15)	1(3)	0.13
ACE inhibitors	n(%)	17(26)	7(26)	10(26)	0.98
Antiarrhythmic drugs	n(%)	15(23)	8(30)	7(18)	0.52

LVOT, left ventricular outflow tract; SCD, sudden cardiac death; NYHA, New York Heart Association Class; PVC, premature ventricular complexes; NSVT, non sustained ventricula tachycardia; SDNN, standard deviation of of RR intervals;SDANN, standard deviation of the average normal to normal QRS intervals calculated over periods of 5 min; pNN50, the number of interval differences of successive NN intervals >50 ms divided by the total number of NN intervals;RMSSD, the square root of the mean squared differences of successive NN intervals.

the presence and extent of LGE, left ventricular (LV) mass index, and maximal LV end-diastolic wall thickness.

Patients and Methods

We enrolled 69 consecutive patients with HCM based on previously reported criteria undergoing a CMR examination. Three patients were excluded for low-quality images, and 1 was excluded for claustrophobia. Thus, the final population consisted of 65 patients (51 males, 49±17 years). The study was approved by the Ethical Committee of Fondazione G.Monasterio-Pisa. All the patients received and signed informed consent.

Clinical evaluation

The presence of established risk factors for sudden death in patients with HCM were evaluated, including a family history of sudden death, extreme LV wall thickness (>30 mm), unexplained syncope, non-sustained ventricular tachycardia on an ambulatory Holter ECG recording (>3 ventricular beats at a heart rate >120 beats per min), and an abnormal or "flat" systolic arterial pressure during an exercise stress test [19]. A complete clinical evaluation was performed on the day of CMR examination. Based on the clinical examination, each patient was assigned a New York Heart Association (NYHA) class on the basis of the presence and severity of dyspnea. Other symptoms (syncope, chest pain, palpitations) were also recorded. A 12-lead resting ECG was recorded on the same day.

Patients also underwent a 24-h ECG recording around the time of CMR examination. Conventional ECG analysis was performed, including the following heart rate variability measurements in the time-domain analysis: standard deviation (SD) of the RR intervals, SD of the average normal to normal QRS (NN) interval calculated over periods of 5 min (SDANN), the number of interval differences of successive NN intervals >50 msec divided by the total number of NN intervals (pNN50), and the square root of the mean squared differences of successive NN intervals (RMSSD) [20,21].

CMR acquisition protocol

CMR was performed using two 1.5 Tesla systems: a Signa Hdx (General Electric Healthcare, Milwaukee, Wisconsin) and a 1.5 Tesla Magnetom Avanto (Siemens, Erlangen, Germany) with cardiac phased array multichannel coils.

Short axis cine images from the mitral plane valve to the LV apex were acquired using a steady-state free precession pulse sequence with the following parameters: 30 phases, slice thickness 8 mm, no gap, views per segment 8, NEX 1, FOV 40 cm, phase FOV 1, matrix 224×224, reconstruction matrix 256×256, 45° flip angle, and a TR/TE equal to 3.5/1.5.

T2-STIR images were acquired using triple inversion recovery T2-weighted pulse sequence in short axis views and 2 long axis views (vertical and horizontal long axis view) using the following parameters: TR = 2 RR, TE ≈ 70 msec, FOV 40 cm, phase FOV 1, matrix 256×256. LGE images were acquired 10 min after the administration of Gd-DTPA (Magnevist, Schering-AG) with a dosage of 0.2 mmol/kg for the short axis views. An inversion recovery T1-weighted gradient- echo (GRE) sequence was used with the following parameters: field of view 40 mm, slice thickness 8 mm, no gap between each slice, repetition time 4.6 msec, echo time 1.3, a flip angle of 20°, matrix 224×224, reconstruction matrix 256×256, and an excitation number of 1. The appropriate inversion time was set to null for normal myocardium (range 250–300 msec).

Images post-processing

A commercially available research software package (Mass Analysis, Leyden, The Netherlands) was used to quantify the functional parameters using conventional methods [22]. LV mass index was considered severely increased when it was >3 SD over the upper limit of normality [23]. Maximal LV end diastolic wall thickness was measured as previously described [24].

T2-STIR images were evaluated using a qualitative visual assessment performed by three expert independent investigators who were blinded to each other's results. The presence of signal abnormalities (HyT2) was established when there was agreement between at least two investigators. Agreement among the three investigators was reached when analyzing the images of 95% patients.

The extent of LGE was measured using a previously validated method [25]. Briefly, the endocardial and epicardial contours in each image were manually traced to identify the LV myocardium in each image. To obtain the SD of the signal noise of the images, a region of interest was placed in the background of the image, near the patient's thoracic wall. The mean signal intensity and SD were measured in this region of interest. Myocardial voxels with a signal intensity higher than the average signal intensity of the

Table 2. CMR parameters.

		Global population	Hy-T2	No-HyT2	p value*
Population:	n(%)	65	27(42)	38(58)	
Septal morphology:					
- Reverse septal	n(%)	30(46)	12(44)	18(47)	0.85
-Sigmoid	n(%)	20(31)	8(40)	12(31)	0.63
-Neutral	n(%)	9(14)	3(11)	6(16)	0.75
-Apical	n(%)	6(9)	2(7)	4(10)	0.65
Maximal Wall thickness (mm)	mean±SD	21±6	25±7	19±5	0.63
LV EDVi (ml/m2)	mean±SD	73±26	76±35	71±16	0.86
LV ESVi (ml/m2)	mean±SD	24±19	28±27	20±9	0.11
LV Mass index (g/m2)	mean±SD	112±40	133±47	98±28	**<0.001**
LV ejection fraction (%)	mean±SD	69±12	66±15	72±8	**<0.05**
RV EDVi (ml/m2)	mean±SD	65±17	62±18	67±17	0.27
RV ESVi (ml/m2)	mean±SD	19±8	18±9	19±7	0.76
RV ejection fraction (%)	mean±SD	70±7	70±9	71±5	0.63
LGE presence	n(%)	55(84)	23(84)	32(84)	0.86
LGE extent (% of LV mass)	mean±SD	11±11	16±12	7±8	**<0.001**

LV, left ventricle; EDVi, end-diastolic volume index; ESVi, end-systolic volume index, RV, right ventricle; LGE, late gadolinium enhancement.

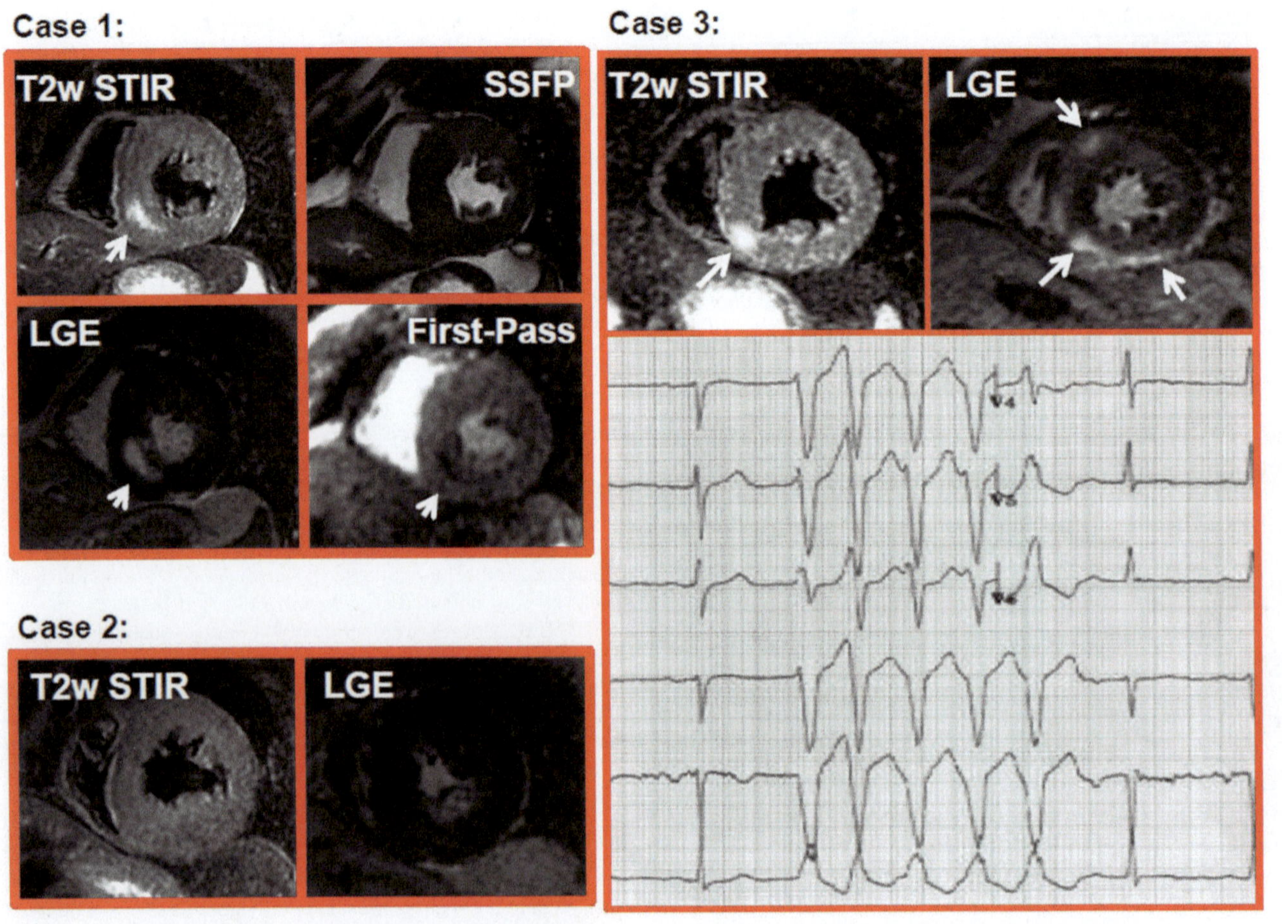

Figure 1. Examples of HCM patients. Case 1: a patient with HCM presenting with HyT2 (arrow in T2-STIR image), myocardial fibrosis (arrow LGE image), and pefusion defect (arrow in the frame of the first pass gadolinium) in the same myocardial segments; Case 2: a patient with HCM having myocardial fibrosis (LGE image) without HyT2 (T2-STIR image); Case 3: a patient with HyT2 (arrow in T2-STIR images) and myocardial fibrosis (arrow in LGE images) having a run of NSVT in the ECG stripe (lower panel).

region of interest plus 6 SD were considered enhanced [26]. The percentage of enhanced voxels in the entire LV myocardium was measured. The extent of LGE was expressed in grams and the percentage of the LV mass.

Statistical analysis

Categorical variables were compared using Pearson's chi-squared test with the continuity correction or Fisher's exact test when appropriate. The Kolmogorov-Smirnov test was used to assess the normality of the data. Pearson's (r) and Spearman's (ρ) correlation coefficients were employed for Gaussian and skewed variables, respectively. One-way analysis of variance (ANOVA) and Kruskal-Wallis test, when appropriate, were employed to compare quantitative variables between groups. Logistic regression analysis was used to explore the impact of each variable in a model, with NSVT upon 24-h Holter ECG monitoring as the dependent variable and myocardial abnormalities on T2-STIR, LGE extent, LV mass index, maximal end-diastolic wall thickness, and number of arrhythmic risk factors (excluding NSVT) as independent variables.

A p-value <0.05 was considered statistically significant. Data are presented as continuous variables and proportions (percentages). Continuous variables are expressed as the mean ± SD or the median and interquartile range (IQR), as indicated.

Results

The clinical characteristics of the HCM population are reported in table 1. All patients were in sinus rhythm; however, previous paroxysmal atrial fibrillation was reported in 16 patients (24%). None of the subjects had severe valvular abnormalities.

Twenty-two subjects (34%) presented with non-sustained ventricular tachycardia on the 24-h ECG recording, 11 (17%) had a family history of sudden death, and 8 (12%) showed a maximal end-diastolic wall thickness ≥30 mm, while none had a significant blood pressure drop during exercise. Thirty-six patients (55%) had no risk factors for sudden death, 18 (28%) presented one risk factor, and 11 (17%) patients had an arrhythmic risk score ≥2.

CMR findings

A summary of the CMR results is reported in table 2. The LV mass index was increased in 44 patients (68%) and severely increased in 23 patients (35%) (24). LV systolic dysfunction (LV ejection <55%) was found in 6 patients (9%), and LV dilation was present in two patients (3%).

LGE was present in 55 patients (84%). Patients with LGE had greater end-diastolic wall thickness ($p=0.05$), and a linear

Table 3. Predictors of NSVT.

Indipendent variables	NSVT	No NSVT	p value	Logistic regression Analysis			
				Coefficient	Odds Ratio	95%-C.I.	p-value
Arrhythmic Risk factors	0.6±0.7	0.14±0.3	0.001				
LV mass index	131±38	103±39	0.007				
HyT2	21(95)	1(5)	<0.001	5.1	165	11–2455	<0.001
Maximal Wall Thickness	25±6	19±6	<0.001	0.12	1.1	1.0–1.3	<0.001
Extent of LGE	18.3±11.9	6.8±7.9	<0.001				

Arrhythmic risk factors: number of arrhythmic risk factors, n ± SD; LV (left ventricular) mass index, expressed in g/m^2± SD; HyT2, presence of myocardial signal hyperintensity in T2-STIR image, expressed as n(%); Maximal wall thickness in mm ± SD; Extent of LGE, late gadolinium enhancement, in % of LV mass.

relationship was found between the extent of LGE and the LV mass index ($\rho = 0.27$, $p = 0.03$).

T2-STIR, clinical variables and CMR parameters

On T2-STIR images, HyT2 was detected in 27 patients (42%), with no sex ($p = 0.62$) or age ($p = 0.10$) differences (Figure 1). The relationships between HyT2 and the clinical and CMR parameters are summarized in tables 1 and 2. As shown in table 2, subjects with HyT2 had a greater LV mass index, lower LVEF and higher extent of LGE than those without HyT2. In addition, the prevalence of HyT2 was higher in patients with severely increased LV mass index (26% vs. 17%, $p = 0.004$), and all patients presenting with systolic dysfunction had HyT2. The extent of HyT2 was significantly lower than that of LGE ($p < 0.001$). In 24 of 27 patients (88%), HyT2 was found in a myocardial region with LGE, whereas HyT2 and LGE were detected in different myocardial regions in 3 subjects.

T2-STIR, and electrical instability

During the 24-h ECG, 22 patients (27%) had episodes of NSVT. As shown in table 3, patients with NSVT had higher LGE extents, greater end-diastolic maximal wall thickness, lower LV ejection fraction (64±15% vs. 72±8%, respectively, $p = 0.006$), greater LV mass index and more arrhythmic risk factors (0.6±0.7 vs. 0.14±0.3, respectively, $p = 0.001$) than those without NSVT. HyT2 was present in 21 (95%) patients with NSVT ($p < 0.001$); conversely, only 6 of 27 (22%) patients with HyT2 had no NSVT (Figure 1). The presence of LGE was not associated with the occurrence of NSVT ($p = 0.35$), as 39 patients with LGE (64%) had no NSVT, while all patients with NSVT showed LGE. The SD of RR interval and SDANN upon ECG 24-h ECG monitoring were significantly lower in patients with HyT2 than those without (110±38 msec vs. 154±64 msec, $p < 0.01$, and 102±21 msec vs. 86±25 msec, $p = 0.02$, respectively). Based on the logistic regression analysis, HyT2 and LGE extent were independent predictors of NSVT upon 24-h Holter ECG recording (table 3).

Discussion

Together, our findings led to the following conclusions: 1) HyT2 was associated with signs of advanced disease, i.e., higher LV mass index, lower ejection fraction and greater LGE extent; 2) HyT2 was associated with a higher arrhythmic risk score, markers of arrhythmic burden (NSVT) and autonomic impairment (decreased heart rate variability), as shown by 24-h ECG recordings; and 3) HyT2 was the best predictor of NSVT among all CMR-derived and clinical parameters. These results suggest that the presence of myocardial edema, which was identified by HyT2 in HCM patients, is linked to disease progression and arrhythmogenesis.

HyT2 was detected in 95% of patients with NSVT during the 24-h ECG recording. Indeed, NSVT detection is considered a relevant arrhythmic risk marker in patients with HCM as well as ischemic and non-ischemic cardiomyopathies [27–29]. The presence of HyT2 was also associated with decreased heart rate variability, which suggests a sympathovagal imbalance, with decreased vagal tone, net sympathetic predominance, and subsequent cardiac electrical instability. Low heart rate variability is generally associated with an increased risk of sudden death in ischemic and non-ischemic heart disease [30–31] and the risk of arrhythmic events in patients with HCM [32]. In addition, the occurrence of NSVT is a risk factor for sudden cardiac death. However, conventional ambulatory ECG recordings, which last up to 24 h, may underestimate the arrhythmic risk of HCM patients or miss NSVT events due to their relatively short duration. Conversely, HyT2 may be detected >1 month after the acute event, and this timing provides a clinical advantage because HyT2 detection may permit the identification of patients with electrical instability, who have a higher arrhythmic risk and require strict clinical surveillance and enhanced therapeutic effort, even when NSVT is absent on ECG recordings.

Although HyT2 is a sign of myocardial edema on CMR, this relationship remains incompletely understood [14]. In ischemic heart disease, myocardial edema occurs secondary to prolonged acute ischemic events [33]. In the setting of acute myocardial infarction, edema highlights the presence of ischemic but viable myocardium surrounding necrotic areas, and the ratio between edema and the extent of necrosis is used to assess the myocardial salvage index [34]. In myocarditis, HyT2 is considered a sign of active inflammation and is usually located in the subepicardial layer or in the midwall [35]. HyT2 usually lasts one month after a myocardial infarction, whereas it may be detected 6 months after myocarditis [36].

In our HCM patients, HyT2 was located in the midwall of hypertrophic myocardial segments and was localized with or without LGE. Previously, Melacini et al. hypothesized that these T2 abnormalities in HCM could be attributed to ischemia caused by microvascular dysfunction, impaired diastolic relaxation, mismatch between capillary density, myocardial tissue interstitial fibrosis and/or myocardial bridging [17]. In this setting, prolonged ischemia involving the hypertrophic myocardial segments may cause small intramural, rather than subendocardial, myocardial damage, which presents on CMR as both HyT2 and LGE. HyT2 may be detectable in the acute/subacute phase but may subsequently disappear, while LGE may persist as a chronic scar [17]. However, Frustaci and colleagues found histopathological evidence of acute myocarditis in biopsies in a significant fraction of their HCM cohort, which was related to the patient's clinical status [37]; therefore, HyT2 may indicate the presence of inflammatory myocardial damage.

The hypothesis that microvascular disease and ischemia result in HyT2 is strongly supported by the observation that the area of HyT2 closely matched the region of hypoperfusion based on the first-pass gadolinium CMR technique [18]. Moreover, a global decrease in myocardial blood flow was previously demonstrated in patients with HCM in CMR and positron emission tomography (PET) studies [15]. Specifically, the extent of LGE was inversely related to the global myocardial blood flow, suggesting a close relationship between ischemic events and chronic myocardial damage [38]. Furthermore, repetitive episodes of ischemia could explain the rapid progression of myocardial fibrosis in HCM, as recently demonstrated [11]. In the current study, we detected HyT2 in 42% of patients with HCM. In particular, patients with HyT2 demonstrated higher LV mass indexes, lower ejection fractions and a greater extent of LGE than those without HyT2. Moreover, patients with HyT2 had more arrhythmic risk factors than those without. Together, these findings suggest the presence of more advanced disease in patients with HyT2. A higher LV mass index has also been associated with microvascular disease [39], a lower blood supply/demand ratio and increased interstitial fibrosis. These findings suggest that, in advanced disease, ischemic events may be more severe and prolonged than in the early stage and may cause myocardial damage, ranging from a reversible injury, such as HyT2, to an irreversible cell loss that eventually produces myocardial fibrosis. Moreover, these factors may represent the substrate for electrical instability, which may be triggered by prolonged ischemic events. As hypothesized in Coumel's triangle theory, myocardial disarray, fibrosis and hypertrophy serve as arrhythmogenic substrates that necessitate a trigger to induce arrhythmic events [40]; these events may finally be elicited by either ischemia or inflammation, which are detected by CMR as HyT2.

The presence of LGE in patients with HCM may be considered relevant in terms of risk stratification, as recent reports have demonstrated that after a clinical follow-up of 3 years, patients with LGE had a worse prognoses than those without [8,9]. However, LGE is usually detected in most HCM patients during the first CMR evaluation, with a reported prevalence of 60–90% [6,41]. Thus, the specificity of LGE as a prognostic marker in HCM should be discussed. Moreover, once cardiac fibrosis develops, its progression is relatively rapid. Indeed, we recently demonstrated that the progression of LGE extent was fast and related to clinical worsening [11]. Thus, features other than LGE extent should be investigated as predictors of sudden cardiac death [42]; for example, the presence of extensive (>15% of LV mass) and diffuse LGE is currently indicated as an emerging new arrhythmic risk factor [43]. However, previous studies showed that an extent of LGE >15% of LV mass was related to depressed systolic function [41], which may contribute to progression to end-stage disease [44]. Other CMR techniques, such as T1 mapping and measurements of the extracellular volume, are currently under evaluation as prognostic factors for HCM.

Some limitations of the current study should be mentioned. First, HyT2 may be detected in conditions other than ischemia and inflammation, and the results of the current study did not allow us to understand the nature and etiology of HyT2 in HCM. Additionally, the mechanism underlying the association between HyT2 and ventricular arrhythmias remains unclear. Second, we assumed that HyT2 in HCM is a sign of acute, transient myocardial damage, although this assumption was based only on the observation of HyT2 in other cardiac diseases. Thus, further studies with serial CMR examinations should be performed to confirm the reversibility of HyT2 and the prognostic role of HyT2 in larger HCM populations.

In conclusion, in patients with HCM, the presence of HyT2 upon CMR examination is associated with more advanced disease, ventricular arrhythmias and signs of electrical instability. HyT2 was detected in 42% of patients with HCM, and it was the best predictor of NSVT during a 24-h Holter ECG recording. HyT2 was associated with decreased heart rate variability and a greater number of arrhythmic risk factors.

Author Contributions

Conceived and designed the experiments: GT GDA. Performed the experiments: GT LP EZ FR AB ADF. Analyzed the data: PP GDA GT LP. Contributed reagents/materials/analysis tools: GT GDA. Contributed to the writing of the manuscript: GT GDA AP ME ML.

References

1. Maron BJ (2002) Hypertrophic cardiomyopathy: a systematic review. JAMA 287: 1308–1320.
2. Elliott PM, Poloniecki J, Dickie S, Sharma S, Monserrat L, et al. (2000) Sudden death in hypertrophic cardiomyopathy: identification of high risk patients. J Am Coll Cardiol 236: 2212–2218.
3. Biagini E, Coccolo F, Ferlito M, Perugini E, Rocchi G, et al. (2005) Dilated-hypokinetic evolution of hypertrophic cardiomyopathy: revalence, incidence, risk factors, and prognostic implications in pediatric and adult patients. J Am Coll Cardiol 46: 1543–1550.
4. Kohorst JJ, Bos JM, Hagler DJ, Ackerman MJ (2013) Sudden Cardiac Arrest in a Young Patient with Hypertrophic Cardiomyopathy and Zero Canonical Risk

Factors: The Inherent Limitations of Risk Stratification in Hypertrophic Cardiomyopathy. Congenit Heart Dis. 9: E51–57.

5. Moon JC, McKenna WJ, McCrohon JA, Elliott PM, Smith GC, et al. (2003) Toward clinical risk assessment in hypertrophic cardiomyopathy with gadolinium cardiovascular magnetic resonance. J Am Coll Cardiol. 41: 1561–1567.
6. Aquaro GD, Masci P, Formisano F, Barison A, Strata E, et al. (2010) Usefulness of delayed enhancement by magnetic resonance imaging in hypertrophic cardiomyopathy as a marker of disease and its severity. Am J Cardiol 105: 392–397.
7. Adabag AS, Maron BJ, Appelbaum E, Harrigan CJ, Buros JL, et al. (2008) Occurrence and frequency of arrhythmias in hypertrophic cardiomyopathy in relation to delayed enhancement on cardiovascular magnetic resonance. J Am Coll Cardiol 51: 1369–1374.
8. O'Hanlon R, Grasso A, Roughton M, Moon JC, Clark S, et al. (2010) Prognostic significance of myocardial fibrosis in hypertrophic cardiomyopathy. J Am Coll Cardiol 56: 867–874.
9. Bruder O, Wagner A, Jensen CJ, Schneider S, Ong P, et al. (2010) Myocardial scar visualized by cardiovascular magnetic resonance imaging predicts major adverse events in patients with hypertrophic cardiomyopathy. J Am Coll Cardiol 56: 875–887.
10. Rubinshtein R, Glockner JF, Ommen SR, Araoz PA, Ackerman MJ, et al. (2010) Characteristics and clinical significance of late gadolinium enhancement by contrast-enhanced magnetic resonance imaging in patients with hypertrophic cardiomyopathy. Circ Heart Fail 3: 51–58.
11. Todiere G, Aquaro GD, Piaggi P, Formisano F, Barison A, et al. (2012) Progression of myocardial fibrosis assessed with cardiac magnetic resonance in hypertrophic cardiomyopathy. J Am Coll Cardiol 60: 922–929.
12. Abdel-Aty H, Zagrosek A, Schulz-Menger J, Taylor AJ, Messroghli D, et al. (2004) Delayed enhancement and T2-weighted cardiovascular magnetic resonance imaging differentiate acute from chronic myocardial infarction. Circulation 109: 2411–2416.
13. Abdel-Aty H, Boyé P, Zagrosek A, Wassmuth R, Kumar A, et al. (2005) Diagnostic performance of cardiovascular magnetic resonance in patients with suspected acute myocarditis: comparison of different approaches. J Am Coll Cardiol.45: 1815–1822.
14. Abdel-Aty H, Cocker M, Strohm O, Filipchuk N, Friedrich MG (2008) Abnormalities in T2-weighted cardiovascular magnetic resonance images of hypertrophic cardiomyopathy: regional distribution and relation to late gadolinium enhancement and severity of hypertrophy. J Magn Reson Imaging 28: 242–245.
15. Cecchi F, Olivotto I, Gistri R, Lorenzoni R, Chiriatti G, et al. (2003) Coronary microvascular dysfunction and prognosis in hypertrophic cardiomyopathy. N Engl J Med 349: 1027–1035.
16. Maron BJ, McKenna WJ, Danielson GK, Kappenberger LJ, Kuhn HJ, et al. (2003) Task Force on Clinical Expert Consensus Documents. American College of Cardiology; Committee for Practice Guidelines. European Society of Cardiology. American College of Cardiology/European Society of Cardiology Clinical Expert Consensus Document on Hypertrophic Cardiomyopathy. A report of the American College of Cardiology Foundation Task Force on Clinical Expert Consensus Documents and the European Society of Cardiology Committee for Practice Guidelines. J Am Coll Cardiol 42: 1687–713.
17. Melacini P, Corbetti F, Calore C, Pescatore V, Smaniotto G, et al. (2008) Cardiovascular magnetic resonance signs of ischemia in hypertrophic cardiomyopathy. Int J Cardiol.128: 364–373.
18. Hen Y, Iguchi N, Machida H, Takada K, Utanohara Y, et al. (2012) High signal intensity on T2-weighted cardiac magnetic resonance imaging correlates with the ventricular tachyarrhythmia in hypertrophic cardiomyopathy.Heart Vessels 28: 742–749.
19. Frenneaux MP (2004).Assessing the risk of sudden cardiac death in a patient with hypertrophic cardiomyopathy. Heart 90: 570–575.
20. Task Force of the European Society of Cardiology and the North American Society of Pacing and Electrophysiology (1996) Heart rate variability. Standards of measurement, physiological interpretation, and clinical use.Eur Heart J 17: 354–381.
21. Goldberger JJ, Cain ME, Hohnloser SH, Kadish AH, Knight BP, et al. (2008) American Heart Association; American College of Cardiology Foundation; Heart Rhythm Society. American Heart Association/American College of Cardiology Foundation/Heart Rhythm Society Scientific Statement on Noninvasive Risk Stratification Techniques for Identifying Patients at Risk for Sudden Cardiac Death. A scientific statement from the American Heart Association Council on Clinical Cardiology Committee on Electrocardiography and Arrhythmias and Council on Epidemiology and Prevention. J Am Coll Cardiol 52: 1179–1199.
22. Sechtem U, Pflugfelder P, Higgins CB (1987) Quantification of cardiac function by conventional and cine magnetic resonance imaging. Cardiovasc Intervent Radiol 10: 365–73.
23. Maceira AM, Prasad SK, Khan M, Pennell DJ (2006) Normalized left ventricular systolic and diastolic function by steady state free precession cardiovascular magnetic resonance. J Cardiovasc Magn Reson 8: 417–426.
24. Rickers C, Wilke NM, Jerosch-Herold M, Casey SA, Panse P, et al. (2005) Utility of cardiac magnetic resonance imaging in the diagnosis of hypertrophic cardiomyopathy. Circulation 112: 855–861.
25. Aquaro GD, Positano V, Pingitore A, Strata E, Di Bella G, et al. (2010) Quantitative analysis of late gadolinium enhancement in hypertrophic cardiomyopathy. J Cardiovasc Magn Reson 12: 21.
26. Harrigan CJ, Peters DC, Gibson CM, Maron BJ, Manning WJ, et al. (2011) Hypertrophic cardiomyopathy: quantification of late gadolinium enhancement with contrast enhanced cardiovascular MR imaging. Radiology 258: 128–133.
27. Adabag AS, Maron BJ, Appelbaum E, Harrigan CJ, Buros JL, et al. (2008) Occurrence and frequency of arrhythmias in hypertrophic cardiomyopathy in relation to delayed enhancement on cardiovascular magnetic resonance. J Am Coll Cardiol 51: 1369–1374.
28. Doval HC, Nul DR, Grancelli HO, Varini SD, Soifer S, et al. (1996) Nonsustained ventricular tachycardia in severe heart failure. Independent marker of increased mortality due to sudden death. GESICA-GEMA Investigators. Circulation 94: 3198–3203.
29. Pelliccia F, Gallo P, Cianfrocca C, d'Amati G, Bernucci P, et al. (1990) Relation of complex ventricular arrhythmias to presenting features and prognosis in dilated cardiomyopathy. Int J Cardiol 29: 47–54.
30. Ikegawa T, Chino M, Hasegawa H, Usuba F, Suzuki S, et al. (1987) Prognostic significance of 24-hour ambulatory electrocardiographic monitoring in patients with dilative cardiomyopathy: a prospective study. Clin Cardiol 10: 78–82.
31. La Rovere MT, Pinna GD, Hohnloser SH, Marcus FI, Mortara A, et al ATRAMI Investigators (2001) Autonomic Tone and Reflexes After Myocardial Infarcton. Baroreflex sensitivity and heart rate variability in the identification of patients at risk for life-threatening arrhythmias: implications for clinical trials. Circulation 103: 2072–2077.
32. Uemura S, Tomoda Y, Fujimoto S, Yamamoto H, Matsukura Y, et al. (1997) Heart rate variability and ventricular arrhythmia in clinically stable patients with hypertrophic cardiomyopathy. Jpn Circ J 61: 819–826.
33. Willerson JT, Scales F, Mukherjee A, Platt M, Templeton GH, et al. (1977) Abnormal myocardial fluid retention as an early manifestation of ischemic injury. Am J Pathol 87: 159–188.
34. Friedrich MG, Abdel-Aty H, Taylor A, Schulz-Menger J, Messroghli D, et al. (2008) The salvaged area at risk in reperfused acute myocardial infarction as visualized by cardiovascular magnetic resonance. J Am Coll Cardiol 51: 1581–1587.
35. Friedrich MG, Sechtem U, Schulz-Menger J, Holmvang G, Alakija P, et al. (2009) International Consensus Group on Cardiovascular Magnetic Resonance in Myocarditis. Cardiovascular magnetic resonance in myocarditis: A JACC White Paper. J Am Coll Cardiol 53: 1475–1487.
36. Aquaro GD, Gabutti A, Meini M, Prontera C, Pasanisi E, et al. (2011) M.Silent myocardial damage in cocaine addicts. Heart 97: 2056–2062.
37. Frustaci A, Verardo R, Caldarulo M, Acconcia MC, Russo MA, et al. (2007) Myocarditis in hypertrophic cardiomyopathy patients presenting acute clinical deterioration. Eur Heart J 28: 733–740.
38. Aquaro GD, Todiere G, Barison A, Strata E, Marzilli M, et al. (2011) Myocardial blood flow and fibrosis in hypertrophic cardiomyopathy. J Card Fail 17: 384–91.
39. Petersen SE, Jerosch-Herold M, Hudsmith LE, Robson MD, Francis JM, et al. (2007) Evidence for microvascular dysfunction in hypertrophic cardiomyopathy: new insights from multiparametric magnetic resonance imaging. Circulation 115: 2418–2425.
40. Coumel P (1993) Cardiac arrhythmias and the autonomic nervous system. J Cardiovasc Electrophysiol; 4: 338–355.
41. Olivotto I, Maron BJ, Appelbaum E, Harrigan CJ, Salton C, et al. (2010) Spectrum and clinical significance of systolic function and myocardial fibrosis assessed by cardiovascular magnetic resonance in hypertrophic cardiomyopathy. Am J Cardiol 106: 261–267.
42. Chan RH, Maron BJ, Olivotto I, Pencina MJ, Assenza GE, et al. (2014) Prognostic value of quantitative contrast-enhanced cardiovascular magnetic resonance for the evaluation of sudden death risk in patients with hypertrophic cardiomyopathy. Circulation 130: 484–495.
43. Maron BJ, Maron MS (2013) Hypertrophic cardiomyopathy. Lancet 381: 242–255.
44. Olivotto I, Cecchi F, Poggesi C, Yacoub MH (2012) Patterns of disease progression in hypertrophic cardiomyopathy: an individualized approach to clinical staging. Circ Heart Fail 5: 535–546.

11

Demonstration of the Effect of Generic Anatomical Divisions versus Clinical Protocols on Computed Tomography Dose Estimates and Risk Burden

Rachael E. Moorin[1,2]*, David A. J. Gibson[2], Rene K. Forsyth[3], Richard Fox[4]

1 Centre for Population Health Research, Curtin University, Perth, Western Australia, Australia, **2** Centre for Health Services Research, School of Population Health, University of Western Australia, Perth Western Australia, Australia, **3** Department of Medical Imaging Science, Curtin University, Perth, Western Australia, Australia, **4** School of Physics, University of Western Australia, Perth, Western Australia, Australia

Abstract

Objective: Choosing to undertake a CT scan relies on balancing risk versus benefit, however risks associated with CT scanning have generally been limited to broad anatomical locations, which do not provided adequate information to evaluate risk against benefit. Our study aimed to determine differences in radiation dose and risk estimates associated with modern CT scanning examinations when computed for clinical protocols compared with those using anatomical area.

Methods: Technical data were extracted from a tertiary hospital Picture Archiving Communication System for random samples of 20–40 CT examinations per adult clinical CT protocol. Organ and whole body radiation dose were calculated using ImPACT Monte Carlo simulation software and cancer incidence and mortality estimated using BEIR VII age and gender specific lifetime attributable risk weights.

Results: Thirty four unique CT protocols were identified by our study. When grouped according to anatomic area the radiation dose varied substantially, particularly for abdominal protocols. The total estimated number of incident cancers and cancer related deaths using the mean dose of anatomical area were 86 and 69 respectively. Using more specific protocol doses the estimates rose to 214 and 138 incident cancers and cancer related deaths, at least doubling the burden estimated.

Conclusions: Modern CT scanning produces a greater diversity of effective doses than much of the literature describes; where a lack of focus on actual scanning protocols has produced estimates that do not reflect the range and complexity of modern CT practice. To allow clinicians, patients and policy makers to make informed risk versus benefit decisions the individual and population level risks associated with modern CT practices are essential.

Editor: Gabriele Multhoff, Technische Universitaet Muenchen, Germany

Funding: This study was supported by a National Medical and Research Council (http://www.nhmrc.gov.au/) project grant (APP 1008394). The funders had no role in study design, data collection and analysis, decision to publish, or preparation of the manuscript.

Competing Interests: The authors have declared that no competing interests exist.

* E-mail: r.moorin@curtin.edu.au

Introduction

Over the four decades since the introduction of Computed Tomography (CT) scanning, diagnostic imaging technological advancements have been a potent factor driving innovations in medicine [1]. Recent concerns about the radiation dose associated with CT scanning have led to guidelines, advising on clinical indications for utilisation and/or reference levels for radiation dose received from each type of examination[2–4]. Recent studies reporting the cancer risks of ionizing radiation [5–9] have spurred intense debate about the risks of diagnostic imaging, and how these risks ought to be incorporated into the decision making process[8–12].

Large scale data capture of CT scanner radiation dose in databases have been proposed to enable institutional benchmarking, optimization of CT protocols, and quality control [9,13]. These data will also enable more accurate patient specific dose estimation than was possible from previously available data sources, enabling more accurate patient specific risk assessment to better inform imaging decisions [9,14].

Estimates of radiation dose and cancer risk from CT scanning were classically undertaken using 'typical' anatomically based CT protocol/machine settings[5,15–17]. However, the enormous technological advance in CT scanning has brought diversification in examination types (protocols) within anatomical locations subsequently affecting the radiation dose and risk [8,9]. Reliance on simplistic anatomical location based radiation dosimetry and derived risk estimates that do not adequately reflect current practice limits the ability of referring clinicians to make informed risk: benefit decisions for their patients.

The aim of our study was to examine the radiation dose associated with modern CT scanning examinations by anatomical location versus actual clinical protocol to demonstrate the degree of variation in radiation dose and its impact on population burden and risk estimates.

Materials and Methods

Study Design and Setting

A cross-sectional, observational, retrospective study design with technical CT data collected from a large metropolitan tertiary/teaching hospital in Western Australia (using two 64-slice CT machines of the same make and model), via the Picture Archiving Communication System (PACS), on adult diagnostic CT scanning protocols (excluding extremities) identified by way of discrete protocol code/naming conventions used by the institution. Prior to collection of the data the study was approved by the Western Australian Department of Health Human Research Ethics Committee, with a waiver of informed consent for the retrospective review of electronic medical records.

Data Sources

A random sample of 20 to 40 cases from each protocol identified was collected on scans performed between 1st January and 30th April 2011. Rarely fewer than twenty cases were identified within the collection period; in this event all cases were included in the study. If the technical parameters appeared particularly variable up to forty cases were collected. A sample of 20 cases is at least double studies using self-report data have used [15], comparable to similar studies [9] and conforms to the European guidelines on the sample required to assess usual patient doses [18]. Protocol information (excluding the scout view) consisted of separate scanning sequences (phases) whenever present. The technical parameters collected included kilovoltage (kV), milliamperage (mA), tube rotation times, collimation widths, pitch, scanning method, anatomical reference start-stop positions, volume weighted CT dose index (CTDIvol) and dose–length product (DLP).

Radiation Dosimetry

Values of CTDIvol (inclusive of automated tube current modulation) and DLP were used to calculate the organ specific dose (mGy) and effective dose (mSv) for each sequence using the ImPACT dosimetry calculation software [19]. This tool allows organ and effective dose to be estimated in a population of patients based on Monte Carlo simulation in an idealized phantom. Justification of this method and its limitations are presented in the discussion section. Scan length was obtained by dividing DLP by CTDIvol present in each case's dose report. Where ImPACT gave slightly different values of CTDIvol to those reported by the machine, the effective dose given by ImPACT was corrected by the ratio of the reported CTDIvol and the ImPACT estimate. Cumulative protocol values of CTDIvol, DLP, organ dose and effective dose were calculated by summation of all sequences reported for each case. The mean, minimum and maximum values for each parameter were reported for each protocol and anatomical area.

Cancer Risk Modelling

The age and gender specific lifetime attributable risk (LAR) inferable from a single exposure was estimated for the mean, lowest and highest dose across protocols and each anatomical area. This was achieved using the protocol specific organ dose and the age/sex-specific risk coefficients from tables 12D-1 and 12D-2 of the BEIR VII report [20]. The LAR of cancer incidence and mortality resulting from radiation dose to the remainder and 'other' organs was calculated using doses for organs not named in the BEIR VII LAR tables but have a weight by International Commission on Radiological Protection (ICRP) 103 [21], or are included in the remainder organs by ICRP 103, and weighting them by the risk attributed by BEIR VII for 'other' organs. This method assumes all such organs contribute equally to risk. The analysis was repeated for all combinations of age (ranging from 18 to 80 years) in yearly increments, using linear interpolation of the BEIR VII risk coefficients from the two nearest tabulated ages when data were not available for a specific age. To estimate the cancer incidence risk and cancer related mortality attributable to CT scanning for persons aged over 80 years the linear interpolation was extended until the estimated number of cancers or mortality reached zero for each protocol using the same method described above. The age and gender specific count of CT scanning procedures performed in Western Australia obtained from Medicare Australia and WA PACS data were used to estimate the number of incident cancers and cancer related mortality attributable to CT.

Results

Radiation Dose Associated with CT Protocols

Table 1 shows a summary of data recorded for each CT scanning protocol in the study. There was wide variation in the radiation dosimetry associated with each protocol not completely attributable to the number of sequences. Protocols for temporal bone, sinuses (non-contrast), abdomen for renal colic, abdomen/pelvis, pelvis (non-contrast), chest/abdo/pelvis, thoracic and lumbar spine CT scanning consistently included only a single sequence. However, the maximum to minimum ratios indicated a large variation in radiation dose. Table 1 also presents the mean and range of radiation dose attributable to CT scanning according to anatomical area, 'all protocols,' where highly variable with maximum to minimum ratios ranging from 4 (CTDIvol for chest/abdo/pelvis) to 91 (DLP for Abdominal CT) were observed.

Figure 1 shows a summary of the mean total and organ specific effective doses attributable to cases collected for the CT scanning protocols included in the study. Note, for simplicity some protocols have been paired (+/− contrast) where no substantive differences were discernible resulting in 25 bars for the total 34 clinical protocols identified in Table 1. Visceral spiral (helical) angiography produced the highest mean effective whole body dose of 31.2 mSv, while CT of the sinuses produced the lowest mean effective dose (0.4 mSv). Of the 34 individual protocols, 11 (32%) produced mean effective doses greater than 10 mSv. Four protocols (12%) produced mean effective doses in excess of 15 mSv while two (6%) produced mean effective doses in excess of 20 mSv. Only seven protocols (20%) produced mean effective doses of less than 2 mSv. Only one protocol (visceral spiral angiography) produced a mean organ specific dose contribution greater than 6 mSv (6.2 mSv to the stomach). This protocol's total effective dose also comprised 5.6 mSv from the colon and 4.1 mSv from the remainder organs. Thoracic spine CT was the only other protocol to include an organ specific dose contribution greater than 5 mSv (5.6 mSv from the lung). Several protocols produced specific organ contributions to effective dose between 4 and 5 mSv, these were: cardiac non-coronary spiral (helical) angiography (4.7 mSv from the breast and 4.6 mSv from the lung), CT of the thoracic spine (4.6 mSv from the breast), and CT of the cervical spine (4.2 mSv from the thyroid). When evaluating the effective doses according to anatomical area a wide variation was observed with the largest variation noted for abdominal protocols and the lowest variation in head closely followed by facial bone protocols.

Table 1. Variation in the number of sequences, dose-length product (DLP) and volume weighted Computed Tomographic dose index (CTDIvol) recorded for selected CT scanning examinations performed in a Western Australian tertiary hospital over a three month period in 2011.

Anatomical location	Protocol Name	Number of cases	Sequences in protocol				Protocol DLP[1]				Protocol CTDIvol[1]			
			Mean	Min	Max	Max:Min	Mean	Min	Max	Max:Min	Mean	Min	Max	Max:Min
Head	Head (Non-contrast)	20	1.5	1	3	3	1207.8	842.3	2699.2	3	64.6	39.5	158.8	4
	Head (Contrast)	17	1.1	1	2	2	1064.9	633.0	1952.3	3	51.2	32.3	112.3	3
	Head Pre and Post Contrast	28	2.0	2	3	2	1928.4	1008.6	3603.5	4	104.3	45.1	166.4	4
	Angiogram Head	20	1.3	1	3	3	734.5	65.8	2027.6	31	37.2	3.8	122.0	33
	Temporal Bones	10	1.0	1	1	1	661.2	501.6	792.3	2	65.9	49.0	69.5	1
	All protocols	**95**	**1.4**	**1**	**3**	**3**	**1119.4**	**65.8**	**3603.5**	**55**	**64.6**	**3.8**	**166.4**	**44**
Facial bones	Facial bones (Non-contrast)	10	1.2	1	2	2	845.2	270.7	3050.0	11	34.5	16.1	115.7	7
	Facial bones (Contrast)	20	1.3	1	4	4	630.7	179.9	2139.2	12	34.7	7.4	130.8	18
	Sinuses (Non-contrast)	10	1.0	1	1	1	157.3	103.7	392.6	4	8.8	6.8	22.7	3
	Sinuses (Contrast)	10	1.1	1	2	2	506.7	345.8	1076.5	3	26.4	17.0	45.1	3
	Sinus and Brain (Non-contrast)	11	1.4	1	2	2	1705.7	391.6	3064.9	8	69.9	22.5	114.2	5
	Orbits and/or Brain (Non-contrast)	10	1.1	1	2	2	299.0	233.2	669.2	3	19.6	15.5	45.1	3
	Orbits and/or Brain (Contrast)	7	1.1	1	2	2	385.5	233.2	503.2	2	23.9	17.0	33.9	2
	All protocols	**78**	**1.2**	**1**	**4**	**4**	**647.1**	**103.7**	**3064.9**	**30**	**31.1**	**6.8**	**130.8**	**19**
Soft tissue neck	Neck (Non-contrast)	20	1.3	1	2	2	521.6	51.6	1526.9	30	17.7	2.8	50.3	18
	Neck (Contrast)	20	1.4	1	3	3	451.9	232.3	937.0	4	22.8	6.9	61.4	9
	Angiogram Neck (Carotid)	20	1.3	1	2	2	633.7	242.3	1579.5	7	23.3	5.9	66.1	11
	All protocols	**60**	**1.3**	**1**	**3**	**3**	**535.7**	**51.6**	**1579.5**	**31**	**21.3**	**2.8**	**66.1**	**24**
Chest	Chest High Res	20	2.1	1	4	4	488.1	131.1	1183.1	9	13.7	3.5	30.9	9
	Chest (Non-contrast)	20	1.2	1	4	4	418.6	135.6	1183.1	9	10.7	3.5	55.6	16
	Chest with Contrast	40	1.1	1	3	3	464.3	175.5	998.5	6	11.8	4.3	44.4	10
	Chest Pulmonary Embolism Study	20	3.6	3	7	2	738.2	41.8	1635.7	39	47.8	14.8	103.7	7
	Angiogram Thoracic Aorta	20	3.8	3	5	2	799.9	192.4	1596.1	8	36.8	20.9	52.3	3
	Angiogram Cardiac (non-coronary)	20	1.5	1	2	2	747.4	141.3	2407.9	17	32.6	9.1	68.5	8
	All protocols	**140**	**2.2**	**1**	**7**	**7**	**609.4**	**41.8**	**2407.9**	**58**	**25.6**	**3.5**	**103.7**	**30**
Abdomen (+/− Pelvis)	Abdomen Renal Colic	20	1.0	1	1	1	149.6	98.6	239.5	2	3.1	2.4	5.3	2
	Angiogram Renal	14	3.3	1	5	5	689.5	361.8	1358.7	4	47.0	15.1	120.1	8
	Abdomen and Pelvis (Non-contrast)	20	1.0	1	1	1	564.5	103.4	1169.1	11	11.0	2.4	22.5	10
	Abdomen and Pelvis (Contrast)	20	1.7	1	3	3	903.4	329.4	1786.7	5	19.7	6.4	39.0	6
	Virtual Colonoscopy	20	2.4	2	3	3	372.3	221.0	1360.5	6	7.4	4.7	25.3	5
	Angiogram Visceral	20	4.3	1	6	6	1895.1	39.6	3599.8	91	60.1	2.4	162.0	69
	All protocols	**114**	**2.3**	**1**	**6**	**6**	**762.4**	**39.6**	**3599.8**	**91**	**24.7**	**2.4**	**162.0**	**69**
Pelvis only	Pelvis (Non-contrast)	20	1.0	1	1	1	657.9	306.8	1189.1	4	21.3	8.8	35.0	4

Table 1. Cont.

Anatomical location	Protocol Name	Number of cases	Sequences in protocol				Protocol DLP[1]				Protocol CTDIvol[1]			
			Mean	Min	Max	Max:Min	Mean	Min	Max	Max:Min	Mean	Min	Max	Max:Min
	Pelvis (Contrast)	20	1.5	1	4	4	997.1	223.8	2036.5	9	29.2	5.5	64.8	12
	All protocols	**40**	**1.3**	**1**	**4**	**4**	**827.5**	**223.8**	**2036.5**	**9**	**25.2**	**5.5**	**64.8**	**12**
Chest/Abdo/Pelvis	Chest/Abdo/Pelvis (Non-contrast)	10	1.0	1	1	1	997.2	463.4	1816.7	4	14.1	7.5	25.2	3
	Chest/Abdo/Pelvis (Contrast)	10	1.0	1	1	1	933.1	307.4	1919.2	6	13.5	7.0	29.0	4
	All protocols	**20**	**1.0**	**1**	**1**	**1**	**965.2**	**307.4**	**1919.2**	**6**	**13.8**	**7.0**	**29.0**	**4**
Spine	Spine Cervical (Non-Contrast)	10	1.3	1	2	2	1117.5	210.5	2832.6	13	48.6	9.5	126.7	13
	Spine Thoracic (Non-Contrast)	10	1.0	1	1	1	1032.3	374.7	1787.9	5	28.8	9.6	48.1	5
	Spine Lumbar (Non-Contrast)	10	1.0	1	1	1	990.9	432.9	2480.4	6	24.4	16.4	36.7	2
	All protocols	**30**	**1.1**	**1**	**2**	**2**	**1046.9**	**210.5**	**2832.6**	**13**	**34.0**	**9.5**	**126.7**	**13**

[1]Where applicable values are generated using summed value for cases where multiple sequences were recorded.

Variation in the LAR (Expressed as a Percentage) of Cancer Incidence and Cancer Related Mortality Across Anatomical Areas

As expected there was a large variation in the estimated risk of incident cancers and cancer related mortality across anatomical areas (Figure 2) driven by differences in the radio-sensitivity of the organs included within the scanning field, the radiation dose generated by the CT protocol and gender. The estimated risk of incident cancers and cancer related mortality was considerably higher in females compared with males, except for CT scanning of the pelvis where the estimated risk of cancer for females was consistently lower than males. The largest difference across genders was consistently observed for chest CT. Using the mean dose protocol, females at age 20 years had a 0.25% risk of cancer compared with 0.09% for males and a 0.12% risk of cancer related death compared with 0.06% for males. The magnitude of this difference is highly subject to the dose scenario evaluated, for example when the protocol giving the maximum dose was evaluated (end of the bars in Figure 2) females at age 20 years were estimated to have a 0.94% risk of incident cancers compared with 0.33% for males and a 0.43% risk of cancer related deaths compared with 0.22% for males.

When anatomical area mean dose was considered (black lines in Figure 2), facial bones CT was attributed the lowest risk of incident cancers and cancer related mortality while chest/abdo/pelvis CT was attributed the highest risk of incident cancers and cancer related mortality. This ranking of anatomical areas varied dependent on both the radiation dose scenario and to a lesser extent age at CT scan.

Impact of the Dose Scenario on Burden of Cancer and Cancer Related Mortality Attributable to CT Scanning

Table 2 shows a demonstration of the number of incident cancers and cancer related mortality attributable to selected CT scanning examinations, using doses derived from anatomical area versus clinical protocols. If the mean dose derived from protocols within each anatomical area was used as the input to the risk modelling, 86 incident cancers and 69 cancer related deaths were estimated to be attributable to the independent effect (unadjusted for competing risk factors not considered in the BEIR VII risk model) of CT scanning radiation dose. However, using actual protocol doses the estimates rose to 214 and 138 incident cancers and cancer related deaths, an increase of a factor of 2.5 and 2.0 respectively. The range of predicted cancers was highly variable for anatomical areas comprising multiple protocols with four anatomical areas providing estimates varying by over 10 (cancers) predicted between the anatomical area estimate and individual protocol estimates. The largest difference in the anatomical area and protocol estimates was in abdomen CT. Large maximum to minimum ratios were also observed in six anatomical areas, with four having a maximum to minimum ratios of greater than 50, one exceeding 600 (abdomen).

Discussion

Decisions regarding whether to undertake a particular diagnostic imaging test should always be made balancing risks against potential benefits. Given the there may be strategies which may incur lower radiation dose while still affording an acceptable level of diagnostic accuracy for the particular clinical circumstance, comprehensive information regarding radiation dose and risk associated with modern CT scanning is required. This is particularly important in patients where the magnitude of the risk burden from ionising radiation is high (ie children, young adults

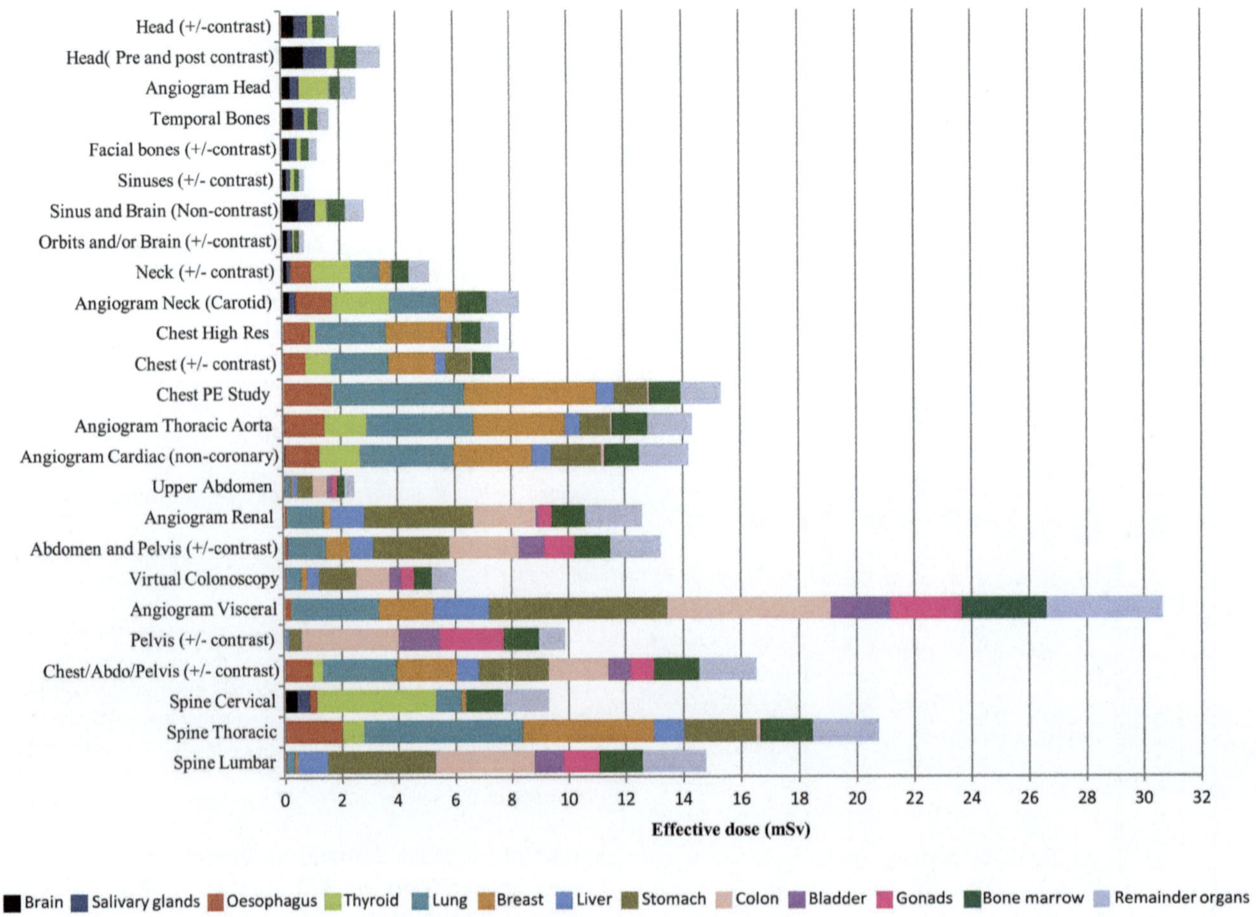

Figure 1. Mean whole body and organ specific effective doses (mSv) for selected CT scanning examinations performed in a Western Australian tertiary public hospital in 2011.

and women). Our study has provided comprehensive information about the radiation dose and risk burden of modern CT scanning in order to facilitate incorporation into clinical decision making.

This study has demonstrated modern CT practice comprises multiple protocols, across most anatomical areas, resulting in a wide range of radiation doses. This variation in radiation dose interacted substantially with the lifetime attributable risk ascribed to ionising radiation, greatly influencing the number of incident cancers and cancer related mortality estimated to be associated with CT scanning. The effective radiation dose, and subsequent risk, resulting from a single CT examination is highly dependent on machine parameters (ie the protocol used) and the radiosensitivity of the anatomical area scanned. Both of these factors need to be considered when dosimetric and risk assessments are undertaken. Using anatomical area for dose and risk estimates does not accurately account for the significant differences between protocols. The end result is an inaccurate perception of risk to individual patients but also the impact of CT radiation burden at a population level.

The majority of authors when reporting CT radiation dose either state a broad range (eg 10 to 100 mGy [22]) or provide a series typical doses for each anatomical area [23], while some authors have quantified differences in effective dose produced in limited scenarios by changing certain technical parameters [24]. However, only a few studies have previously published limited range of protocol specific dose observations, either using survey data or directly collected from PACS dose reports [8,9]. Our study has also demonstrated variation in intra-protocol dose suggesting patient specific modification of technical settings occurs, most likely based on either clinical requirements or patient habitus. This finding is welcome in response to concerns in the literature over the lack of modification of standard protocols with respect to body habitus and thus potential over-exposure of patients [4]. While we cannot definitively determine the intra-protocol variation observed in our study was due to patient characteristics, it is a plausible explanation for our observations.

A limitation of our study is that our method of estimating effective and organ dose did not include size specific dose estimation (SSDE) methods since information regarding the body habitus of the patients included in the study were not available. However, for this study the use of SSDE would not change the (numerical) deviation between the two methods because it concerns the same patient groups. In addition, while it is very important to account for patient size when estimating individual patient radiation dose [25], effective dose is intended to represent the dose to a population of patients (as we have done in our study) not individual patient dose [26]. This is an important distinction since effective dose is derived from measurements in an idealized phantom that integrates the relative weighting of the radiosensitive organs exposed and does not reflect the morphometrics of an individual patient [26]. All estimates of radiation dose have limitations, for example SSDE does not take into account

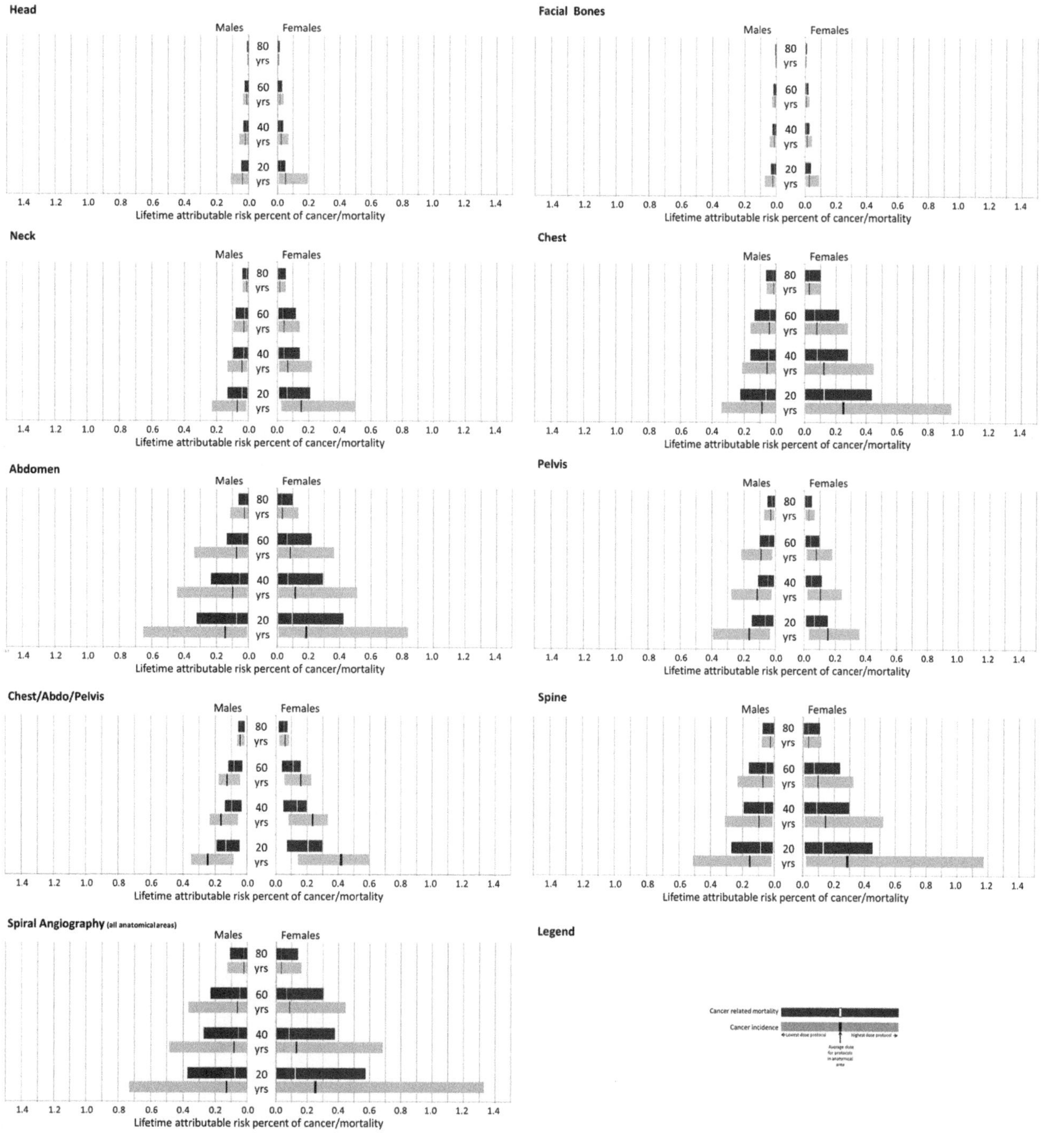

Figure 2. Variation in the lifetime attributable risk percent of cancer incidence (light bars) and mortality (dark bars) according to gender and age at a single exposure from CT scanning protocols grouped according to anatomical location.

variations in dose based on variations in scan length, assumes patients are centred in the CT gantry so that magnification effects are minimized and cannot be used for estimation of organ dose, and thus cannot be used to estimate effective dose [26]. Thus while SSDE is recommended and appropriate for estimating individual patient radiation dose it is not suitable when organ and effective dose estimates are required and is not necessary when estimating the average radiation dose characteristics of a particular examination ie examination specific rather than patient specific dosimetry is required.

In our study we aimed to estimate the average effective radiation dose for each adult CT protocol using a random sample of adult patients. The use of random sampling methodology was used to capture any underlying variation in doses produced for each scanning protocol, comparable to other published research [9], and avoid recall or selection bias associated with the use of survey methods. Additionally, the use of actual scan parameters and dosimetry information recorded at the time of imaging rather than reliance on self-selected mean doses, 'standard' protocols or phantoms facilitate a more accurate representation of actual dose

Table 2. Estimated number of incident cancers and cancer related mortality attributable to selected CT scanning undertaken in WA during 2010/11 and 2011/12 using protocol and anatomical area based risk modelling.

Anatomical location	CT scanning protocol	Incident cancers					Cancer related mortality				
		n	min[1]	max[2]	range[3]	max:min	n	min[1]	max[2]	range[3]	max:min
Head	Head (+/− Contrast)	12.1					7.2				
	Temporal Bones	0.8					0.5				
	Angiogram Head	0.1					0.1				
	Average Head	**4.3**	**0.1**	**12.1**	**11.9**	**95.5**	**2.6**	**0.1**	**7.2**	**7.2**	**102.1**
Facial bones	Facial bones OR Sinuses (+/− Contrast)	2.5					1.4				
	Sinus and Brain (Non-Contrast)	0.7					0.4				
	Orbits and/or Brain (+/− Contrast)	0.1					0.0				
	Average Sinuses/Facial bones	**1.1**	**0.1**	**2.5**	**2.4**	**40.0**	**0.6**	**0.0**	**1.4**	**1.4**	**38.6**
Soft tissue neck	Neck (+/− Contrast)	3.8					2.7				
	Angiogram Neck (Carotid)	0.6					0.5				
	Average Soft tissue neck	**2.2**	**0.6**	**3.8**	**3.2**	**6.2**	**1.6**	**0.5**	**2.7**	**2.2**	**6.0**
Chest	Chest (+/− Contrast) including High Res	19.5					15.6				
	Chest PE Study	3.8					3.0				
	Angiogram Thoracic Aorta	0.6					0.5				
	Angiogram Cardiac (Non-Coronary)	0.2					0.2				
	Average Chest	**6.0**	**0.2**	**19.5**	**19.3**	**100.0**	**4.8**	**0.2**	**15.6**	**15.5**	**100.7**
Abdomen	Abdomen +/− Pelvis (+/− Contrast)	63.4					38.9				
	Virtual Colonoscopy	0.2					0.1				
	Angiogram Renal	0.1					0.1				
	Angiogram Visceral	0.9					0.6				
	Average Abdomen	**16.2**	**0.1**	**63.4**	**63.3**	**679.4**	**9.9**	**0.1**	**38.9**	**38.8**	**619.9**
Pelvis	Pelvis (+/− Contrast)	1.8					0.9				
	Average Pelvis	**1.8**	**1.8**	**1.8**	**0.0**	**1.0**	**1.8**	**1.8**	**1.8**	**0.0**	**1.0**
Chest/Abdo/Pelvis	Chest/Abdo/Pelvis (+/− Contrast)	38.4					28.0				
	Average Chest/Abdo/Pelvis	**38.4**	**38.4**	**38.4**	**0.0**	**1.0**	**38.4**	**38.4**	**38.4**	**0.0**	**1.0**
Spine	Spine Cervical (+/− Contrast)	9.6					5.7				
	Spine Thoracic (+/− contrast)	3.2					2.4				
	Spine Lumbar (+/− Contrast)	40.8					22.4				
	Spine Multiple Areas (+/− Contrast)	2.4					1.4				
	Average Spine	**14.0**	**2.4**	**40.8**	**38.4**	**16.9**	**8.0**	**1.4**	**22.4**	**21.1**	**16.6**
Spiral Angiography[4]	Angiogram Head	0.1					0.1				
	Angiogram Neck (Carotid)	0.6					0.5				
	Angiogram Thoracic Aorta	0.6					0.5				

Table 2. Cont.

Anatomical location	CT scanning protocol	Incident cancers					Cancer related mortality				
		n	min[1]	max[2]	range[3]	max:min	n	min[1]	max[2]	range[3]	max:min
	Angiogram Cardiac (Non-Coronary)	0.2					0.2				
	Chest PE Study	3.8					3.0				
	Angiogram Renal	0.1					0.1				
	Angiogram Visceral	0.9					0.6				
	Angiogram Unspecified	7.2					5.1				
	Angiogram Cardiac (Coronary)	1.3					1.0				
	Average Spiral Angiography	**1.6**	**0.1**	**7.2**	**7.1**	**76.8**	**1.2**	**0.1**	**5.1**	**5.0**	**80.6**
Total	**Based on anatomical areas**	**85.6**			**128.3**	**2.5**	**68.8**			**69.6**	**2.0**
	Based on protocols	**213.9**					**138.4**				

n = Number of estimated incident cancers/cancer related mortality based on cancer risk modelling from the mean radiation dose of the cases collected in protocols included in the study.
[1]number based on the minimum dose protocol within the anatomical area.
[2]number based on the maximum dose the protocol within the anatomical area.
[3]Range = number based on the maximum dose protocol - number based on the minimum dose protocol.
[4]Spiral angiography also included within each anatomical location for the public providers. Note separation of spiral angiography codes are not available for private providers except coronary angiography and hence is excluded.

in practice. Our data source and sampling method provide a more rigorous picture of real CT practice, rather than idealised or theoretical CT doses and practices.

Detailed information regarding patient numbers according to CT protocols from routinely captured administrative data has allowed for cancer and cancer related mortality attributable to CT scanning to be estimated, for individual protocols and by anatomical area. The risk estimates reported in this study are not based on epidemiological data of actual malignancies in populations of patients receiving CT scans (such information is unavailable). The estimates are extrapolations of the attributable cancer risk models developed in the BEIR VII report [20] using standard Monte Carlo methods modelling photon transport in CT. This study employs previously used methods to estimate risk and are the best available given available data [16]. Our estimation of the number of incident cancers and cancer related mortality attributable to CT scanning assumed all providers would give identical doses. Similar assumptions have been used in these types of estimates previously [27]. However, the focus of this study was not to estimate the actual risk of cancer and cancer related mortality but to demonstrate the impact on risk estimates from inter-protocol variation versus aggregation of CT protocols to anatomical areas.

While the BEIR VII report provides a framework for estimating age, sex and organ specific cancer risks from a radiation exposure it does not fully account for underlying pathology and life expectancy. The BEIR VII risks should be considered representative of the independent effect of radiation dose and can only be said to account for competing risks included in the original BEIR VII models. The estimated number of incident cancers and cancer related mortality are presented here as a demonstration of the magnitude of the effect on risk estimates of using protocol rather than anatomic area dose. There is substantial difficulty in estimating population cancer risk as noted by the International Organization for Medical Physics (IOMP) [28]. In our study the imprecision is equally applied to both dose scenarios (anatomical and protocol) hence the magnitude of the effect of using a simplistic generalised method (ie anatomic based) over a more comprehensive and clinically realistic model (protocol based) is not affected by the concerns of the IOMP. These concerns primarily rest with debate regarding acceptance of the 'linear, no-threshold theory' for ionising radiation exposure risk. The linear, no-threshold theory forms the foundation for radiation protection recommendations by international and national committees [20,21,29]. Criticism of the linear, no-threshold theory rest on statistical uncertainty for the relationship between radiation exposure and cancer incidence at low doses (less than 100 mSv) [12,21]. However, current biological evidence does not support a threshold model where exposure to sub-100 mSv radiation doses represent no risk [20,29,30]. Additionally, other studies estimating the cancer incidence resulting from the independent effects of CT radiation exposure have been published using the linear, no-threshold theory and BEIR-VII LAR estimates [6,8]. Therefore our study has employed conservative, clinically representative, peer-reviewed and internationally recognised methodology for dose and risk estimation.

Conclusion

Radiation dose and risks associated with CT scanning have commonly been presented using broad anatomical locations without consideration for the diversity of modern CT examinations performed within each region. This leaves referring clinicians and patients with limited or simplistic information to evaluate risk against benefit. Our study demonstrated the insufficiency of presenting radiation dose according to anatomical areas, rather than specific CT protocols, using rigorous CT technical data sources and established risk estimation methods. Lack of focus on actual clinical scanning protocols has produced dose estimates that do not reflect current clinical practice, therefore to improve risk versus benefit decision making differentiation of the associated radiation dose resulting from the variety of services present in modern CT is essential.

Author Contributions

Conceived and designed the experiments: RM DG R. Fox. Performed the experiments: DG R. Forsyth. Analyzed the data: RM R. Forsyth. Contributed reagents/materials/analysis tools: RM DG. Wrote the paper: RM DG R. Forsyth R. Fox.

References

1. Zweifel P, Ferrari M (1992) Is there a Sisyphus Syndrome in health care? In: Zweifel P, Frech III H, editors. Health Economics Worldwide. Dordrecht, NL: Kluwer.
2. Shrimpton PC, Wall BF (1995) The increasing importance of x-ray computed tomography as a source of medical exposure. Radiation Protection Dosimetry 57: 413–415.
3. Wall BF (2005) Implementation of DRLs in the UK. Radiation Protection Dosimetry 114: 183–187.
4. Golding SJ, Shrimpton PC (2002) Radiation Dose in CT: are we meeting the challenge? The British Journal of Radiology 75: 1–4.
5. Pearce MS, Little MP, McHugh K, Lee C, Kim KP, et al. (2012) Radiation exposure from CT scans in childhood and subsequent risk of leukaemia and brain tumours: a retrospective cohort study. The Lancet Published online June 7 DOI: 10.1016/S0140-6736(12)60815-0.
6. Mathews JD, Forsythe AV, Brady Z, Butler MW, Goergen SK, et al. (2013) Cancer risk in 680 000 people exposed to computed tomography scans in childhood or adolescence: data linkage study of 11 million Australians. British Medical Journal 346: f2360.
7. Berrington De Gonzalez A, Darby S (2004) Risk of cancer from diagnostic x-rays: estimates for the UK and 14 other countries. The Lancet 363: 345–351.
8. Berrington De Gonzalez A, Mahesh M, Kim KP, Bhargavan M, Lewis R, et al. (2009) Projected Cancer Risks From Computed Tomographic Scans Performed in the United States in 2007. Arch Intern Med 169: 2071–2077.
9. Smith-Bindman R, Lipson J, Marcus R, Kim KP, Mahesh M, et al. (2009) Radiation dose associated with common computed tomography examinations and the associated lifetime attributable risk of cancer. Archives of Internal Medicine 169: 2078–2086.
10. Redberg RF (2009) Cancer Risks and Radiation Exposure From Computed Tomographic Scans. Arch Intern Med 169: 2049–2050.
11. Schroeder AR, Redberg RF (2013) The Harm in Looking. JAMA Pediatr Published Online June 10 2013: E1–3.
12. Hendee WR, O'Connor MK (2012) Radiation Risks of Medical Imaging: Separating Fact from Fantasy. Radiology 264: 312–321.
13. Sodickson A, Warden GI, Farkas CE, Ikuta I, Prevedello LM, et al. (2012) Automated anatomy-specific CT radiation exposure extraction for quality assurance and radiation monitoring. Radiology 264: 397–405.
14. Sodickson A (2013) CT radiation risks coming into clearer focus. British Medical Journal 346: f3102.
15. Shrimpton PC, Hillier MC, Lewis MA, Dunn M (2006) National survey of doses from CT in the UK:2003. The British Journal of Radiology 79: 968–980.
16. Einstein AJ, Henzlova MJ, Rajagopalan S (2007) Estimating risk of cancer associated with radiation exposure from 64-Slice Computed Tomography Coronary Angiography. JAMA 298: 317–323.
17. Moorin R, Forsyth R, Gibson D, Fox R (2013) Radiation dosimetry assessment of routine CT scanning protocols used in Western Australia. Journal of Radiological Protection 33: 295–312.
18. European Commission: Dose Datamed Project (2008) European Guidance on Estimating Population Doses from Medical X-Ray Procedures, Radiation Protection No.154. Chilton, Didcot, Oxfordshire: Health Protection Agency.
19. Imaging and Performance and Assessment of CT scanners (ImPACT) (2001) CT patient dosimetry Excel spreadsheet. Imaging and Performance and Assessment of CT scanners evaluation centre of the DH Medicines and Healthcare products Regulatory Agency (MHRA), http://www.impactscan.org. Accessed 2014 May 6.
20. Committee to Assess Health Risks from Exposure to Low Levels of Ionizing Radiation (2006) Health risks from exposure to low levels of ionizing radiation: BEIR VII-Phase 2. Board on Radiation Effects Research, Division on Earth and Life Studies, National Research Council.
21. International Commission on Radiological Protection (2007) Recomendations of the International Commission on Radiological Protection publication number 103. ICRP.
22. International Commission on Radiological Protection (2000) Managing patient dose in computed tomography. International Commission on Radiological Protection Publication 87. Annals of the ICRP 30.
23. Brenner DJ, Hall EJ (2007) Computed Tomography: An increasing source of radiation exposure. The New England Journal of Medicine 357: 227–2284.
24. Mayo JR, Aldrich J, Muller NL (2003) Radiation exposure at chest CT: A statement of the Fleischner Society. Radiology 228: 15–21.
25. Christner JA, Braun NN, Jacobsen MC, Carter RE, Kofler JM, et al. (2012) Size-specific dose estimates for adult patients at CT of the torso. Radiology 265: 841–847.
26. Brink JA, Morin RL (2012) Size-specific dose estimation for CT: Howe should it be used and what does it mean? Radiology 265: 666–668.
27. Clarke JC, Cranley K, Kelly BE, Bell K, Smith PHS (2001) Provision of MRI can significantly reduce CT collective dose. The British Journal of Radiology 74: 926–931.
28. Hendee WR (2013) Policy statement of the international organization for medical physics. Radiology 267: 326–327.
29. United Nations Scientific Committee on the Effects of Atomic Radiation (2000) Sources and effects of ionizing radiation. New York: United Nations.
30. Little MP, Wakeford R, Tawn EJ, Bouffler SD, Berrington De Gonzalez A (2009) Risks associated with low doses and low dose rates of ionizing radiation: why linearity may be (almost) the best we can do. Radiology 251: 6–12.

12

Prospective Screening of Family Members with Moyamoya Disease Patients

Cong Han[1]✉, Hui Feng[2]✉, Yi-Qin Han[1], Wei-Wei Liu[3], Zheng-Shan Zhang[1], Wei-Zhong Yang[1], Lian Duan[1]*

1 Department of Neurosurgery, 307 Hospital, PLA, Beijing, China, **2** Department of Ultrasound, 302 Hospital, PLA, Beijing, China, **3** Consulting centre of biomedical statistics, academy of military medical sciences, PLA, Beijing, China

Abstract

Background: Genetic factors play an important role in the pathogenesis of moyamoya disease (MMD). Previous studies concentrated on familial MMD patients. In this study, we focused on family members of sporadic MMD patients, and aimed to gain a clearer understanding of the role that genetic factors play in MMD.

Methods: The immediate family members of MMD patients were initially screened by transcranial Doppler sonography (TCD) and positive cases were verified by magnetic resonance angiography (MRA).

Results: From July 2011 to March 2013, there were 527 MMD patients managed in our hospital, including 38 familial MMD cases. In this study, 285 immediate family members of 245 sporadic MMD patients were screened. Another 41 cases of familial MMD cases were identified, which included 21 family members and 20 corresponding sporadic MMD patients who had family members confirmed positive with MMD. As a result, the proportion of familial MMD patients increased from 7% (38/527) to 15% (79/527) in this period. For the main segments of the circle of Willis, Kappa values between TCD and MRA for the anterior cerebral arteries, middle cerebral arteries and posterior cerebral arteries were 0.91, 0.72, and 0.47, respectively. Familial cases confirmed by our screening showed a significantly higher percentage of asymptomatic patients (57%) compared with 9% from the control group who had a clear family history before.

Conclusions: Familial MMD patients may account for a higher percentage among all cases than previously thought. Some family members of MMD patients may also have MMD, but not have any obvious symptoms. Routine screening should be implemented for all family members of MMD patients to improve the detection rate for this part of the patient base. TCD has a high diagnostic agreement with MRA for MMD. TCD may be the preferred choice for screening because it is inexpensive and safe.

Editor: Kai Wang, Anhui Medical University, China

Funding: This study was supported by grant from National Natural Science Foundation of China (81171083, www.nsfc.gov.cn). The funders had no role in study design, data collection and analysis, decision to publish, or preparation of the manuscript.

Competing Interests: The authors have declared that no competing interests exist.

* E-mail: duanlian307@sina.com

✉ These authors contributed equally to this work.

Introduction

Moyamoya disease (MMD) is a chronic cerebrovascular disorder, characterized by progressive stenosis and/or occlusion of the intracranial internal carotid artery and its proximal branches, with development of a basal collateral network. Previous studies have suggested that genetic factors play an important role in the pathogenesis of MMD [1]. Approximately 6–12% of MMD patients have a family history [2–3]. However, no screening of family members for sporadic MMD cases has been reported. Therefore, in this study, we screened the family members of MMD patients who do not have an established family history. Our result may help further clarify the role that genetic factors play in MMD. In addition, we also aimed to evaluate the effectiveness of transcranial Doppler sonography (TCD) in MMD screening.

Subjects and Methods

Patient Selection

From July 2011 to March 2013, there were 527 MMD patients managed in our hospital, including 38 familial MMD cases. In this study, 38 confirmed familial cases (from 17 families) were chosen as control group. For the other sporadic MMD patients, 4 family members of 2 MMD patients were excluded for absent temporal bone windows to screen with TCD, and other family members of 242 patients refused to participate for a variety of reasons. Therefore, 285 immediate family members (first degree relative only) of 245 sporadic MMD patients were enrolled. None of the family members had a previous diagnosis history of MMD or any other cerebrovascular disease. Subjects who had other basic diseases, such as arteriosclerosis, autoimmune disease, meningitis, Down syndrome, and so on, were excluded from the study, in accordance with the guidelines for diagnosis and treatment of MMD in 2012 [4].

Examination

All family members were initially screened with TCD. A transcranial Doppler instrument (DWL Doppler-Box, Germany) was used to examine the subjects according to a previously published standard protocol [5–6]. All of the screening was performed by an experienced sonographer in TCD. When a suspected case occurred, magnetic resonance angiography (MRA) was performed to validate the diagnosis of MMD by the 3-dimensional time-of-flight method with a 1.5 T superconducting magnet (Signa, GE Medical Systems). The diagnostic criteria of MRA was based on the guidelines recommended by the Research Committee on the Pathology and Treatment of Spontaneous Occlusion of the Circle of Willis in 2012 [4].

Statistical Analyses

Data are shown using frequencies and percentages for categorical variables, and means and standard deviations for continuous variables. The consistency between the results of TCD and MRA was calculated by the chi-square test and Kappa testing. Comparisons between family members (screened group) and the control group was evaluated using the chi-square test and t test. The factors analyzed included sex, age, family relationship, and clinical symptoms. Statistical analyses were performed with SAS 9.2 (SAS Institute Inc, Cary, NC). Statistical significance was set at $P<0.05$.

Ethics Statement

This study was approved by the local ethical committee (the Ethics Committees of 307 Hospital, PLA), and written informed consent forms were obtained directly from patients and the immediate family members.

Results

Abnormal results were found in 33 subjects from 285 immediate family members by TCD screening, with an 11.6% detection rate. 21 of the 33 subjects underwent a MRA to make a definite diagnosis. The other 12 subjects refused to have further examinations (Figure 1). In the 21 cases who were examined further, the accordant rate between TCD and MRA was 100%. 11 cases were diagnosed with typical bilateral MMD, and the other 10 cases were diagnosed with unilateral MMD. We also evaluated the parameters of the 3 main intracranial arterial segments - the anterior cerebral arteries (ACA), middle cerebral arteries (MCA) and posterior cerebral arteries (PCA) in the circle of Willis - in all 21 cases (32 sides). Table 1 shows contingency tables for the categorical variables used for the assessment of stenosis. The results of TCD and MRA were highly consistent. Kappa values for the comparison of TCD and MRA were 0.92 for the ACA, 0.72 for the MCA, and 0.47 for the PCA. Such high Kappa values in the ACA and MCA indicated substantial agreement between the two methods, and TCD findings matched MRA findings in 94 of 96 arterial segments (94.8%). The sensitivity and specificity of TCD were 96.3% and 92.9% respectively, compared with MRA.

Prior to our study, the proportion of familial MMD in our hospital was 7.2% (38/527) from July 2011 to March 2013. In this screening, we found that 21 family members and 20 corresponding index MMD patients (the index patients are the confirmed MMD cases whose family members were screened in this study) also had family heredity of MMD. Therefore, the proportion of familial MMD increased to 15.0% (79/527). In all 21 positive cases, the male/female ratio was 11/10, and the age ranged from 7 to 55 years old, with a mean age of 35 years old. The genetic relationships between the screened subjects and index patients were 6 father-offspring pairs, 7 mother-offspring pairs and 8 sibling pairs. The clinical symptoms of the positive screened cases included TIA (transient ischemic attack, 5 cases), cerebral infarction (4 cases), and the other 12 cases were asymptomatic. There were no significant differences in age, sex, or genetic relationship between the screened groups and the control group. However, a significantly higher percentage (57%, 12/21) of asymptomatic cases was observed in the screened group compared with the confirmed familial MMD group (9%, $P<0.001$). In addition, the proportion of those presenting with severe symptoms, including infarction and hemorrhage, was higher in the confirmed familial MMD group than in the screened group (Tables 2).

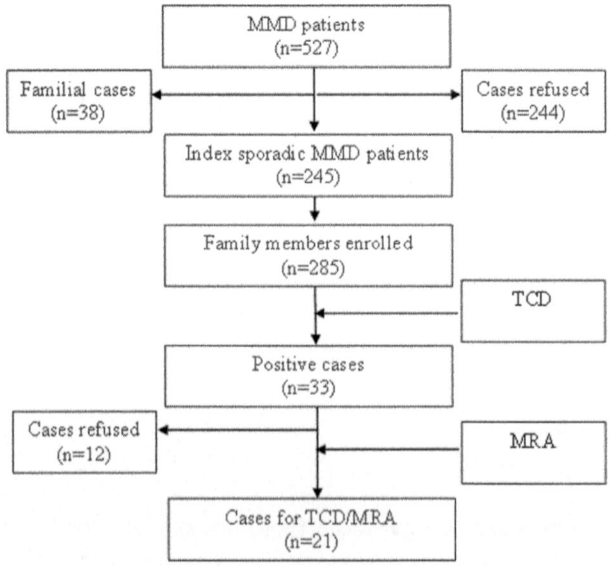

Figure 1. Diagram of Family members with MMD included in this study.

Table 1. Main results of TCD compared to MRA.

TCD		ACA		MCA		PCA	
	MRA	P	N	P	N	P	N
P		24	0	27	2	1	1
N		1	7	0	3	1	29
K value		0.92		0.72		0.47	

(ACA = anterior cerebral arteries, MCA = middle cerebral arteries, PCA = posterior cerebral arteries, TCD = transcranial Doppler sonography, MRA = magnetic resonance angiography, P = positive, N = negative, K = Kappa).

Discussion

MMD used to be considered a rare cerebrovascular disorder and the number of cases reported is scarce. With the development of noninvasive diagnostic tools such as MRA and growing awareness by clinicians, the detection rate of MMD has dramatically improved. A nationwide epidemiological survey in 2003 showed that the prevalence and incidence of MMD in Japan was 6.03 and 0.54 per 100 000, respectively [2]. An even higher prevalence has been shown by some regional surveys at 9.1–10.5 per 100,000 [7–8].

Table 2. Characteristics of family members screened for moyamoya disease.

Characteristics	Cases		Significance (P value)
	family members screened	control	
Confirmed cases	21	38	
Male/Female	11:10	23:15	0.5444
Age (years)	35±12	32±16	0.4086
Relationship			
father–offspring	6	9	0.3232
mother–offspring	7	3	
siblings	8	9	
Clinical symptoms			
asymptomatic	12	2	0.0001
headache	0	7	
TIA	5	12	
infarction	4	13	
hemorrhage	0	4	

(TIA = Transient Ischemic Attack).

The exact etiology and pathogenesis of MMD remain unknown, but various evidence has indicated that genetic factors play a major role [1,3]. A total of 12.1% of patients have a family history of MMD according to a Japanese epidemiological survey [2], and 6% were reported in the USA [3]. However, all of the previous data for familial occurrence were based upon well-defined familial patient groups, and there has been no study focusing on family screening of sporadic cases. In our study, we prospectively examined 285 immediate family members of 245 MMD patients using TCD. We found that 7.4% (21/285) of cases were confirmed as positive for MMD. Consequently, the proportion of familial MMD in our hospital increased from 7.2% (38/527) to 15.0% (79/527). Because the index patients for this study only comprised 245 out of the 527 MMD cases in this period, the proportion may be higher than 15%. Therefore, the proportion of familial MMD may be higher than previously thought. Further prospective studies may be necessary to finalize management guidelines for family screening of sporadic MMD cases.

We also compared the clinical features between screened familial MMD cases in this study and confirmed familial MMD cases with a clear MMD family history in the past. We found that the majority of screened cases were asymptomatic (12/21) compared with the control group (2/38). This asymptomatic phenomenon might be the reason why some familial MMD patients are easily missed. Our findings also suggest that the incidence of asymptomatic MMD and the nature history of MMD need to be re-evaluated. Asymptomatic MMD patients have not previously received enough attention, they are often hard to detect and the nature history was unknown. However, increasing evidence suggests that disease progression for these patients is severer than previously considered. A multicenter questionnaire survey including 33 asymptomatic MMD patients showed that, in the conservatively treated group (28 patients), 2 patients died from intracranial bleeding and 4 patients experienced TIA during follow-up period of an average of 44 months [9]. Another multicenter survey included 34 non-surgically treated asymptomatic patients, 3 patients experienced TIA, 1 patient had ischemic stroke and 3 patients had intracranial bleeding at follow-up. The annual risk for all kinds of strokes was 3.2% during follow-up period [10]. These previous results show that asymptomatic MMD is not a silent disorder, and disease progression might occur silently or continue to be undetected until it presents with serious neurological deficits. Asymptomatic MMD patients should be carefully monitored for disease progression before a serious cerebrovascular event occurs. Therefore, we recommend that all immediate family members of MMD patients should be screened by neuroimaging, regardless of their family medical history. Such a routine vascular screening may lead to early surgical intervention and prevention of significant neurological complications. Because the financial cost of routine screening may be significant, TCD is a cost effective choice.

Digital subtraction angiography (DSA) is still the golden standard for the diagnosis of MMD at present, but MRA findings are also recognized as a diagnostic criteria [4,11,12]. In addition, TCD is another diagnostic tool, which is widely used to identify different intracranial vascular abnormalities. Many studies have reported the diagnostic value of TCD compared with MRA, computed tomographic angiography (CTA), and DSA [13–14], but a limited number of studies have investigated its application in MMD. Lee et al [5] detected 45 adult MMD patients with TCD, while all the patients were diagnosed with MRA or DSA. They showed that changes in TCD parameters can reflect the severity of MMD, and TCD results can be coordinated with MRA findings. In our study, the Kappa statistic showed high consistency between these two methods in the ACA and MCA. The sensitivity and specificity of TCD was 96.3% and 92.9%, respectively. Therefore, our study and previous studies show that TCD is an effective method for MMD screening.

However, TCD has some limitations. First, in MMD, lesions are limited to the circle of Willis, which has confluent flowing from the internal carotid arteries and the basilar artery. The hemodynamics in this area are significantly different anatomically from normal branching, such as the distal branches of the MCA or PCA. Especially in the ACA, the results are usually affected by the contralateral ACA through the anterior communicating artery. A great deal of experience of operators is required to identify it. Second, TCD examinations depend on the cranial "window" where the ultrasound beam can penetrate without being excessively dampened, but some cases do not have a corresponding "window". Therefore, currently, TCD cannot replace DSA or MRA. However, in terms of screening a high-risk population, TCD shows a number of advantages over other available methods because it is non-invasive, non-ionizing, inexpensive, portable, and safe.

In conclusion, our study shows that a considerable portion of family members of sporadic MMD patients also have MMD. The proportion of familial MMD patients may be higher than previously thought and this issue requires re-evaluation. Because this part of MMD patients is asymptomatic or only presents with mild symptoms, sufficient attention and in-depth analysis have not been applied in the past. Routine vascular screening with necessary follow-ups for all immediate family members of MMD patients is highly recommended. These processes may lead to early detection and prevention of severe complications. TCD is considered a good choice as a screening method because it is cost effective, and is non-invasive with good acceptance, among other advantages. Because no reliable criteria for TCD parameters have been set for the diagnosis of MMD, all suspected cases detected by TCD currently require further examinations to confirm the diagnosis and severity.

Acknowledgments

We sincerely thank all the patients and health care workers who participated in this study.

Author Contributions

Conceived and designed the experiments: LD. Performed the experiments: CH HF YQH. Analyzed the data: HF ZSZ. Contributed reagents/materials/analysis tools: WWL WZY. Wrote the paper: CH.

References

1. Liu W, Morito D, Takashima S, Mineharu Y, Kobayashi H, et al. (2011) Identification of RNF213 as a susceptibility gene for moyamoya disease and its possible role in vascular development. PLoS One 6: e22542.
2. Kuriyama S, Kusaka Y, Fujimura M, Wakai K, Tamakoshi A, et al. (2008) Prevalence and clinicoepidemiological features of moyamoya disease in Japan: findings from a nationwide epidemiological survey. Stroke 39: 42–47.
3. Scott RM, Smith ER (2009) Moyamoya disease and moyamoya syndrome. N Engl J Med 360: 1226–1237.
4. Research Committee on the Pathology and Treatment of Spontaneous Occlusion of the Circle of Willis, Health Labour Sciences Research Grant for Research on Measures for Intractable Diseases (2012) Guidelines for diagnosis and treatment of moyamoya disease (Spontaneous Occlusion of the Circle of Willis). Neurol Med Chir (Tokyo) 52: 245–266.
5. Lee YS, Jung KH, Roh JK (2004) Diagnosis of moyamoya disease with transcranial Doppler sonography: correlation study with magnetic resonance angiography. J Neuroimaging 14: 319–323.
6. Alexandrov AV, Sloan MA, Wong LK, Douville C, Razumovsky AY, et al. (2007) American Society of Neuroimaging Practice Guidelines Committee: Practice standards for transcranial Doppler ultrasound: Part I – test performance. J Neuroimaging 17: 1811–1817.
7. Baba T, Houkin K, Kuroda S (2008) Novel epidemiological features of moyamoya disease. J Neurol Neurosurg Psychiatry 79: 900–904.
8. Im SH, Cho CB, Joo WI, Chough CK, Park HK, et al. (2012) Prevalence and epidemiological features of moyamoya disease in Korea. J Cerebrovasc Endovasc Neurosurg 14: 75–78.
9. Yamada M, Fujii K, Fukui M (2005) Clinical features and outcomes in patients with asymptomatic moyamoya disease–from the results of nation-wide questionnaire survey. No Shinkei Geka 33: 337–342.
10. Kuroda S, Hashimoto N, Yoshimoto T, Iwasaki Y (2007) Research Committee on Moyamoya Disease in Japan: Radiological findings, clinical course, and outcome in asymptomatic moyamoya disease: results of multicenter survey in Japan. Stroke 38: 1430–1435.
11. Houkin K, Nakayama N, Kuroda S, Nonaka T, Shonai T, et al. (2005) Novel magnetic resonance angiography stage grading for moyamoya disease. Cerebrovasc Dis 20: 347–354.
12. Li Z, Zhou P, Xiong Z, Ma Z, Wang S, et al. (2013) Perfusion-Weighted Magnetic Resonance Imaging Used in Assessing Hemodynamics following Superficial Temporal Artery-Middle Cerebral Artery Bypass in Patients with Moyamoya Disease. Cerebrovasc Dis 35: 455–460.
13. Suwanwela NC, Phanthumchinda K, Suwanwela N (2002) Transcranial Doppler sonography and CT angiography in patients with atherothrombotic middle cerebral artery stroke. AJNR Am J Neuroradiol 23: 1352–1355.
14. Zhao L, Barlinn K, Sharma VK, Tsivgoulis G, Cava LF, et al. (2011) Velocity criteria for intracranial stenosis revisited: an international multicenter study of transcranial Doppler and digital subtraction angiography. Stroke 42: 3429–3434.

Common Carotid Intima Media Thickness and Ankle-Brachial Pressure Index Correlate with Local but Not Global Atheroma Burden: A Cross Sectional Study Using Whole Body Magnetic Resonance Angiography

Jonathan R. Weir-McCall[1,2]*, Faisel Khan[3], Matthew A. Lambert[1], Carly L. Adamson[4], Michael Gardner[4], Stephen J. Gandy[5], Prasad Guntur Ramkumar[2], Jill J. F. Belch[1], Allan D. Struthers[1], Petra Rauchhaus[6], Andrew D. Morris[1], J. Graeme Houston[1,2]

1 Division of Cardiovascular and Diabetes Medicine, Medical Research Institute, University of Dundee, Dundee, United Kingdom, **2** NHS Tayside Clinical Radiology, Ninewells Hospital, Dundee, United Kingdom, **3** Vascular & Inflammatory Diseases Research Unit, Medical Research Institute, University of Dundee, Dundee, United Kingdom, **4** University of Dundee, Ninewells Hospital & Medical School, Dundee, United Kingdom, **5** NHS Tayside Medical Physics, Ninewells Hospital, Dundee, United Kingdom, **6** Dundee epidemiological and biostatistics unit, University of Dundee, Dundee, United Kingdom

Abstract

Background: Common carotid intima media thickness (CIMT) and ankle brachial pressure index (ABPI) are used as surrogate marker of atherosclerosis, and have been shown to correlate with arterial stiffness, however their correlation with global atherosclerotic burden has not been previously assessed. We compare CIMT and ABPI with atheroma burden as measured by whole body magnetic resonance angiography (WB-MRA).

Methods: 50 patients with symptomatic peripheral arterial disease were recruited. CIMT was measured using ultrasound while rest and exercise ABPI were performed. WB-MRA was performed in a 1.5T MRI scanner using 4 volume acquisitions with a divided dose of intravenous gadolinium gadoterate meglumine (Dotarem, Guerbet, FR). The WB-MRA data was divided into 31 anatomical arterial segments with each scored according to degree of luminal narrowing: 0 = normal, 1 = < 50%, 2 = 50–70%, 3 = 70–99%, 4 = vessel occlusion. The segment scores were summed and from this a standardized atheroma score was calculated.

Results: The atherosclerotic burden was high with a standardised atheroma score of 39.5±11. Common CIMT showed a positive correlation with the whole body atheroma score (β 0.32, p = 0.045), however this was due to its strong correlation with the neck and thoracic segments (β 0.42 p = 0.01) with no correlation with the rest of the body. ABPI correlated with the whole body atheroma score (β −0.39, p = 0.012), which was due to a strong correlation with the ilio-femoral vessels with no correlation with the thoracic or neck vessels. On multiple linear regression, no correlation between CIMT and global atheroma burden was present (β 0.13 p = 0.45), while the correlation between ABPI and atheroma burden persisted (β −0.45 p = 0.005).

Conclusion: ABPI but not CIMT correlates with global atheroma burden as measured by whole body contrast enhanced magnetic resonance angiography in a population with symptomatic peripheral arterial disease. However this is primarily due to a strong correlation with ilio-femoral atheroma burden.

Editor: Angelo Scuteri, INRCA, Italy

Funding: Funding for the study was provided by Wyeth TMRC. JRWM is supported by the Wellcome Trust through the Scottish Translational Medicine and Therapeutics Initiative (Grant no. WT 085664) in the form of a Clinical Research Fellowship. The authors have declared that no competing interests exist. The funders had no role in study design, data collection and analysis, decision to publish, or preparation of the manuscript.

Competing Interests: The authors have declared that no competing interests exist.

* E-mail: j.weirmccall@dundee.ac.uk

Introduction

Common carotid intima media thickness (CIMT), ankle brachial pressure index (ABPI) and whole body magnetic resonance angiography (WB-MRA) are all markers of atherosclerosis.

Common carotid intima media thickness is a measure of early atherosclerosis and vascular remodelling which correlates highly with standard cardiovascular risk factors. This has been acknowledged by the FDA who have approved it as a marker of atherosclerosis [1]. A reduction of CIMT thickness to lipid lowering agents has also been shown [2,3]. These factors have led to the conclusion that it meets the criteria as a surrogate for CV disease endpoints [4,5], and can therefore be used as a primary outcome in clinical trials to allow for more rapid assessment and development of more effective treatments at lower cost [3,6]. However its success in predicting risk of future cardiovascular events has been mixed with a recent meta-analysis showing it to add little benefit over the Framingham risk score in predicting future cardiovascular events [1,7–9]. Additionally while some studies have shown good response of CIMT with statins, the ENHANCE trial showed a rise in CIMT with statins and ezetemide despite improved biochemical markers [3,10].

The ankle brachial pressure index has primarily been used for the diagnosis and follow-up of lower extremity arterial disease, and has been shown to correlate with future cardiovascular events in groups with and without established peripheral arterial disease [11]. Thus this has been suggested as a surrogate marker for systemic atherosclerosis [12].

Whole body contrast-enhanced magnetic resonance angiography provides visualisation of the arterial tree from the skull vertex to the pedal arteries following the intravenous injection of a gadolinium based contrast agent. It can be used to quantify atheroma burden by scoring and summating the extent of stenosis in the arterial territories of the entire body [13]. As atherosclerosis is a body wide process, an advantage of WB-MRA is that both symptomatic and asymptomatic lesions throughout the arterial tree can be detected and quantified, potentially providing more information about future vascular risk. Studies have shown WB-MRA to produce reproducible high quality images of the arterial tree [14–16], and that the extent of atherosclerosis demonstrated on WB-MRA correlates with traditional Framingham risk factors, severity of coronary artery disease and prediction of major adverse cardiovascular events (MACE) [13,17–19].

To better understand the role of common CIMT and ABPI as markers of global atherosclerosis, it is important to know what features of atherosclerosis they accurately reflect. CIMT has been shown to correlate highly with arterial stiffness but not endothelial function [20], while ABPI has been shown to correlate with aortic stiffness and weakly with endothelial dysfunction [21,22]. While studies have looked into the relationship between coronary angiography findings and CIMT [23,24], and ABPI [25,26], the correlation between these and an objective measurement of the global stenotic atheroma burden throughout the body has not been reported. Therefore we set out to assess the correlation between CIMT and ABPI and whole body atheroma burden as demonstrated on WB-MRA.

Methodology

Ethical approval was granted by the East of Scotland Research Ethics Committee. Fifty consecutive patients with symptomatic peripheral artery disease referred for magnetic resonance angiography of their lower limbs were recruited to the study with written informed consent obtained from all participants. Disease severity was classified using the Fontaine scoring system. All patients underwent WB-MRA, ankle-brachial pressure index (ABPI), exercise tolerance testing, and CIMT measurement. These were performed on the same day, with the operators and image readers blinded to the patients' clinical status and results of the other tests.

WB-MRA

Each patient underwent whole body contrast enhanced MRI angiography using a 1.5T MRI unit (Siemens Magnetom Avanto Erlangen, Germany). Patients were imaged head first and supine in the magnet bore, with surface coils used to cover the entire body, using separate head matrix, neck matrix, spine matrix, two body matrix coils and a peripheral angiography coil. 4 stations were imaged: station 1 covered the vessels of the head and neck; station 2 the vessels of the abdomen; station 3 the upper legs; and station 4 the lower legs.(See Figure 1) Each station was acquired using a 3D TurboFLASH sequence pre and post contrast, Table 1 describes the acquisition parameters used for each of the four stations. 0.05M Intravenous gadolinium gadoterate meglumine (Dotarem, Guerbet, FR) was administered via a 20G venflon in the antecubital fossa using a two-injection contrast technique. Each injection involved a 20 ml bolus of contrast followed by 20 mls of normal saline at 1 ml/s by an injector pump. Prior to the first injection, pre-contrast images were acquired of station 1 and 4. After this the first injection was administered a Care bolus sagittal-oblique fluoroscopic image through the aortic arch was used to manually trigger image acquisition as contrast reached the aortic arch. Following acquisition of station 1, station 4 acquisition immediately began. Three sequential TurboFLASH sequences were performed of station 4 to optimise acquisition of peak contrast enhancement of the calf vessels. A 10 minute delay occurred between the end of image acquisition and the second contrast injection to allow contrast washout and minimise venous contamination [27]. After the second injection of contrast, a Care bolus coronal oblique fluoroscopic image was used to guide triggering, starting image acquisition for station 2 when contrast reached the proximal abdominal aorta. TurboFLASH sequence of station 3 was acquired immediately following this.

The resulting images were analysed by dividing the arterial tree into 31 distinct anatomical segments. See figure 1 for a description of the stations and anatomical segments. All images were analysed using the raw data, with the aid of multiplanar reformats and maximum intensity projections on a Kodak Carestream workstation (PACS Client Suite Version 10.1 sp1, Rochester, NY, USA). Each segment was scored using a 5-point scoring system:

- 0: Normal vessels
- 1: <50% stenosis
- 2: 50–70% stenosis
- 3: >70% stenosis
- 4: Completely occluded vessel

Each segment was scored according to the maximum stenosis present at any point along the length of the vessel. Arterial segments that were not visualised with sufficient clarity for grading of the degree of stenosis were not analysed. To account for this, the final score was divided by the number of segments that had been successfully analysed to produce a normalised whole body atheroma score. The 'standardised atheroma score' (SAS) was calculated using equation [1]; standardisation was achieved by dividing by the maximum potential vessel score of 4.

$$SAS = \left[\left(\frac{\sum MRAscore}{n}\right) \div 4\right] \times 100 \qquad (1)$$

For regional atheroma assessment the arterial tree was split into 4 distinct regions with a standardised atheroma score calculated for each of these:

Thoracic – Carotids, vertebrals, subclavians, brachiocephalic and thoracic aorta;

Abdominal – Abdominal aorta, coeliac, superior and inferior mesenteric arteries and renal arteries;

Pelvic/thighs – Iliacs, femoral and femoral profundas;

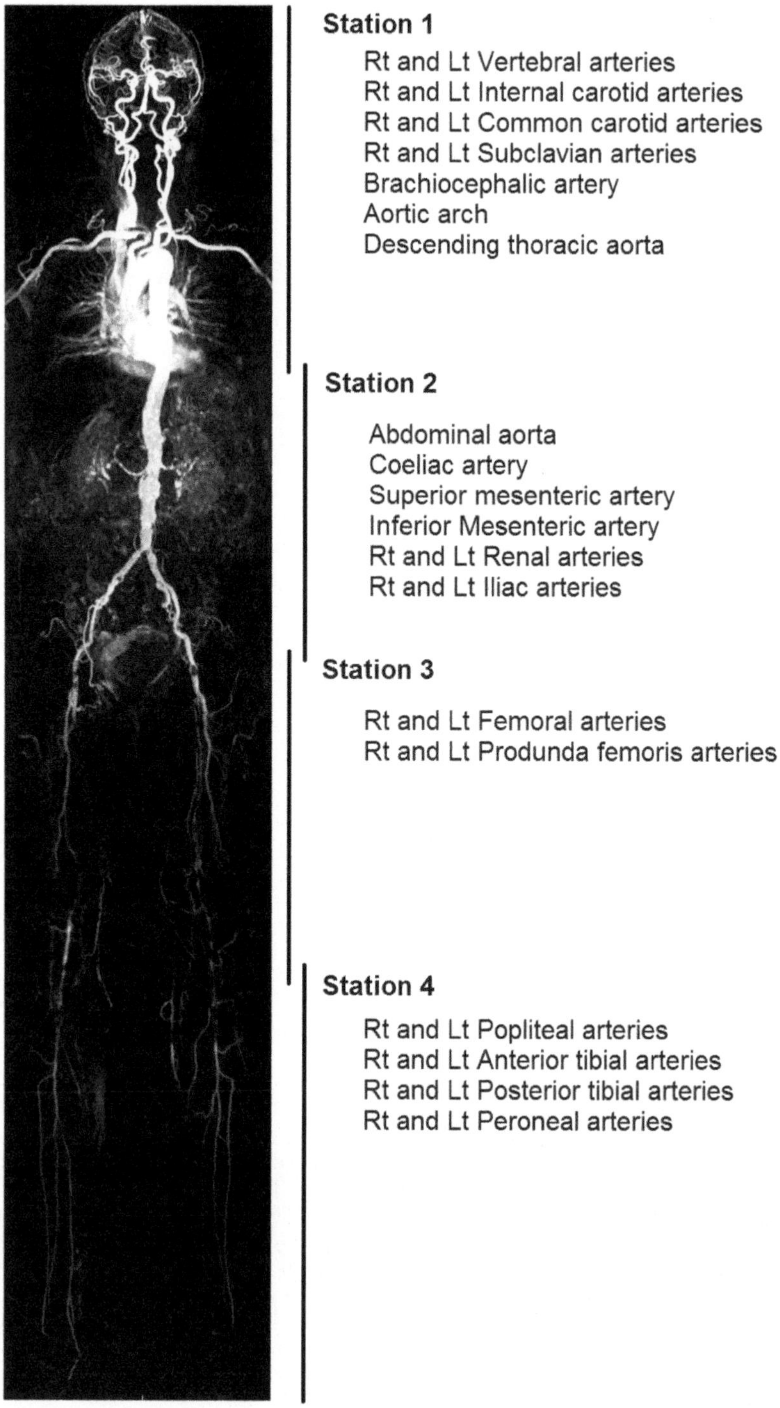

Figure 1. Diagram of the whole body magnetic resonance angiography stations and arterial segments. Maximum intensity projection image derived from the whole body angiogram from a typical patient in the study lies on the far left. To the right of this are the 4 overlapping 3D volume acquisitions acquired with a breakdown of the 31 arterial segments according to which station they are acquired in.

Lower limb – Popliteals, anterior tibials, posterior tibials and peroneals.

Carotid Intima Media Thickness

Ultrasound imaging of the common carotid artery (CCA) was acquired using an Acuson Sequoia with a 6 MHz Linear transducer. All scans were performed by a single operator. For the measurements the patient was lying supine on the couch. The participant was rested for at least 10 minutes in a supine position and at an environmental temperature of 25°C before any measurements were taken. A plastic arch with degrees of angulation marked on it was placed around the neck. The head was slightly extended and held in a straight position. The common carotid artery (CCA) was assessed from the clavicle to the bulb

Table 1. The different sequence parameters used for the 4 stations of WB-MRA.

PARAMETER	STATION 1	STATION 2	STATION 3	STATION 4
Repetition Time (ms)	3.15	3.23	3.23	3.23
Echo Time (ms)	1.06	1.1	1.08	1.1
Flip angle (°)	25	25	25	25
Bandwidth (Hz/px)	450	450	450	450
Field of View	500×375	500×335	500×335	500×335
Number of slices	104	80	80	72
Matrix	384×307	384×345	384×326	384×345
Voxel size (mm^3)	1.3×1.2×1.2	1.3×1.0×1.4	1.3×1.0×1.4	1.3×1.0×1.4
GRAPPA factor	2	2	2	2
k-space ordering	centric	linear	centric	Centric
Imaging Time (s)	18	16	16	46

both in transverse and longitudinal section. In order to provide reproducibility the CCA was assessed at a point 1 cm central to the bulb in the longitudinal position. An image was deemed acceptable if a length of greater than 1 cm of continuous IMT could be visualised. The angle of the transducer to the skin at this point was recorded using the plastic arch. Images were recorded continuously for 10 seconds, stored in the DICOM (Digital Imaging and Communications in Medicine) file format, and subsequently analysed using the Vascular Tools Carotid Analyzer for Research software (Medical Imaging Applications LLC, Coralville, USA). The IMT of the far wall was measured using a semi-automatic technique. A user-defined region of interest was selected in a 10 mm segment of the distal wall of the common carotid artery 10 mm central to the bulb in an area without any focal plaque. The software then automatically detected the intima-media borders within this region and calculated a mean CIMT. Both carotids were measured in this manner and each side was measured twice. A mean CIMT thickness was then calculated from the four measures, as previously described [28].

Ankle brachial pressure index

The resting pressure was taken after the patient had been supine for 10 minutes to ensure a true resting pressure. A sphygmomanometer cuff was placed around each arm in turn and each leg in turn. Arm: A continuous wave (CW) pencil probe Doppler is placed over the brachial artery in the cubital fossa. Once the signal is heard the cuff is inflated to occlude the brachial artery. It is then slowly released and the pressure at which the signal returns is recorded. This is repeated for the other arm. Legs: The cuff is place around each leg, just above the level of the malleolus. Both the Posterior Tibial Artery (PTA) and Dorsalis Pedis (DP) are insonated with the CW probe. The cuff and systolic measurements are recorded in the same manner as the brachial arteries.

The ABPI was calculated as:

$$\text{ABPI} = \text{Ankle pressure(PT or DP)/Highest brachial pressure(right or Left)}.$$

Both the American Heart Association method of using the highest of the two ankle pressures [29], and a modified technique of using the lowest ankle pressure were used [12,30].

Exercise treadmill test

The patient is subsequently exercised on the treadmill at a speed of 4 Kph and a gradient of 10% for one minute. After this they return immediately to the examination couch and the highest ankle pressure on each side together with the arm with the highest resting brachial pressure is re assessed. A post exercise ABPI is recorded. The lowest of the right and left post-exercise ABPI was used for analysis.

Statistical analysis

All statistical analyses were performed with IBM SPSS Statistics for Windows, version 21.0 (IBM Corp., Armonk, NY, USA). Normality of continuous variables was tested with the Kolmogorov-Smirnov test. Where a variable failed normality testing, a standard transformation of the variable was performed using a quadratic, reciprocal or logarithmic transformation as appropriate. Data are presented as frequencies or percentages for categorical variables, as means ± SD for normally distributed continuous variables, and as median with interquartile range (IQR; 25–75th percentile) for skewed variables. Correlations were performed between WB-SAS, CIMT, ABPI and population demographic metrics using the Pearson product-moment correlation coefficient. Univariate linear regression analysis was performed between the whole body atheroma score and each of the demographic variables and CIMT and ABPI. All variables with a $p<0.3$ were entered into a multiple linear regression with the Standardised Atheroma Score as the dependant variable and the remainder as independent variables. A p-value of <0.05 was considered significant.

Results

Demographic data

Fifty consecutive patients were recruited to the study. Four patients were excluded due to inability to complete the MRI examination due to claustrophobia, leaving 46 participants in the final analysis. Of these, 65% (n = 30) were male and 35% (n = 16) females, with a mean age of 64.9±10 years. 41 participants were smokers or ex smokers with a 35 (IQR 20–50) pack year history. A summary of demographic data is provided in Table 2.

In terms of symptomatic peripheral arterial disease severity, 2 patients were Fontaine 1, 2 were Fontaine IIa, 35 were Fontaine IIb, 5 were Fontaine III and 2 were Fontaine IV. A significant proportion of patients were on medications for risk factor modification (see Table 2).

Table 2. Demographic data of the study population.

Characteristic	Study cohort (n = 46)
Age (yrs)	64.9±10
Sex	30 male; 16 female
Systolic BP (mmHg)	146±17
Diastolic BP (mmHg)	78±12
BMI(kg/m^2)	27.7 (IQR 25–30)
Smoking	35 (IQR 20–50)
Diabetes (n)	12
IHD (n)	18
Previous CVA (n)	10
Medications	
Antiplatelet	37 (80)
Statin	35 (76)
Antihypertensive agents:	33 (72)
1	12
2	13
≥3	8
Anti-claudicant	2 (4)
Anti-anginal	7 (15)

WB-MRA

Forty-six of the fifty participants were able to complete the study. Thus there were a potential 1,426 segments for analysis. Of the 1,426 possible segments, 1395 (98%) were of sufficient quality for analysis. Of the 1,395 analysed segments, 628 were normal (45%), 346 had <50% stenosis (25%), 160 had 50–70% stenosis (12%), 169 had >70% stenosis (12%), and 77 were occluded (6%). Total atheroma burden was high, with a mean WB-SAS of 39.48±10.96.

WB-SAS increased as the clinical severity of the disease increased (see Table 3) apart from in the most severely symptomatic group.

CIMT

It was not possible to obtain technically adequate images in six of the fifty patients leaving 44 for analysis. The mean common CIMTs were raised bilaterally. The CIMT was 0.98 mm (IQR 0.7–1.25) on the right and 1.02 mm (IQR 0.66–1.38) on the left. Right and left cIMT correlated highly with one another (correlation co-efficient 0.57; p<0.001). Mean CIMT was 1.00 mm (IQR 0.72–1.27). In a sub cohort of 15 individuals scanned on two different days by the same operator, the coefficient of variation of the mean CIMT was 5%.

Ankle Brachial Pressure Index

The ABPI in the observed population was low. Using the AHA technique, the highest ABPI was 0.87±0.33, while the alternate ABPI measurement using the lower of the two ankle resulted in a median ABPI of 0.79 (IQR 0.48–1.1). On exercising the ABPI further fell to 0.52 (IQR 0.19–0.85). Table 3 documents the ABPI according to clinical severity as measured by the Fontaine classification.

Correlation with WBAS

Common CIMT showed correlation (β 0.32 p = 0.045) with the whole body atheroma score on the univariate analysis. When this was looked at on a regional basis, CIMT only correlated with the thoracic and neck station (β 0.42 p = 0.011) with no correlation with any other anatomical region. WBAS correlated highly with age but no other demographic factor (Table 4). On multiple linear regression adjusting for confounding factors (age, systolic and diastolic blood pressure, diabetic status, and statin usage) this significance disappeared for both the whole body (β 0.13 p = 0.45) with a non-significant trend towards association with the thoracic atheroma burden (β 0.33 p = 0.07). (See table 5)

ABPI significantly correlated with the whole body SAS. The AHA method of using the higher ankle pressure correlated better with the whole body SAS (β −0.39 p = 0.012) than using the lower ankle pressure (β −0.34 p = 0.03). This improved correlation continued when assessing the regional distribution, and strengthened on the multivariate analysis (β −0.45 p = 0.005 for highest ABPI, vs. β −0.31 p = 0.05 for the lowest ABPI). ABPI only correlated with the ilio-femoral vessels on regional analysis, with no correlation with any other anatomical region. Post exercise ABPI also showed significant correlation with the WBAS (β −0.48 p = 0.003) on univariate analysis, however on multivariate analysis this became insignificant (β −0.17 p = 0.17).

Discussion

In our study we found a significant correlation between CIMT and whole body atheroma burden, however this was entirely reliant on atheroma burden within the local vessels, and this link was lost when common confounding factors were accounted for. ABPI correlated with the whole body atheroma burden, but this was mediated by a strong correlation with the iliofemoral vessels with no correlation seen with distal anatomical regions. Unlike CIMT, this correlation persisted on multivariable linear regression.

Table 3. Comparison of whole body standardised atheroma score (WB-SAS) and ankle-brachial pressure index (ABPI) by Fontaine Score.

Fontaine Score	WB-SAS	ABPI resting	ABPI exercise
I	11.5±3.7	1.38±0.63	1.08 (0.33–1.16)
IIa	21.4±5.1	1.04±0.01	0.46 (0.34–0.57)
IIb	26.8±10	0.81±0.27	0.27 (0.08–0.68)
III	38.3±12.7	0.85±0.22	0.26 (0.19–0.33)
IV	19.8±2.9	1.08±0.4	0.77 (0.53–1)

WB-SAS and ABPI rest is given as mean ± SD. ABPI exercise is given as median (IQR).

Table 4. Univariate linear regression analysis of variables against whole body atheroma score.

Variable	B-coefficient	p-value
Age	0.51	<0.0001
Sex	0.15	0.31
Systolic blood pressure	0.19	0.22
Diastolic blood pressure	−0.31	0.04
Diabetes	0.18	0.24
Statin therapy	0.19	0.24
BMI	0.07	0.96
Smoking status	0.05	0.77
CIMT	0.32	0.045
ABPI - rest	−0.34	0.03
ABPI – exercise	−0.48	0.003

The lack of evidence of correlation between common CIMT and global atherosclerotic burden seen in our study suggests that intima media thickening may not correlate with luminal stenosis secondary to plaque formation. Given that this is the key feature of the pathophysiological process of atherosclerotic disease that guides treatment and risk stratification of coronary artery disease, cerebrovascular disease and peripheral arterial disease this lack of correlation may explain the lack of additional benefit to traditional scoring methods [9]. This correlates well with a recent study showing atherosclerotic burden as measured by WB-MRA to correlate with future major adverse cardiovascular events (MACE) in an elderly patient population (aged 70 years), with no correlation seen between CIMT and MACE [18]. In this study by Lundberg et al. addition of CIMT to the WB-MRA atheroma score improved prediction, suggesting that while CIMT is not indicative of body wide atheroma burden, it may still provide additional useful data about the underlying health of the arteries and as a marker of disease. The correlation with the thoracic atheroma burden in our study may explain the previous observation that CIMT better predicts strokes than it does coronary heart disease [31,32]. Previous studies have shown both CIMT and WB-MRA to correlate with cardiovascular risk factors, major adverse cardiovascular events and arterial stiffness but not endothelial function, itself a risk factor for cardiovascular disease [33], thus suggesting they all represent different stages and processes in the multifaceted disorder that is atherosclerosis [20,34,35]. Thus CIMT may provide information on local arterial remodelling but not plaque formation, which may account for the observed improved risk stratification when added to the WBAS.

WB-MRA has been shown to accurately delineate the site and severity of peripheral arterial disease and in the current study, ABPI correlated highly with both the whole body and ilio-femoral regional atheroma score [36]. Use of the higher ABPI provided greater prediction of the atheroma burden than use of the lower ABPI. While previous studies have suggested the use of the lower threshold due to increased sensitivity for high risk patients [12,30], our results suggest this method over diagnoses the extent of atherosclerosis. This is in support of the current recommendations from the AHA, which advise that use of the lower value leads to reduced specificity and lower risk prediction by decreasing the threshold for diagnosis of significant atherosclerotic disease [29]. The correlation observed in our population between ABPI and WBAS is in keeping with that observed by Lehrke et al. in patients with coronary artery disease but without peripheral arterial disease [17].

The correlation of CIMT and ABPI with local stenotic disease but not with disease in other areas of the body suggests a complimentary role for these two techniques in the assessment of the arterial tree. Indeed the Rotterdam study showed improvement in the risk stratification from the combination of these techniques [37]. Further work is required to assess the complimentary or exclusive role of WB-MRA with CIMT and ABPI in risk stratification and prediction.

Limitations of the study include the patient selection, which examined patients with symptomatic peripheral vascular disease, a group at a very advanced stage of the cardiovascular disease spectrum. Further work is thus warranted to look at the ability of CIMT and ABPI to predict atheroma burden in a healthier population. The population was predominantly Fontaine type IIb patients, which is not surprising as these are the patients most likely to be considered for intervention, and therefore for vascular imaging, however this group may have skewed results. 78% of the participants were on statin therapy. Some studies have shown CIMT to improve with statin therapy [3], and that statins have been shown to replace the fibrofatty component of plaques with calcific plaque without reducing plaque volume [38]. Given that plaque volume is the key contributor to the degree of stenosis used to calculate the WBAS, this may have confounded the results. However, a separate study by groups have found no reduction in

Table 5. Relationships between standardised atheroma scores by region and common carotid intima media thickness (CIMT) and rest ankle-brachial pressure index (ABPI).

Region	Unadjusted model		Adjusted model*	
	CIMT	ABPI	CIMT	ABPI
Whole body	0.32‡	−0.39‡	0.13	−0.45‡
Thoracic	0.42‡	−0.17	0.33	−0.45
Abdomen	0.27	−0.30‡	0.2	−0.47‡
Ilio-femoral	0.09	−0.52‡	0.1	−0.56‡
Distal run-off	0.06	−0.13	0.19	−0.62

The ABPI values used for this analysis are the higher of the two lower limb measurements.
* Adjusted model accounts for all factors with a $p>0.3$ in the univariate analysis. Thus the model was adjusted for age, systolic and diastolic blood pressure, presence of diabetes and prescription of statins. Results expressed as β co-efficient.
‡ $p<0.05$.

CIMT with statin therapy [10], and a study using MRI volumetric plaque analysis showed statins to reduce plaque volume in the carotid arteries despite no change in the CIMT [39]. Thus the impact of statin therapy on the current results is uncertain.

In the current study we used common CIMT as this is the most established technique for assessing IMT, however the internal CIMT and carotid plaque dimensions on ultrasound have both been suggested as more discerning alternatives to common CIMT [40,41].

Additionally WB-MRA does not assess the coronary vessels. Coronary MRA is still someway off routine clinical practice although this is a promising area with several studies showing accurate assessment of the proximal vessels and integration of this in the future is a possibility [42].

In conclusion, CIMT and ABPI are markers of local atherosclerotic stenotic plaque burden but not systemic plaque burden in a population with peripheral arterial disease. Thus the techniques may be complimentary in their assessment of the vascular system.

Author Contributions

Conceived and designed the experiments: JRWM FK SJG PGR PR JJFB ADS ADM JGH. Performed the experiments: JRWM FK MAL MG SJG PGR JGH. Analyzed the data: JRWM PR FK MAL CLA MG SJG PGR JJFB ADS ADM JGH. Contributed reagents/materials/analysis tools: FK PR SJG JJFB ADS ADM JGH. Wrote the paper: JRWM FK MAL CLA MG SJG PGR PR JJFB ADS ADM JGH.

References

1. Lorenz MW, Schaefer C, Steinmetz H, Sitzer M (2010) Is carotid intima media thickness useful for individual prediction of cardiovascular risk? Ten-year results from the Carotid Atherosclerosis Progression Study (CAPS). Eur Heart J 31: 2041–2048. Available: http://www.ncbi.nlm.nih.gov/pubmed/20530503. Accessed 2013 Dec 29.
2. Crouse JR, Raichlen JS, Riley WA, Evans GW, Palmer MK, et al. (2007) Effect of rosuvastatin on progression of carotid intima-media thickness in low-risk individuals with subclinical atherosclerosis: the METEOR Trial. JAMA 297: 1344–1353. Available: http://www.ncbi.nlm.nih.gov/pubmed/17384434. Accessed 2013 Dec 29.
3. Espeland MA, O'leary DH, Terry JG, Morgan T, Evans G, et al. (2005) Carotid intimal-media thickness as a surrogate for cardiovascular disease events in trials of HMG-CoA reductase inhibitors. Curr Control Trials Cardiovasc Med 6: 3. Available: http://www.pubmedcentral.nih.gov/articlerender.fcgi?artid = 555546&tool = pmcentrez&rendertype = abstract. Accessed 2013 Dec 29.
4. Fitch KV, Stavrou E, Looby SE, Hemphill L, Jaff MR, et al. (2011) Associations of cardiovascular risk factors with two surrogate markers of subclinical atherosclerosis: endothelial function and carotid intima media thickness. Atherosclerosis 217: 437–440. Available: http://www.pubmedcentral.nih.gov/articlerender.fcgi?artid = 3146552&tool = pmcentrez&rendertype = abstract. Accessed 2013 Dec 29.
5. Peters SAE, Grobbee DE, Bots ML (2011) Carotid intima–media thickness: a suitable alternative for cardiovascular risk as outcome? Eur J Cardiovasc Prev Rehabil 18: 167–174. Available: http://www.ncbi.nlm.nih.gov/pubmed/21568017. Accessed 2013 Dec 29.
6. Bots ML, Evans GW, Riley WA, Grobbee DE (2003) Carotid intima-media thickness measurements in intervention studies: design options, progression rates, and sample size considerations: a point of view. Stroke 34: 2985–2994. Available: http://www.ncbi.nlm.nih.gov/pubmed/14615619. Accessed 2013 Dec 29.
7. Costanzo P, Perrone-Filardi P, Vassallo E, Paolillo S, Cesarano P, et al. (2010) Does carotid intima-media thickness regression predict reduction of cardiovascular events? A meta-analysis of 41 randomized trials. J Am Coll Cardiol 56: 2006–2020. Available: http://www.ncbi.nlm.nih.gov/pubmed/21126642. Accessed 2013 Dec 29.
8. Helfand M, Buckley DI, Freeman M, Fu R, Rogers K, et al. (2009) Emerging risk factors for coronary heart disease: a summary of systematic reviews conducted for the U.S. Preventive Services Task Force. Ann Intern Med 151: 496–507. Available: http://www.ncbi.nlm.nih.gov/pubmed/19805772. Accessed 2013 Dec 13.
9. Den Ruijter HM, Peters S a E, Anderson TJ, Britton AR, Dekker JM, et al. (2012) Common carotid intima-media thickness measurements in cardiovascular risk prediction: a meta-analysis. JAMA 308: 796–803. Available: http://www.ncbi.nlm.nih.gov/pubmed/22999719. Accessed 2013 Dec 18.
10. Kastelein JJP, Akdim F, Stroes ESG, Zwinderman AH, Bots ML, et al. (2008) Simvastatin with or without ezetimibe in familial hypercholesterolemia. N Engl J Med 358: 1431–1443. Available: http://www.ncbi.nlm.nih.gov/pubmed/18376000. Accessed 2013 Dec 30.
11. Fowkes FGR, Murray GD, Butcher I, Heald CL, Lee RJ, et al. (2008) Ankle brachial index combined with Framingham Risk Score to predict cardiovascular events and mortality: a meta-analysis. JAMA 300: 197–208. Available: http://www.pubmedcentral.nih.gov/articlerender.fcgi?artid = 2932628&tool = pmcentrez&rendertype = abstract. Accessed 2014 Feb 2.
12. Espinola-Klein C, Rupprecht HJ, Bickel C, Lackner K, Savvidis S, et al. (2008) Different calculations of ankle-brachial index and their impact on cardiovascular risk prediction. Circulation 118: 961–967. Available: http://www.ncbi.nlm.nih.gov/pubmed/18697822. Accessed 2014 Feb 2.
13. Hansen T, Ahlström H, Wikström J, Lind L, Johansson L (2008) A total atherosclerotic score for whole-body MRA and its relation to traditional cardiovascular risk factors. Eur Radiol 18: 1174–1180. Available: http://www.ncbi.nlm.nih.gov/pubmed/18270716. Accessed 2014 Feb 4.
14. Fenchel M, Scheule AM, Stauder NI, Kramer U, Tomaschko K, et al. (2006) Atherosclerotic disease: whole-body cardiovascular imaging with MR system with 32 receiver channels and total-body surface coil technology–initial clinical results. Radiology 238: 280–291. Available: http://www.ncbi.nlm.nih.gov/pubmed/16304083. Accessed 2013 Dec 29.
15. Ruehm SG, Goehde SC, Goyen M (2004) Whole body MR angiography screening. Int J Cardiovasc Imaging 20: 587–591. Available: http://www.ncbi.nlm.nih.gov/pubmed/15856646. Accessed 2013 Dec 29.
16. Goehde SC, Hunold P, Vogt FM, Ajaj W, Goyen M, et al. (2005) Full-body cardiovascular and tumor MRI for early detection of disease: feasibility and initial experience in 298 subjects. AJR Am J Roentgenol 184: 598–611. Available: http://www.ajronline.org/doi/abs/10.2214/ajr.184.2.01840598. Accessed 2013 Dec 19.
17. Lehrke S, Egenlauf B, Steen H, Lossnitzer D, Korosoglou G, et al. (2009) Prediction of coronary artery disease by a systemic atherosclerosis score index derived from whole-body MR angiography. J Cardiovasc Magn Reson 11: 36. Available: http://www.pubmedcentral.nih.gov/articlerender.fcgi?artid = 2758875&tool = pmcentrez&rendertype = abstract. Accessed 2013 Dec 19.
18. Lundberg C, Johansson L, Barbier CE, Lind L, Ahlström H, et al. (2013) Total atherosclerotic burden by whole body magnetic resonance angiography predicts major adverse cardiovascular events. Atherosclerosis 228: 148–152. Available: http://www.sciencedirect.com/science/article/pii/S0021915013001251. Accessed 2013 Dec 19.
19. Bamberg F, Parhofer KG, Lochner E, Marcus RP, Theisen D, et al. (2013) Diabetes Mellitus: Long-term Prognostic Value of Whole-Body MR Imaging for the Occurrence of Cardiac and Cerebrovascular Events. Radiology 269: 730–737. Available: http://www.ncbi.nlm.nih.gov/pubmed/24023074. Accessed 2013 Dec 19.
20. Lind L, Andersson J, Hansen T, Johansson L, Ahlström H (2009) Atherosclerosis measured by whole body magnetic resonance angiography and carotid artery ultrasound is related to arterial compliance, but not to endothelium-dependent vasodilation - the Prospective Investigation of the Vasculature in Uppsala Seniors (PIV. Clin Physiol Funct Imaging 29: 321–329. Available: http://www.ncbi.nlm.nih.gov/pubmed/19486081. Accessed 2013 Jun 14.
21. Matsumae T, Abe Y, Murakami G, Ishihara M, Ueda K, et al. (2007) Determinants of arterial wall stiffness and peripheral artery occlusive disease in nondiabetic hemodialysis patients. Hypertens Res 30: 377–385. Available: http://www.ncbi.nlm.nih.gov/pubmed/17587749. Accessed 2014 Apr 18.
22. Brevetti G, Silvestro A, Schiano V, Chiariello M (2003) Endothelial dysfunction and cardiovascular risk prediction in peripheral arterial disease: additive value of flow-mediated dilation to ankle-brachial pressure index. Circulation 108: 2093–2098. Available: http://www.ncbi.nlm.nih.gov/pubmed/14530195. Accessed 2014 Apr 18.
23. Coskun U, Yildiz A, Esen OB, Baskurt M, Cakar MA, et al. (2009) Relationship between carotid intima-media thickness and coronary angiographic findings: a prospective study. doi:10.1186/1476-7120-7-59.
24. Kwon T-G, Kim K-W, Park H-W, Jeong J-H, Kim K-Y, et al. (2009) Prevalence and significance of carotid plaques in patients with coronary atherosclerosis. Korean Circ J 39: 317–321. doi:10.4070/kcj.2009.39.8.317.
25. Sadeghi M, Heidari R, Mostanfar B, Tavassoli A, Roghani F, et al. (2011) The Relation Between Ankle-Brachial Index (ABI) and Coronary Artery Disease Severity and Risk Factors: An Angiographic Study. ARYA Atheroscler 7: 68–73. Available: http://www.pubmedcentral.nih.gov/articlerender.fcgi?artid = 3347847&tool = pmcentrez&rendertype = abstract. Accessed 2014 Feb 7.
26. Papamichael CM, Lekakis JP, Stamatelopoulos KS, Papaioannou TG, Alevizaki MK, et al. (2000) Ankle-brachial index as a predictor of the extent of coronary atherosclerosis and cardiovascular events in patients with coronary artery disease. Am J Cardiol 86: 615–618. Available: http://www.ncbi.nlm.nih.gov/pubmed/10980210. Accessed 2014 Jan 31.
27. Waugh SA, Ramkumar PG, Gandy SJ, Nicholas RS, Martin P, et al. (2009) Optimization of the contrast dose and injection rates in whole-body MR

angiography at 3.0T. J Magn Reson Imaging 30: 1059–1067. Available: http://www.ncbi.nlm.nih.gov/pubmed/19856438. Accessed 2013 Dec 19.
28. Engelen L, Ferreira I, Stehouwer CD, Boutouyrie P, Laurent S (2013) Reference intervals for common carotid intima-media thickness measured with echotracking: relation with risk factors. Eur Heart J 34: 2368–2380. Available: http://www.ncbi.nlm.nih.gov/pubmed/23186808. Accessed 2014 Apr 17.
29. Aboyans V, Criqui MH, Abraham P, Allison M a, Creager M a, et al. (2012) Measurement and interpretation of the ankle-brachial index: a scientific statement from the American Heart Association. Circulation 126: 2890–2909. Available: http://www.ncbi.nlm.nih.gov/pubmed/23159553. Accessed 2014 Feb 3.
30. Nead KT, Cooke JP, Olin JW, Leeper NJ (2013) Alternative ankle-brachial index method identifies additional at-risk individuals. J Am Coll Cardiol 62: 553–559. Available: http://www.ncbi.nlm.nih.gov/pubmed/23707317. Accessed 2014 Feb 2.
31. Lorenz MW, Markus HS, Bots ML, Rosvall M, Sitzer M (2007) Prediction of clinical cardiovascular events with carotid intima-media thickness: a systematic review and meta-analysis. Circulation 115: 459–467. Available: http://www.ncbi.nlm.nih.gov/pubmed/17242284. Accessed 2014 Apr 23.
32. Folsom AR, Kronmal RA, Detrano RC, O'Leary DH, Bild DE, et al. (2008) Coronary artery calcification compared with carotid intima-media thickness in the prediction of cardiovascular disease incidence: the Multi-Ethnic Study of Atherosclerosis (MESA). Arch Intern Med 168: 1333–1339. Available: http://www.pubmedcentral.nih.gov/articlerender.fcgi?artid = 2555989&tool = pmcentrez&rendertype = abstract. Accessed 2014 Apr 23.
33. Lerman A, Zeiher AM (2005) Endothelial function: cardiac events. Circulation 111: 363–368. Available: http://www.ncbi.nlm.nih.gov/pubmed/15668353. Accessed 2013 Dec 31.
34. De Simone G, McClelland R, Gottdiener JS, Celentano A, Kronmal RA, et al. (2001) Relation of hemodynamics and risk factors to ventricular-vascular interactions in the elderly: the Cardiovascular Health Study. J Hypertens 19: 1893–1903. Available: http://www.ncbi.nlm.nih.gov/pubmed/11593112. Accessed 2014 Apr 18.
35. Yeboah J, Burke GL, Crouse JR, Herrington DM (2008) Relationship between brachial flow-mediated dilation and carotid intima-media thickness in an elderly cohort: the Cardiovascular Health Study. Atherosclerosis 197: 840–845. Available: http://www.ncbi.nlm.nih.gov/pubmed/17804000. Accessed 2014 Apr 18.
36. Wikström J, Hansen T, Johansson L, Ahlström H, Lind L (2009) Lower extremity artery stenosis distribution in an unselected elderly population and its relation to a reduced ankle-brachial index. J Vasc Surg 50: 330–334. Available: http://www.ncbi.nlm.nih.gov/pubmed/19446989. Accessed 2013 Dec 30.
37. Van der Meer IM, Bots ML, Hofman A, del Sol AI, van der Kuip D a M, et al. (2004) Predictive value of noninvasive measures of atherosclerosis for incident myocardial infarction: the Rotterdam Study. Circulation 109: 1089–1094. Available: http://www.ncbi.nlm.nih.gov/pubmed/14993130. Accessed 2014 Apr 23.
38. Nozue T, Yamamoto S, Tohyama S, Umezawa S, Kunishima T, et al. (2012) Statin treatment for coronary artery plaque composition based on intravascular ultrasound radiofrequency data analysis. Am Heart J 163: 191–9.e1. Available: http://www.ncbi.nlm.nih.gov/pubmed/22305836. Accessed 2013 Dec 30.
39. Migrino RQ, Bowers M, Harmann L, Prost R, LaDisa JF (2011) Carotid plaque regression following 6-month statin therapy assessed by 3T cardiovascular magnetic resonance: comparison with ultrasound intima media thickness. J Cardiovasc Magn Reson 13: 37. Available: http://www.pubmedcentral.nih.gov/articlerender.fcgi?artid = 3166901&tool = pmcentrez&rendertype = abstract. Accessed 2013 Dec 19.
40. Polak JF, Pencina MJ, Pencina KM, O'Donnell CJ, Wolf PA, et al. (2011) Carotid-wall intima-media thickness and cardiovascular events. N Engl J Med 365: 213–221. Available: http://www.pubmedcentral.nih.gov/articlerender.fcgi?artid = 3153949&tool = pmcentrez&rendertype = abstract. Accessed 2013 Dec 18.
41. Inaba Y, Chen JA, Bergmann SR (2012) Carotid plaque, compared with carotid intima-media thickness, more accurately predicts coronary artery disease events: a meta-analysis. Atherosclerosis 220: 128–133. Available: http://www.ncbi.nlm.nih.gov/pubmed/21764060. Accessed 2013 Dec 30.
42. Sakuma H (2011) Coronary CT versus MR angiography: the role of MR angiography. Radiology 258: 340–349. Available: http://www.scopus.com/inward/record.url?eid = 2-s2.0-79952398815&partnerID = 40&md5 = d8e12db65df5edd617bfaa06afd7e11e. Accessed 2013 Dec 30.

14

Multidimensional Compressed Sensing MRI Using Tensor Decomposition-Based Sparsifying Transform

Yeyang Yu*, Jin Jin, Feng Liu, Stuart Crozier

School of Information Technology and Electrical Engineering, the University of Queensland, St Lucia, Queensland, Australia

Abstract

Compressed Sensing (CS) has been applied in dynamic Magnetic Resonance Imaging (MRI) to accelerate the data acquisition without noticeably degrading the spatial-temporal resolution. A suitable sparsity basis is one of the key components to successful CS applications. Conventionally, a multidimensional dataset in dynamic MRI is treated as a series of two-dimensional matrices, and then various matrix/vector transforms are used to explore the image sparsity. Traditional methods typically sparsify the spatial and temporal information independently. In this work, we propose a novel concept of tensor sparsity for the application of CS in dynamic MRI, and present the Higher-order Singular Value Decomposition (HOSVD) as a practical example. Applications presented in the three- and four-dimensional MRI data demonstrate that HOSVD simultaneously exploited the correlations within spatial and temporal dimensions. Validations based on cardiac datasets indicate that the proposed method achieved comparable reconstruction accuracy with the low-rank matrix recovery methods and, outperformed the conventional sparse recovery methods.

Editor: Xi-Nian Zuo, Institute of Psychology, Chinese Academy of Sciences, China

Funding: The authors have no funding or support to report.

Competing Interests: The authors have declared that no competing interests exist.

* E-mail: yeyang.yu@uqconnect.edu.au

Introduction

Dynamic MRI (dMRI) plays a vital role in many clinical applications, such as cardiac, perfusion and functional brain imaging. In these applications, high spatial-temporal resolution is desired to reveal anatomical details and physiological dynamics. Conventionally, the data is acquired in chronological order adhering to Nyquist sampling theorem, making MRI a relatively slow imaging modality. Routine methods speed up the MRI acquisition using a combination of fast gradient and Radio Frequency (RF) pulsing with full *k*-space sampling [1,2]. However, owing to hardware and physiological constraints, achieving high spatiotemporal resolutions with hardware intensive sequences is technologically challenging.

Instead of increasing the data sampling rate, various approaches, including Compressed Sensing (CS) [3], have attempted to reconstruct full field-of-view (FOV) images from sub-Nyquist acquisitions. CS has been recently applied to MRI to accelerate the data collecting process. The pioneering work of applying CS to MRI to accelerate the data collecting process can be found in [4,5]. CS states that a faithful reconstruction of the signal is achievable with a sampling rate far lower than the Nyquist limit, provided that the signal has a sparse representation in some transform basis (called the 'sparsity basis'), which must be incoherent with the sensing matrix (i.e., Fourier transform in MRI) [3,6]. In static MRI and dMRI, the incoherence between the sensing basis and the sparsity basis can be achieved by randomly acquiring data in the *k*-space or *k-t* space [3,7]. Both the predefined sparsity bases [8] and the data-dependent (also called data-derived) transforms [9,10] have provided successful reconstructions in static MRI applications.

CS has also been applied to dMRI, where the data sets are naturally higher-order tensors (for instance, a *third*-order tensor for a cine MRI and a *fourth*-order tensor for a volume dMRI). Conventionally, 2D/1D sparsity bases were used to account for the spatial and temporal sparsity. When the method *k-t* SPARSE [4] was applied to the cine cardiac data, the 2D wavelet transform was first applied in the spatial domain, followed by the 1D Fourier transform along the temporal dimension. The non-linear conjugate gradient algorithm [11] was then used to reconstruct the sparsity coefficients. This is a practical and straightforward extension of the SPARSE MRI [8] as used in the static scenario. However, using 2D wavelet transforms may generate smooth/blurry reconstructions at the image boundaries. Alternatively, the *k-t* FOCUSS method [12,13] applied different transforms to sparsify diverse MRI signals and explored the temporal sparsity by employing Principle Component Analysis and Fourier transform for the aperiodic and periodic/pseudo-periodic data, respectively. Then the recursively weighted minimum norm reconstruction algorithm (called 'FOCUSS') [14,15] was used to reconstruct the sparsity coefficients. Also using the FOCUSS algorithm, the *k-t* ISD [16] improved the CS reconstruction by exploiting the support information from the *x-f* space. Recent methods studied the anatomical structures or features [17,18] to further improve the reconstruction. Extending the application of sparsity, theoretical works [19–25] have investigated the low-rank matrix completion/recovery for more efficient signal recovery. The applications of the low-rank matrix structure have demonstrated merits in exploring the spatial-temporal signal redundancy in dMRI. For example, the methods described in [26–34] used sparse sampling schemes for data acquisition, and then generated basis functions for low-rank regularisation or to model the dMRI signals. The function bases in methods [26–28] were tailored from the training data of the objects, they were more capable of capturing the correlations among the dynamic image series. The quality of the reconstructions achieved by these methods, however, relied heavily on the quality of the training data. Some other methods [29–34] used the combination of sparse sampling and low-rank regularisation without training data.

Essentially, most of the existing CS-dMRI methods intend to use 2D/1D transforms to solve 3D or even higher-dimension problems. They either treat the 3D/4D data as a series of 2D images and then employ 2D/1D sparsifying transforms to explore spatial/temporal sparsity [4,12,13] or, unfold the higher-order dataset into a 2D matrix to explore the spatiotemporal redundancy [29–31,35]. Intuitively, using matrix/vector transforms in dMRI data, being a higher-order tensor in nature, may not simultaneously explore the inherent data redundancy. To investigate the possibilities of preserving the higher-dimensional data format, this work proposes a novel concept of tensor sparsity for dMRI. Inspired by a recent application of the *second*-order Singular Value Decomposition (SVD) [9,10] in exploiting in-plane sparsity, the Tucker model based Higher-order Singular Value Decomposition (HOSVD) [36,37] was employed as a practical example for the current investigation. Tensor sparsity or tensor rank, is a powerful multidimensional signal processing tool that has been successfully applied in various areas. For instance in the area of pattern recognition/computer vision, HOSVD has been used to extract the features of the training dataset to recognise/classify future images (such as face verification) [38,39]. Recently, a low n-rank tensor approach has also been successfully applied to dMRI to achieve high quality image reconstruction for parallel and dMRI [33]. Instead of regularising the global low-rank structure, improved reconstruction accuracy and resolution were achieved by exploiting the local low-rank structure for multidimensional MR signals, where the unknown values of the image matrices were locally estimated by considering the correlation among neighbour pixels or voxels [32,34]. Comprehensive reviews of the applications of tensor decomposition, are provided in [40,41]. The HOSVD in the current study takes advantage of the fact that the signals in dMRI scenario are higher-order tensors. The presented approach sparsifies the dMRI signals in their original tensor format instead of the matrix format. Three experiments were designed to present the comparisons of the performances between this tensor sparsity basis and matrix transforms. In the first and the second experiments, the *third*-order SVD (3D-SVD) was used to sparsify the cine cardiac data (two spatial dimensions plus one temporal dimension). These experiments aim to compare the performance of the proposed method for pseudo-periodical data with two existing methods in dMRI. In the third experiment, the *fourth*-order SVD (4D-SVD) was applied as sparsity basis for the dynamic volume cardiac data (three spatial dimensions plus one temporal dimension), where the feasibility of the proposed sparsity basis in 4D application is demonstrated.

The remainder of this article is organised as follows. Section 2 explains the theoretical background of the proposed method. Section 3 describes the materials and methods used for validations. Section 4 presents the comparisons of the reconstruction results between the proposed method and the existing methods. Section 5 discusses additional properties of the proposed sparsity basis. Section 6 concludes the contribution of this work.

Theory

In this section the general formulation of dMRI reconstruction in CS framework is first introduced. Then, the construction of a key component, the spasifying transform using tensor decomposition, is described.

2.1. Formulation of Compressed Sensing in Dynamic MRI (CS-dMRI)

To assist the discussion, the notations of scalars, vectors, matrices (*second*-order tensors) and tensors are denoted by lowercase letters (a, b, …), capital letters (A, B, …) and calligraphic letters ($\mathcal{A}$, $\mathcal{B}$, …), respectively. Letter i and j are used to index row and column vectors, respectively. $(A)_j = A_j = a_j$, for example, denotes the jth column vector of matrix A. Hence, $A = (A_1, A_2, \ldots, A_J)$, where J is reserved for the index upper bounds, as is I. $(A)_{ij}$, also symbolised as a_{ij}, denotes the element with a row index i and a column index j.

Suppose an Nth-order tensor $\mathcal{A} \in \mathbb{C}^{I_1 \times I_2 \times \ldots \times I_N}$ is used to represent the spatial-temporal behaviour of the imaged object. Without losing generality, the first $M = N$-1 dimensions of the tensor are used to describe the spatial information (for example $M = 2$ for 2D slice or $M = 3$ for 3D volume), which is collected at I_N time instances. The CS-dMRI problem can be solved using the following optimisation procedure:

$$\begin{aligned} &Minimise : \|\Psi(\mathcal{A})\|_0 \\ &s.t. \|\Phi_F(\mathcal{A}) - y\| < \epsilon \end{aligned} \tag{1}$$

where y is the k space measurements collected from the MRI scanner; ε represents the data-fidelity tolerance between the optimisation result and the measurements; Ψ is a transform that sparsifies the tensor $\mathcal{A}$ (the imaging object), and Φ_F is a combination of operations, that is, the 2D Fourier transform for the in-plane data followed by a random under-sampling.

Equation (1) minimises the l_0-norm to enforce the sparsity of the object $\mathcal{A}$, and uses the l_2-norm as a constraint to guarantee the data-fidelity in the sampling domain. The optimisation problem in equation (1) is NP-hard (Non-deterministic Polynomial-time hard). The common solution for this problem is to relax the l_0 norm to l_1 norm, its nearest convex constraint [42]. Thus, the problem in equation (1) can be restated as:

$$\begin{aligned} &Minimise : \|\Psi(\mathcal{A})\|_1 \\ &s.t. \|\Phi_F(\mathcal{A}) - y\| < \epsilon \end{aligned} \tag{2}$$

However, as has been extensively studied [43–48], replacing the l_1 norm with an l_p quasi-norm ($0<p<1$) problem can reduce the amount of measurements needed for reconstruction or, can improve the reconstruction quality given the same amount of measurements. Therefore, in this work, we adopt the l_p norm as a constraint to enforce the sparsity of the images. Thus, the NP-hard problem in equation (1) can be replaced by solving a problem as follows:

$$\begin{aligned} &Minimise : \|\Psi(\mathcal{A})\|_p^p \\ &s.t. \|\Phi_F(\mathcal{A}) - y\| < \epsilon \end{aligned} \tag{3}$$

where $0<p<1$. Section 3 will describe in detail the algorithm adopted to solve the non-convex problem in the form of equation (3).

2.2. Construction of the Sparsity Basis Ψ using Higher-order Singular Value Decomposition

In this section, the general framework of HOSVD [37] and the applications of HOSVD as sparsifying transform in CS-dMRI will be introduced. Several higher-order tensor operations will be introduced first to pave the way for the discussion of HOSVD. The HOSVD sparsity basis was obtained from the inverse Fourier transform of the zero-filled under-sampled *k* space (denoted as $\mathcal{A}_0$), therefore no training data is required in this method.

Definition 1: Matrix unfolding-unfolding a tensor into matrices [37].

For the *Nth*-order tensor $\mathcal{A}_0 \in \mathbb{C}^{I_1 \times I_2 \times \ldots \times I_N}$, the unfolded matrix $\boldsymbol{A_{0(n)}}$ contains the element $a_{0_{i_1 i_2 \ldots i_n}}$ at the position with a row number i_n and a column number equal to

$$(i_{n+1}-1)I_{n+2}I_{n+3}\ldots I_N I_1 I_2 \ldots I_{n-1}+$$
$$(i_{n+2}-1)I_{n+3}I_{n+4}\ldots I_1 I_2 \ldots I_{n-1}+\ldots+$$
$$(i_N-1)I_1 I_2 \ldots I_{n-1}+(i_2-1)I_3 I_4 \ldots I_{n-1}+\ldots+i_{n-1}$$

Figure 1(a) exemplifies the process of unfolding a 3D tensor. There are three matrix representations (horizontal, lateral, and frontal) of the 3D tensor $\mathcal{A}_0 \in \mathbb{C}^{I_1 \times I_2 \times I_3}$ in which all the slices are stacked one after another. The lateral matrix representation $A_{0(1)} \in \mathbb{C}^{I_1 I_3 \times I_2}$ is defined as $[A_{0(1)}]_{(i_1-1)I_3+i_3,i_2} = a_{0_{i_1 i_2 i_3}}$; the frontal matrix representation $A_{0(2)} \in \mathbb{C}^{I_2 I_1 \times I_3}$ is defined as $[A_{0(2)}]_{(i_2-1)I_1+i_1,i_3} = a_{0_{i_1 i_2 i_3}}$; and

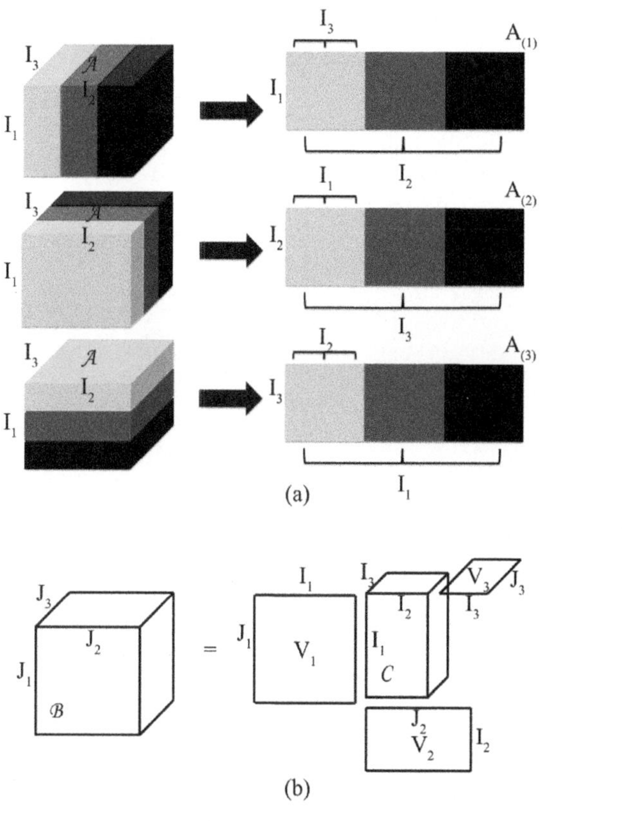

Figure 1. Visualisation of matrix unfolding of a tensor. (a) Visualises the matrix unfolding of a *third*-order tensor and, (b) visualises a *third*-order tensor multiplied by matrix.

the horizontal matrix representation $A_{0(3)} \in \mathbb{C}^{I_3 I_2 \times I_1}$ is defined as $[A_{0(3)}]_{(i_3-1)I_2+i_2,i_1} = a_{0_{i_1 i_2 i_3}}$.

Definition 2: Multiplication of a higher-order tensor by matrices [37].

The *n-mode* product of the tensor $\mathcal{A}_0 \in \mathbb{C}^{I_1 \times I_2 \times \ldots \times I_N}$ by a matrix $U \in \mathbb{C}^{J_n \times I_n}$, denoted as $\mathcal{A}_0 \times_n U$ is an $(I_1 \times I_2 \times \ldots \times I_{n-1} \times J_n \times I_{n+1} \times \ldots \times I_N)$ tensor, of which the entries are given by

$$(\mathcal{A}_0 \times_n U)_{i_1 i_2 \ldots i_{n-1} j_n i_{n+1} \ldots i_N} \overset{def}{=} \sum_{i_n} a_{0_{i_1 i_2 \ldots i_{n-1} i_n i_{n+1} \ldots i_N}} u_{j_n i_n}$$

Figure 1(b) visualises the multiplication of a 3D tensor by matrix, where $\mathcal{B} = \mathcal{C} \times_1 V_1 \times_2 V_2 \times_3 V_3$ $(\mathcal{B} = \mathbb{C}^{J_1 \times J_2 \times J_3}, \mathcal{C} = \mathbb{C}^{I_1 \times I_2 \times I_3})$. In figure 1(b) we can see that there are three multiplications of a 3D tensor by matrix. The *1-mode* product of the tensor $\mathcal{C} = \mathbb{C}^{I_1 \times I_2 \times I_3}$ by a matrix $V_1 \in \mathbb{C}^{J_1 \times I_1}$ is defined as $(\mathcal{C} \times_1 V_1)_{j_1 i_2 i_3} \overset{def}{=} \sum_{i_1} c_{i_1 i_2 i_3} v_{j_1 i_1}$, which is a $J_1 \times I_2 \times I_3$ sized tensor; the *2-mode* product of $\mathcal{C} = \mathbb{C}^{I_1 \times I_2 \times I_3}$ by a matrix $V_2 \in \mathbb{C}^{J_2 \times I_2}$ is defined as $(\mathcal{C} \times_2 V_2)_{i_1 j_2 i_3} \overset{def}{=} \sum_{i_2} c_{i_1 i_2 i_3} v_{j_2 i_2}$, which is a $I_1 \times J_2 \times I_3$ sized tensor; similarly, the *3-mode* product of $\mathcal{C} = \mathbb{C}^{I_1 \times I_2 \times I_3}$ by a matrix $V_3 \in \mathbb{C}^{J_3 \times I_3}$ is defined as $(\mathcal{C} \times_3 V_3)_{i_1 i_2 j_3} \overset{def}{=} \sum_{i_3} c_{i_1 i_2 i_3} v_{j_3 i_3}$, which is an $I_1 \times I_2 \times J_3$ sized tensor.

With these two operations defined, any *Nth*-order tensor $\mathcal{A}_0 \in \mathbb{C}^{I_1 \times I_2 \times \ldots \times I_N}$ can now be decomposed, in the HOSVD framework, by

$$a_{0_{i_1 i_2 i_3 \ldots i_N}} = \sum_{j_1}^{I_1} \sum_{j_2}^{I_2} \ldots \sum_{j_N}^{I_N} s_{j_1 j_2 \ldots j_N} u^{(1)}_{i_1 j_1} u^{(2)}_{i_2 j_2} \ldots u^{(N)}_{i_N j_N} \quad (4)$$

where $u^{(n)}_{i_n j_n}, n = 1,2,\ldots,N$, are the entries of the unitary matrices $U_n, n = 1,2,\ldots,N$, and $s_{j_1 j_2 j_3 \ldots j_N}$ are the entries of $\mathcal{S} \in \mathbb{C}^{I_1 \times I_2 \ldots \times I_N}$ which is a complex tensor of size $I_1 \times I_2 \times \ldots \times I_N$. To facilitate the understanding of the properties of HOSVD, we first retrospect to the matrix SVD, which was used as a sparsity basis for static MRI [9,10]. For any complex matrix $M \in \mathbb{C}^{I_1 \times I_2}$, we can decompose it into product as

$$M = USV^H = S \times_1 U \times_2 V^H = S \times_1 U_1 \times_2 U_2 \quad (5)$$

where $U_n, n = 1,2$, are $I_n \times I_n, n = 1,2$, sized unitary matrices, and S is an $I_1 \times I_2$ sized matrix with the properties of [37]:

(i) pseudo-diagonality: $S = diag(\sigma_1, \sigma_2, \ldots, \sigma_{\min(I_1, I_2)})$
(ii) ordering: $\sigma_1 \geq \sigma_2 \geq \ldots \geq \sigma_{\min(I_1, I_2)} \geq 0$

where σ_i are called the singular values of M.

Likewise, in higher-order situation, we can decompose any complex *Nth*-order tensor $\mathcal{A}_0 \in \mathbb{C}^{I_1 \times I_2 \times \ldots \times I_N}$ as

$$\mathcal{A}_0 = \mathcal{S} \times_1 U_1 \times_2 U_2 \times_3 \ldots \times_N U_N, \quad (6)$$

where the unitary matrices $U_n \in \mathbb{C}^{I_n \times I_n}, n = 1,2,\ldots,N$ are called the *n-mode* singular matrices. Tensor $\mathcal{S} \in \mathbb{C}^{I_1 \times I_2 \times \ldots \times I_N}$ has the following properties:

(i) all-orthogonality: two sub-tensors $\mathcal{S}_{i_n=\alpha}$ and $\mathcal{S}_{i_n=\beta}$ are orthogonal for all possible n, α and β subject to $\alpha \neq \beta$, which means $\langle \mathcal{S}_{i_n=\alpha}, \mathcal{S}_{i_n=\beta} \rangle = 0$ when $\alpha \neq \beta$,

(ii) ordering: $\|\mathcal{S}_{i_n=1}\| \geq \|\mathcal{S}_{i_n=2}\| \geq \ldots \geq \|\mathcal{S}_{i_n=I_n}\| \geq 0$ for all possible n,

where the Frobenius-norms $\|\mathcal{S}_{i_n=i}\|$, symbolised by $\sigma_i^{(n)}$, are called the *n-mode* singular values of $\mathcal{A}_0$.

As demonstrated in [37], given a *Nth*-order tensor $\mathcal{A}_0$, the *n-mode* singular matrix U_n in equation (6) is actually the left singular matrix of the correlated *n-mode* matrix unfolding of $\mathcal{A}_0$ (as per Definition 1 and 2). Therefore the computation of the HOSVD in equation (6) eventually leads to N different matrix SVD operations on the unfolded tensor. Therefore, the tensor $\mathcal{S}$ can be computed as

$$\mathcal{S} = \mathcal{A}_0 \times_1 U_1^H \times_2 U_2^H \times_3 \ldots \times_N U_N^H \tag{7}$$

For example, U_1 can be obtained by performing the matrix SVD on the *1-mode* unfolding matrix $A_{0(1)}$ as:

$$S_1 = U_1 A_{0(1)} V_1 \tag{8}$$

Generally, $U_n, n = 1,2,\ldots,N$, can be obtained by performing the matrix SVD on the *n-mode* unfolding matrix $A_{0(n)}$ as:

$$S_n = U_n A_{0(n)} V_n. \tag{9}$$

With the unitary matrices obtained, we can then construct the tensor sparsifying transform as:

$$\Psi(\mathcal{A}_0) = \mathcal{A}_0 \times_1 U_1^H \times_2 U_2^H \times_3 \ldots \times_N U_N^H \tag{10}$$

where the sparsity basis $U_n, n = 1,2,\ldots,N$ is obtained from the inverse Fourier transform of the zero-filled under-sampled k space $\mathcal{A}_0$.

The inverse sparsifying transform is then obtained as:

$$\Psi^{-1}(\mathcal{S}) = \mathcal{S} \times_1 U_1 \times_2 U_2 \times_3 \ldots \times_N U_N \tag{11}$$

Figure 2(a) visualises the decomposition of a *third*-order tensor $\mathcal{A}_0 \in \mathbb{C}^{I_1 \times I_2 \times I_3}$ as

$$\mathcal{A}_0 = \mathcal{S} \times_1 U_1 \times_2 U_2 \times_3 U_3 \tag{12}$$

The unitary matrices $U_n, n = 1,2,3$, in equation (12) can be obtained from equation (9). The properties of all-orthogonality and ordering [37] guarantee that most of the energy of tensor $\mathcal{S}$ accumulates around one vertex, and little energy distributes to the broad area away from this region. Therefore, tensor $\mathcal{S}$ has a sparse representation (refer to figure 2(a) for illustration). Likewise, figure 2(b) presents an example of the HOSVD in the *fourth*-order tensor case. It should be noted that the tensor $\mathcal{S}$ is shown in logarithmic scale to assist the presentation, because $\mathcal{S}$ is too sparse to be easily visible. It is clearly shown that in both 3D and 4D cases the coefficients with large values are highly concentrated in one voxel (light blue colour), while the vast majority of the elements in the $\mathcal{S}$ tensor are close to zero (deep blue colour).

Materials and Methods

To test the possibility of employing HOSVD as higher-order sparsifying transform in CS-dMRI applications, three experiments are designed: two cine cardiac MRI schemes and one dynamic volume cardiac MRI series.

3.1. Datasets

3.1.1. 3D-SVD: Application in cine cardiac MRI. Two sets of cine cardiac MRI data were used to validate the proposed method. The first dataset (Dataset A) was acquired at the University of Utah, which was used in the method k-t SLR [30]. 70 frames of k-space were acquired on a 3T Siemens scanner with the spatial resolution of 90×190 (phase encoding×frequency encoding). The cardiac data was obtained with a saturation recovery sequence (TR/TE = 2.5/1 ms, saturation recovery time = 100 ms). The second dataset (Dataset B) was acquired at Yonsei University Medical Center, which was used in the method k-t FOCUSS [12,13]. 25 frames of full k-space data was acquired using a 1.5T Philips system with an in-plane spatial resolution of 256×256. The cine cardiac data was obtained using steady-state free precession (SSFP) sequence with a flip angle of 50 degree and TR = 3.45 msec. The FOV was 345 mm×270 mm. The slice thickness was 10 mm. A few frames from both Dataset A and Dataset B are shown in figure 3(a, b).

3.1.2. 4D-SVD: Application in volume dynamic cardiac MRI. The third experiment investigated the possibility of employing the proposed HOSVD sparsifying transform for 4D dynamic cardiac MRI. The images of the this dataset (Dataset C) were of one subject, arbitrarily chosen from a total of 33 available subjects [49]. The measurements were acquired from a GE Genesis Signa MR scanner using the FIESTA protocol. The dimension of the subject data is 256×256×10×20 (phase encoding×frequency encoding×z position×time). It is noted that Dataset C is in DICOM (Digital Imaging and Communications in Medicine) format. Using the real-valued images, instead of the complex-valued k-space data, has made the reconstruction of the 4D experiment easier. A few frames from Dataset C are shown in figure 3(c).

3.2. Reconstruction

3.2.1. Optimisation algorithm. The l_p quasi-norm in equation (3) poses a non-convex optimisation problem. Theoretical work [44,46] has demonstrated that this non-convex problem is solvable and, the local minima can be avoided in practice [43,50]. The applications in the medical imaging context [30,45,47,48,51–55], have already demonstrated the practicability and advances of non-convex optimisation. In this work, we adopt the algorithms used in [30,47] to solve the optimisation problem stated in equation (3). In [47], Chartrand used both wavelet transform and discrete gradient to enforce the sparsity of the MR images. In [30], Lingala et al. used the combination of rank property and signal sparsity for reconstruction. In this work we use only the HOSVD for sparsity enforcement. Therefore we herein briefly state the modified optimisation process as follows.

We begin with the definition of a variable splitting operator:

$$\Theta(\mathcal{A}) \stackrel{def}{=} Minimise: \|\Psi(\mathcal{B})\|_p^p + \beta\|\mathcal{A}\text{-}\mathcal{B}\|_2 \tag{13}$$

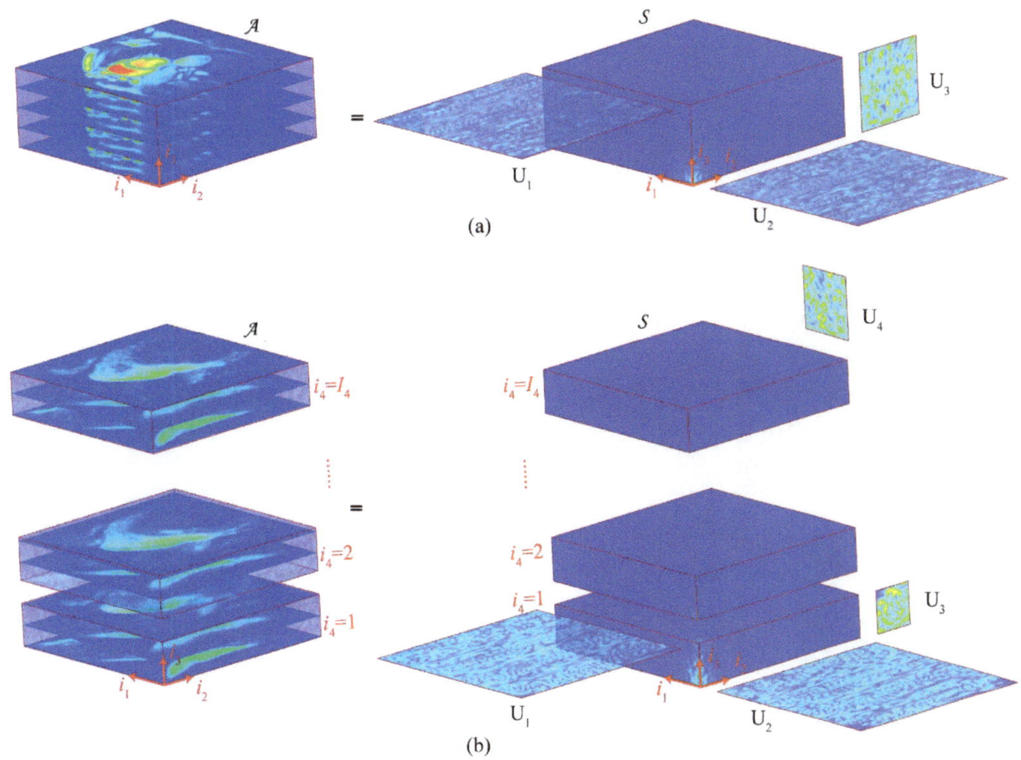

Figure 2. Visualisation of HOSVD. (a) Shows HOSVD on a *third*-order tensor and, (b) shows HOSVD on a *fourth*-order tensor. The left of (b) shows a four dimensional cardiac dataset denoted as **A**. The four dimensions are labelled as i_1, i_2, i_3 and i_4. The right of (b) presents tensor **S** and the unitary matrices U_1 U_2 U_3 and U_4, that were obtained by performing HOSVD operation on **A**. **S** is also a *fourth*-order tensor, the dimensions of which are marked as i_1, i_2, i_3 and i_4.

where $\beta > 0$ is a constant. It is noted that $\Theta(\mathcal{B})$ is forced to approach $\|\Psi(\mathcal{B})\|_p^p$ when $\beta \to \infty$.

We rewrite the problem in equation (3) as into its Lagrange's form as:

$$Minimise: \|\Phi_F(\mathcal{A}) - y\|_2 + \lambda\|\Psi(\mathcal{A})\|_p^p \quad (14)$$

where λ is a constant to balance the weighting between the data fidelity and the signal sparsity. Then the splitting operator was applied on equation (14), arriving at:

$$Minimise: \|\Phi_F(\mathcal{A}) - y\|_2 + \lambda\Theta(\mathcal{A}) \quad (15)$$

which can be expanded as:

$$Minimise: \|\Phi_F(\mathcal{A}) - y\|_2 + \beta\|\mathcal{A}\text{-}\mathcal{B}\|_2 + \lambda\|\Psi(\mathcal{B})\|_p^p \quad (16)$$

We can then solve the problem above by iteratively solving the variables $\mathcal{A}$ and $\mathcal{B}$ in turn. In this way the problem in equation (16) is decomposed into two simple sub-problems. The two sub-problems are decoupled, making it computational efficient. By setting $\beta \to \infty$, the solution of equation (16) approaches that of equation (14).

To solve the sub-problem with respect to variable $\mathcal{A}$, we can fix variable $\mathcal{B}$ and adopt the conjugate gradient algorithm as used in [30]:

$$Minimise: \|\Phi_F(\mathcal{A}) - y\|_2 + \beta\|\mathcal{A}\text{-}\mathcal{B}\|_2 \quad (17)$$

To solve the sub-problem with respect to variable $\mathcal{B}$, we fix variable $\mathcal{A}$ and apply p-shrinkage operator to each pixel of $\Psi(\mathcal{B})$. As explained in [47] the p-shrinkage operator is executed as:

$$S_\alpha^p(b) = max\{|b| - \alpha|b|^{p-1}, 0\}b/|b| \quad (18)$$

To choose an appropriate value for the parameter β, we initialised it with a relatively small value and then geometrically increased it as proposed in [56]. To enforce the data-fidelity, the residual of each sub-problem was added back to the data at each iteration as proposed in [57]. For a summary of the optimisation, please refer to figure 4.

3.3. Comparison Validations

The proposed method was compared with one of the recent low-rank image reconstruction methods, *k-t* SLR, and a classic CS method, *k-t* SPARSE. For fair comparison, we ensure that firstly all the methods used the same sampling pattern of *k-t* space; secondly, the parameters for all the methods were adjusted appropriately so that both the signal to error ratio (SER) and the averaged signal intensity for all methods were optimised; and thirdly the optimisations for all the methods share the same stopping criterion, that is the optimisations ceased when the gradient magnitude of the object function reached 1×10^{-4} or the

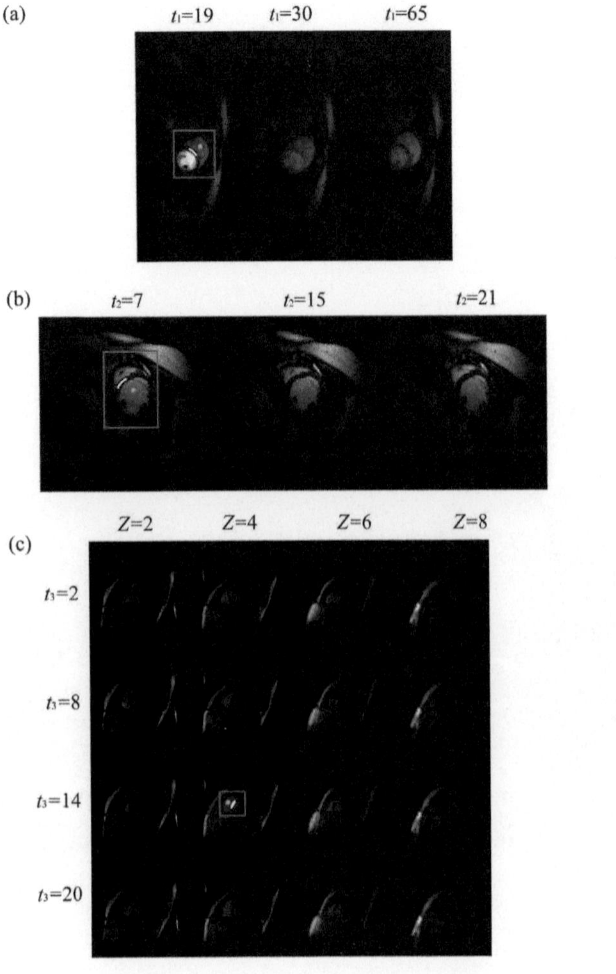

Figure 3. Several frames of the datasets obtained at different time instants (as indicated). From top to bottom: (a) Dataset A, (b) Dataset B and, (c) Dataset C. In (c), images obtained at four time instants (as indicated by t_3) are presented row by row, and images obtained at four z positions (as indicated by z, along axial direction (base-apex)) are presented column by column. The regions of interest of each dataset are marked within the red rectangles and, the regions of myocardial and blood pool used for averaged signal intensity comparison are marked with yellow and light blue colours, respectively.

number of iterations reached 300. All the evaluations were implemented using Matlab 2011a (MathWorks, Natick, MA) on a Mac OS X Lion operation system, with a dual-core 2.4 GHz Intel processor and 4 GB of memory. The SER was calculated as:

$$SER = -10\log_{10}\frac{\|A_{res}-A_{full}\|_F}{\|A_{full}\|}, \qquad (19)$$

where A_{res} is the result of the reconstruction, A_{full} is the fully sampled dynamic images, and $\|\cdot\|_F$ denotes the Frobenius norm. A greater SER value correlates to a better image quality.

The method *k-t* SLR employs two regularisations: the low-rank structure and the sparsity of the signal. To exploit the low-rank structure, *k-t* SLR reshaped the 3D dataset into a large 2D matrix $\mathbf{\Gamma}$. More specifically, the 2D images in a dynamic sequence were firstly vectorised and then concatenated to form the matrix $\mathbf{\Gamma}$. To exploit the sparsity of the signal, the total variation (TV) was used as an extra regularisation. Moreover, instead of using convex

```
Input: k-t space data y, parameters λ, β_1
---------------------------------------------------------
Initialisation: A_1 = Φ_F^{-1}(y), b_1 = 0
for n = 1: the number of outer iterations do
    while the stopping criterion is NOT satisfied do
        m = 1;
        update A_m to A_{m+1} by solving equation (17);
        apply shrinkage operator Ψ(B_{m+1}) = S^p_α(Ψ(A_{m+1}) + b_m);
        b_{m+1} = b_m + Ψ(B_{m+1});
        A_{m+1} = B_{m+1};
        m = m + 1;
    end
    β_{n+1} = β_n × INCREASE_PARAMETER;
end
---------------------------------------------------------
Output: A_m
```

Figure 4. Outline of the reconstruction algorithm.

penalties to regularise the low rank property and the sparsity, *k-t* SLR adopted some of the recent algorithms on the non-convex regularisation [43,47,48] for the optimisation, further improving the reconstruction result. In [30], the combination of the constraints provided better image quality than the variants of the *k-t* SLR, which rely on either matrix SVD or TV constraint alone. Therefore in this work, we only compare the proposed method with *k-t* SLR, where both SVD and the TV regularisations were used in the optimisation. The method *k-t* SPARSE is a classic CS-dMRI method. It uses the wavelet transform (Daubechies 4 was used as the mother wavelet in this work) for in-plane sparsity and the Fourier transform for temporal sparsity, assuming that the change of the heartbeat is periodical. All the methods compared in this work are flexible to account for arbitrary non-Cartesian *k*-space sampling schemes; we adopt the radial trajectory with uniform angular spacing as used in [30]. The trajectory was randomly rotated with a small angle for each frame to implement random sampling.

Results

4.1. 3D Application

Figure 5 and 6 show the reconstruction of Dataset A at reduction factors 6 and 11 respectively. When the reduction factor was 6 (reduction factor *n* means only *1/n* of the full *k*-space measurements were obtained), the SER values achieved by the proposed method, the *k-t* SLR and the *k-t* SPARSE, were 8.9 dB, 8.7 dB and, 7.7 dB, respectively. Figure 5 shows the reconstruction of Dataset A when the reduction factor was 6. As shown in figure 5(b), all the methods provided comparable averaged signal intensity for the blood pool area (normalised to the maximum grey level of the region of interest, figures 6, 7, 8, and 9 are normalised in the same fashion). However, when comparing at the myocardial

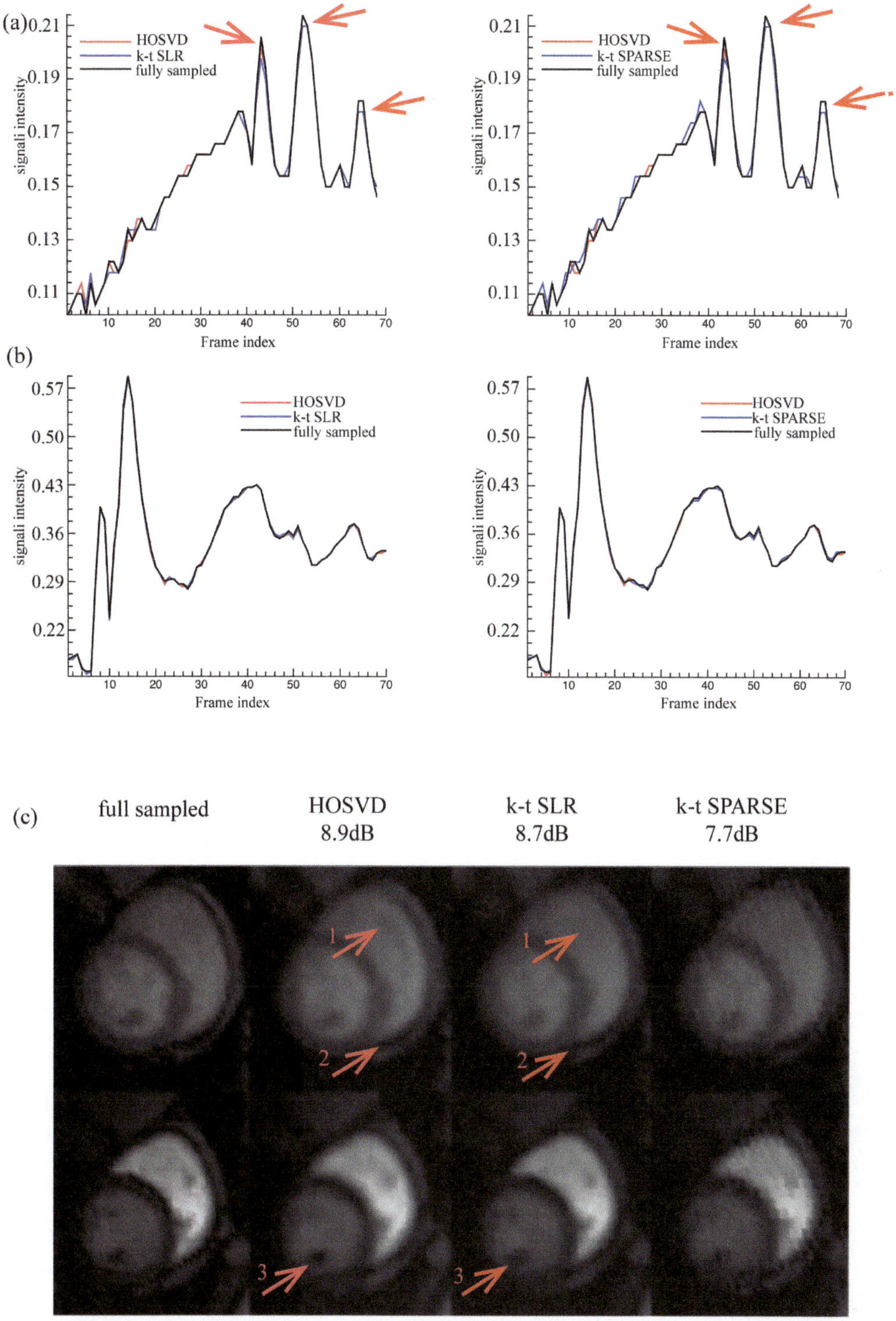

Figure 5. Reconstructions of Dataset A at reduction factor 6. (a) and (b) show the averaged normalised signal intensity at the myocardial and blood pool regions, respectively, and (c) shows the images (region of interest only) at the peak signal intensity of myocardial (the 54th frame, top row) and blood pool (the 14th frame bottom row). The left of (a) and (b) shows the averaged signal intensity of the fully sampled images (black line), *k-t* SLR reconstruction (blue line) and, the reconstruction of the proposed method (red line); the right of (a) and (b) shows the averaged signal intensity of the fully sampled images (black line), the *k-t* SPARSE reconstruction (blue line) and, the reconstruction of the proposed method (red line).

signal intensity, both the proposed method and *k-t* SLR obviously outperformed *k-t* SPARSE, especially at the frames where the averaged signal intensity changed rapidly (as marked with red arrows in figure 5(a)). The region of interest (as marked in figure 3(a)) of the 54th and the 14th frames, where the myocardial and the blood pool signal intensities reached their peak values, are presented on the top and the bottom rows of figure 5(c), respectively. In figure 5(c), it appears that Dataset A contains

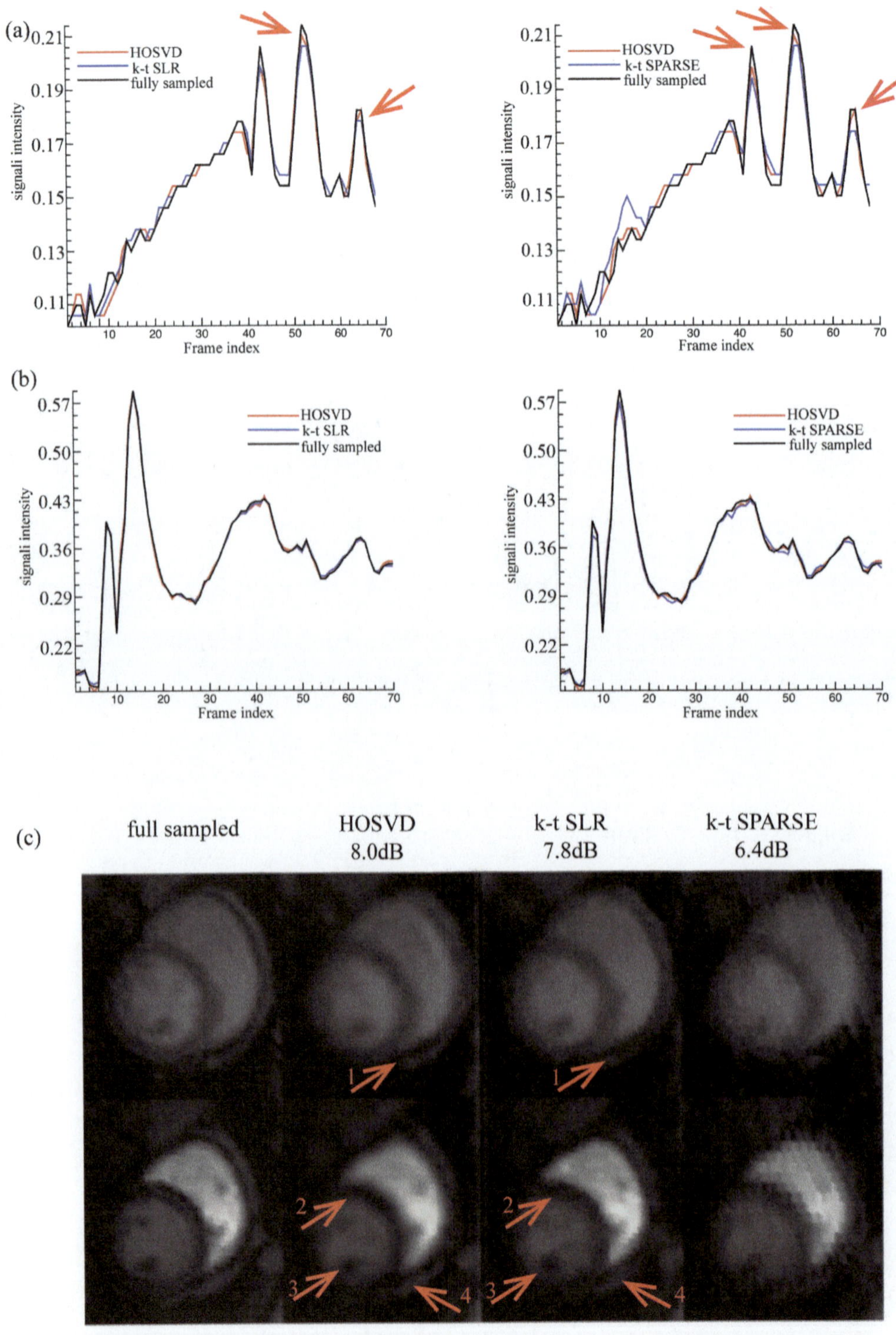

Figure 6. Reconstructions of Dataset A at reduction factor 11. (a) and (b) show the averaged normalised signal intensity at the myocardial and blood pool regions, respectively, and (c) shows the images (region of interest only) at the peak signal intensity of myocardial (the 54th frame, top row) and blood pool (the 14th frame bottom row). The left of (a) and (b) shows the averaged signal intensity of the fully sampled images (black line), *k-t* SLR reconstruction (blue line) and, the reconstruction of the proposed method (red line); the right of (a) and (b) shows the averaged signal intensity of the fully sampled images (black line), the *k-t* SPARSE reconstruction (blue line) and, the reconstruction of the proposed method (red line).

visible white noise, and some of the residual noise was maintained in the result of the method *k-t* SPARSE. The images recovered by the proposed method and the *k-t* SLR successfully supressed the white noise. Both the proposed method and the *k-t* SLR provided comparable overall image quality at the low reduction factor. When the reduction factor was 11, the SER values achieved by the proposed method, the *k-t* SLR and the *k-t* SPARSE, were 8.0 dB, 7.8 dB and, 6.4 dB, respectively. As shown in figure 6(b), all the

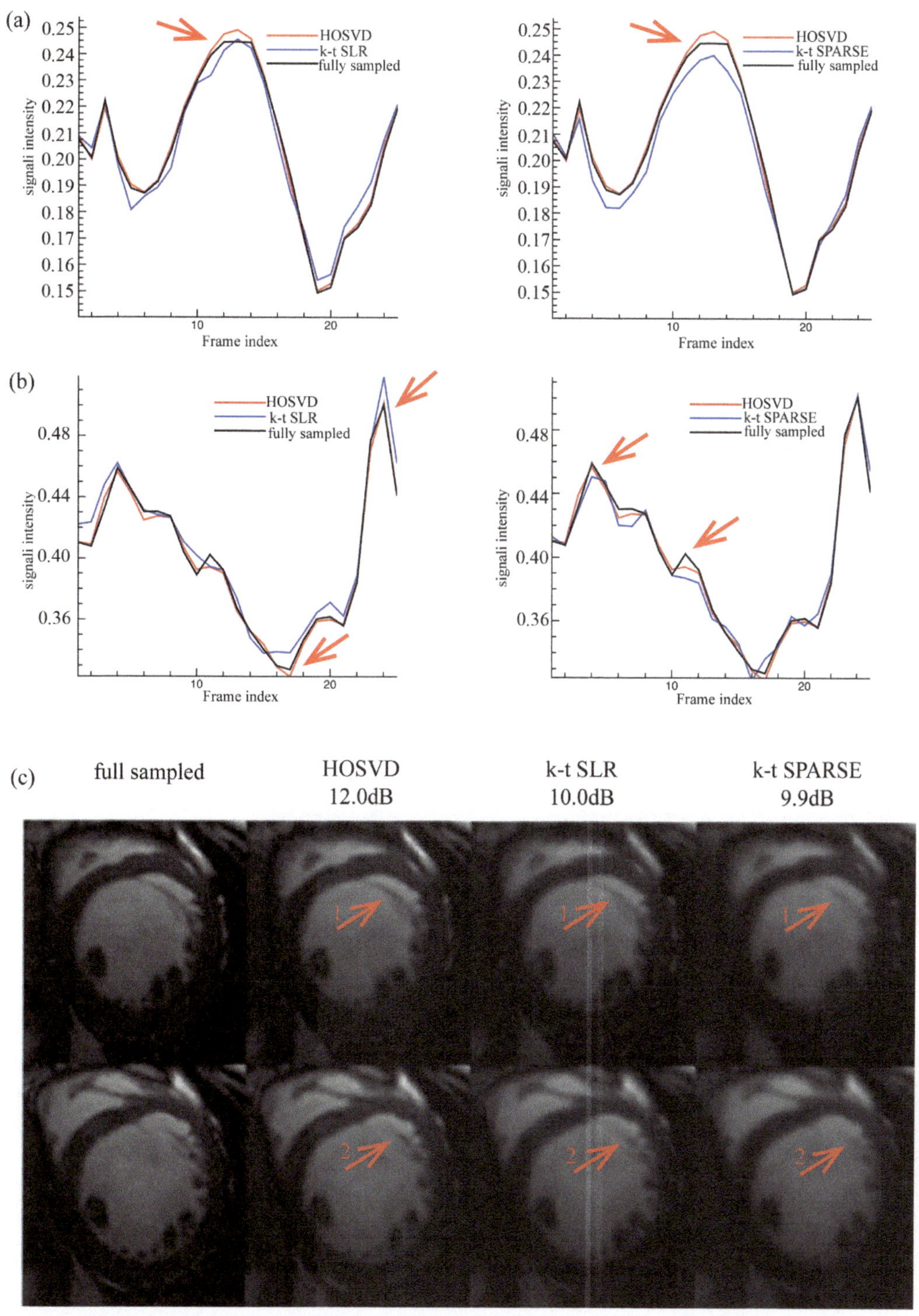

Figure 7. Reconstructions of Dataset B at reduction factor 6. (a) and (b) show the averaged normalised signal intensity at the myocardial and blood pool regions, respectively, and (c) shows the images (region of interest only) at the peak signal intensity of myocardial (the 13th frame, top row) and blood pool (the 24th frame bottom row). The left of (a) and (b) shows the averaged signal intensity of the fully sampled images (black line), *k-t* SLR reconstruction (blue line) and, the reconstruction of the proposed method (red line); the right of (a) and (b) shows averaged the signal intensity of the fully sampled images (black line), the *k-t* SPARSE reconstruction (blue line) and, the reconstruction of the proposed method (red line).

methods recovered comparable averaged signal intensity of the blood pool area. However, when comparing the myocardial area, the proposed method and the *k-t* SLR outperformed the *k-t* SPARSE more obviously, especially at the frames where the signal changes quickly (as indicated by the red arrows in figure 6(a)). The region of interest of the 54th and the 14th images are presented on the top and the bottom row of figure 6(c), respectively. The *k-t* SPARSE was severely affected by the white noise at this high reduction factor, while both the *k-t* SLR and the proposed method were still robust to noise. In *k-t* SLR, TV regularisation provided

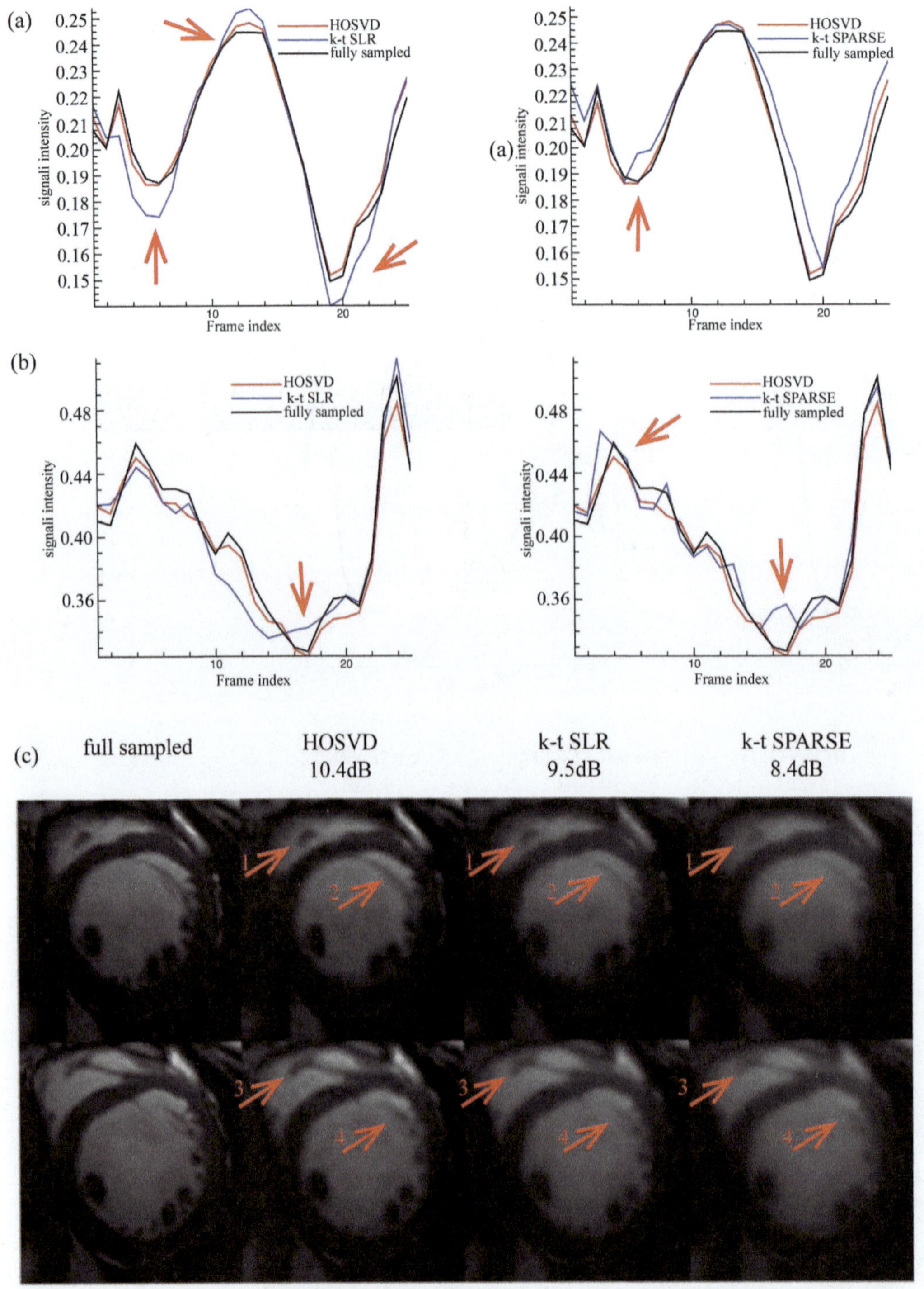

Figure 8. Reconstructions of Dataset B at reduction factor 11. (a) and (b) show the averaged normalised signal intensity at the myocardial and blood pool regions, respectively, and (c) shows the images (region of interest only) at the peak signal intensity of myocardial (the 13th frame, top row) and blood pool (the 24th frame bottom row). The left of (a) and (b) shows the averaged signal intensity of the fully sampled images (black line), *k-t* SLR reconstruction (blue line) and, the reconstruction of the proposed method (red line); the right of (a) and (b) shows the averaged signal intensity of the fully sampled images (black line), the reconstruction of *k-t* SPARSE (blue line) and, the reconstruction of the proposed method (red line).

slightly better reconstruction for large contours or boundaries of the images. However, it also generated a cartoon-like/over-smooth effect on local fine details (also observed in [30]). This effect is more obvious at reduction factor 11 (see figure 6(c)). Compared with TV regularised *k-t* SLR, the proposed method provided slightly better reconstruction of local fine details (see the red arrows in figure 6(c)). The evaluation of all the methods based on Dataset A indicates that the proposed tensor sparsity basis outperformed the conventional matrix sparsity basis. Moreover, even when comparing with *k-t* SLR that combines the low-rank

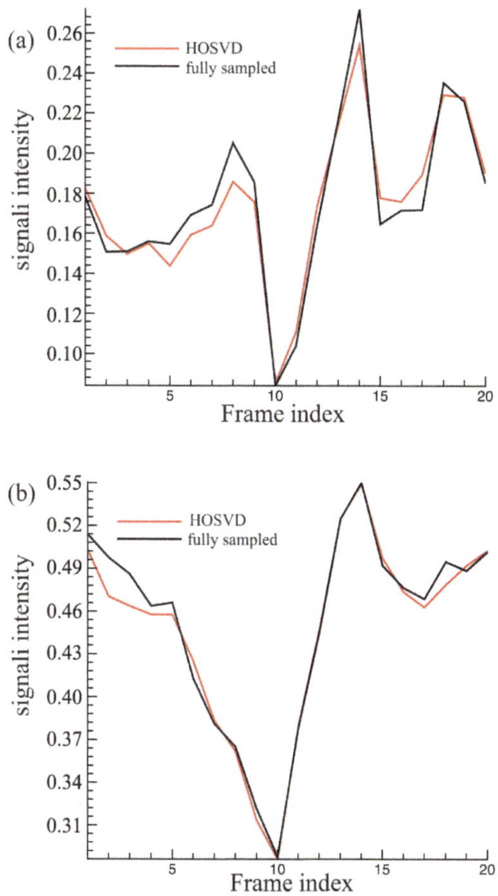

Figure 9. The averaged normalised signal intensity achieved by the proposed method at reduction factor 11. (a) The myocardial signal intensity of the fully sampled images and the reconstructed images provided by the proposed method; (b) the blood pool signal intensity of the fully sampled images and the reconstructed images provided by the proposed method.

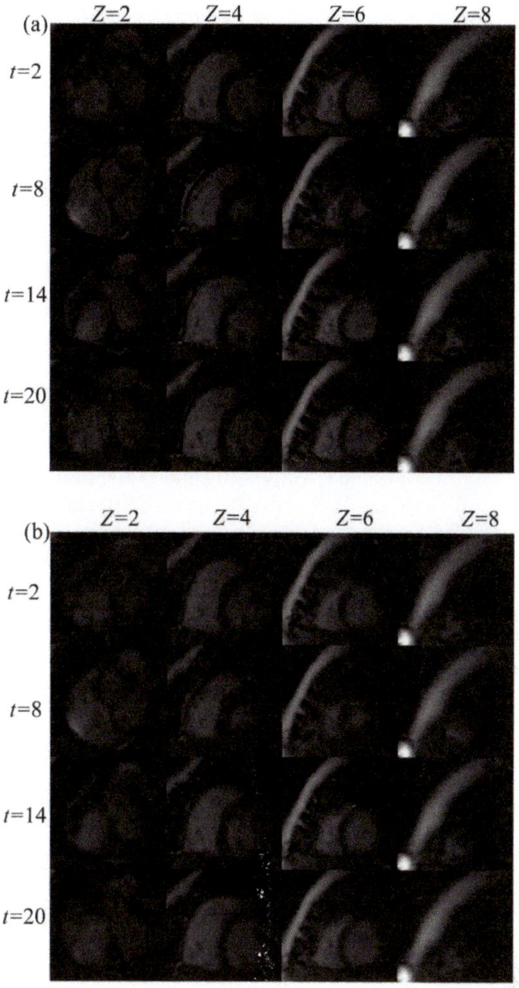

Figure 10. The reconstruction of Dataset C (region of interest only) achieved by the proposed method at reduction factor 11. (a) Presents several fully sampled images, and (b) presents the corresponding reconstructed images. In (a), images obtained at four time instants (indicated by *t*) are present row by row; and images obtained at four *z* positions (indicated by *z* along axial direction (base-apex)) are presents column by column. Likewise, (b) presents the reconstructed images at the corresponding time instants (indicated by *t*) and *z* positions (indicated by *z*).

matrix recovery and the sparsity constraint, the proposed method was still able to provide comparable overall reconstruction accuracy.

Figure 7 and 8 show the reconstruction of Dataset B provided by all the methods at reduction factors of 6 and 11, respectively. When the reduction factor was 6, the proposed method, the *k-t* SLR and the *k-t* SPARSE achieved the SER values of 12dB, 10dB and, 9.9dB, respectively. The averaged signal intensity comparison, as shown in figure 7(a, b), demonstrates that the proposed method was more capable of capturing the dynamic features of the signal (see the red arrows in figure 7(a, b)) than *k-t* SPARSE. The 13th and the 24th frames (region of interest only, as marked in figure 3(b)), where the peak averaged signal intensity of myocardial and blood pool areas were reached, are presented on the top and the bottom rows of figure 7(c), respectively. As shown in figure 7 (c), Dataset B contains more local details than Dataset A and, it has little visible white noise. All the methods succeeded in recovering the coarse features of Dataset B; meanwhile, the proposed method and the *k-t* SLR captured more fine details (see the red arrows in figure 7(c)). When the reduction factor was 11, the SER values achieved by the proposed method, the *k-t* SLR and the *k-t* SPARSE, were 10.4 dB, 9.5 dB and, 8.4 dB, respectively. The averaged signal intensity of the myocardial and the blood pool was compared in figure 8(a, b). The proposed method achieved comparable reconstruction with the *k-t* SLR and, better overall reconstructions as compared to *k-t* SPARSE. And the visual evaluation in figure 8(c) shows consistent results with those of the averaged signal intensity comparison, as indicated by the red arrows. The quantitative and visual evaluations of Dataset B were also consistent with those of Dataset A.

4.2. 4D Application

As shown in figure 2, the HOSVD method can be applied straightforwardly to higher order datasets. In this work, we present the application of HOSVD in the dynamic volume cardiac imaging, where the dataset is a 4D tensor. At reduction factor 11, the SER of the reconstructed 4D images achieved by the proposed method was 12.1 dB. The averaged signal intensity at the myocardial and the blood pool areas is presented in figure 9. As illustrated in figure 9, at the high reduction factor of 11 the proposed method was still able to recover the dynamic features of the signal without noticeable error. Several fully sampled and the reconstructed images (region of interest only, as marked in figure 3(c)) are shown in figure 10(a) and (b), respectively. As shown in figure 10(b), the proposed method successfully recovered the coarse features of the object and, most of the fine details were also recovered, which demonstrated the feasibility of the proposed sparsifying transform for the 4D application.

Discussions

5.1. The Tucker Model Based HOSVD

This work takes the Tucker model based HOSVD as an example to demonstrate the potential of tensor decomposition in the exploration of higher-order signal sparsity. The Tucker model based HOSVD decomposes a dense tensor into a sparse tensor multiplied by matrices along individual modes (as shown in figure (1–2)). The *k-t* SLR actually used solely the *mode-2* unfold of the tensor structure to explore the low rank properties. However, this work does not explore the low-rank structure of the reshaped tensor. Instead, it explores the sparsity in a tensor structure. In addition to HOSVD, there are a broad range of tensor decomposition techniques for future investigation, such as the CANDECOMP/PARAFAC decomposition [58,59] and its variants, which can be used to explore the tensor rank minimisation.

5.2. Computational Cost

In this work, when the same stopping criteria was set, the computation time for the proposed method in the 3D application was, on average, 28 and 29 minutes for Dataset A and B respectively. The *k-t* SLR method used 21 minutes for Dataset A and 29 minutes for Dataset B. As for the *k-t* SPARSE, it took 29 minutes on average for Dataset A and 40 minutes for Dataset B. In dealing with *third*-order tensor, the proposed method performs SVD three times (once per equation (8–10)), while *k-t* SLR needs only one SVD computation. The proposed method involves only one regularisation, while the *k-t* SLR involves two regularisations. Therefore, though the computing time of the HOSVD basis function is three times that of the SVD basis function, the overall optimisation time of the proposed method was only approximately 30% more than that of the *k-t* SLR. The sparsifying transform in the *k-t* SPARSE involves multiple times of wavelet transforms for each frame and one Fourier transform for the temporal dimension therefore, it was slightly slower than the proposed method.

5.3. Parameter Setting

The balance between the data fidelity in *k*-space and the sparsity of the images has become a common concern in many the CS approaches. This issue becomes more complicated when more than one regularisation terms are involved in the optimisation, such as in the method *k-t* SLR. Although the setting of the regularisation parameters has been discussed within the CS-MRI framework [6060,61], it is believed that further investigation is still required for specific applications. As far as we have observed, when using the same sparsifying transform, the image artefacts increase as the amount of *k*-space acquisitions decreases. Therefore, the weighting of the sparsity constraint needs to be slightly increased. With the same reduction factor, different sparsifying transforms provide significantly different values of the l_p quasi-norm, while the values of the l_2 norm (the data-fidelity in *k*-space) stay relatively stable. Therefore it would be inappropriate if the values of λ are identical for different sparsifying transforms. Instead they should be optimised case by case.

Conclusion

This work proposes a novel concept of tensor sparsity for Compressed Sensing in dynamic MRI, and presents the Tucker model based Higher-order Singular Value Decomposition as a practical example. The tensor decomposition based method derives the sparsity basis adaptively and directly from the zero-filled under-sampled *k-t* space measurements, and does not require extra scan time to obtain training data. The proposed tensor sparsity basis provides improved image reconstruction quality when compared to the classic sparsity basis. The reconstruction quality is similar to that with a stronger constraint–low rank property of matrix.

Author Contributions

Conceived and designed the experiments: YY FL. Performed the experiments: YY. Analyzed the data: YY JJ. Contributed reagents/materials/analysis tools: YY JJ FL. Wrote the paper: YY JJ FL SC.

References

1. Haase A (1990) Snapshot flash mri. applications to t1, t2, and chemical-shift imaging. Magnetic Resonance in Medicine 13: 77–89.
2. Stehling MK, Turner R, Mansfield P (1991) Echo-planar imaging: magnetic resonance imaging in a fraction of a second. Science 254: 43–50.
3. Donoho DL (2006) Compressed sensing. IEEE Transactions on Information Theory 52: 1289–1306.
4. Lustig M, Santos JM, Donoho DL, Pauly JM (2006) kt SPARSE: High frame rate dynamic MRI exploiting spatio-temporal sparsity. Proceedings of the 13th Annual Meeting of ISMRM, Seattle. 2420.
5. Lustig M, Donoho DL, Santos JM, Pauly JM (2008) Compressed sensing MRI. IEEE Signal Processing Magazine 25: 72–82.
6. Candes EJ, Romberg J (2007) Sparsity and incoherence in compressive sampling. Inverse Problems 23: 969.
7. Candes EJ, Romberg J, Tao T (2006) Robust uncertainty principles: exact signal reconstruction from highly incomplete frequency information. IEEE Transactions on Information Theory 52: 489–509.
8. Lustig M, Donoho D, Pauly JM (2007) Sparse MRI: The application of compressed sensing for rapid MR imaging. Magnetic Resonance in Medicine 58: 1182–1195.
9. Hong M, Yu Y, Wang H, Liu F, Crozier S (2011) Compressed sensing MRI with singular value decomposition-based sparsity basis. Physics in Medicine and Biology 56: 6311–6325.
10. Yu Y, Hong M, Liu F, Wang H, Crozier S (2011) Compressed sensing MRI using Singular Value Decomposition based sparsity basis. Engineering in Medicnie and Biology Society, EMBC, 2011 Annual International Conference of the IEEE on. Boston USA. Aug. 30 2011-Sept. 3 2011. 5734–5737.
11. Leonid R, Stanley O, Emad F (1992) Nonlinear total variation based noise removal algorithms. Phys D 60: 259–268.
12. Jung H, Ye JC, Kim EY (2007) Improved k-t BLAST and k-t SENSE using FOCUSS. Physics in medicine and biology 52: 3201–3226.
13. Jung H, Sung K, Nayak KS, Kim EY, Ye JC (2009) k-t FOCUSS: A general compressed sensing framework for high resolution dynamic MRI. Magnetic Resonance in Medicine 61: 103–116.
14. Gorodnitsky IF, George JS, Rao BD (1995) Neuromagnetic source imaging with FOCUSS: a recursive weighted minimum norm algorithm. Electroencephalography and clinical neurophysiology 95: 231–251.
15. Gorodnitsky IF, Rao BD (1997) Sparse signal reconstruction from limited data using FOCUSS: a re-weighted minimum norm algorithm. Signal Processing, IEEE Transactions on 45: 600–616.
16. Liang D, DiBella EVR, Chen R-R, Ying L (2011) K-T ISD: Compressed sensing with iterative support detection for dynamic MRI. Biomedical Imaging: From Nano to Macro, 2011 IEEE International Symposiumon: IEEE. 1264–1267.
17. Akçakaya M, Basha TA, Goddu B, Goepfert LA, Kissinger KV, et al. (2011) Low-dimensional-structure self-learning and thresholding: Regularization beyond compressed sensing for MRI Reconstruction. Magnetic Resonance in Medicine 66: 756–767.
18. Prieto C, Usman M, Wild JM, Kozerke S, Batchelor PG, et al. (2012) Group sparse reconstruction using intensity-based clustering. Magnetic Resonance in Medicine 69: 1169–1179.
19. Candès EJ, Recht B (2009) Exact matrix completion via convex optimization. Foundations of Computational mathematics 9: 717–772.

20. Meka R, Jain P, Dhillon IS (2009) Guaranteed rank minimization via singular value projection. arXiv preprint arXiv: 09095457.
21. Candes EJ, Plan Y (2010) Matrix completion with noise. Proceedings of the IEEE 98: 925–936.
22. Keshavan RH, Montanari A, Oh S (2010) Matrix completion from noisy entries. The Journal of Machine Learning Research 99: 2057–2078.
23. Dai W, Milenkovic O (2010) SET: an algorithm for consistent matrix completion. Acoustics Speech and Signal Processing (ICASSP), 2010 IEEE International Conference on. Dallas USA. 3646–3649.
24. Lee K, Bresler Y (2010) Admira: Atomic decomposition for minimum rank approximation. Information Theory, IEEE Transactions on 56: 4402–4416.
25. Recht B, Fazel M, Parrilo PA (2010) Guaranteed minimum-rank solutions of linear matrix equations via nuclear norm minimization. SIAM review 52: 471–501.
26. Brinegar C, Wu YJL, Foley LM, Hitchens TK, Qing Y, et al. (2008) Real-time cardiac MRI without triggering, gating, or breath holding; 20–25 Aug. 2008. 3381–3384.
27. Brinegar C, Haosen Z, Wu YJL, Foley LM, Hitchens TK, et al (2009) Real-time cardiac MRI using prior spatial-spectral information. Engineering in Medicnie and Biology Society, EMBC, 2009 Annual International Conference of the IEEE on. Minneapolis USA. 3–6 Sept. 2009. 4383–4386.
28. Pedersen H, Kozerke S, Ringgaard S, Nehrke K, Kim WY (2009) k-t PCA: Temporally constrained k-t BLAST reconstruction using principal component analysis. Magnetic Resonance in Medicine 62: 706–716.
29. Haldar JP, Liang Z-P (2010) Spatiotemporal imaging with partially separable functions: a matrix recovery approach. Biomedical Imaging: From Nano to Macro, 2010 IEEE International Symposium on. Rotterdam Netherlands. 716–719.
30. Lingala SG, Hu Y, DiBella E, Jacob M (2011) Accelerated dynamic MRI exploiting sparsity and low-rank structure: k-t SLR. IEEE Transactions on Medical Imaging 30: 1042–1054.
31. Haldar JP, Liang Z-P (2011) Low-rank approximations for dynamic imaging. Biomedical Imaging: From Nano to Macro, 2011 IEEE International Symposium on. Chicago USA. 1052–1055.
32. Trzasko J, Manduca A, Borisch E (2011) Local versus global low-rank promotion in dynamic MRI series reconstruction. Proceeding of the 19th Annual Meeting of ISMRM. Montréal, Canada. 4371.
33. Trzasko J, Manduca A (2013) A Unified Tensor Regression Framework for Calibrationless Dynamic, Multi-Channel MRI Reconstruction; 2013; Salt Lake City, USA.
34. Trzasko JD (2013) Exploiting local low-rank structure in higher-dimensional MRI applications. International Society for Optics and Photonics. Proc. SPIE 8858, Wavelets and Sparsity XV, 885821 (September 26, 2013). doi:10.1117/12.2027059.
35. Liang Z-P (2007) Spatiotemporal imaging with partially separable functions. Noninvasive Functional Source Imaging of the Brain and Heart and the International Conference on Functional Biomedical Imaging, 2007. NFSI-ICFBI 2007. Joint Meeting of the 6th International Symposium on. Hangzhou China. 181–182.
36. Tucker LR (1966) Some mathematical notes on three-mode factor analysis. Psychometrika 31: 279–311.
37. De Lathauwer L, De Moor B, Vandewalle J (2000) A multilinear singular value decomposition. SIAM Journal on Matrix Analysis and Applications 21: 1253–1278.
38. Wang S-J, Yang J, Sun M-F, Peng X-J, Sun M-M, et al. (2012) Sparse tensor discriminant color space for face verification. Neural Networks and Learning Systems, IEEE Transactions on 23: 876–888.
39. Wang S-J, Sun M-F, Chen Y-H, Pang E-P, Zhou C-G (2012) STPCA: sparse tensor principal component analysis for feature extraction. Pattern Recognition (ICPR), 2012 21st International Conference on. Tsukuba Japan. 2278–2281.
40. Comon P (2002) Tensor decompositions. Mathematics in Signal Processing V: 1–24.
41. Kolda TG, Bader BW (2009) Tensor decompositions and applications. SIAM review 51: 455–500.
42. Candes EJ, Romberg JK, Tao T (2006) Stable signal recovery from incomplete and inaccurate measurements. Communications on Pure and Applied Mathematics 59: 1207–1223.
43. Chartrand R (2007) Exact Reconstruction of Sparse Signals via Nonconvex Minimization. Signal Processing Letters, IEEE 14: 707–710.
44. Chartrand R, Staneva V (2008) Restricted isometry properties and nonconvex compressive sensing. Inverse Problems 24 035020 doi:10.1088/0266-5611/24/3/035020.
45. Fischer A, Breuer F, Blaimer M, Seiberlich N, Jakob PM (2008) Introduction of a nonconvex compressed sensing algorithm for MR imaging. Proceeding of the 16th Annual Meeting of ISMRM. Toronto Canada.
46. Saab R, Chartrand R, Yilmaz O (2008) Stable sparse approximations via nonconvex optimization. Acoustics, Speech and Signal Processing, 2008. ICASSP 2008. IEEE International Conference on. Las Vegas USA. 3885–3888.
47. Chartrand R (2009) Fast algorithms for nonconvex compressive sensing: MRI reconstruction from very few data. Biomedical Imaging: From Nano to Macro, 2009. ISBI '09. IEEE International Symposium on. Boston USA. 262–265.
48. Majumdar A, Ward RK (2011) An algorithm for sparse MRI reconstruction by Schatten p-norm minimization. Magnetic Resonance Imaging 29: 408–417.
49. Andreopoulos A, Tsotsos JK (2008) Efficient and generalizable statistical models of shape and appearance for analysis of cardiac MRI. Medical Image Analysis 12: 335–357.
50. Chartrand R, Wotao Y (2008) Iteratively reweighted algorithms for compressive sensing. Acoustics, Speech and Signal Processing, 2008. ICASSP 2008. IEEE International Conference on. Las Vegas USA. 3869–3872.
51. Trzasko J, Haider C, Manduca A (2009) Practical nonconvex compressive sensing reconstruction of highly-accelerated 3D parallel MR angiograms. Biomedical Imaging: From Nano to Macro, 2009. ISBI '09. IEEE International Symposium on. Boston USA. 274–277.
52. Majumdar A, Ward RK (2010) Under-determined non-cartesian MR reconstruction with non-convex sparsity promoting analysis prior. Medical Image Computing and Computer-Assisted Intervention–MICCAI 2010: Springer. 513–520.
53. Ramirez-Giraldo J, Trzasko J, Leng S, Yu L, Manduca A, et al. (2011) Nonconvex prior image constrained compressed sensing (NCPICCS): Theory and simulations on perfusion CT. Medical Physics 38: 2157.
54. Trzasko JD, Haider CR, Borisch EA, Campeau NG, Glockner JF, et al. (2011) Sparse-CAPR: Highly accelerated 4D CE-MRA with parallel imaging and nonconvex compressive sensing. Magnetic Resonance in Medicine 66: 1019–1032.
55. Majumdar A, Ward RK, Aboulnasr T (2012) Non-convex algorithm for sparse and low-rank recovery: Application to dynamic MRI reconstruction. Magnetic resonance imaging 31: 448–455.
56. Shiqian M, Wotao Y, Yin Z, Chakraborty A (2008) An efficient algorithm for compressed MR imaging using total variation and wavelets. Computer Vision and Pattern Recognition, 2008. CVPR 2008. IEEE Conference on. Anchorage USA. 1–8.
57. Osher S, Burger M, Goldfarb D, Xu J, Yin W (2005) An Iterative Regularization Method for Total Variation-Based Image Restoration. Multiscale Modeling & Simulation 4: 460–489.
58. Hitchcock FL (1927) Multiple invariants and generalized rank of a p-way matrix or tensor. Journal of Mathematics and Physics 7: 39–79.
59. Hitchcock FL (1927) The expression of a tensor or a polyadic as a sum of products. Journal of Mathematics and Physics 6: 164–189.
60. ElShahaby FEA, Landman BA, Prince JL (2011) Effect of regularization parameter and scan time on crossing fibers with constrained compressed sensing. Proceedings-Society of Photo-Optical Instrumentation Engineers: Image Processing. 79624J. doi:10.1117/12.878382.
61. Miao J, Huang F, Wilson D (2011) Investigation on Compressed Sensing Regularization Parameter using Case-PDM. Proceeding of the 19th Annual Meeting of ISMRM. Montréal, Canada.

Image Quality and Radiation Dose of Lower Extremity CT Angiography Using 70 kVp, High Pitch Acquisition and Sinogram-Affirmed Iterative Reconstruction

Li Qi[1], Felix G. Meinel[2], Chang Sheng Zhou[1], Yan E. Zhao[1], U. Joseph Schoepf[1,2], Long Jiang Zhang[1]*, Guang Ming Lu[1]*

1 Department of Medical Imaging, Jinling Hospital, Clinical School of South Medical University, Nanjing, Jiangsu, China, **2** Department of Radiology and Radiological Science, Medical University of South Carolina, Charleston, South Carolina, United States of America

Abstract

Objectives: The purpose of this study was to assess image quality and radiation dose of lower extremity CT angiography (CTA) with 70 kVp, high pitch acquisition and sinogram-affirmed iterative reconstruction (SAFIRE).

Methods: Lower extremity CTAs were performed on 44 patients: 22 patients were examined using protocol A (120 kVp, pitch of 0.85 and 120 ml of contrast agent on a first-generation dual-source CT) (120 kVp group) and 22 patients were evaluated with protocol B (70 kVp, pitch of 2.2 and 80 ml of contrast agent on a second-generation dual-source CT) (70 kVp group). Images from the 120 kVp group were reconstructed with filtered back projection (FBP) and images from the 70 kVp group with SAFIRE. The attenuation, image noise, signal-to-noise ratio (SNR) and contrast-to-noise ratio (CNR) were calculated. Two radiologists subjectively assessed image quality of lower extremity arteries, plantar arterial enhancement and venous contamination of all patients. Radiation dose was compared between the two groups.

Results: Higher mean intravascular attenuation was obtained in the 70 kVp group (70 vs. 120 kVp group, 555.4±83.4 HU vs. 300.9±81.4 HU, $P<0.001$), as well as image noise (20.0±2.8 HU vs. 17.5±3.2 HU, $P=0.010$), SNR (32.0±7.0 vs. 19.1±6.9, $P<0.001$) and CNR (28.1±6.6 vs 15.9±6.3, $P<0.001$). No difference in subjective image quality and plantar arterial enhancement was found between 120 kVp group and 70 kVp group (all $P>0.05$). The venous contamination score was 1.5±0.8 for 120 kVp group while no venous contamination was found in 70 kVp group. The inter-observer agreement was moderate to good for both groups (0.515~1, $P<0.001$). The effective dose was lower in 70 kVp group (0.3±0.1 mSv) than in 120 kVp group (1.6±0.7 mSv)($P<0.001$).

Conclusions: Lower extremity CTA using 70 kVp, high pitch acquisition and SAFIRE, except increasing imaging noise, allows for lower radiation dose and contrast material volume without compromising image quality.

Editor: Zhuoli Zhang, Northwestern University Feinberg School of Medicine, United States of America

Funding: This work was all supported by the Program for New Century Excellent Talents in University (NCET-12-0260). The funders had no role in study design, data collection and analysis, decision to publish, or preparation of the manuscript.

Competing Interests: UJS is a consultant for and receives research support from Bayer, Bracco, GE, Medrad, and Siemens. The other authors have no conflicts of interest to declare.

* E-mail: kevinzhlj@163.com (LJZ); cjr.luguangming@vip.163.com (GML)

Introduction

Peripheral arterial disease (PAD) is a common, chronic and progressive health problem. It is reported that the overall prevalence of PAD was 16.7% in Chinese patients with type 2 diabetes and 27.5% in Chinese patients with hypertension [1,2]. The mortality rates in patients with PAD average 2% per year and the rates of nonfatal myocardial infarction, stroke, and vascular death are 5% to 7% per year [3]. Early diagnosis and appropriate medical interventions can mitigate limb-specific symptoms, improve quality of life, and decrease systemic cardiovascular risk [4].

CT angiography (CTA), as a non-invasive and safe examination, has been widely used in clinical practice to diagnose PAD and acute lower-extremity vascular injury with high accuracy [5–8]. However, the radiation exposure to the patients and the relatively high dose of contrast medium necessary to perform lower extremity CTA due to the wide scan range from the abdomen to the feet have raised concerns. A previous study has shown that the weighted CT dose index (CTDIw) of lower extremity CTA could be as high as 12.2 mGy and the volume of contrast material could be as much as 140 ml [5]. With the rapid refinement of CT technology, various strategies of reducing radiation dose and dosage of contrast medium have been developed. The technique of lowering tube voltage is most often used among various dose-reducing strategies. The tube voltage of 80 kVp has been verified to be feasible for lower extremity CTA with substantial reduction of radiation dose [9,10]. Most recently, Duan et al have reduced radiation dose to 1.94 mSv and contrast medium volume to 1.2 mL/kg when a tube voltage of 70 kVp was used in lower extremity CTA [11]. However, further reducing radiation dose of low extremity CTA appears to be feasible. For example, high pitch CTA acquisition has been used to evaluate deep vein thrombosis [12]. The combination of 70 kVp and high-pitch acquisition technique holds potential to further reduce radiation dose. In addition, sinogram-affirmed iterative reconstruction (SAFIRE), a raw-data-based IR algorithm, has the potential to improve image quality and reduce image noise which benefits for the radiation dose saving [13]. However, to the best of our knowledge, no study has been performed on lower extremity CTA using 70 kVp combined with high pitch acquisition and iterative reconstruction. The aim of our study was therefore to investigate the feasibility, image quality and radiation dose of lower extremity CTA using 70 kVp combined with dual-source high pitch acquisition and iterative reconstruction.

Materials and Methods

Study subjects

This retrospective study was approved by Jinling Hospital, Clinical School of South Medical University, Nanjing, China and informed consent was waived. The inclusion criteria for the enrollment was the utilization of the two special scan protocols (120 kVp scan protocol and 70 kVp, high-pitch scan protocol) for lower extremity CTA. Subjects were excluded when severe beam hardening artifacts were present because of metal stents. Finally, a total of 44 patients (32 male and 12 female; mean age 60±20 years; age range 19–90 years) undergoing lower extremity CTA because of known tumors ($n=5$), injury ($n=12$), or suspected arterial occlusive disease ($n=27$) were included in the study.

Among these patients, 22 patients (16 male and 6 female; mean age 56±22 years; age range 19–90 years) who had undergone CTA of the lower extremities at 120 kVp on a first-generation dual-source CT system between December 2012 and November 2013 were selected as the control (120 kVp group). Of these 22 patients, one patient had soft tissue tumors, 8 patients had traumatic lower extremity injury and 13 patients had peripheral artery disease.

Another 22 patients (16 male and 6 female; mean age 63±18 years; age range 20–86 years) underwent lower extremity CTA using 70 kVp combined with high pitch (2.2) acquisition and iterative reconstruction on a second-generation dual-source CT system (70 kVp group). These studies were performed between July 2013 and October 2013 because of known tumors ($n=4$), traumatic lower extremity injury ($n=4$) and suspected peripheral artery disease ($n=14$).

CT protocol and contrast medium infusion protocols

All patients in the 120 kVp group were examined on a first-generation dual-source CT (Somatom Definition; Siemens Medical Solutions, Germany). For the patients in the 70 kVp group, a second-generation dual-source CT system (Definition Flash, Siemens Medical Solutions, Forchheim, Germany) with an integrated circuit detector was used. The acquisition parameters in the 120 kVp group were tube voltage, 120 kVp; pitch, 0.85; collimation, 64×0.6 mm; slice thickness, 1.0 mm; reconstruction increment, 0.7 mm. The acquisition parameters in the 70 kVp group were tube voltage, 70 kVp; pitch, 2.2; collimation, 128×0.6 mm; slice thickness, 1.0 mm; reconstruction increment, 1 mm. Automatic tube current modulation (ATCM, CARE Dose 4D; Siemens Medical Solutions, Germany) was used in both acquisitions with a quality reference tube current-time product of 150 mAs for the 120 kVp group and a reference tube voltage of 100 kVp and a reference tube current-time product of 370 mAs for the 70 kVp group. The mean acquisition time was recorded for each patient. Each acquisition was performed in the craniocaudal direction from the abdominal aortic bifurcation to the feet.

In all patients, iopromide (300 mg I/mL, Bayer Schering, Berlin, Germany) was delivered via an 18-gauge intravenous cannula placed into a superficial vein positioned in the antecubital fossa. Contrast enhancement was achieved by injecting 120 mL of contrast material (first 80 mL at 4 mL/s and then 40 mL at 2 mL/s) for the 120 kVp group and 80 mL (first 60 mL at 4 mL/s and then 20 mL at 2 mL/s) for the 70 kVp group, followed by a 30 mL saline flush at 2 mL/s, which were designed according to our clinical experience. The bolus-tracking technique was used in both groups. In the 120 kVp group, a region of interest (ROI) was positioned in the aortic bifurcation and image acquisition automatically started 14 seconds after the signal attenuation of ROI reached the predefined threshold of 100 Hounsfield Units (HU). In order to adapt timing to the high-pitch scanning, image acquisition in 70 kVp group started with a 6-second delay after the signal attenuation of the proximal popliteal artery rather than the abdominal aortic bifurcation had reached the predefined threshold of 100 HU.

Image reconstruction

CT data from the 120 kVp group was constructed with filtered back projection (FBP, Siemens Healthcare, Forchheim, Germany), and data from the 70 kVp group was constructed with sinogram-affirmed iterative reconstruction (SAFIRE, Siemens Healthcare, Forchheim, Germany). For the SAFIRE algorithm, five presets (strength 1–5) are available for adapting the noise model and controlling image impression and noise reduction [14]. As recommended by the manufacturer, a medium strength level of 3 was used.

Image analysis

All data sets were transferred to a dedicated workstation (Syngo.via; Siemens Medical Solutions, Forchheim, Germany). The anteroposterior and transverse diameters of each patient were measured at the level of the aortic bifurcation on axial CT images as a metric of body habitus. Effective diameter, defined as the square root of the anteroposterior diameter times the transverse diameter, was calculated for each patient. Maximum intensity projections (MIP) and curved planar reformations (CPR) were generated for each patient. To evaluate objective image quality, the intravascular attenuation was measured in five locations (aortic bifurcation, iliac bifurcation, proximal and middle femoral artery and proximal popliteal artery) on axial CT images. The measurements were averaged to derive a mean intravascular attenuation. Moreover, the attenuation of the muscle and the noise within subcutaneous fat (standard deviation of the CT attenuation) at the same slice of the measurement of intravascular attenuation of the five locations were also measured to calculate signal-to-noise ratio (SNR) and contrast-to-noise ratio (CNR) of each arterial segment. The image noise was defined as the mean value of the five SDs in subcutaneous fat. The attenuations were measured in a region of interest (ROI) within the vessels which was defined to be as large as possible while avoiding calcifications, plaques and stenoses. The SNR and CNR were calculated as follows:

SNR = attenuation of the vessel lumen/SD of subcutaneous fat

CNR = (attenuation of the vessel lumen - attenuation of muscle)/SD of subcutaneous fat

In order to evaluate subjective image quality, all CT images (axial images, MIP and CPR images) were independently reviewed by two radiologists (with 5 and 2 years of reading experience, respectively) blinded to patients' information and CTA protocols.

Before image evaluation, the observers were instructed to divide vascular structures into three segments (the aorto-iliac area, the femoro-popliteal region, and the lower leg segment) and to then score the image quality in these segments using a 4-point scale according to the degree of noise artifacts, the presence of streak artifacts and graininess of the images. The scoring criteria were as follows [15]: Poor (grade 1): graininess or streak artifacts were significant and did not provide sufficient information for the diagnosis; Adequate (grade 2): the examination provided acceptable information but unsatisfactory image quality; Good (grade 3): image quality was satisfactory enough to provide the information necessary to make an adequate radiological diagnosis; Excellent (grade 4): image quality provided optimal information for a radiological diagnosis. In addition, because the plantar vessels were too small to measure their attenuations, the enhancement of plantar arteries was subjectively scored using a 4-point scale: 1, not visible; 2, poor, visible but insufficient arterial enhancement for diagnosis; 3, moderate, enough arterial enhancement for diagnosis; 4, optimal arterial enhancement for diagnosis. Venous contamination was also graded on a three-point scale: 1, not visible; 2, visible but does not affect diagnostic interpretation; 3, present and definitely compromises diagnostic interpretation. In the event of observer disagreement, another reading session was convoked to reach an agreement.

Radiation dose estimation

For an estimation of the radiation dose, the volume CT dose index (CTDIvol) and the dose length product (DLP) of each patient were recorded. We also calculated the effective radiation dose delivered for the pelvic and hip regions, since the exposure of the extremities contributes only minimally to the overall effective dose and the conversion factors for legs are not available [11,16]. The distance from the pelvic crest to the proximal third of the thighs, including the testicles in men and vulva in women, was measured in each patient. The effective dose (ED) was calculated by multiplying the product of CTDIvol and the distance of the pelvic crest to the proximal third of the thighs by a conversion factors of 0.015 [17]. In addition, the acquisition length of the abdominal aorta and runoff arteries was calculated by dividing the DLP by the CTDIvol.

Statistical analysis

Statistical analyses were performed using the SPSS software version 16.0 (SPSS Inc. Chicago, IL, USA). Quantitative variables were expressed as mean ± SD, while categorical variables were expressed as frequencies or percentages. The Mann-Whitney test was used to compare categorical characteristics and the independent-sample t test was used to compare continuous variables. Kappa analysis was used to assess the inter-observer agreement of the subjective image quality rating. A k value of less than 0.20 indicates poor agreement; a k value of 0.21–0.40, fair agreement; a k value of 0.41–0.60, moderate agreement; a k value of 0.61–0.80, good agreement; and a k value of 0.81–1.00, very good agreement. $P<0.05$ was considered to indicate a statistically significant difference.

Result

There were no statistically significant differences in age (56±22 years vs. 63±18 years, $P=0.216$), sex (male, 72.7% vs. 71.4%, $P=0.925$), anteroposterior body diameter (18.8±2.5 cm vs. 19.8±2.7 cm, $P=0.297$), transverse diameter (31.2±2.8 cm vs. 30.3±2.8 cm, $P=0.218$), effective diameter (24.1±2.4 cm vs. 24.4±2.6 cm, $P=0.708$) and acquisition range (108.6±10.9 cm vs. 113.1±5.8 cm, $P=0.010$) between the 120 kVp group and the 70 kVp group. The mean acquisition time was 3.8 seconds in the 70 kVp group and 32.9 seconds in 120 kVp group ($P<0.001$).

The attenuations measured in all above-mentioned locations were shown in Table 1. The mean intravascular attenuation was 300.9±81.4 HU for the 120 kVp group and 555.4±83.4 HU for the 70 kVp group ($P<0.001$), indicating an 84.6% increase in the attenuation. Furthermore, the image noise in the 120 kVp group was lower than that in the 70 kVp group (17.5±3.2 HU vs. 20.0±2.8 HU, respectively, $P=0.010$), as were the SNR (19.1±6.9 vs. 32.0±7.0, respectively, $P<0.001$) and CNR (15.9±6.3 vs. 28.1±6.6, respectively, $P<0.001$).

A total of 254 segments in 44 patients were assessed for subjective image quality, while 10 segments were excluded because of vascular occlusion. The kappa values for image quality, enhancement of plantar arteries and venous contamination were 0.605, 0.672, 0.707 for 120 kVp group and 0.690, 0.515, 1 for 70 kVp group (all $P<0.001$). There was found no significant difference in the image quality score (120 vs. 70 kVp group, 3.5±0.5 vs. 3.5±0.4, $P=0.981$) and plantar arterial enhancement score (120 vs. 70 kVp group, 2.9±0.6, 2.7±1.1, $P=0.576$) between the two groups. The image quality scores of the three segments were displayed in Table 2. Figures 1–4 show some representative cases with different scores using 120 kVp and 70 kVp protocols. Venous contamination was not found in any patient of 70 kVp group. The venous contamination score was 1.5±0.8 for 120 kVp group.

The radiation dose estimation for both groups was summarized in Table 3. The DLP and CTDIvol of the abdominal aorta and runoff arteries were significantly lower in 70 kVp group when compared with the 120 kVp group ($P<0.001$). The mean distance from pelvic crest to the proximal third of the thighs was 26.9±2.9 cm for 120 kVp group and 26.4±2.0 cm for 70 kVp group ($P=0.509$). The mean DLP of the distance from pelvic crest to the proximal third of the thighs was 109.4±47.7 mGy×cm for 120 kVp group and 19.5±2.1 mGy×cm for 70 kVp group, resulting in a mean ED of 1.6±0.7 in 120 kVp group and 0.3±0.1 mSv in 70 kVp group.

Discussion

The present study demonstrates the feasibility of lower extremity CTA using 70 kVp combined with high pitch acquisition and iterative reconstruction on a second-generation dual-source CT system with an integrated circuit detector. Moreover, this protocol resulted in an 81.3% radiation dose reduction and a 33.3% decrease in the volume of contrast material compared to our standard protocol with 120 kVp on a first-generation dual-source CT without compromising image quality.

Lowering tube voltage is an effective method to reduce radiation dose because of the exponential relationship between kilovoltage and radiation dose [18]. Lowering tube voltage from 120 kVp to 80 kVp has been reported to result in a 30% reduction in radiation dose for lower extremity CTA [9]. In our study, a tube voltage of 70 kVp was used, which has been verified to be feasible and accurate in Duan's study [11]. In addition, increasing pitch is another method to reduce radiation dose by shortening image acquisition time [19]. Amacker et al reported that the mean radiation dose decreased by 20% and 42% when the pitch was increased from 1 to 3.2 for routine chest and abdominal CT scans [20]. The two strategies have been widely used in combination for coronary CTA [21,22] but rarely in lower extremity CTA. Our study applied the two radiation dose reducing strategies to lower extremity CTA and revealed that the radiation dose of lower

Table 1. Objective image quality evaluation of lower extremity CTA.

Parameter	120 kVp group	70 kVp group	*P* value
Aortic bifurcation			
Mean CT value (HU)	312.9±84.9	504.7±102.7	<0.001
SNR	17.1±8.1	22.5±8.6	0.040
CNR	14.5±7.6	19.6±8.0	0.038
Iliac bifurcation			
Mean CT value (HU)	298.8±75.0	504.61±100.0	<0.001
SNR	17.7±6.6	24.4±8.3	0.005
CNR	14.8±6.1	21.3±7.8	0.004
Proximal femoral artery			
Mean CT value (HU)	295.2±82.8	544.0±87.9	<0.001
SNR	16.1±8.1	28.5±9.3	<0.001
CNR	13.7±7.5	25.1±8.8	<0.001
Middle femoral artery			
Mean CT value (HU)	299.3±88.9	578.7±90.4	<0.001
SNR	23.6±13.3	35.3±11.8	0.004
CNR	19.7±11.8	31.2±11.0	0.002
Proximal popliteal artery			
Mean CT value (HU)	292.9±70.3	620.3±100.3	<0.001
SNR	23.8±10.9	47.0±16.0	<0.001
CNR	19.6±9.6	41.5±14.6	<0.001
Mean			
Mean CT value (HU)	300.9±81.4	555.4±83.4	<0.001
SNR	19.1±6.9	32.0±7.0	<0.001
CNR	15.9±6.3	28.1±6.6	<0.001
Noise (HU)	17.5±3.2	20.0±2.8	0.010

SNR = signal-to-noise ratio; CNR = contrast-to-noise ratio.

extremity CTA could be reduced by 81.3% with the 70 kVp high-pitch CTA protocol. The radiation dose of our low extremity CTA is lower than that of Duan's study using 70 kVp for low extremity CTA (1.94 mSv) [11].

Moreover, lowering tube voltage and raising pitch are not only the strategies to reduce radiation dose but also the strategies to reduce contrast material requirements. Lowering tube voltage effectively increases attenuation of the iodinated contrast agent, which offers a potential of reducing the dose of iodine. It has been

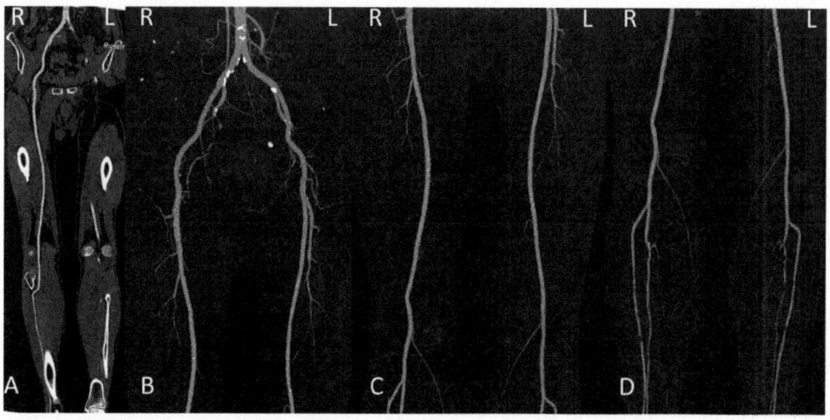

Figure 1. Lower extremity CTA using 120 kVp protocol in a 76-year-old man with PAD. A, curved planar reformatted image and B–D, maximum intensity projection images. The image quality was visually classified as score 4 (excellent) in the aortoiliac (B), femoropopliteal (C) and lower leg segments (D).

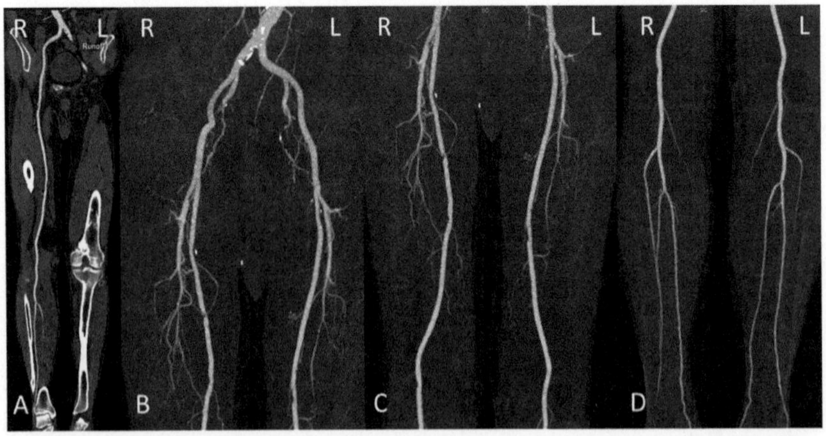

Figure 2. Lower extremity CTA using 70 kVp protocol in a 75-year-old man with PAD. A, curved planar reformatted image and B–D, maximum intensity projection images. The image quality was visually classified as score 4 (excellent) in the aortoiliac (B), femoropopliteal (C) and lower leg segments (D).

reported that a reduction of tube voltage from 120 kVp to 80 kVp allows reducing the volume of contrast medium from 1.8 mL/kg to 1.2 mL/kg without deterioration of vascular enhancement for lower extremity CTA [9]. Additional, long scan time of lower extremity CTA requires high dose of contrast medium injection to ensure the contrast enhancement peak is high and wide enough. However, the shortened acquisition time in high-pitch acquisition requires only a short temporal window of vascular enhancement and the CT acquisition can "ride the bolus", which can reduce the volume of contrast material. Yang et al reported that dual-source CT coronary angiography using a pitch of 3.4 can be performed with 30 ml of contrast medium without affecting vessel enhancement [23]. In combination with lowering tube voltage and high pith, lower extremity CTA can be performed with 80 mL of contrast material with a mean CT value of 555.4 HU, which was statistically higher than that of standard 120 kVp group. Our finding of obtaining more than 500 HU of peripheral arteries when using 70 kVp and the high pitch technique indicates the possibility of further lowering the contrast material volume in this CTA protocol. However, for the long scan range of lower extremity CTA, pitch affect the enhancement of distal vessels. In our study, we choose the proximal popliteal artery rather than the abdominal aortic bifurcation as the monitoring position to adapt the high-pitch scan of 70 kVp group, which resulted in no difference in the plantar arterial enhancement when compared with 120 kVp group. Additional, no venous contamination was found in patient of 70 kVp group.

However, the major disadvantage of both strategies for reducing radiation dose and contrast material is the increase in image noise, which may impair diagnostic interpretability. To counteract this problem, sinogram-affirmed iterative reconstruction (SAFIRE) was used in the 70 kVp group to reduce image noise. SAFIRE is a noise-modeling technique which compares reconstructed and measured data in the raw data domain and iteratively corrects the images to reduce noise and improve image quality [24,25]. Several studies have shown the benefit of SAFIRE algorithm for various clinical applications [26–28]. Han has reported that low-dose pediatric cardiac CT images constructed with SAFIRE had a 34% decrease in noise when compared with images constructed with the standard weighted filtered back projection [26]. Besides, the new integrated circuit detector used in the second-generation 128-section dual-source CT system (SOMATOM Definition Flash with an integrated circuit detector; Siemens Healthcare, Forchheim, Germany) has the capability to reduce electronic noise and improve spatial resolution compared with previous detector technology. Spiczak et al have demonstrated that a significantly

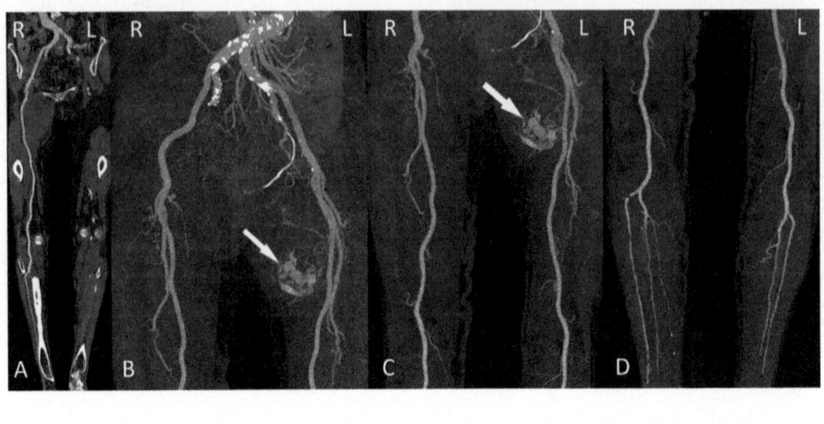

Figure 3. Lower extremity CTA using 70 kVp protocol in a 64-year-old woman with tumor. A, curved planar reformatted image and B–D, maximum intensity projection images. The image quality was visually classified as score 3 (good) in the aortoiliac (B), femoropopliteal (C) and lower leg segments (D). Note abnormal hypervascular mass (myxofibrosarcoma) in the left thigh (arrow in panels B and C).

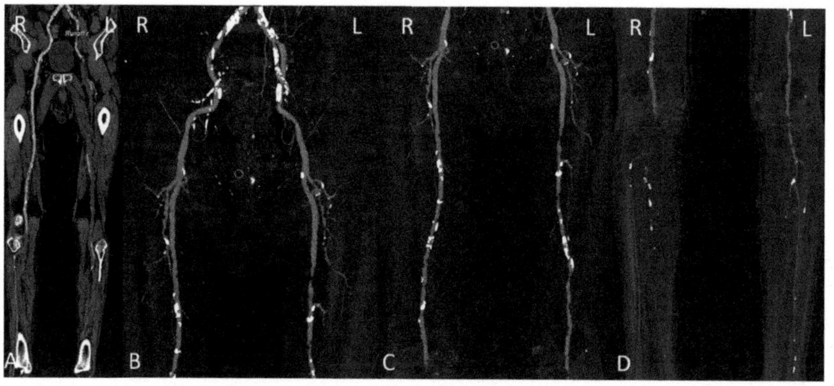

Figure 4. Lower extremity CTA using 120 kVp protocol in a 83-year-old man with PAD. A, curved planar reformatted image and B–D, maximum intensity projection images. The image quality was visually classified as score 3 (good) in the aortoiliac (a) and femoropopliteal (b) and score 2 (adequate) in the lower leg segments (c) because of poor visualization. Note extensive calcification of bilateral arteries of low extremity.

lower image noise was observed in data sets scanned with integrated detector compared to data sets scanned with conventional detector [29]. Although these two strategies were used to decrease noise in the 70 kVp group, the image noise in the 70 kVp group was still higher than in the 120 kVp group. Baumueller's study [30] showed that image noise at 80 kVp reconstructed with SAFIRE was significantly lower than that in datasets acquired at 100 kVp and reconstructed with FBP. The difference probably resulted from the more pronounced reduction in tube potential and the simultaneous increase in pitch in our study. Another possible interpretation is that the strength level of 3 for SAFIRE may not be sufficient for 70 kVp data compared with 80 kVp data, this hypothesis merits further studies. Although the image noise in the 70 kVp group was higher than that in the 120 kVp group, the image quality was still diagnostic with a mean subjective image quality score of 3.5. No statistically significant difference was found for subjective image quality evaluation between the two groups.

There are certain limitations to our study that must be acknowledged. First, patients' body mass index was not compared between the two groups because the height and weight were not recorded when patients underwent CTA examinations and were thus not available in this retrospective study. However, as an alternative anthropometric parameter to gauge body habitus, we measured the anteroposterior and transverse diameter in the CT images and calculated effective diameter of each study subject, which showed no significant difference between the two groups. Second, because of the retrospective design of this study, it was impossible to exactly control several parameters influencing radiation dose and image quality, such as the collimation. Additionally, selection bias because of the nature of retrospective study may occur in our study. Therefore, a prospective study is required. Third, a relatively small sample size of 44 patients was investigated in this feasibility study. A further study with a larger sample should be performed to confirm the results of our single-center study. Fourth, the diagnostic accuracy of lower extremity

Table 2. Subjective image quality scores of three arterial segments of the lower extremities.

Score	120 kVp group	70 kVp group	*P* value
Aorto-iliac area			
Reader 1	3.6±0.5	3.7±0.5	0.366
Reader 2	3.6±0.5	3.5±0.6	0.766
Both	3.6±0.5	3.7±0.5	0.598
Femoro-popliteal region			
Reader 1	3.7±0.5	3.6±0.5	0.511
Reader 2	3.7±0.5	3.6±0.6	0.629
Both	3.6±0.6	3.7±0.5	0.762
lower leg segment			
Reader 1	3.1±0.7	3.4±0.6	0.156
Reader 2	3.1±0.5	3.3±0.8	0.140
Both	3.3±0.7	3.1±0.6	0.316
Mean			
Reader 1	3.5±0.4	3.6±0.4	0.313
Reader 2	3.5±0.4	3.5±0.5	0.391
Both	3.5±0.5	3.5±0.4	0.981

Table 3. Radiation dose comparison of two lower extremity CTA protocols.

Parameters	120 kVp group	70 kVp group	*P* value
DLP (mGy×cm)	434.5±164.1	83.7±7.4	<0.001
CTDIvol (mGy)	4.0±1.4	0.7±0.1	<0.001
ED (mGy)	1.6±0.7	0.3±0.1	<0.001

DLP = dose-length product; CTDIvol = volume CT dose index; ED = effective dose.

CTA using 70 kVp and high pitch acquisition was not assessed, since in most patients invasive angiography as the reference standard was not available. A further study assessing the diagnostic accuracy of lower extremity CTA using this protocol is required.

In conclusion, lower extremity CTA using 70 kVp, high pith acquisition and iterative reconstruction is feasible and allows for lowering radiation dose and contrast material without compromising image quality when compared with a standard 120 kVp CTA protocol.

Author Contributions

Conceived and designed the experiments: GML. Performed the experiments: LQ CSZ YEZ LJZ GML. Analyzed the data: LQ CSZ YEZ LJZ GML. Wrote the paper: LQ FGM CSZ YEZ UJS LJZ GML.

References

1. Li J, Hasimu B, Yu J, Wang J, Hu D (2012) Prevalence of peripheral arterial disease and risk factors for the low and high ankle-brachial index in Chinese patients with type 2 diabetes. J HEALTH SCI 2006; 52(2): 97
2. Luo YY, Li J, Xin Y, Zheng LQ, Yu JM, et al.(2007) Risk factors of peripheral arterial disease and relationship between low ankle brachial index and mortality from all-cause and cardiovascular disease in Chinese patients with hypertension. JJ Hum Hypertens 21(6): 461–466
3. Foley WD, Stonely T (2010) CT angiography of the lower extremities. Radiol Clin North Am 2010; 48(2):367–396
4. Hirsch AT, Criqui MH, Treat-Jacobson D, Regensteiner JG, Creager MA, et al. 2001; (2001) Peripheral arterial disease detection, awareness, and treatment in primary care. JAMA 286(11):1317–1324
5. Catalano C, Fraioli F, Laghi A, Napoli A, Bezzi M, et al. (2004) Infrarenal aortic and lower-extremity arterial disease: diagnostic performance of multi-detector row CT angiography. Radiology 231(2):555–563
6. Romano M, Mainenti PP, Imbriaco M, Amato B, Markabaoui K, et al. (2004) Multidetector row CT angiography of the abdominal aorta and lower extremities in patients with peripheral arterial occlusive disease: diagnostic accuracy and interobserver agreement. Eur J Radiol 50(3):303–308
7. Huang SY, Nelson RC, Miller MJ, Kim CY, Lawson JH, et al. (2012) Assessment of vascular contrast and depiction of stenoses in abdominopelvic and lower extremity vasculature: comparison of dual-energy MDCT with digital subtraction angiography. Acad Radiol 19(9):1149–1157
8. Redmond JM, Levy BA, Dajani KA, Cass JR, Cole PA. (2008) Detecting vascular injury in lower-extremity orthopedic trauma: the role of CT angiography. Orthopedics. 31(8):761–767
9. Utsunomiya D, Oda S, Funama Y, Awai K, Nakaura T, et al. (2010) Comparison of standard- and low-tube voltage MDCT angiography in patients with peripheral arterial disease. Eur Radiol; 20(11):2758–2765
10. Lezzi R, Santoro M, Marano R, Di Stasi C, Dattesi R, et al. (2012) Low-dose multidetector CT angiography in the evaluation of infrarenal aorta and peripheral arterial occlusive disease. Radiology; 263(1):287–298
11. Duan Y, Wang X, Yang X, Wu D, Cheng Z, et al. (2013) Diagnostic efficiency of low-Dose CT angiography compared with conventional angiography in peripheral arterial occlusions. AJR Am J Roentgenol 201(6):W906–914
12. Park CK, Choo KS, Jeon UB, Baik SK, Kim YW, et al. (2013) Image quality and radiation dose of 128-slice dual-source CT venography using low kilovoltage combined with high-pitch scanning and automatic tube current modulation. Int J Cardiovasc Imaging; 29 Suppl 1:47–51.
13. Grant K, Raupach R. SAFIRE: Sinogram Affirmed Iterative Reconstruction. (2013)
14. Baumueller S, Winklehner A, Karlo C, Goetti R, Flohr T, et al. Low-dose CT of the lung: potential value of iterative reconstructions[J]. Eur Radiol 2012; 22(12):2597–2606
15. Fraioli F, Catalano C, Napoli A, Francone M, Venditti F, et al. (2006) Low-dose multidetector-row CT angiography of the infra-renal aorta and lower extremity vessels: image quality and diagnostic accuracy in comparison with standard DSA. Eur Radiol 16:137–146
16. Napoli A, Anzidei M, Zaccagna F, Cavallo Marincola B, Zini C, et al. (2011) Peripheral arterial occlusive disease: diagnostic performance and effect on therapeutic management of 64-section CT angiography. Radiology; 261(3):976–986
17. Shrimpton P. (2004) Assessment of patient dose in CT. In: European Commission. European guidelines for multislice computed tomography. Luxembourg: European Commission.
18. Gunn ML, Kohr JR (2010) State of the art: technologies for computed tomography dose reduction. Emerg Radiol; 17(3):209–218
19. De Zordo T, von Lutterotti K, Dejaco C, Soegner PF, Frank R, et al. (2012) Comparison of image quality and radiation dose of different pulmonary CTA protocols on a 128-slice CT: high-pitch dual source CT, dual energy CT and conventional spiral CT. Eur Radiol; 22(2):279–286
20. Amacker NA, Mader C, Alkadhi H, Leschka S, Frauenfelder T. (2012) Routine chest and abdominal high-pitch CT: an alternative low dose protocol with preserved image quality. Eur J Radiol 2012; 81(3):e392–397
21. Schuhbaeck A, Achenbach S, Layritz C, Eisentopf J, Hecker F, et al. (2013) Image quality of ultra-low radiation exposure coronary CT angiography with an effective dose <0.1mSv using high-pitch spiral acquisition and raw data-based iterative reconstruction. Eur Radiol; 23(3):597–606
22. Achenbach S, Goroll T, Seltmann M, Pflederer T, Anders K, et al. (2011) Detection of coronary artery stenoses by low-dose, prospectively ECG-triggered, high-pitch spiral coronary CT angiography. JACC Cardiovasc Imaging; 4(4):328–337
23. Yang WJ, Chen KM, Liu B, Pang LF, Zhang H, et al. (2013) Contrast media volume optimization in high-pitch dual-source CT coronary angiography: feasibility study. Int J Cardiovasc Imaging; 29(1):245–252
24. Baumueller S, Winklehner A, Karlo C, Goetti R, Flohr T, et al. (2012) Low-dose CT of the lung: potential value of iterative reconstructions. Eur Radiol;2 22(12):2597–2606
25. Nie P, Li H, Duan Y, Wang X, Ji X, et al. (2014) Impact of sinogram affirmed iterative reconstruction (SAFIRE) algorithm on image quality with 70 kVp-tube-voltage dual-source CT angiography in children with congenital heart disease. PloS one, 9(3): e91123
26. Han BK, Grant KL, Garberich R, Sedlmair M, Lindberg J, et al. (2012) Assessment of an iterative reconstruction algorithm (SAFIRE) on image quality in pediatric cardiac CT datasets. J Cardiovasc Comput Tomogr 6(3):200–204
27. Winklehner A, Karlo C, Puippe G, Schmidt B, Flohr T, et al. (2011) Raw data-based iterative reconstruction in body CTA: evaluation of radiation dose saving potential. Eur Radiol; 21(12): 2521–2526
28. Yang WJ, Yan FH, Liu B, Pang LF, Hou L, et al. (2013) Can sinogram-affirmed iterative (SAFIRE) reconstruction improve imaging quality on low-dose lung CT screening compared with traditional filtered back projection (FBP) reconstruction? J Comput Assist Tomogr; 37(2):301–305
29. von Spiczak J, Morsbach F, Winklhofer S, Frauenfelder T, Leschka S, et al. (2013) Coronary artery stent imaging with CT using an integrated electronics detector and iterative reconstructions: first in vitro experience. J Cardiovasc Comput Tomogr; 7(4):215–222
30. Baumueller S, Winklehner A, Karlo C, Goetti R, Flohr T, et al. (2012) Low-dose CT of the lung: potential value of iterative reconstructions. Eur Radiol 2012; 22(12):2597–2606

16

Value of Prominent Flow Voids without Cord Edema in the Detection of Spinal Arteriovenous Fistulae

Lea M. Alhilali*, Arich R. Reynolds, Saeed Fakhran

Department of Radiology, University of Pittsburgh Medical Center, Pittsburgh, Pennsylvania, United States of America

Abstract

Purpose: To determine the prevalence of spinal dural arteriovenous fistulae (SDAVF) in patients presenting with prominent vascular flow voids on imaging without other imaging findings suggestive of SDAVF.

Methods: We retrospectively identified patients from January 1, 2005 to March 1, 2012 who underwent spinal angiography for suspected SDAVF with prominent vascular flow voids on prior imaging. We excluded patients with other major spinal pathology or other imaging findings of SDAVF including cord hyperintensity, enhancement, or expansion. We calculated the proportion of patients with positive findings for SDAVF on angiography and evaluated the prevalence of SDAVF for this finding alone and in correlation with clinical findings.

Results: 18 patients underwent spinal angiography for prominent flow voids on imaging without other spinal pathology or imaging findings of SDAVF. Three had a SDAVF detected on angiography. The prevalence of SDAVF in this population was low, only 17% (95% CI 6-39%). All of the patients with positive angiography findings had myelopathy, increasing the prevalence to 100% if the additional clinical finding of myelopathy was present.

Conclusions: Prominent flow voids without other imaging findings suggestive of SDAVF is poorly predictive of the presence of a SDAVF, unless myelopathy is present clinically.

Editor: Jeroen Hendrikse, University Medical Center (UMC) Utrecht, Netherlands

Funding: These authors have no support or funding to report.

Competing Interests: The authors have declared that no competing interests exist.

* E-mail: alhilalilm@upmc.edu

Introduction

Although spinal dural arteriovenous fistulae (SDAVF) account for approximately 70% of all spinal vascular malformations, they still remain a relatively rare entity [1,2]. The symptomatology associated with SDAVF is nonspecific and may mimic much more common pathologies including degenerative disc disease, radiculopathy, spinal stenosis and peripheral neuropathy [3–6]. Early detection is key, as prognosis depends on the duration of symptoms [1]. With its nonspecific clinical presentation, conventional imaging may be the first to suggest a SDAVF as the causative pathology. T2 hyperintensity within the cord has been shown to be 100% sensitive for detection of SDAVF[7,8], but may be a later finding, as it indicates edema and hypoxia which are long-term sequelae resulting due to venous hypertension from the SDAVF [3].

Dilated intradural veins, seen as dilated flow voids on T2 weighted imaging, may be an earlier sign of venous hypertension and are occasionally seen before venous hypertension causes cord signal changes. Abnormal intradural vasculature without cord signal abnormality is usually seen in patients with milder disability, which is the ideal detection time-point, as greater initial disability is correlated with poorer outcome [9]. Recently, a case-series has reported that abnormal flow voids without cord signal changes have been used to detect essentially incidental SDAVFs, where all the SDAVFs detected with this isolated sign were asymptomatic [10]. However, there is overlap between the appearance of flow voids in SDAVF and the appearance of flow voids in normal patients [11,12]. Additionally, prior studies evaluating the diagnostic value of flow voids in patients with SDAVF have included patients both with flow voids and abnormal cord signal [7], which when seen together may increase the specificity of the flow voids in diagnosing SDAVF, as compared to flow voids as an isolated finding. The purpose of our study was to determine the prevalence of SDAVF in patients with prominent flow voids as the only imaging finding suggestive of SDAVF on MR, using catheter angiography as the gold standard. We further sought to determine if there were any specific imaging or clinical findings that distinguished patients with prominent flow voids and positive angiographic findings from those with a negative angiogram.

Materials and Methods

Ethics Statement

Our institutional review board approved this study, with waiver of informed consent. All imaging and angiographic examinations included in this study were performed as standard of care and the results were retrospectively reviewed.

Patient Selection and Image Acquisition

We searched our enterprise-wide electronic medical record, encompassing 20 academic and community hospitals, including a free-standing pediatric hospital, in an effort to identify patients who underwent spinal angiography for suspected SDAVF between January 1, 2005 to March 1, 2012. All spinal angiography reports were searched using the key-words "spinal dural arteriovenous fistula", "SDAVF," "spinal fistula," "spinal dural AVF," and "spinal dural AV fistula,". Additionally, MR reports were searched with the keywords "dilated vasculature," "dilated vessels," "abnormal vasculature," "abnormal vessels," "prominent flow voids," and "abnormal flow voids." Patients were excluded if age was less 18 years, prior cross-sectional imaging or spinal angiography was not available for review (8 patients), if there was evidence of spinal pathology other than a SDAVF on imaging excluding minor degenerative findings based upon review by a fellowship-trained neuroradiologist both with certificates of added qualification (2 patients with hypervascular metastases), or angiography was performed more than 30 days after cross-sectional imaging (1 patient). Pediatric patients were not included in this study, as the pathology of spinal vascular malformations in children is significantly different than in the adult population, consisting of vascular malformations both with and without a nidus and are often associated with syndromes such as Weber-Osler-Rendu, Parkes Weber, Klippel-Trenaunay, and Cobb syndrome [13]. Additionally patients were excluded if there were other imaging findings of SDAVF including cord hyperintensity, enhancement, or expansion based upon review by a fellowship-trained CAQ certified neuroradiologist (30 patients). At our institution, MR examinations of the spine are interpreted by fellowship-trained neuroradiologists. Although the current study was a retrospective review, the determination of prominent vasculature for this study utilized the prospective interpretation by the initial interpreting neuroradiologist. Demographic data collected included age and sex. Clinical data collected included presenting symptoms, imaging and angiography results, and post-imaging clinical management.

MR examinations were performed on a 1.5T system (GE Healthcare, Milwaukee, Wisconsin) with neutral positioning using a standard spine coil. Sagittal sequences were obtained with 24 cm FOV and 256×192 matrix for the cervical and lumbar spines and a 32 cm FOV and 512×224 matrix for the thoracic spine as follows: sagittal spin echo T1-weighted (TR, 500 msec; TE, min; section thickness, 3 mm; number of acquisitions, 3), sagittal fast spin echo T2-weighted fat saturation (TR, 3500 msec; TE, 84-102 msec; section thickness, 3 mm; number of acquisitions, 3). Axial images were obtained with 22 cm FOV and 256×192 matrix for the cervical and lumbar spine and 24 cm FOV and 256×224 matrix for the lumbar spine as follows: axial spine echo T1-weighted (TR, 500 msec; TE, min; section thickness, 3 mm; number of acquisitions, 2), fast spin echo T2-weighted images (TR, 3500; TE 102–120 msec; section thickness, 3mm; number of acquisitions, 2). Additional axial 3D gradient echo images (TR, 35 msec; TE, 13 msec; flip angle 5; section thickness, 2 mm; number of acquisitions, 1) were obtained with a 22 cm FOV and 256×192 matrix in the cervical spine. If contrast enhanced T1-weighted images were obtained, post-contrast imaging was performed with 0.1 mmol/kg gadolinium-based contrast material (Multihance: Bracco, Milan, Italy) using typical T1-weighted parameters as described above. At our institution, post contrast imaging of the spine is performed immediately (<1 minute) after contrast administration.

Digital subtraction angiograms were performed within 30 days of the MR examinations. At our institution, the standard protocol is to inject all segmental arteries from the level of the vertebral arteries to the level of the internal iliac arteries. Segmental arteries were injected with approximately 3 cc of iohexol (Omnipaque, GE Healthcare, Milwaukee, Wisconsin; 300 mg of iodine/mL). Images were obtained at a rate of 2–4 frames/sec with a 1024×1024 matrix. Identification of the anterior spinal artery occurred in all cases. All segmental arteries were selectively catheterized and injected in all patients.

Image Analysis

All MR examinations that were prospectively interpreted by a fellowship-trained neuroradiologist as having prominent vasculature were re-reviewed in consensus by 2 additional fellowship-trained, neuroradiologists with certificates of additional qualification and more than 2 years of experience. Images were re-evaluated for findings that have previously been found to be suggestive of abnormal vasculature on conventional imaging [11,14,15,16]: (1) flow voids spanning more than 3 vertebral body levels; (2) serpentine appearance of the vessels; (3) largest size > 2 mm; (4) detection of more than two vessels. Inter-rater agreement for these imaging findings was determined utilizing Cohen's kappa: two fellowship-trained neuroradiologists were separately asked to determine the presence or absence of each of the four imaging findings indicative of abnormal vasculature for each study, blinded to both the clinical and angiographic findings as well as the other's interpretation. Kappa results were interpreted according to Altman (1.0 = perfect agreement, 0.80–0.99 = very good agreement, 0.60–0.79 = good agreement, 0.40–0.59 = moderate agreement, 0.20–0.39 = fair agreement, and less than 0.20 = poor agreement) [17]. Studies were then scored in consensus by the two neuroradiologists using these findings and given 1 point for each finding, for a maximum total score of 4. Additonally, the number of vertebral body levels spanned by any abnormal vasculature was recorded.

Data Analysis

Comparison of proportions in the demographic and imaging analysis data was performed using Fisher's exact test. Comparison of continuous variables in the demographic and imaging analysis data was performed with a two-tailed unpaired t-test. Confidence intervals for the prevalence were calculated using the interval estimation for a binomial proportion [18]. Comparison of the number of vertebral body levels spanned by the abnormal vasculature between patients with and without SDAVF was performed with a two-tailed unpaired t-test. P values were two-tailed and p values less than 0.05 were considered significant.

Results

18 patients (8 male, 10 female; mean age 49 years, range 2–88) underwent spinal angiography for suspected SDAVF with prominent flow voids as the only relevant imaging finding suggestive of SDAVF. The majority of patients presented with back pain (12 patients, 67%); three patients presented with myelopathy (17%).

Inter-rater agreement for the finding of flow voids spanning more than 3 vertebral body levels was perfect (kappa = 1.0, 95% CI 1.00–1.00), while agreement was very good for determining serpentine appearance of the vessels (kappa = 0.83, 95% CI 0.65-1.00) or the detection of more than two vessels (kappa = 0.89, 95% CI 0.74-1.00). Inter-rater agreement was good for the finding of largest size >2 mm (0.67, 95% CI 0.43–0.99). The average score for imaging findings suggestive of abnormal vasculature in these patients was 2.4 (median 2, range 1–4). Ten patients had abnormal

Table 1. Demographic and clinical characteristics of patients undergoing myelography with prominent flow voids as the only imaging finding suggestive of SDAVF.

Patient No.	Age	Sex	Presenting Symptom	Angiography Findings
1	39	F	Myelopathy[1]	SDVAF from right T6 and T7 radicular arteries
2	63	F	Post-laminectomy syndrome	Negative
3	73	M	Thoracolumbar pain	Negative
4	26	F	Back pain	Negative
5	27	F	Bilateral lower extremity pain	Negative
6	43	M	Back pain	Negative
7	20	F	Chiari Malformation	Negative
8	63	F	Back pain	Negative
9	53	F	Bilateral lower extremityweakness, myelopathy[2]	SDVAF arising from the left L1 radicular artery
10	51	F	Lower extremity pain	Negative
11	60	M	Back pain	Negative
12	59	M	Back pain	Negative
13	45	M	Back pain	Negative
14	42	F	Back pain	Negative
15	64	M	Bilateral lower extremity pain	Negative
16	60	M	Back pain	Negative
17	88	F	Back pain	Negative
18	47	M	Back pain and myelopathy[3]	SDVAF arising from the right T12 radicular artery

[1]Myelopathic symptoms of progressive loss of strength and sensation in the lower extremities.
[2]Myelopathic symptoms of urinary retention and constipation.
[3]Myelopathic symptoms of abnormal sensation in the lower extremities.

vessels spanning more than 3 vertebral levels (56%); eleven had serpentine vessels (61%); only six had vessels greater than 2 mm in size (33%); and the large majority had more than 2 vessels detected (16 patients, 89%). Demographic and clinical characteristics are summarized in Table 1.

Three patients had a spinal angiogram positive for a SDAVF (1 male, 2 females; mean age 46.3, range 39–53). All three patients had type 1 SDAVF according to the Ansler and Spetlzer criteria [19] and were treated with embolization without findings of residual SDAVF on subsequent catheter angiography.

The prevalence of SDAVF in our population with only prominent flow voids was 17% (95% CI 6-39%). Figure 1 shows a comparison of images between three patients with prominent flow voids on MR, one with a positive angiogram and two without findings on angiography.

Of the 15 patients with negative angiography results, seven continued to be followed for non-specific back pain by a primary care physician. Presenting symptoms were ascribed to intracranial pathology without spinal involvement in three patients (1 melanoma brain metastases, 1 multiple sclerosis, and 1 normal pressure hydrocephalus). In two patients, the presenting symptom of pain was felt to be related to diabetic neuropathy and in one it was attributed to restless legs syndrome. One patient underwent spinal decompression for epidural lipomatosis as the presumed etiology of the presenting symptoms. In the remaining patient, the presenting pain was felt to be related to a prior cervical cord injury that was not imaged and the patient was treated with an intrathecal catheter.

There was no significant difference in the demographic characteristics between patients with and without positive angiography findings. Similarly, no significant difference was seen in the scores for findings suggestive of abnormal vasculature or in the presence of vessels spanning more than 3 vertebral body levels, serpentine vessels, vessels larger than 2 mm, or more than 2 detected vessels. The average extent of the abnormal vasculature between patients with and without SDAVF trended towards, but did not reach statistical significance (mean number of vertebral body levels spanned by abnormal vasculature = 6.0 and 3.7, range 1–7 and 4–8, respectively, $p = 0.07$).

Of note, all three patients with positive angiography findings had myelopathy present clinically and no patients with a negative angiogram had clinical myelopathy ($p = 0.001$). No patients with a score less than 3 had a positive angiogram. Comparison of the demographic and imaging data between the two groups is summarized in Table 2.

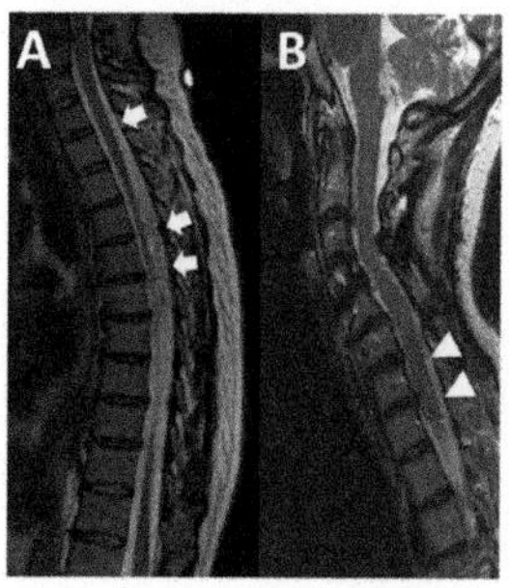

Figure 1. Abnormal flow voids without cord signal are seen in both patients with and without SDAVF. Sagittal T2-weighted images show prominent flow voids in (a) a patient with a positive spinal angiogram (arrows) and (b) a patient with negative angiography results (triangular arrowheads).

Table 2. Comparison of demographic and imaging data for patients with and without positive findings on angiography.

	Patients with Negative Angiogram	Patients with Positive Angiogram	p value
Number	15	3	N/A
Number male (%)	7 (47%)	1 (33%)	0.6
Age (yrs, mean, range)	49.7 (20–88)	46.3 (39–53)	0.61
Score for findings suggesting abnormal vessels (mean, range)	2.2 (1–4)	3.3 (3–4)	0.2
Vessels spanning more than 3 levels (number, percent)	7 (47%)	3 (100%)	0.22
Serpentine vessels (number, percent)	8 (53%)	2 (66%)	1
Vessel >2 mm size (number, percent)	5 (33%)	2 (66%)	0.53
Detection of more than 2 vessels (number, percent)	13 (87%)	3 (100%)	1
Presence of myelopathy (number, percent)	0 (0%)	3 (100%)	0.001

Discussion

Prominent flow voids without other imaging findings of SDAVF were found to be poorly predictive of the presence of a SDAVF, unless myelopathy was present clinically. No patients with less than three of the four imaging findings previously found to be suggestive of abnormal vasculature had a positive angiogram.

Previous studies evaluating the value of flow voids in the diagnosis of SDAVF have included patients with both flow voids and abnormal cord signal [3,7,10,20], therefore obscuring the value of this finding in isolation. A recent study has indicated the importance of suggesting the diagnosis of SDAVF in the setting of prominent flow voids, even in the absence of other imaging findings suggestive of SDAVF or myelopathic symptoms, given the possibility of detecting a SDAVF before it becomes symptomatic [10]. However, this study only retrospectively evaluated patients with positive angiographic findings and did not evaluate the prevalence of prominent flow voids in patients with negative angiographic studies. Thus, radiologists have been left with the impression that they may potentially miss a curable spinal myelopathy if SDAVF is not routinely mentioned in the setting of prominent flow voids. However, our results would suggest such an approach would result in a very high number of false positive studies. False positives are significant in the workup of a SDAVF, as they can result in catheter angiography, which has significant risks, even in the hands of experienced practitioners, as well as the potential for nephrotoxicity associated with use of iodinated contrast [3].

Our study is the first to evaluate for SDAVF in all patients with prominent vasculature as the only finding of SDAVF on conventional imaging, with catheter angiogram for definitive diagnosis. Previous studies examining prominent flow voids without abnormal cord signal have only evaluated its value in populations with known SDAVFs [10,21]. No study has yet evaluated this finding in the general population to determine its associated false positive rate for diagnosing a SDAVF. In contradistinction to the prior case series [10], we did not find any patients with a SDAVF with only prominent flow voids on imaging and without myelopathy on clinical examination. The presence of myelopathy without abnormal cord signal in our patients may reflect venous hypertension high enough to cause decreased cord perfusion and myelopathy, but not substantial or long-standing enough to cause edema and abnormal cord signal [3]. This correlates with the known lack of association between cord signal and symptoms after treatment of the SDAVF [22]. Lack of both abnormal cord signal and myelopathy suggests the prominent vasculature does not reflect venous hypertension but rather anatomic variation, except perhaps in rare, reportable cases [10]. Therefore, in patients with prominent vascular flow voids but no abnormal cord signal, given the relative rarity of SDVAF in this population, correlation for a history of myelopathy should be undertaken.

None of the patients with less than three of the four imaging findings previously found to be suggestive of abnormal vasculature had a SDAVF. The presence of any one of the four findings may result in a subjective appearance of prominent vasculature on imaging. However, based on our findings, we would advise that determination of abnormal vasculature should not be based on a simple overall impression, which may be influenced by only one or two of the flow void findings. Rather, if there is a suspicion that the vasculature may be abnormal, a dedicated evaluation for the known four imaging findings of flow voids in SDAVF should be undertaken as well as a search of the medical record, or discussion with the referring physician, for a history of myelopathy. Additionally, a further workup to assess for subtle myelopathic findings on physical examination or subtle imaging findings of a SDAVF, including possible MR angiography, may be helpful [23]. Furthermore, a higher number of vertebral body levels spanned by the abnormal vasculature showed a trend towards significance, and has previously been correlated with the degree of myelopathy in patients with SDAVF [24]. Larger studies may be helpful to confirm this finding as a way to determine truly abnormal vasculature.

The principal limitation to this study is that our institution does not routinely perform spinal MR angiograms (spinal MRA). While, spinal MRA has emerged as a useful, noninvasive, tool in which to localize arterial feeders and venous drainage patterns in patients with high clinical imaging suspicion for, and corroborative imaging findings strongly suggestive of, SDAVF [25,26], it has not been shown to improve sensitivity or specificity in detection of SDAVF in patients with equivocal conventional MR findings, such as lack of abnormal cord signal [11]. As a result, our spinal angiographers, believe that spinal MRA, in patients with such equivocal MR findings, to be of insufficient negative predictive value to preclude spinal angiography, and hence do not routinely order them in this subset of patients.

Additional limitations of this study include its retrospective nature and small sample size. However, SDAVF itself is a rare disease, and prominent flow voids and lack of abnormal T2 signal is an even rarer imaging presentation of the disease [9,25,26]. In selecting for patients only with a definitive angiographic study, we further decreased our potential patient population, as it rare to undertake invasive angiography with only a single imaging finding. However, we feel that this further strengthens our finding, as the patients included in our study underwent angiography either because the radiologist felt very strongly about the flow void appearance or there was strong clinical concern. The poor correlation between flow voids and SDAVF in this population with either high imaging confidence or clinical suspicion further supports that prominent flow voids without cord signal abnormality should not be considered abnormal on a routine basis.

Conclusion

In conclusion, the prevalence of SDAVF in patients with prominent flow voids as the only imaging finding suggestive of SDAVF is low, particularly in patients without myelopathy and in those with less than three imaging findings to suggest abnormal vasculature.

Author Contributions

Conceived and designed the experiments: LA SF. Performed the experiments: LA SF. Analyzed the data: LA SF AR. Contributed reagents/materials/analysis tools: LA SF AR. Wrote the paper: LA SF AR.

References

1. Krings T, Geibprasert S. Spinal dural arteriovenous fistulas (2009) AJNR Am J Neuroradiol 30: 639–48.
2. Jellema K, Tijssen CC, Sluzewski M, van Asbeck FW, Koudstaal PJ, et al. (2006)Spinal dural arteriovenous fistulas—an underdiagnosed disease. A review of patients admitted to the spinal unit of a rehabilitation center. J Neurol 253: 159–62.
3. Marcus J, Schwarz J, Singh IP, Sigounas D, Knopman J, et al. (2013) Spinal dural arteriovenous fistulas: a review. Curr Atheroscler Rep 15: 335.
4. Jellema K, Tijssen CC, van Gijn J (2006)Spinal dural arteriovenous fistulas: a congestive myelopathy that initially mimics a peripheral nerve disorder. Brain 129: 3150–64.
5. Symon L, Kuyama H, Kendall B (1984) Dural arteriovenous malformations of the spine. Clinical features and surgical results in 55 cases. J Neurosurg 60: 238–47.
6. Rosenblum DS, Myers SJ (1991)Dural spinal cord arteriovenous malformation. Arch Phys Med Rehabil. 72: 233–6.
7. Toossi S, Josephson SA, Hetts SW, Chin CT, Kralik S, et al. (2012) Utility of MRI in spinal arteriovenous fistula. Neurology 79: 25–30.
8. Hartman J, Rabinstein AA (2012) Can we rule out a spinal arteriovenous fistula using only MRI? Yes, we can. Neurology 79: 15–6.
9. Muralidharan R, Saladino A, Lanzino G, Atkinson JL, Rabinstein AA (2011) The clinical and radiological presentation of spinal dural arteriovenous fistula. Spine (Phila Pa 1976) 36: E1641–7.
10. van Rooij WJ, Nijenhuis RJ, Peluso JP, Sluzewski M, Beute GN, et al. (2012) Spinal dural fistulas without swelling and edema of the cord as incidental findings. AJNR Am J Neuroradiol. 33: 1888–92.
11. Saraf-Lavi E, Bowen BC, Quencer RM, Sklar EM, Holz A, et al. (2002) Detection of spinal dural arteriovenous fistulae with MR imaging and contrast-enhanced MR angiography: sensitivity, specificity, and prediction of vertebral level. AJNR Am J Neuroradiol 23: 858–67.
12. Aghakhani N, Parker F, David P, Lasjaunias P, Tadie M (2008) Curable cause of paraplegia: spinal dural arteriovenous fistulae. Stroke 39: 2756–9.
13. Hacein-Bey L, Konstas AA, Pile-Spellman J (2014)Natural history, current concepts, classification, factors impacting endovascular therapy, and pathophysiology of cerebral and spinal dural arteriovenous fistulas. Clin Neurol Neurosurg. Jan 31. [Epub ahead of print]
14. Bowen BC, Pattany PM (2000) Contrast-enhanced MR angiography of spinal vessels. Magn Reson Imaging Clin N Am 8: 597–614.
15. Gulliver D, Noakes J (1988) Myelographic differentiation of spinal cord arteriovenous malformations from the normal population. Australas Radiol 32: 57–64.
16. Mascalchi M, Ferrito G, Quilici N, Mangiafico S, Cosottini M, et al. (2001) Spinal vascular malformations: MR angiography after treatment. Radiology 219: 346–53.
17. Altman DG (1991) Practical Statistics for Medical Research. London, England: Chapman and Hall, p.404
18. Brown LD, Cai TT, DasGupta A (2001) Interval estimation for a binomial proportion. Statistical Science 16: 101–103.
19. Anson JA, Spetzler RF (1992) Interventional neuroradiology for spinal pathology. Clin Neurosurg. 39: 388–417.
20. Donghai W, Ning Y, Peng Z, Shuo X, Xueen L, et al. (2013) The Diagnosis of Spinal Dural Arteriovenous Fistulas. Spine (Phila Pa 1976) Feb 1. [Epub ahead of print]
21. Sato K, Terbrugge KG, Krings T (2012) Asymptomatic spinal dural arteriovenous fistulas: pathomechanical considerations. J Neurosurg Spine. 16(5): 441–6.
22. Muralidharan R, Mandrekar J, Lanzino G, Atkinson JL, Rabinstein AA, et al. (2013) Prognostic value of clinical and radiological signs in the postoperative outcome of spinal dural arteriovenous fistula. Spine (Phila Pa 1976) 38: 1188–93.
23. Hetts SW, Moftakhar P, English JD, Dowd CF, Higashida RT, et al. (2012) Spinal dural arteriovenous fistulas and intrathecal venous drainage: correlation between digital subtraction angiography, magnetic resonance imaging, and clinical findings. J Neurosurg Spine. 16(5): 433–40.
24. Mull M, Nijenhuis RJ, Backes WH, Krings T, Wilmink JT, et al. (2007) Value and limitations of contrast-enhanced MR angiography in spinal arteriovenous malformations and dural arteriovenous fistulas. AJNR Am J Neuroradiol. 28(7): 1249–58.
25. Masaryk TJ, Ross JS, Modic MT, Ruff RL, Selman WR, et al. (1987) Radiculomeningeal vascular malformations of the spine: MR imaging. Radiology 164: 845–9.
26. Hurst RW, Grossman RI (2000) Peripheral spinal cord hypointensity on T2-weighted MR images: a reliable imaging sign of venous hypertensive myelopathy. AJNR Am J Neuroradiol 21: 781–6.

Computer Simulation of Magnetic Resonance Angiography Imaging: Model Description and Validation

Artur Klepaczko*, Piotr Szczypiński, Grzegorz Dwojakowski, Michał Strzelecki, Andrzej Materka

Medical Electronics Division, Institute of Electronics, Lodz University of Technology, Lodz, Poland

Abstract

With the development of medical imaging modalities and image processing algorithms, there arises a need for methods of their comprehensive quantitative evaluation. In particular, this concerns the algorithms for vessel tracking and segmentation in magnetic resonance angiography images. The problem can be approached by using synthetic images, where true geometry of vessels is known. This paper presents a framework for computer modeling of MRA imaging and the results of its validation. A new model incorporates blood flow simulation within MR signal computation kernel. The proposed solution is unique, especially with respect to the interface between flow and image formation processes. Furthermore it utilizes the concept of particle tracing. The particles reflect the flow of fluid they are immersed in and they are assigned magnetization vectors with temporal evolution controlled by MR physics. Such an approach ensures flexibility as the designed simulator is able to reconstruct flow profiles of any type. The proposed model is validated in a series of experiments with physical and digital flow phantoms. The synthesized 3D images contain various features (including artifacts) characteristic for the time-of-flight protocol and exhibit remarkable correlation with the data acquired in a real MR scanner. The obtained results support the primary goal of the conducted research, i.e. establishing a reference technique for a quantified validation of MR angiography image processing algorithms.

Editor: Oscar Deniz Suarez, Universidad de Castilla-La Mancha, Spain

Funding: This paper was supported by the Polish National Science Centre under grants no. N N519 650940 and 2013/08/M/ST7/00943. The funders had no role in study design, data collection and analysis, decision to publish, or preparation of the manuscript.

Competing Interests: The authors have declared that no competing interests exist.

* E-mail: aklepaczko@p.lodz.pl

Introduction

Magnetic Resonance Angiography (MRA) is a powerful technique for visualization of blood vessels. Within the MRA setting, there exist both non-invasive imaging protocols, such as e.g. Time-Of-Flight (ToF) [1–3] or Phase Contrast Angiography (PCA) [4], and sequences that rely on application of contrast agent [5]. In this paper we focus on the ToF sequence.

Direct examination of the measured ToF images provides essentially qualitative description of the vessel system. Nonetheless, the quantitative information about the defects of vascularity of a visualized organ can help decide on the appropriate treatment. Such data can only be obtained with the use of specialized MRA image processing algorithms. If conducted properly, a quantitative analysis can increase objectivity and correctness of the medical diagnosis. For instance, the methods for vessels segmentation and tracking [6–9] enable an automatic identification of occlusions, pathological narrowings and hyper- or neovascularizations.

However, prior to the introduction of an image-based decision supporting system to clinical practice, it must be verified in a series of experiments involving a large number of test images, how reliable and accurate particular methods are. A statistically credible validation is difficult due to relatively high costs of collecting images solely for the research purposes. Additionally, MR scanners are extensively used in clinics and therefore are rarely accessible for experimentation. In consequence, the number of images available for evaluation studies is too low and there appears a need for a technique to generate synthetic images.

The problem of simulating the magnetic resonance imaging (MRI) has been studied over the last two decades and several computer simulators have been designed. The proposed solutions differ in the approach to model tissue of the imaged objects, in the routines of MR image synthesis, and in the degree to which different artifactual or undesired phenomena (like noise, chemical shift, ringing or Gibbs phenomenon, partial volume effect etc.) are taken into account.

In the approach proposed in [10], the imaged objects are defined as parameter maps. The maps visualize distribution of T_1 (spin-lattice relaxation time constant), T_2 (spin-spin relaxation) and ρ (proton density) values within the object. These values are calculated from real images. Formation of new images is performed using different repetition and echo times. On the other hand, in paper [11] the virtual organ object is modeled using the concept of spin density. By the use of inverse Fourier Transform, the simulator constructs the image representation in the spatial-frequency domain (k-space formalism). Simulation of the signal sampling phase and specific imaging sequence is accomplished through appropriate selection of the k-space elements and their amplitude and phase alteration. Separate simulation phases are required for each of the modeled tissues. This fact introduces a significant obstacle if a voxel contains more than one tissue leading to a partial volume effect.

In comparison with other approaches, more realistic simulation effects are achieved by solutions proposed in [12–15]. The models of the used imaged organs require that for each object voxel and every tissue component, relaxation times T_1 and T_2, proton density ρ, as well as value of the frequency offset linked to chemical shift artifact are defined. Consequently, to deal with the partial volume effect it is sufficient to determine the volume of particular tissue in a voxel.

It must be underlined that the simulators proposed so far can be used to synthesize only anatomical images, where the flow effects, suppressed by the imaging protocol parameters (echo and repetition times and RF pulse flip angle) are neglected. However, when it comes to MR angiography, beside nuclear phenomena, it is the motion of the hydrogen nuclei that produces the measured signal. Since none of the currently available simulators can be employed for MRA image synthesis, this paper presents an original computer system for simulation of the 3D ToF sequence.

Methods

The design of the MRA simulator decomposes into the following tasks:

1. geometry definition of a vessel or a set of vessel branches (i.e. vascularity of an organ, hereafter shortly referred to as a *vascularity object*),
2. simulation of blood flow through the vessels,
3. modeling of stationary tissues which surround vessels (i.e. an *organ*),
4. simulation of magnetic resonance imaging sequences.

At first the blood flow and a vessel model is described. Since the aim of the research is a validation of the designed simulator, the focus is narrowed to relatively simple virtual phantoms of vascularity objects. Geometry of these models was adjusted to match real flow phantoms manufactured by Shelley Medical Imaging Technologies [16] (see Fig. 1) for the purpose of MR scanners calibration. This approach is motivated by the idea of reconstructing similar, corresponding to each other sets of images both in a simulator and a real MR scanner. The quantified degree of such correspondence enables an objective verification of the synthesized images from the point of view how realistic they are. The flow model description is succeeded by a presentation of the stationary tissue model and MR image formation procedures.

Eventually, details of real MRA image acquisitions are provided. Apart from the physical phantoms, the experimental apparatus consisted of the MR compatible, high-precision flow pump, CompuFlow 1000 MR, also manufactured by Shelley [17]. The pump is capable of forcing the flow at wide range of rates (from 0.1 ml/s to 35 ml/s) characteristic of human vessel system. It is also possible to generate a specific pulsatile flow waveforms, choosing either between one of the typical physiological courses

Table 1. BMF physical parameters.

Parameter	Value
Density d	1020 kg/m^3
Viscosity ν	4.1 mPa s
Proton density ρ (water relative)	1.00
T_1 @ 1.5 T	850 ms
T_2 @ 1.5 T	170 ms

(like common carotid or femoral waveforms) or a user-defined function. In the described experiments, however, only a steady flow option was used. It simplifies comparison of real and simulated images by removing additional factor causing potential discrepancies resulting from imperfect reproduction of the same pulsatile waveform in a flow simulation software. The pump is constructed mainly from non-ferromagnetic materials and is thus allowed to operate at high magnetic fields such as in the MR environment for the purpose of MR scanners calibration.

Furthermore, to achieve realistic conditions of the experiments, the medium used with the flow phantoms was Shelley's blood mimicking fluid (BMF). It is essentially a water solution of glycerol in proportion 6:4. The physical properties of the fluid are presented in Table 1. All further computer simulations, with respect to flow and MR image formation, were performed using the same ν,d,ρ,T_1, and T_2 parameters.

Blood flow and vessel model

A simulation of flow is performed in COMSOL Multiphysics software. The routines implemented therein solve Navier-Stokes equations for the incompressible fluid. A laminar flow, known also as stratified flow, assumes that fluid moves in parallel layers [18]. Each layer has its own speed and slides past one another with no lateral mixing. Blood flows in one direction with the parabolic velocity profile reaching the greatest value in the middle of the cylinder and it decreases towards vessel walls. The model is sufficiently accurate for simulating blood flow in a straight tube of relatively large diameter. However, in case of more complex structures with stenoses and bifurcations the flow behavior locally changes and turbulences and frictional forces should be taken into consideration [19]. Therefore, in the presented study the flow simulation is conducted in the turbulent regime using the RANS k-ϵ equation [20].

Among other available options, fluid motion in a vessel can be forced by determining pressure difference between the inlet and outlet surfaces. From the physiological point of view, the

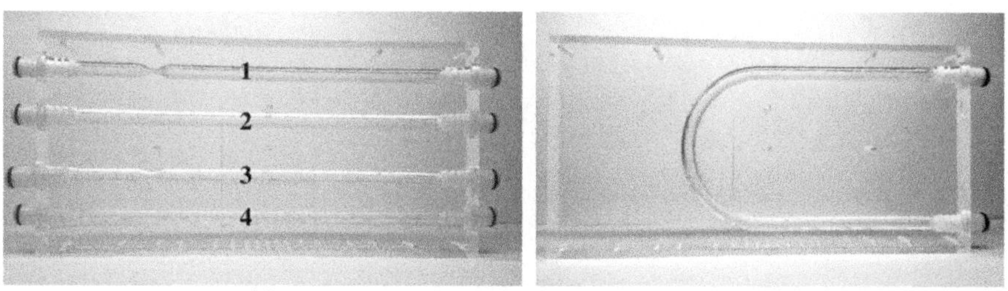

Figure 1. Flow phantoms used in the study. Channel diameters: 8 mm (1, 2, 3 and U-bend) and 5 mm (channel 4). Stenoses: channel 1 (75% of the diameter), channel 3 (50% of the diameter). Straight channels length: 207 mm. Curvature radius of the U-bend channel: 44 mm.

reasonable rates of peak velocity of blood for medium and large arteries(such as those modeled by the Shelley phantoms) range from 30 to 100 cm/s and the pressure values must be adjusted accordingly. Figure 2 presents a simulated distribution of pressure and velocity inside digitally reconstructed phantoms, where input and output pressure values were set to 11448 Pa and 11148 Pa respectively. Additionally, vessel walls are assumed solid, which prevents leakage.

It is important to note that COMSOL splits the domain of interest (in our case – the fluid) into a mesh of 3D geometrical primitives – tetrahedral nodes – of some finite volume. Velocity vectors are calculated for every mesh node. A crucial issue, is how to transfer this information in a usable form into the virtual MR scanner. A direct approach involves an operation on the COMSOL-generated mesh but it breeds a problem, referred to as numerical diffusion [21,22]. An example of fluid motion in Fig. 3, showing positions of a portion of blood in 3 subsequent time steps illustrates the problem. If the flow channel is decomposed into a mesh of regular square-shaped nodes (in fact, any shape of mesh primitives entails similar consequences) it seems that in step 2, only half of the fluid volume shifts from node 1 to node 2. Thus, any further mesh-based calculations would require a division of fluid volume of this particular blood portion into 2 fractions, each for nodes 1 and 2. In step 3, these fractions move on: a part of blood residing in node 2 is transported to node 3, and again only a fraction of node 1 volume shifts towards node 2. Apparently, a sample of blood which initially occupied only one mesh node, spilled over 3 nodes. Clearly, this leads to an ambiguous localization of fluid portions – an error which accumulates in subsequent time steps. Moreover, this problem affects simulation of magnetic resonance, where subsequent image formation procedures (selective excitation, spatial encoding etc.) are invoked in discrete time moments and applied to portions of fluids at specific locations. Hence, a numerical diffusion may cause misinterpretation of true position of some blood samples.

To avoid the above described problem another COMSOL toolbox, namely the Particle Tracing for Fluid Flow module [23] is used. Based on the laminar and turbulent flow solution, the group of particles fed into a tube at an inlet is transported to its outlet. Each spherically-shaped particle is described by its density and diameter. Furthermore, the simulation is configured in such a manner, that there is no particle-fluid interaction. On the other hand, fluid forces particles to move along a vessel and by tracing their locations in subsequent time steps it is possible to find a bundle of trajectories which represent the motion of blood (see Fig. 4). These particle trajectories define the input to the MRA simulator.

It is instructive to analyze the velocities achieved by the particles, as they move along a vessel, and compare them with the values obtained in a fluid flow simulation. Figure 5 presents time courses of the velocity magnitude plotted for four randomly picked particles in the experiment inside the 50%-stenosis tube. It has been observed that the velocities remain constant until particles reach the narrowing, where they experience rapid acceleration, then they slow down and finally flow out from the vessel. The initial velocity value and the moment of its increase differ between the particles, depending on their position relative to central axis of the channel. Figures 6a–b depict locations of the same four particles in two cross-sections of the vessel situated either at 100 mm from the inlet or in the middle of stenosis. Also, velocity magnitudes, as calculated by the fluid flow simulation, are shown. Clearly, particle velocities presented in the time courses remain close to the values obtained using the plots in Fig. 6. It demonstrates the equivalence between a standard flow simulation and particle traces.

MRA Imaging Simulation

The main software modules of the designed simulator are presented in Fig. 7 and described below.

Digital phantom. The input to the MRA simulator is a model composed of particle trajectories as described above. These trajectories are defined by a series of particle coordinates at subsequent flow simulation time steps Δt. In fact, the coordinates can be easily interpolated in time domain, which in turn allows the selection of any other time step for the purpose of the subsequent stages of the simulation. In other words, in both stages i.e. in the simulation of flow and in the simulation of magnetic resonance effects, the discretization of time domain can be adjusted independently.

In the MRA simulation, the whole volume of a vascularity object has to be filled with particles. Furthermore, every particle corresponds to a portion of the fluid so that the sum of all these

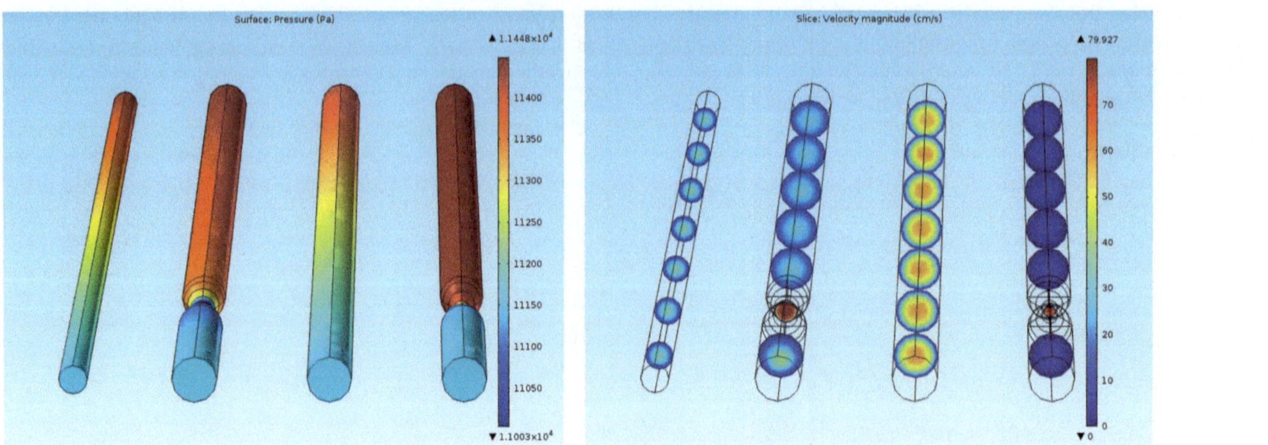

(a) (b)

Figure 2. Blood flow simulation in the 4 straight tubes phantom. Simulated pressure (a) and velocity magnitude (b) distribution. Pressure difference (300 Pa) between channel inlets and outlets is made equal for every tube. Note the rapid increase in the velocity value and simultaneously pressure drop in the area of stenoses.

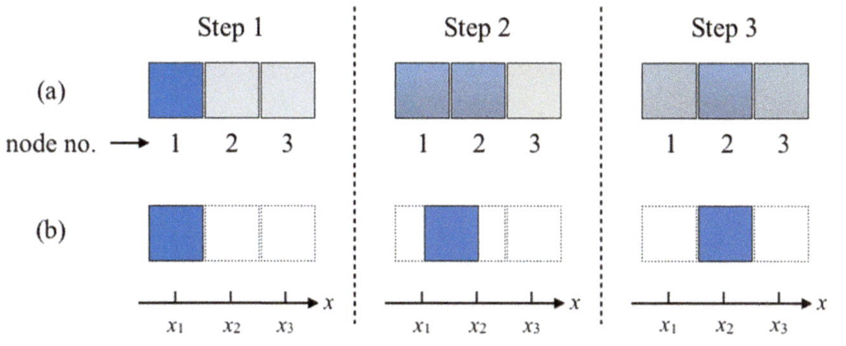

Figure 3. Illustration of the numerical diffusion problem. Fluid transportation in the case of a fixed mesh (a) and actual translation of a fluid portion along the x coordinate (b). In the former case, a fluid portion originally occupying node no. 1 spills over three consequtive nodes at time step 3 although in fact during this time period it has only and entirely moved from position x_1 to x_2.

portions constitute the total volume of the blood flowing through the vessels. Therefore, in the proposed method every trajectory is populated by particles according to the following strategy.

Firstly, the area of a tube inlet, which should be perpendicular to the course of trajectories, is tessellated by means of the Voronoi decomposition (Fig. 8a). It divides the inlet area into regions, so that every region corresponds with the individual trajectory. As a result, every trajectory is assigned an area Δs_j, where the j indicates a particular trajectory. In consequence, contributions from trajectories sparsely scattered are balanced with respect to those which are distributed more densely. Secondly, let us consider a right prism in which an individual Voronoi cell constitutes a base polygon and the distance between the two base polygons is equal to Δl_j (Fig. 8b). The volume of such prism is a product of the base face area Δs_j and the distance Δl_j. Therefore, in case of a straight tube, i in which the fluid speed along the trajectory is stable and

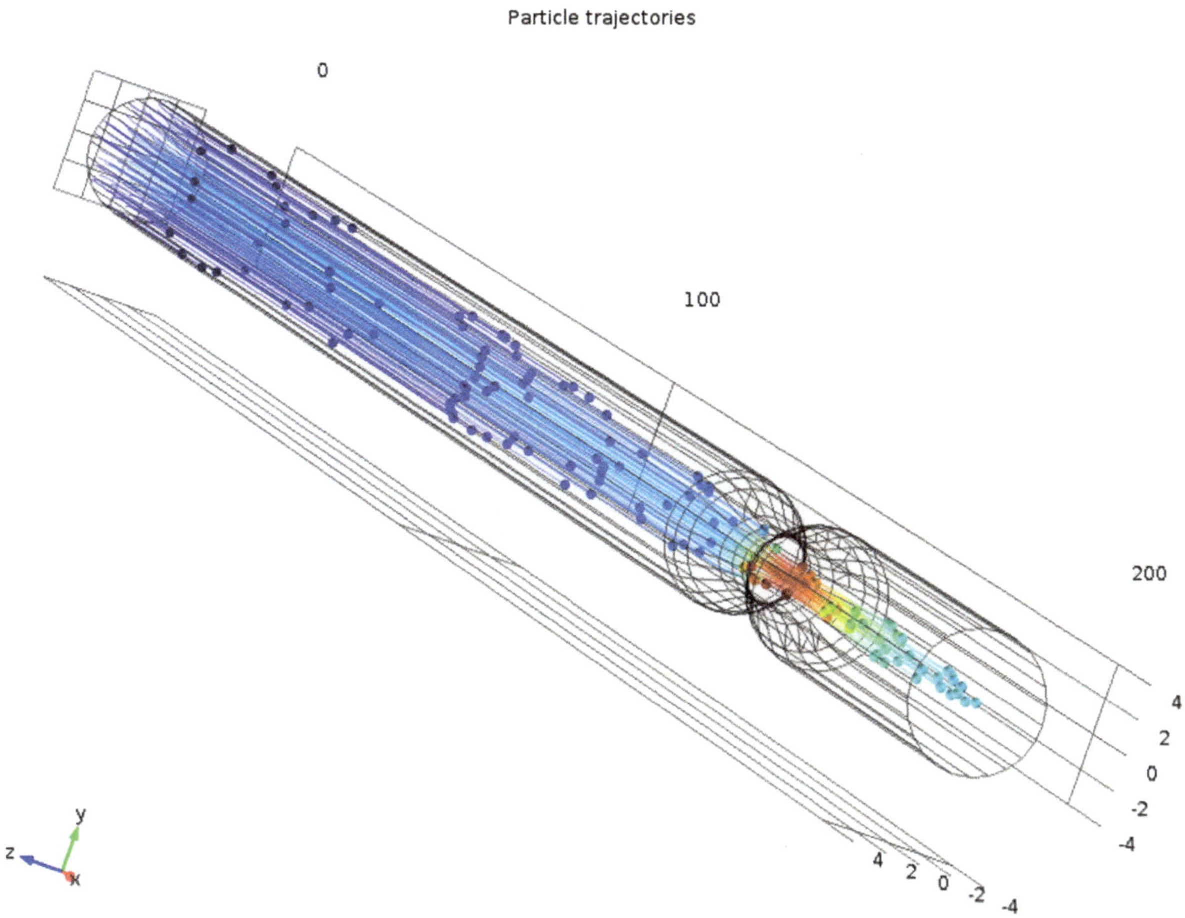

Figure 4. Particle trajectories as determined by the Particle Tracing Module. Simulated trajectories at a time step $t > t_0$, where t_0 indicates initiation of flow. The fastest particles move close to the main axis of the tube.

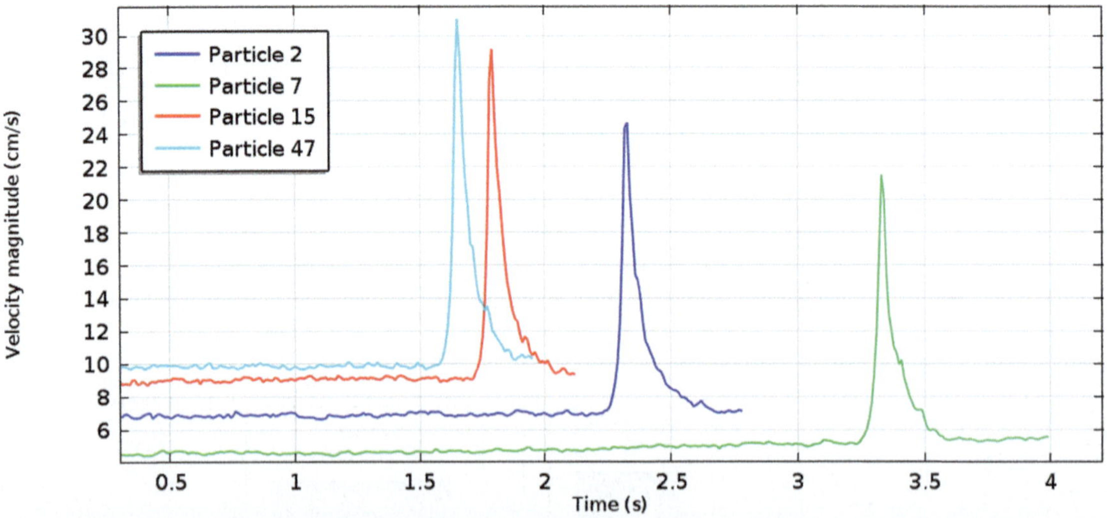

Figure 5. Time courses of velocity magnitude plotted for 4 randomly picked particles. Simulation performed for the 50%-stenosis tube with the flow rate of 2.5 ml/s. Particle which move faster (labeled 15 and 47) reach the narrowing earlier and gain larger peak velocity in the stenosis region than particles 2 and 7.

the tube's cross-section remains constant, the trajectory is populated with particles equally spaced by the distance Δl_j. The volume associated with every such particle is equal to the volume of the right prism mentioned above.

As the MRA simulation advances, the particles move along the associated trajectories toward the tube outlets and finally, as they pass through the outlet, they disappear from the simulation. At the same time new particles must be introduced at the inlet of the tube, as the vascularity object should be filled with particles at all times of the simulation. The new particles are introduced at a specific time rate Δt_j (not to be confused with the flow simulation time step Δt) equal to the ratio of the distance Δl_j and speed of the fluid along the corresponding trajectory. Therefore, every particle introduced at the inlet is distant from the preceding one by the Δl_j and represents the same amount of the volume equal to $\Delta s_j \cdot \Delta l_j$. The Δl_j and consequently Δt_j can be adjusted individually for each trajectory. In our approach, by default they are chosen so that the distances between adjacent particles on the same trajectory are comparable to the distances between the neighboring trajectories, giving an even distribution of particles in all three dimensions. These values however, can be manipulated to achieve a desired number of particles along trajectories.

Note that in a narrowing particles move faster and the distance Δl_j becomes larger. At the same time the area of vessel cross-section shrinks, Δs_j decreases with inverse proportion to the increase of Δl_j and as a result the volume corresponding with the

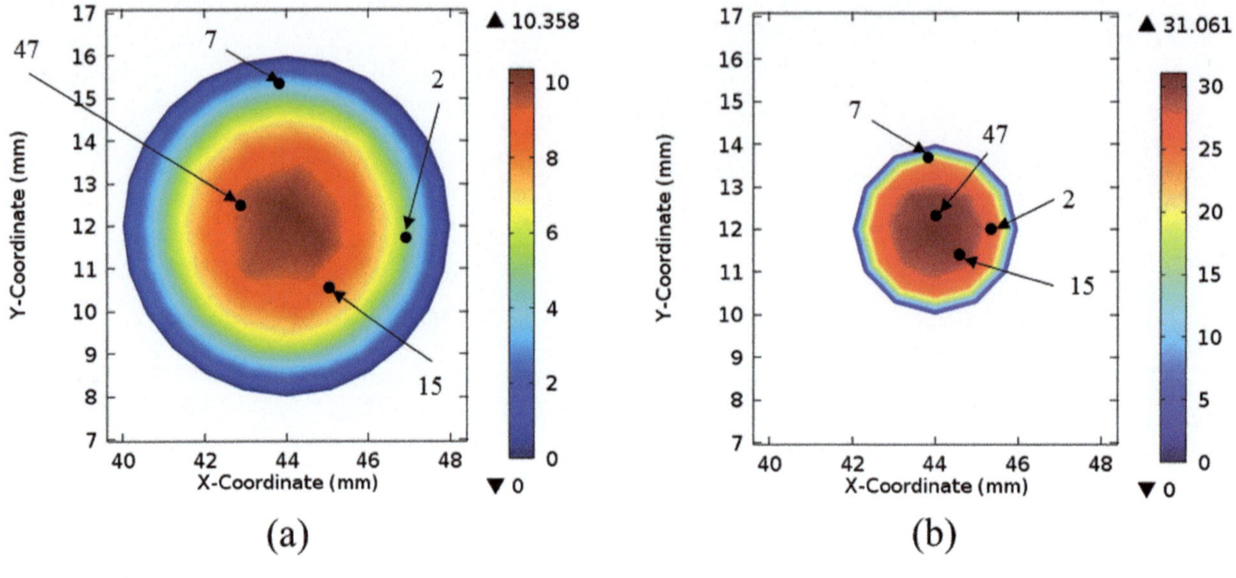

Figure 6. Distribution of velocity magnitude at two cross-sections of the 50%-stenosis tube [cm/s]. Fluid flow rate equals to 2.5 ml/s. Black dots depict approximated locations of 4 particles whose velocity time courses are shown in Fig. 5 The selected cross-sections are situated a) 100 mm from the vessel inlet and b) in the middle of stenosis.

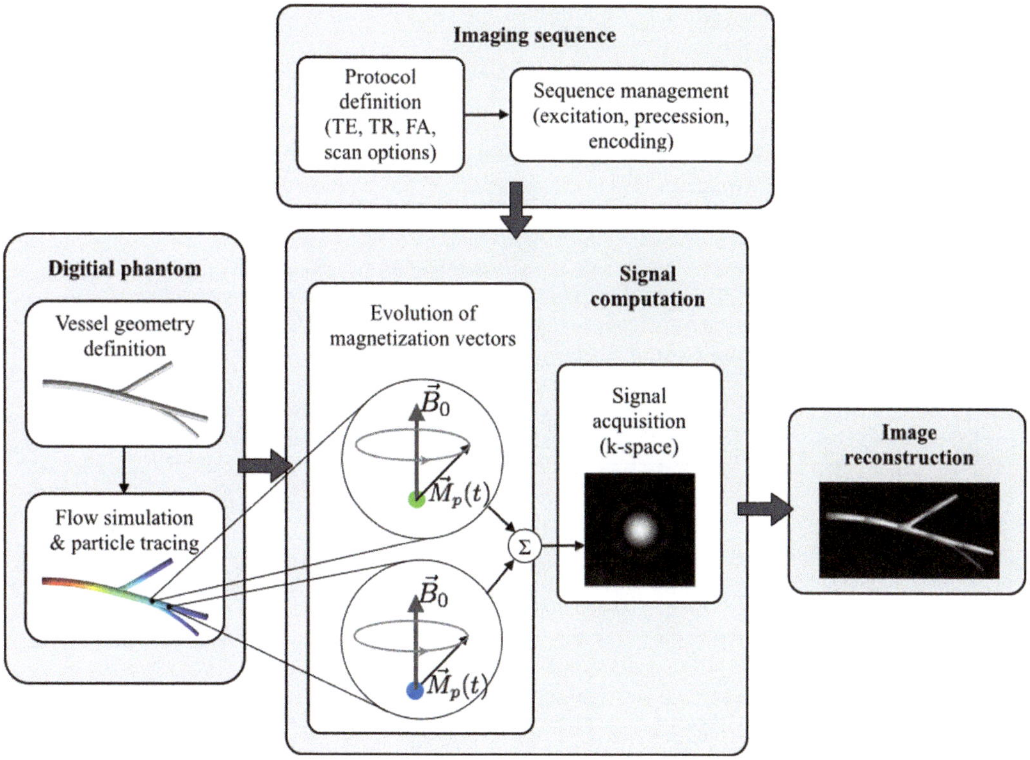

Figure 7. Main modules of the designed MRA simulator. The simulator is decomposed into 4 integral parts: 1) virtual object description, 2) sequence management, 3) signal computation and 4) image reconstruction.

particle remains constant.As the particles on different trajectories convey various portions of blood, the associated volume is used to weight the MR signal originating from its corresponding particle. It is important that information on exact shape of boundaries limiting the volume is not further required. In consequence, there is no need for exact tessellation of the three dimensional volume of the vascularity object, which in turn simplifies the simulator implementation.

As indicated above, the time step of MRA simulation δt generally differs from the step used in flow simulation Δt and also from the steps Δt_j used to fill trajectories with particles. The system finds position of a particle at time $t = n\Delta t + k\delta t$ by interpolating its coordinates corresponding to two locations, one at time $n\Delta t$ and the other at $(n+1)\Delta t$, where n and k are respectively the flow and MRA simulation step numbers. This solution enables performing image synthesis at arbitrary temporal resolution.

Apart from volume and parameters related to their motion, particles are assigned T_1 and T_2 relaxation times and proton density value ρ. Eventually, each particle on a trajectory obtains a unique identification label allowing to trace it during image

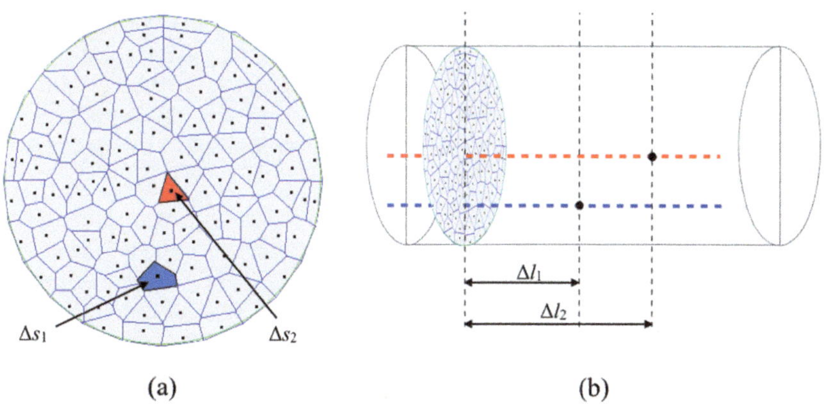

Figure 8. Calculation of particles cell volume. a) The result of Voronoi tessellation of a tube cross-section. Particles (black dots) cast on the selected surface serve as seed points. The blue and red polygons are example base faces of particle-associated cells. b) Lengths Δl_1 and Δl_2 denote distances traveled by particles on trajectories 1 (blue line) and 2 (red line), both during the same time interval Δt. $\Delta l_2 > \Delta l_1$ as velocity on the red trajectory is larger.

formation. A description of the digital phantom is completed by the information about physical size of an imaged organ and position of the vessels within it.

In the performed experiments the number of trajectories in a single tube was set to 256. Furthermore, the particle-associated volumes were adjusted to achieve the ratio of 3 particles per millimeter of a vessel length. It gives the value of about 20 particles per cubic millimeter or about 12 particles per final voxel. We found this ratio as optimal to obtain realistic images, while avoiding computational overload. In lower resolution images, also the number of trajectories may be decreased.

Stationary tissue which surrounds vessels – for clarity not shown in Fig. 7 – is modeled by a set of particles similarly to flowing spins but a position of the stationary particle is fixed for the entire scope of simulation. The definition of the stationary tissue requires setting of the shape and size of the organ. Then, the number of stationary particles is adjusted to match the density of their distribution to the ratio obtained for the moving ones. Tissue particles are uniformly distributed within the imaged volume except for the regions occupied by vessel branches. Furthermore, particles are assigned their T_1, T_2 and ρ values. Eventually, there can be several tissue types present in the imaging volume. Every component is simulated separately, and the final image is reconstructed from the sum of signals acquired for each tissue. Moreover, the chemical shift between fat and water components can be defined to simulate spatial misregistration of fat protons caused by magnetic shielding of the electron shell altering their effective resonant frequency. Nevertheless, the effect of chemical shift is not considered in the experiments reported in this study.

Imaging sequence. *Protocol definition.* An image synthesis procedure is controlled by a group of parameters constituting a sequence type and output image contents. The latter refers both to the image resolution (k-space size) and to the position and size of the field of view (FOV). By default, FOV embraces a whole object, but it can be reduced to only a part of it and its center can be shifted to any object point. It is important to keep a record of the FOV center offset and its location relative to gradients isocenter, since it directly affects the field strength value experienced by each particle.

The sequence definition is mainly determined by the sequence type. The Time-of-Flight protocol utilizes the Spoiled Gradient Echo sequence (SPGR) [2]. The SPGR sequence leads to saturation of the stationary spins which in turn produce much lower signal than fresh unsaturated molecules flowing into the imaging volume. The degree of inflow enhancement depends on velocity of blood spins and the orientation of vessels relative to the acquisition slice.

As for MR experiment, the program requires a specification of the echo and repetition times (TE and TR accordingly) and also the flip angle (FA). The sequence type also includes information whether the target image is 2- or 3-dimensional. For the 2D image the slice position and orientation should be specified. In case of volumetric acquisitions it must be also defined whether the whole FOV is scanned as one thick volume, or as a series of thin slabs (MOTSA – multiple overlapping thin slabs acquisition technique) [24]. Moreover, for 3D ToF it must be determined whether the ramped RF pulses, with spatially varying ip angle parallel to the direction of ow, are to be used. This technique, sometimes called TONE (tilted optimized non-saturating excitation) [25,26], reduces the effect of signal suppression from molecules which have traversed long distances within a slab and thus have been saturated by multiple RF pulses. Finally, the signal sampling window is determined by the readout time parameter which must ensure that the resulting sampling frequency meets the Nyquist-Shanon theorem.

Sequence management. An event management module is responsible for invoking subsequent steps of computations based on the current simulation stage. It begins with establishing the initial magnetization of particle spins by allowing them to freely precess in the presence of the main external magnetic field B_0. This procedure is later repeated for any new particles replacing those which flow out from vessel outlets. Then, the particles magnetization states are altered by an application of an RF pulse, free precession, and an application of phase encoding gradients. As for volumetric acquisitions and an in-plane flow in 2D, flow compensation gradients are included in the sequence design. These gradients account for a phase dispersion effect, taking place if spins of different speed flow through a voxel during the signal acquisition. Such spins have different phase and cause the signal from the voxel to fade away. By applying additional compensation gradients along the direction of flow, it is possible to partially eliminate this unwelcome effect.

After the phase encoding and – optional – velocity compensation steps, the frequency encoding gradient is applied and the signal acquisition step is executed. Eventually, numerical spoiling of the transverse magnetization is accomplished. At each step the MRI kernel is invoked with the appropriate parameters.

Signal computation. *Evolution of the magnetization vector.* The core of the system routines implements the discrete time analytic solution to the Bloch equation [27]. This approach relies on the assumptions of constant field $\vec{B}$ and that the shape of an RF excitation pulse is rectangular or it can be approximated by the set of such pulses. Thus, the simulation is limited to time-invariant gradient fields during excitation. In the generic case of arbitrarily shaped RF pulses, no analytical solution exists and numerical approach is required.

The analytical solution uses the rotation matrices and exponential scaling to modify magnetization vector of a particle (either moving or stationary) in accordance to specified sequence events. Hence, the magnetization vector $\vec{M}$ of a particle p is given by

$$\vec{M}_p(t+\delta t) = Rot_z(\theta_g) Rot_z(\theta_i) R_{\text{relax}} R_{\text{RF}} \vec{M}_p(t), \quad (1)$$

where $Rot_z(\theta)$ rotates the magnetization vector around the z-axis in reply to the phase encoding gradient (θ_g) and as a consequence of the main magnetic field inhomogeneity (θ_i). Note, that for the proper evaluation of the Bloch equation, position $\vec{r}_p = [x_p, y_p, z_p]^T$ of a particle relative to gradient isocenter must be determined first. For a stationary component, each particle has constant coordinates. In contrast, a moving particle changes position in time. Thus, a magnetization vector must be updated at time intervals which ensure reasonable trade-off between precision of the flow simulation, MR modeling and computational burden. Too high values of t introduce unacceptable discontinuity in evolution of the effective Larmor frequency experienced by a particle. On the other hand, very short δt results in significant increase in simulation time. In our approach, δt is adjusted to match sampling frequency of the signal acquisition phase, i.e. it is set to sampling window duration divided by the number of k-space points in the frequency encoding direction.

The R_{relax} rotation matrix is responsible for the relaxation effects and is calculated as

$$R_{\text{relax}}=\begin{pmatrix} e^{-\frac{\delta t}{T_2(\vec{r})}} & 0 & 0 \\ 0 & e^{-\frac{\delta t}{T_2(\vec{r})}} & 0 \\ 0 & 0 & 1-e^{-\frac{\delta t}{T_1(\vec{r})}} \end{pmatrix}. \quad (2)$$

The last term in (1) is the R_{RF} operator. In the general case, where the local field differs from B_0 due to field inhomogeneity or chemical shift artifact, the resonance frequency ω_{RF} deviates from ω_0 implied by B_0. Hence, the effective precessional frequency is

$$\omega_{\text{eff}}=\sqrt{\Delta\omega_0^2+\omega_1^2}, \quad (3)$$

where $\Delta\omega_0$ measures the frequency offset. Consequently, a $\vec{B}_1$ pulse of duration τ_p which is assumed to knock over $\vec{M}$ by angle α from $\vec{B}_0$ yields the effective flip angle

$$\alpha_{\text{eff}}=\tau_p\omega_{\text{eff}}=\tau_p\sqrt{\Delta\omega_0^2+\left(\frac{\alpha}{\tau_p}\right)^2}. \quad (4)$$

In the off-resonance condition spins experience not only the $\vec{B}_1$ pulse directed (assuming rotating frame of reference) along the x axis, optionally with a phase angle φ, but also residual field $\Delta\omega_0/\gamma$ – where γ is gyromagnetic ration – which points along $\vec{B}_0$. Therefore, the effective $\vec{B}_{\text{eff}}$ field forms an angle θ relative to the main magnetic field direction. Hence, the R_{RF} is eventually determined by

$$R_{\text{RF}}=Rot_z(\varphi)Rot_y(\theta)Rot_x(\alpha_{\text{eff}})Rot_y(-\theta)Rot_z(-\varphi). \quad (5)$$

It is important to note, that τ_p has to be divided into time intervals δt as in the other simulation phases (relaxation, gradient application). The blood particles move during RF pulse application and may not acquire sufficient energy to get excited. Thus, at each δt step the particle magnetization vectors are flipped only partially by angle α/n_{ts}, where $n_{ts}=\tau_p/\delta t$. Moreover, in the case of TONE protocol, the equation (4) resolves to

$$\alpha_{\text{eff}}=\tau_p\sqrt{\Delta\omega_0^2+\left(\frac{\alpha+\alpha_{\text{T}}(z)}{\tau_p}\right)^2}, \quad (6)$$

where $\alpha_{\text{T}}(z)$ is the extra flip angle dependent on a particle z-position and which adds to the base angle set for the entry slice.

Signal acquisition. A signal acquisition phase fills one line of k-space per TR. A single data point is calculated through numerical integration of transverse components of particle magnetization vectors over the whole imaging volume according to equation

$$s(t)=\sum_{p=1}^{n_p}\vec{M}_p(t)\vec{x}+j\sum_{p=1}^{n_p}\vec{M}_p(t)\vec{y}, \quad (7)$$

where n_p denotes number of particles.

Sampling frequency is determined by user-defined length of the sampling time frame and the desired number of voxels in the frequency encoding direction. Upon completion of one k-space point acquisition the system is allowed to alter its state - due to blood flow on one side, and relaxation phenomena on the other. After updating particles position and their magnetization vectors, next data point is calculated.

Note that because blood particles are subjected to flow, some of them may leave a vessel between two subsequent signal measurement times. New particles replacing those that have disappeared have no transverse magnetization as they did not receive any RF excitation pulse. As a result, they do not produce any signal until next echo cycle. This shows up in the resulting image as dark voxels in the slices where blood particles of high velocity enter imaging volume.

Image reconstruction. The last stage of image formation procedure consists in transformation of the raw data in the spatial-frequency domain (K-space) into image intensity domain. This stage is accomplished by the fast Fourier transform, followed by calculation of the magnitude of – complex transformation output. Before application of the FFT routine, it may be necessary to filter the raw data to reduce the phase mismapping artifact appearing in the phase encoding direction due to the motion of blood particles. We decided to port the filtering routine and FFT-based image reconstruction to the Matlab environment to enable any kind of low-pass digital filter available in the Signal Processing Toolbox [28] to be used.

Implementation. Apart from the image reconstruction module, the designed system has been implemented as a custom computer program. The source code was written in the ANSI-C language and compiled for the Mac OS X 10.7 platform (the OS X-native *clang* compiler was used). Moreover, the program was parallelized using Open MPI library [29]. The algorithm execution is divided into a set of computing agent-nodes, each responsible for handling a given bunch of trajectories. After calculation of the MR signal from its assigned trajectories, an agent sends the results to the master node who adds the received data to the signals simulated by other agents. If there are trajectories still waiting for assignment, an agent who completed its job is employed to handle another portion of data. This procedure ensures high efficiency as more powerful processing resources can be utilized more often. In our experiments the system was installed on the computer grid composed of one iMac desktop (Intel Core i7 3.4 GHz) and 10 MacMini units (10 × Intel Core i5 2.5 GHz) which is equivalent to 24 CPU cores. Additionally, if hyperthreading feature is taken into account, the execution can be distributed among 48 processing slots. The computers were connected over the local ethernet network and communicated on the SSH layer. The details of the SSH- and Open MPI-based grid setup are outlined in [30], where a heterogeneous computing environment extended on a Linux and legacy OS X (version 10.5) server is employed.

Measurements

Image acquisition was performed on the GE Signa HDxt 1.5 T system for various flow rates and sequence parameters. In every case, the 3D images were acquired using MOTSA and TONE techniques, and with flow compensation option switched on in each dimension. Tables 2 and 3 summarize the experimental setup. Note that in TONE technique, the FA parameter is the nominal flip angle set in the middle of the slab and it linearly decreases or increases along the z coordinate. On the other hand, simulation experiments are restricted to the two tubes with stenoses and the U-bend phantom, as their geometry seems to be more explanatory in quantitative inference.

In addition to flow phantoms, the experimental set is completed by three agarose gel slabs which are placed within the magnet together with the phantoms, as illustrated in Fig. 9a. The purpose of these layers is to increase load for the RF coils and to enhance

Table 2. Flow rates and corresponding image acquisition parameters.

Study #	Flow rate [ml/s]	TE/TR/FA [ms/ms/–]	Slab width/slab overlap [mm]	FOV (x/y/z) [cm]
1	2.5	4.7/40/20°	44/8	17.5/13.4/14.4
2	2.5	4.7/40/15°	44/8	17.5/13.4/14.4
3	4.6	4.6/27/15°	44/8	17.5/13.4/22.4
4	10	4.6/27/15°	25/5	17.5/13.4/24.5

signal quality. Also they can be used to estimate noise level and perform background correction.

Both phantoms were simultaneously put into the scanner and the phantoms were interconnected as viewed schematically in Fig. 9b. In this setting, the fluid first enters the 75%-stenosis tube, then returns through the U-bend phantom to the pump. The phantoms inside the magnet bore were oriented in such a manner that the flow channels were placed parallel to the z axis i.e. parallel to the main magnetic field, and vertically to the transverse plane, thus maximizing the effect of inflow enhancement. In the transverse plane, the data space was sampled with 224 and 160 of respectively frequency and phase encoding steps. The measured k-space slices were then null padded to 256×256–pixel images. A field of view size was adjusted to entirely cover a cross-sectional area of the phantom set, while slabs depth, their number and consequently FOV along the z axis varied depending on the study (cf. Table 2). Eventually, the imaging protocol included spatial presaturation option. In such a protocol spins flowing against the direction of B_0 field enter a saturation band located above an imaging slab. They receive additional RF pulses and are saturated, thus giving no or a reduced signal during acquisition. The goal of this action is to separate signals of arterial and venous origin.

Results

In order to validate the designed simulator system, a series of experiments using the above described physical phantoms imaged in a real MR scanner, was performed. On the other hand we synthesized equivalent images using our simulation framework forcing the same flow and imaging sequence parameters. A comparison of these two groups of images – real and synthetic ones – allows a comprehensive verification of correct implementation of the designed system. Figures 10–13 present the obtained real and their corresponding synthesized images.

Simulation results – qualitative analysis

A visual inspection of the results reveals that the highest degree of similarity between these two sorts of data has been obtained for the lower and medium flow rates. First of all, in both types of images a characteristic signal void near the entry layers of each slab is observed. This effect is caused by the spins flowing faster which are flushed out from the area of their initial excitation and produce a signal deeper in the slab. Slower spins receive more RF pulses and become saturated before reaching the end of the slab. Consequently, image brightness decreases more quickly near the channel walls, when compared to its central tracts, giving a parabolic profile of the image intensity.

Next, it can be noticed that a signal from the return section of the U-bend phantom is low relative to the inlet channel. In this case the mechanism responsible for signal suppression is spatial presaturation. Apparently, the signal close to channel borders is brighter than that observed in the middle. This can be explained by the fact, that it takes same time for spins to travel from the saturation band to an imaging slab. Those spins which move slower i.e. near channel borders, have time to recover some portion of their longitudinal magnetization and thus produce a measurable signal. This effect is better visible in the real images, however still observable in the synthetic ones.

Moreover, image intensity at locations where the fluid only exits, immediately after passing a narrowing and close to central axis rather than channel walls, is significantly larger. It is especially manifested in the 75%-stenosis tube. The main flux – as it can be judged from the brightest voxels bundle – visible after stenosis is asymmetric relative to the tube axis. This fact is reflected in the synthesized images, although the deviation from the symmetry axis is slightly different. It seems to be a result of complex and chaotic flow patterns which appear after a narrowing. Hence, the need to take into account both laminar and turbulent models in the simulation of flow, becomes evident.

Also, one can compare images acquired for the same – 2.5 ml/s – flow rate, but for different nominal flip angle (i.e. 15° or 20°), see Study 1 and 2. As to a larger flip angle, the wash out effect on slab entries is reduced and also channels with reverse direction of flow (i.e. against B_0 field) produce slightly higher signal in the channel

Table 3. Common image acquisition parameters.

Parameter	Value
Magnetic field strength	1.5 T
Protocol	Brain Vascular
Coil	1-channel transmit/receive bird-cage head coil
Scanning sequence	SPGR
Scanning options	Flow compensation, Variable flip angle (TONE), Spatial saturation, MOTSA
Slice thinckness	1 mm

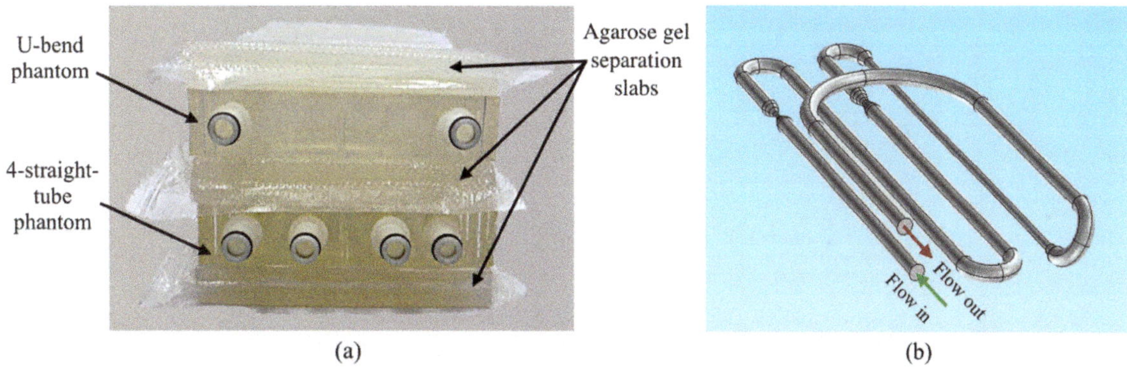

Figure 9. Assembly of the physical phantom set. (a) The stack of flow phantoms and separating agar gel layers. (b) Schematic of flow channel connections.

lumen (observed for the U-bend phantom – Fig. 10). The same effects can be observed for the synthesized images.

On the other hand, images synthesized in Study 4 (with flow rate of 10 ml/s) appear less realistic. For example, in the case of the 50%-stenosis tube simulation intensity jumps between neighboring slabs are clearly visible, although in the real image they can hardly be noticed.

Simulation results – quantitative analysis

Validation methodology. In the analysis described in this section we aim at comparing two sets of images – real and synthesized – objectively, i.e. in the quantitative manner. In order to accomplish this task we propose the following methodology. First, we select volumes of interest (VOIs) in each examined 3D image, which contain isolated tubes with stenosis and the U-bend phantom. Figure 14 shows outline of two exemplar VOIs selected in real images for the 75%-stenosis and the U-bend tubes. VOIs selection was performed manually simply by appropriate indexing of the image data loaded to the MATLAB workspace. As for the tubes with stenoses, the size of the subvolumes are $20 \times 20 \times 152$ voxels, while the U-bend phantom was cropped to a region of size $100 \times 20 \times 152$ voxels. The determined VOI depth ensures that a vessel is embraced at its entire length, while width and height are adjusted to account for oblique vessels orientation. The observed distance range between all voxels from a single tube projected onto an axial plane does not exceed the value of 20 points. Similar VOIs were selected both in the real and synthetic images.

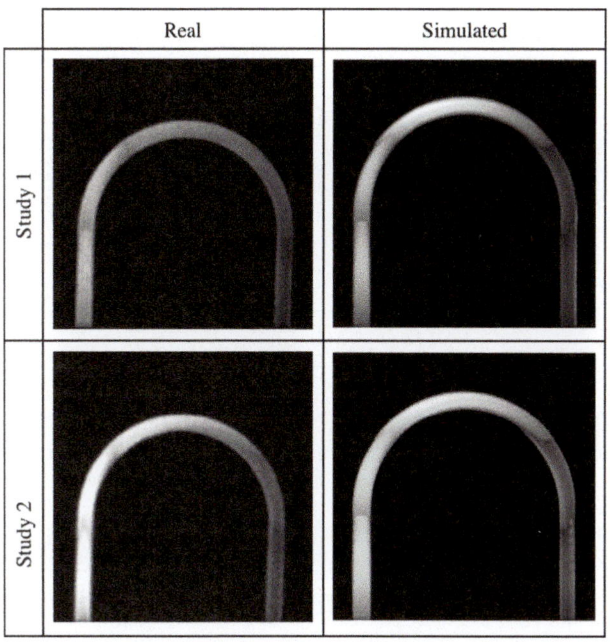

Figure 10. U-bend phantom images – Studies 1 and 2. Real (left panel) and simulated (right panel) acquisitions.

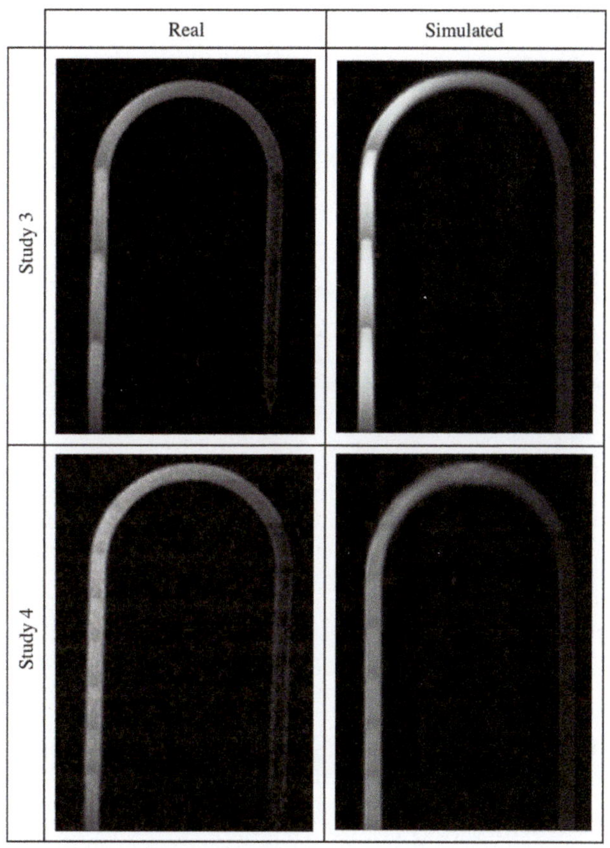

Figure 11. U-bend phantom images – Studies 3 and 4. Real (left panel) and simulated (right panel) acquisitions.

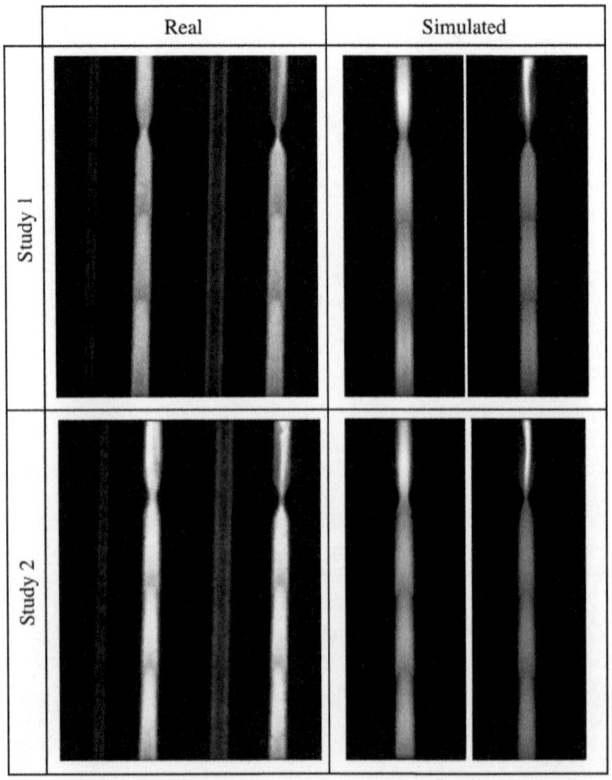

Figure 12. Straight tubes phantom images - Studies 1 and 2. Real (left panel) and simulated (right panel) acquisitions.

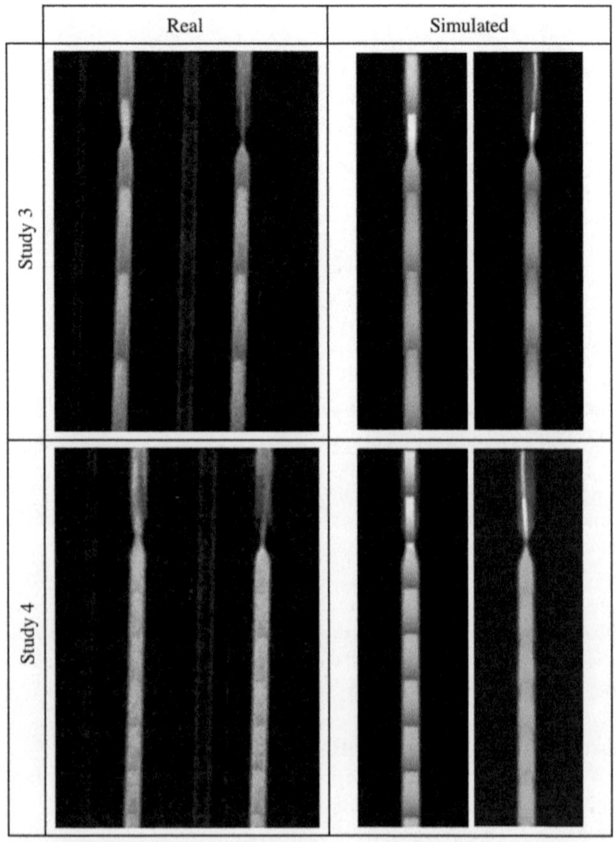

Figure 13. Straight tubes phantom images - Studies 3 and 4. Real (left panel) and simulated (right panel) acquisitions.

Note that the flow channel axes in the real images are neither perfectly parallel to the z axis of the image space coordinate system, nor vertical to the transverse plane. Thus, in order to compare them with the simulation results on the voxel-by-voxel basis, the real and synthetic images must be registered. We perform this procedure within respective VOIs using MATLAB Image Processing Toolbox [31]. The employed algorithm matches two volumetric data sets by performing rigid transformation of a synthesized image and optimizing their mutual information. Having registered VOIs, we calculate correlation coefficients and also – after scaling intensity values to span the same range in both data sets – root mean squared errors between corresponding images.

Image denoising. It must be noted that real images contain noise component, not included in the synthesized images. Noise degrades quality of images which hampers their visual examination and affects their quantitative analysis. Voxel-based calculations and comparisons involving different MR volumes require estimation of the true noise-free signal to ensure reliable, unbiased inference. Also, registration algorithms often suffer from misleading information inherent in the noisy data [32].

Therefore, before the registration step, all analyzed images are submitted to 3-dimensional noise-removal routine. Denoising of MR magnitude images using standard image noise removal techniques is generally not fully justified, since thermal noise adds to raw data space and after its Fourier transform it has no more additive characteristics. It is best modeled by the Rician distribution, in fact. However, for higher SNR ratios (i.e. SNR > 3)) it can be well approximated by the Gaussian function [32,33]. In the case of the available images, SNR ranges from around 16 to 23. Therefore, in this study we perform denoising of the real data assuming the Gaussian model of noise.

The noise removal procedure is accomplished using the non-local means (NLM) filter. Its exact definition is omitted here as it exceeds the scope of this paper. Instead, the reader is suggested to review references [34–36]. The principle of the algorithm operation consists in calculation of an output (denoised) pixel value based on the weighted mean of all other image pixels. Weights for a given pixel are determined by distances between this pixel neighborhood and neighborhoods of other image pixels. A neighborhood is defined as a set of all adjacent image points of a given pixel, excluding this pixel itself, while the distance is calculated as the L2 norm between relevant neighborhood pixel intensities. In our experiments we employ custom made implementation of the NLM algorithm extended to 3D.

Calculation results. The calculated correlation coefficients between simulated and real images are presented in Table 4. The upper and lower bounds for each coefficient assuming 95% confidence interval are also given. The correlation coefficients for Studies 1–3 range from 0.86 to 0.92 and for Study 4 the minimum correlation exists between 50%-stenosis tubes and equals to 0.78. The p-value remains below 0.001 in any case which proves validity of the designed simulation framework and its ability to synthesize realistic MRA images. It is observed that the largest local differences (exceeding the level of 30% of maximum brightness in the real image) appear near the vessel walls as well as in the region after the narrowing, where the main flux of the laminar flow deviates from long axis of the vessel. The calculated RMS error, however, falls into the range (11.5,16.8), below the value of

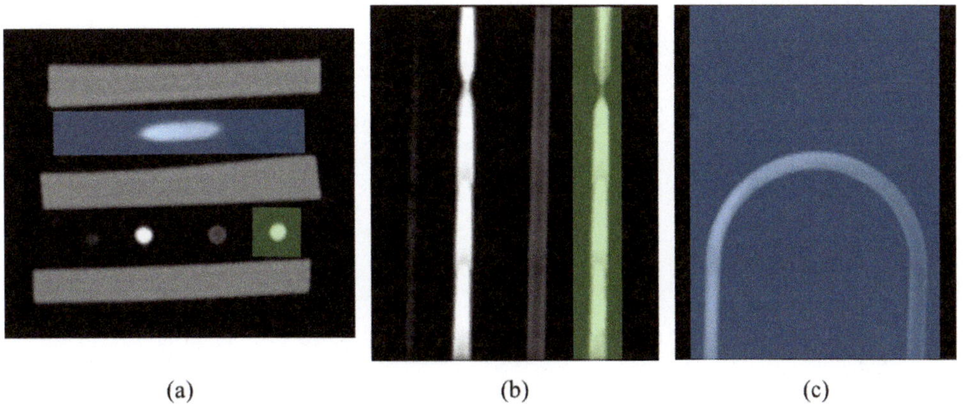

Figure 14. Examples of selected volumes of interest. Axial (a) and coronal (b and c) cross-sections of delineated VOIs embracing U-bend phantom (blue region) and 75%-stenosis tube (green region). Note that it is only a conceptual figure – the actual VOI selection was performed automatically in the MATLAB environment.

standard deviation of both the denoised real images (45–61) and the synthetic ones (32–41).

Performance evaluation. The problem of computational efficiency of any complex and data-exhaustive system deserves individual and thorough analysis and it exceeds the scope of this work. Therefore, in this study, which is primarily concerned with the proposed MRA imaging model validation, we provide only partial evaluation of the execution performance. The following considerations refer solely to image synthesis, and the blood flow modeling, which precedes MRA-related routines, is not taken into account.

The MRA simulation time depends mostly on two factors – the k-space size ($n_x \times n_y \times n_z$) and the number of particles n_p. Table 5 presents simulation times measured for different values of these factors and for various grid configurations. The experiments were accomplished for the 50%-stenosis tube and – if not indicated otherwise – on the previously described computing grid (1 iMac and 10 MacMini computers).

The measured execution times span from single minutes to approximately 1 h for the most complicated case. These results show efficiency of the system implementation. The duration of a single image synthesis process allows for collecting of their relatively large database in a reasonable time period. This is crucial since large data sample is required for statistically significant evaluation of image processing algorithms.

A comparison of individual measurements reveals that the computational complexity is $O(n_x n_y n_z n_p)$. For example, experiments in rows 1–3 were performed on the same image size but various number of particles n_p. As it can be seen, the dependence on the execution time is linear. Similarly, the change on n_z (measurements 6 and 7) in relation 1:1.76 (25:44) results in the equivalent increase of the simulation time (in seconds 794:1419). Furthermore, it can be observed (rows 4 and 5) that using hyper-threading technology leads to improved efficiency, although this benefit is lower than the apparent increase in the number of parallel processing slots would suggest.

It must be underlined that the achieved high performance is in part guaranteed by the model itself. Image formation procedures involving the greatest computational burden iterate over particles i.e. actual sources of MR signal but not over every element of the imaged volume (potentially containing the air) as in the other simulators.

Table 4. Correlation coefficients between simulated and real images.

Phantom	Study ID	Correlation coefficient	Lower bound	Upper bound	RMS error
U-bend	1	0.927	0.926	0.929	11.52
	2	0.927	0.925	0.929	11.68
	3	0.904	0.902	0.906	11.57
	4	0.811	0.809	0.814	13.24
50%-stenosis	1	0.918	0.919	0.921	12.01
	2	0.893	0.889	0.895	12.67
	3	0.911	0.909	0.912	11.89
	4	0.781	0.779	0.784	16.75
75%-stenosis	1	0.897	0.896	0.898	13.05
	2	0.881	0.879	0.884	13.52
	3	0.901	0.899	0.903	12.06
	4	0.875	0.877	0.879	13.97

Table 5. Performance eveluation for the 50%-stenosis tube.

Image size	Number of trajectories	Total number of particles	Number of processing slots	Using hyperthreading	Simulation time
128×128×25	128	71 967	48	Yes	6 m 15 s
		149 386	48	Yes	11 m 24 s
		298 651	48	Yes	23 m 56 s
192×192×44	256	202 141	48	Yes	53 m 59 s
192×192×44			24	No	1 h 5 m 53 s
128×128×44			48	Yes	23 m 39 s
128×128×25			48	Yes	13 m 14 s
128×128×25			24	No	15 m 52 s
128×128×25			16[a]	No	22 m 29 s
128×128×25			10[b]	No	36 m 25 s

[a]Grid composed of 1 iMac desktop and 6 MacMini units.
[b]Grid composed of 1 iMac desktop and 3 MacMini units.

Towards simulation of anatomical models

A comparative study presented above constitutes a formal approach to evaluate the designed system. The ultimate goal is to employ the simulator to collect a series of images for statistical analysis of vessel segmentation algorithms. Therefore, it is required that the produced images contain vessel geometries visible in actual MRA examinations. In this section we demonstrate capabilities of the technique in synthesizing images for structures anatomically more realistic than straight phantom tubes. In particular, Fig. 15a–c show the obtained images – coronal slices from 3D acquisitions – for a stenosed bifurcation, a vessel with fusiform aneurysm and a vessel with side-branches. The observed signal attenuation at stenosis and around aneurysm are characteristic for real MRA studies. These artefacts are caused in part by spin dephasing due to large local differences in flow velocity, especially near stenosis, and becuase of saturation of some molecules which slow down in the area of aneurysm. Note also the lower image intensity in a thinner side branch of a vessel in Fig. 15c. This intensity drop reflects the lower flow rate and signal averaging in a voxel covering both the edge and central axis of the vessel.

Finally, Fig. 15d presents a 2D image synthesized for a 4-tube digital phantom surrounded by two virtual tissue types. The stationary particles were assigned magnetic properties characteristic for gray and white matter. As expected, the signal produced by the moving spins is significantly enhanced relative to the stationary tissues.

Discussion

The above presented comparisons constitute preliminary results of our research into the problem of designing versatile MRA simulation system. he obtained images contain many realistic details although some results fail to meet expectations. Most importantly this concerns the issue of too large intensity drops on the slab borders visible in images synthesized for the 10 ml/s flow rate (Fig. 13). This effect might be caused by an inappropriate adjustment of the excitation pulses. Real scanning systems implement various optimization procedures, which control – in the way hidden for the user – the inclination of a ramped flip angle. The exact dependence of FA from the z coordinate may not be strictly linear on the entire length of the slab. From the synthesized image it is clear that the range of the flip angle used in simulation (20◦ around nominal FA) has been too large to produce balanced signal for the whole slab. However, reducing this range would affect images of the other channels. Also, the U-bend phantom simulated in Study 4 (Fig. 11) deviates from its real counterpart, especially in the arc section. Undoubtedly, in case of larger flow rates, further research is needed into tuning of the simulation parameters in order to achieve closer resemblance to the true data acquisition procedures.

The Time-Of-Flight protocol in spite of its simplicity is quite demanding for computer modeling – both with respect to the underlying physical processes, as well as from the efficient implementation viewpoint. We approached the latter problem by decomposition of a single simulation experiment into a series of acquisitions, each concerned with its dedicated bundle of particle trajectories. Here, a very important advantage of our solution based on particle tracing becomes visible. A possible alternative approach to combined flow and MR simulation would utilize fixed lattice of nodes, where information about fluid flowing in and out is somehow stored and transferred to neighboring nodes. As for the distributed computing it would involve additional message passing between various computing grid agents. In our solution, the only communication events take place between the master and the agent computer and it happens at the beginning of simulation, when agent receives identifiers of trajectories to handle, and then after computations are done, when an agent sends the calculated signals to the master.

The designed system will be further developed to account for phenomena which are now disregarded. The problems which need to be addressed in the future can be grouped into two major issues corresponding to separate physical phenomena, i.e. blood flow simulation and MR physics. The first group of issues includes modeling of blood transport within a body part which is itself subject to motion. A blood particle position is then determined by two processes – hemodynamics and physiological displacement of an organ. It concerns important clinical applications of MRA such as diagnosis of cardiac anatomy, liver or kidney. Moreover, modeling of blood flow in the present study assumes fluid behavior which is either laminar or – in narrowed or bending regions – turbulent. Even in the latter case, however, it is a simplified model. The blood motion in such situations is chaotic and shear stress tensor should be estimated to account for non-Newtonian flow.

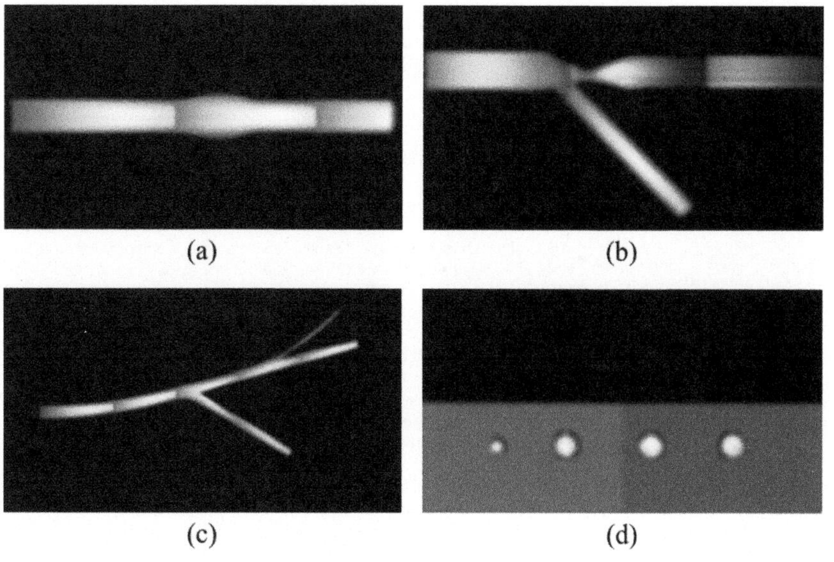

Figure 15. Sample images of realistic structures. A vessel with fusiform aneurysm (a), eccentric shape of stenosis at bifurcation (b) a vessel with side-branches (c) and stationary tissue around 4-vessel phantom (d). a–c) 3D acquisitions using both MOTSA and TONE options (TR/TE/FA = 27/4.6/15°), d) a 2D sequence (TR/TE/FA = 40/4.7/15°).

Finally, more complex, anatomical topologies of the vessel system, as well as pulsatile flow will be considered in order to obtain more realistic MRA data sets.

Within the MRI part of the simulator, future efforts will be directed at including the effect of magnetization transfer used to maximize signal suppression from stationary tissue. Another issue that needs investigation is the consequence of using a special case analytic solution to the Bloch equation instead of a numerical solver. Redesigning the simulator to calculate exact solution of a differential equation will not only allow usage of time-varying gradient pulses, but also it will give an opportunity to quantitatively evaluate the degree of measurement error induced by analytical solution. The images synthesized in this study are noise-free. This assumption is justified in experiments where the goal is to solely verify the simulator operation. However, as far as the validation of MRA image processing algorithms is concerned, the simulation results should be corrupted by noise, so that the applied methods meet the same impediments characteristic for real images. Commonly the noise in MRI simulations is modeled as white Gaussian ergodic process added directly to the calculated k-space.

Nonetheless, the achieved results are satisfactory and meet the initial specification of system. The synthesized images contain much of information found in the real ones. The most important image features reproduced in the performed simulations are as follows:

- parabolic profile of the signal in regions of laminar flow,
- signal void on slab borders,
- specific flow patterns after stenoses,
- signal attenuation due to saturation, both in the stationary tissue and in fluid passing through a saturation band,
- higher signal on vessel walls than in the lumen in the channels with reverse flow direction.

In conclusion, these results encourage a follow-up study on quantitative validation of vessel segmentation algorithms applied to the MRA synthesized images.

Acknowledgments

The authors express their gratitude towards Scanlab Medical Diagnostics Centre Lodz and Dr. Pawel Majewski for their cooperation in conducting experiments with real phantoms and MRI scanners.

Author Contributions

Conceived and designed the experiments: AK AM. Performed the experiments: AK GD MS. Analyzed the data: AK. Contributed reagents/materials/analysis tools: AK PS AM. Wrote the paper: AK. Designed the softwate tools used in the study: AK PS. Arranged experiments with the real MR scanner: MS. Performed flow simulation in the COMSOL software: AK GD. Designed the experiment with the physical phantoms: AM. Overall research coordination and management: AK.

References

1. Arlat I, Bongartz G, Marchal G (2002) Magnetic Resonance Angiography. Berlin: Springer Verlag.
2. Bernstein MA, King KF, Zhou XJ (2004) Handbook of MRI Pulse Sequences. Amsterdam, The Netherlands: Academic Press.
3. Haacke EM, Brown RW, Thompson MR, Venkatesan R (1999) Magnetic resonance imaging: physical principles and sequence design. New York: Wiley-Liss.
4. Stamm AC, Wright CL, Knopp MV, Schmalbrock P, Heverhagen JT (2013) Phase contrast and time-of-ight magnetic resonance angiography of the intracerebral arteries at 1.5, 3 and 7 T. Magn Reson Imaging 31: 545–549.
5. Schneider G, Prince MR, Meaney JF, Ho VB (2005) Magnetic Resonance Angiography. Techniques, Indications and Practical Applications. Milan: Springer-Verlag Italia.
6. Eiho S, Qian Y (1997) Detection of coronary artery tree using morphological operator. Proc Comput Cardiol 7: 525–528.
7. Frangi AF, Niessen WJ, Vincken KL, Viergever MA (1998) Multiscale vessel enhancement filtering. In: Wells WM, Colchester A, Delp S, editors, Medical Image Computing and Computer-Assisted Interventation MICCAI'98, Springer Berlin Heidelberg, volume 1496 of *Lecture Notes in Computer Science*. pp. 130–137.

8. Kirbas C, Quek F (2004) A review of vessel extraction techniques and algorithms. ACM Comput Surv 36: 81–121.
9. Materka A, Strzelecki M, Szczypiński P, Kociński M, Deistung A, et al. (2009) Arteries tracking in simultaneous ToF-SWI MR images: image characteristics and preliminary results. In: Image and Signal Processing and Analysis, 2009. ISPA 2009. Proceedings of 6th International Symposium on. IEEE, pp. 748–753.
10. Simmons A, Arridge SR, Barker GJ, Williams SC (1996) Simulation of MRI cluster plots and application to neurological applications. Magn Reson Imaging 14: 73–92.
11. Petersson J, Christoffersson J, Golman K (1993) MRI simulation using the k-space formalism. Magn Reson Imaging 11: 557–568.
12. Benoit-Cattin H, Collewet G, Belaroussi B, Saint-Jalmes H, Odet C (2005) The SIMRI project: a versatile and interactive MRI simulator. J Magn Reson Imaging 173: 97–115.
13. Kwan RS, Evans A, Pike G (1999) MRI simulation-based evaluation of image-processing and classification methods. IEEE Trans Med Imaging 18: 1085–1097.
14. Stoecker T, Vahedipour K, Pugfelder D, Shah NJ (2010) High-performance computing MRI simulations. Magn Reson Med 64: 186–193.
15. Yoder DA, Zhao Y, Paschal CB, Fitzpatric JM (2004) MRI simulator with object-specific field map calculations. Magn Reson Imaging 22: 315–328.
16. Shelley Medical Imaging Technologies (2013) MRI Quality Assurance Flow Phantom Set. Available: http://www.simutec.com/. Accessed February 2014.
17. Holdsworth DW, Rickey DW, Drangova M, Miller DJM, Fenster A (1991) Computer-controlled positive displacement pump for physiological ow simulation. Med Biol Eng Comput 29: 565–570.
18. Anderson JD (1995) Computational Fluid Dynamics. The Basics with Applications. New York: McGraw-Hill.
19. Kwak D, Kiris CC (2011) Computation of Viscous Incompressible Flows. Springer.
20. Wilcox DC (2006) Turbulence Modeling for CFD. DCW Industries.
21. Hokr M, Maryska J (2005) Inuence of mesh geometry to numerical diffusion in upwind scheme for porous media solute transport. In: Proceedings of algoritmy. pp. 123–131.
22. Holleman R, Fringer O, Stacey M (2013) Numerical diffusion for ow-aligned unstructured grids with application to estuarine modeling. Int J Numer Methods Fluids 72: 1117–1145.
23. Comsol AB (2014) COMSOL Multiphysics Version 4.3, Particle Tracing User's Guide, Comsol AB, Stockholm, Sweden.
24. Parker DL, Yuan C, Blatter DD (1991) MR angiography by multiple thin slab 3D acquisition. Magn Reson Med 17: 434–451.
25. Carr J, Carroll T (2012) Magnetic Resonance Angiography: Principles and Applications. New York: Springer Science+Business Media.
26. Kim SE, Parker DL (2012) Time-of-Flight Angiography,chapter 2. New York: Springer Science+Business Media. pp. 39–50.
27. Liang ZP, Lauterbur PC (2000) Principles of Magnetic Resonance Imaging: A Signal Processing Perspective. New York: IEEE Press.
28. The MathWorks,Inc. (2013) MATLAB and Signal Processing Toolbox Release 2013a, The MathWorks, Inc., Natick, Massachusetts, United States.
29. Gabriel E, Fagg GE, Bosilca G, Angskun T, Dongarra JJ, et al. (2004) Open MPI: Goals, concept, and design of a next generation MPI implementation. In: Proceedings, 11th European PVM/MPI Users' Group Meeting. Budapest, Hungary, pp. 97–104.
30. Klepaczko A, Szczypiński P, Dwojakowski G, Kociński M, Strzelecki M (2012) Computer simulation of magnetic resonance angiography imaging. Parallel implementation in heterogeneous computing environment. In: New Trends in Audio and Video Signal Processing: Algorithms, Architectures, Arrangements and Applications, NTAV/SPA 2012. Proceedings of the Joint Conference. pp. 43–48.
31. The MathWorks, Inc. (2013) MATLAB and Image Processing Toolbox Release 2013a, The MathWorks, Inc., Natick, Massachusetts, United States.
32. Coupé P, Manjón JV, Gedamu E, Arnold D, Robles M, et al. (2010) Robust Rician noise estimation for MR images. Med Image Anal 14: 483–493.
33. Nowak R (1999) Wavelet-based Rician noise removal for magnetic resonance imaging. IEEE Trans Image Process 8: 1408–1419.
34. Buades A, Coll B, Morel JM (2005) A review of image denoising algorithms, with a new one. Multiscale Model Simul 4: 490–530.
35. He L, Greenshields IR (2009) A Nonlocal Maximum Likelihood estimation method for Rician noise reduction in MR images. IEEE Trans Image Process 28: 165–172.
36. Zuo XN, Xing XX (2011) Effects of non-local diffusion on structural MRI preprocessing and default network mapping: Statistical comparisons with isotropic/anisotropic diffusion. PLoS One 6: e26703.

Association of Serum Uric Acid and Coronary Artery Disease in Premenopausal Women

Jian-wei Zhang[1], Ling-jie He[2], Shu-jun Cao[3], Qing Yang[1], Shi-wei Yang[1], Yu-jie Zhou[1]*

1 Department of Cardiology, Beijing Anzhen Hospital, Capital Medical University, Beijing Institute of Heart Lung and Blood Vessel Disease, The Key Laboratory of Remodeling-related Cardiovascular Disease, Ministry of Education, Beijing, China, **2** Department of Emergency, Beijing Friendship Hospital, Capital Medical University, Beijing, China, **3** Department of Cardiology, Beijing Daxing Hospital, Capital Medical University, Beijing, China

Abstract

Objective: To date, no study in the published literature has investigated the role of various serum uric acid (SUA) concentrations in the development of angiographically-proven coronary artery disease (CAD) in premenopausal women. Therefore, the aim of this study was to investigate the role SUA levels may play in the prevalence, severity, and prognosis of CAD in premenopausal women.

Methods: This cross-sectional retrospective study included 607 premenopausal women who had undergone coronary angiography. The CAD diagnosis was based upon stenosis affecting ≥50% of the luminal diameter. Association of the SUA levels with CAD prevalence, severity, and clinical outcomes were assessed by statistical analysis.

Results: In total, 369 (60.8%) of the patients were diagnosed with CAD. The CAD patients had significantly higher SUA levels than those without CAD (5.3±1.9 vs. 4.8±1.7 mg/dL, $P = 0.001$). The SUA levels were found to be significantly associated with CAD prevalence ($P = 0.013$). Patients with higher levels of SUA also showed increased rates of multivessel disease and composite end-points, such as major adverse cardiac events. Furthermore, multivariate analysis identified abnormally high levels of uric acid (hyperuricemia) as an independent risk factor for CAD (OR 1.51 (1.11–2.53), $P < 0.05$).

Conclusions: The SUA levels are significantly associated with the prevalence of CAD. The SUA levels may be a predictor for incidence of major cardiovascular events in premenopausal women.

Editor: Fengfeng Zhou, Shenzhen Institutes of Advanced Technology, China

Funding: This work was supported by grants from the Beijing Municipal High-Level Talent Foundation of Health System (No. 2011-1-5), the Beijing Municipal Administration of Hospitals' Clinical This work was supported bu Medicine Development of Special Funding Support (No. ZY201303), and the National Key Clinical Specialty Construction Project. The funders had no role in study design, data collection and analysis, decision to publish, or preparation of the manuscript.

Competing Interests: The authors have declared that no competing interests exist.

* Email: azzyj12@163.com

Introduction

Menopausal women are at a greater risk of developing coronary artery disease (CAD) than their premenopausal counterparts, a result of the loss of hormone protection that accompanies menopause [1–3]. Recently, however, there has been an increase in the number of premenopausal women suffering from angina and myocardial infarction [4]. Due to the scarcity of data available for premenopausal women diagnosed with CAD, little is known of the characteristics, mechanism, prognosis, and risk factors of these patients.

Hyperuricemia, an abnormally high level of uric acid in the blood, was identified as a novel risk factor for the development of CAD [5]. Levels of uric acid, the final product of nucleic acid metabolism, are controlled by a multitude of different factors, including dietary intake, renal excretion, and rate of cell turnover. However, the role of uric acid in CAD remains largely unknown. Recent studies have demonstrated an independent association between serum uric acid (SUA) and CAD [6–7]. Moreover, several studies have also demonstrated a strong association of SUA levels with cardiovascular disease (CVD) in women, as compared with their male counterparts [5,8,9]. These studies, however, did not evaluate the relationship between levels of SUA and incidence of CAD in premenopausal women. Hence, our study was designed to investigate the role SUA may play in the prevalence, severity, and prognosis of CAD in premenopausal women.

Methods

Study design and patient population

A total of 607 premenopausal women, from three major hospitals in Beijing, China (Beijing Anzhen Hospital, Beijing Daxing Hospital, and Beijing Friendship Hospital, Capital Medical University), were included in this study. Women were considered premenopausal if they were between 20 and 50 years of age with a history of regular menstruation of 3–7 days every 22 to 35 days. All of the women had undergone coronary angiography for the first time to address the chest discomfort they were experiencing at the time. Our study obtained the approval from Ethics Committee at the following institutions: Beijing Anzhen Hospital, Beijing Daxing Hospital, and Beijing Friendship Hospital, Capital Medical University. Written informed consent was obtained from each participant or their legal representatives during hospitalization. This study was conducted from January 2007 to May 2012. The data for the study participants were stratified for cross-sectional comparison of patients with and without angiographically-confirmed CAD.

During the study, all of the study's participants had their blood samples taken on the first day of admission, which was used for SUA analysis by automated biochemical analyzer (Hitachi 747 Biochemical Analyzer; Tokyo, Japan). Outcome/survival data were collected by telephone surveys once a year, for an average of 3.5 years after the initial admission. A total of 13 of the original CAD patients were lost to follow-up due to change in contact information or residence. Based on previously published guidelines, those participants whose SUA level was >6.0 mg/dL were diagnosed with hyperuricemia [4].

Definition of metabolic syndrome (MS)

The International Diabetes Federation definition of the metabolic syndrome (MS) was used to diagnose participants of the study with this syndrome. Participants had to have a central obesity defined as a waist circumference of ≥80 cm in women based on the Asia-Pacific consensus. In addition, two or more of the following criteria had to be matched: 1) a triglyceride level of ≥1.69 mmol/L (150 mg/dL), 2) an HDL-C level of < 1.29 mmol/L (50 mg/dL) in women, 3) systolic/diastolic blood pressure of ≥130/85 mm Hg or previously diagnosed hypertension, and 4) the fasting plasma glucose level of ≥5.6 mmol/L (100 mg/dL) or a previous diagnosis of type-2 diabetes mellitus.

Coronary angiography

The interventional cardiologist assessment was performed using the standard Judkins technique of angiography. Luminal diameter narrowing of ≥50% in any of the major epicardial coronary arteries was considered sufficient for CAD diagnosis. Participants were assessed during the initial coronary angiography for the presence of multivessel disease, defined as the presence of ≥2 major epicardial coronary arteries or their major branches with stenosis of ≥50%.

Exclusion criteria

Potential candidates for study enrollment were excluded according to the following parameters: previous history of diuretics usage for antihypertensive medication, cardiomyopathy, valvular heart disease, cardiac surgery, aortic dissection, acute myocardial infarction, or renal insufficiency. In addition, any patients with previously diagnosed CAD were excluded from the study.

Study end points and definitions in follow-up

Major adverse cardiovascular events (MACE) were cardiac mortality, angina with electrocardiogram changes, acute myocardial infarction, and repeated revascularization.

Statistical analysis

Categorical data were presented as frequencies (percentages), while continuous data were presented as a mean value ± standard deviation. Differences between the means were compared by unpaired t-test when the variables showed normal distribution or by the Mann-Whitney U test when they did not. For the comparison of categorical variables, either the Chi-square test or the Fisher's exact test was used. The significant variables in the univariate analysis were introduced in a multivariate logistical regression model to obtain the predictive variables for CAD. The receiver-operating characteristic (ROC) curve analysis was performed to define the sensitivity and specificity of SUA as a discriminator of CAD prevalence. A P value of <0.05 (two-sided) was considered significant. Data were analyzed with the SPSS statistical software, version 21.0 (Chicago, Illinois, USA).

Results

Based on both the inclusion and exclusion criteria, 607 premenopausal women who underwent coronary angiography for the diagnosis or exclusion of CAD were enrolled in the study. Coronary angiographic test results were used to stratify the study participants into a CAD group and a non-CAD group. Baseline characteristics of study subjects are presented in Table 1. The angiographic test diagnosed 369 (60.8%) patients with CAD (≥ 50% cardiac artery narrowing); the remaining 238 (39.2%) patients composed the non-CAD group.

The frequencies of hyperuricemia in the CAD and non-CAD groups were 23.3% and 16%, respectively. Both hypercholesterolemia and MS were more prevalent in the CAD group than in the non-CAD group (34.7% vs. 23.1% and 32.8% vs. 24.4%, respectively). Furthermore, the CAD group had a more extensive elevation in high-sensitivity C-reactive protein (hs-CRP), greater levels of low-density lipoprotein-cholesterol (LDL-C) and fasting blood sugar, lower level of HDL-C, and a higher level of SUA (5.3±1.9 vs. 4.8±1.7, P = 0.001). The other potential risk factors analyzed (age, triglyceride level, total cholesterol level, body mass index, hypertension, smoking, family history, diabetes mellitus, and obesity) were not associated with CAD in our particular group of coronary angiography newly-diagnosed CAD premenopausal women.

Clinical value of SUA

The SUA quartiles used in this study were as follows: Q1, 1.74–3.58 mg/dL; Q2, 3.59–4.72 mg/dL; Q3, 4.73–5.85 mg/dL; Q4, 5.86–10.52 mg/dL. Based on the univariate analysis, 51.66% of the participants with SUA levels in Q1 had CAD. The patients with levels of SUA in Q2, Q3 and Q4, who also had CAD represented 58.17%, 64.47% and 68.87%, respectively (P = 0.04) (Fig. 1 and Table 2). Collectively, these data suggest that increased SUA levels are associated with increasing prevalence of CAD.

Univariate analysis showed that the risk factors of hs-CRP, LDL-C, fasting blood sugar, hypercholesterolemia, MS, and hyperuricemia played a significant role in CAD (P<0.05). In comparison, the traditional coronary risk factors of hypertension, obesity, and diabetes mellitus were not found to be significantly or independently related to CAD.

The logistic regression analysis model of CAD risk factors further showed that hs-CRP, LDL-C, hypercholesterolemia, and hyperuricemia were all significant risk factors of CAD (P<0.05) (Table 3). The ROC curve analysis showed that the SUA sensitivity as a discriminator of CAD prevalence was 79.0% while the specificity was 62.8%. The area under the curve was 0.770 (95% CI: 0.696, 0.855) (Figure 2).

The angiographic findings, which indicated involvement of a single vessel, double vessels, triple vessel, main stem, and multivessel, were assessed for the women with CAD according to their SUA quartile (Table 4). In addition, follow-up results regarding cardiac mortality, angina, acute myocardial infarction, repeated revascularization, and composite MACE were assessed for all of the women according to their SUA quartile (Table 4). Analysis of the angiographic findings revealed that events of multivessel disease increased as the concentration of SUA increased (Q1: 34.8%, Q2: 41.9%, Q3: 48.9%, Q4: 56.5%; P = 0.022). In contrast, single vessel disease events decreased as the

Table 1. Comparison of clinical findings between the non-CAD and CAD groups.

Factors	CAD group (n = 369)	Non-CAD group (n = 238)	t/χ^2	*P*
Age (years)	42.5±8.6	41.8±9.1	0.957	0.339
WBC counts (10^9/L)	7.2±2.1	7.0±1.9	1.545	0.123
Serum creatinine (mmol/L)	63.4±14.1	64.2±20.2	−0.574	0.566
hs-CRP (mg/L)	3.48±2.15	3.04±1.92	2.565	0.011
Triglyceride (mg/dL)	161±97	146±106	1.793	0.074
HDL-C (mg/dL)	43±15	46±13	−2.532	0.009
LDL-C (mg/dL)	108.4±46.5	100.6±42.7	2.083	0.038
Total cholesterol (mg/dL)	192.1±62.7	185.9±56.8	1.234	0.218
Uric acid (mg/dL)	5.3±1.9	4.8±1.7	3.297	0.001
Fasting blood sugar (mmol/L)	6.3±3.1	5.8±1.9	2.232	0.014
BMI (kg/m^2)	24.7±4.2	25.3±4.6	−1.655	0.096
Left ventricular EF %	64.3±8.1	63.2±7.8	1.657	0.098
Hyperuricemia, n (%)	86 (23.3)	38 (16.0)	4.795	0.029
Traditional coronary risk factor, n (%)				
Hypercholesterolemia	128 (34.7)	55 (23.1)	9.211	0.002
Hypertension	130 (35.2)	81 (34.0)	0.091	0.762
Current smoking	25 (6.8)	17 (7.1)	0.031	0.862
Family history	58 (15.7)	30 (12.6)	1.131	0.288
Obesity	75 (20.3)	45 (18.9)	0.183	0.669
Diabetes mellitus	75 (20.3)	45 (18.9)	0.183	0.669
Metabolic syndrome	121 (32.8)	58 (24.4)	4.935	0.026

Data given as mean ± SD or n (%).
CAD, coronary artery disease; BMI, body mass index; EF, ejection fraction; HDL-C, high density lipoprotein cholesterol; hs-CRP, high-sensitivity C-reactive protein; LDL-C, low-density lipoprotein cholesterol; WBC, white blood cell.

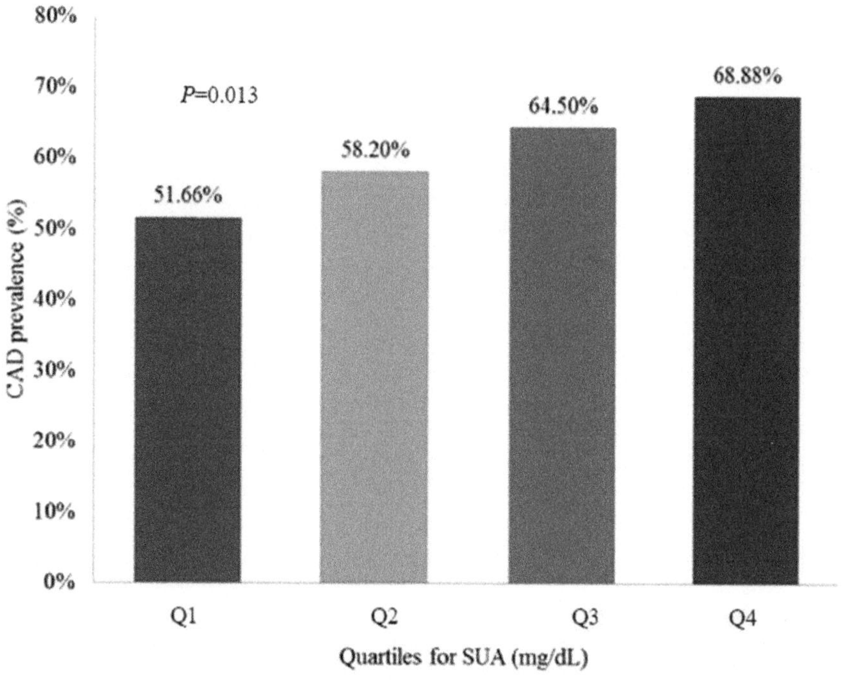

Figure 1. Prevalence of coronary artery disease in premenopausal women as a function of serum uric acid levels.

Table 2. Comparison of quartile levels of serum uric acid between the CAD group and the non-CAD group.

Quartiles	CAD group (n = 369)	Non-CAD group (n = 238)	χ^2	P
Q1: 1.74–3.58 mg/dL	78 (51.7)	73 (48.3)	10.732	0.013
Q2: 3.59–4.72 mg/dL	89 (58.2)	64 (41.8)		
Q3: 4.73–5.85 mg/dL	98 (64.5)	54 (35.5)		
Q4: 5.86–10.52 mg/dL	104 (68.9)	47 (31.1)		

Data given as n (%).

concentration of SUA increased (Q1: 64.1%, Q2: 55.9%, Q3: 46.0%, Q4: 40.0%; $P = 0.036$). Analysis of the follow-up results showed that patients in Q4 had a higher rate of composite MACE compared to all other three quartiles (Q1: 15.6%, Q2: 22.5%, Q3: 23.9%, Q4: 33.7%; $P = 0.041$). All other parameters measured in the follow-up period showed no strong association with CAD across the four quartiles.

Discussion

The principal finding of our study was the demonstration that SUA levels are markedly related to the prevalence of CAD in premenopausal women. Our results strongly suggest that hyperuricemia is an independent risk factor for CAD in this specific target group. The current literature does not provide a consensus on the SUA role in the CAD development. However, a study published in 2013 suggested that SUA was not predictive of either CVD or CVD death and that SUA did not increase patient's risk in conjunction with the traditional CVD risk factors [10]. However, multiple studies have shown that SUA levels are associated with risk of CAD and adverse cardiac events, especially in women. Calvo and colleagues reported a study of postmenopausal Caucasian and Filipino women, in which they identified SUA as a marker of CAD progression [8]. Similarly, Lin and colleagues showed that in a 3.1 year median follow-up elevated SUA could predict the rate of both cardiac and all-cause mortality among patients with angiographically-proven CAD [11]. Ndrepepa and colleagues showed that in subjects with Type 2 diabetes mellitus and confirmed CAD, elevated SUA could predict mortality independently of known traditional cardiovascular risk factors [7].

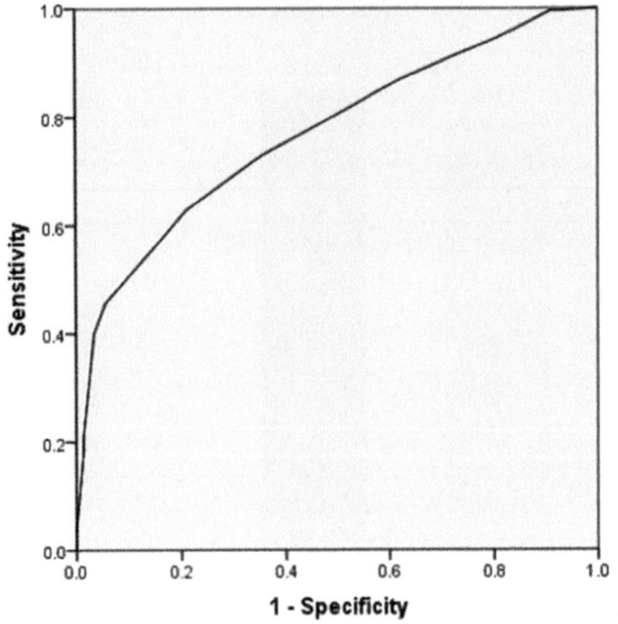

Figure 2. The receiver operating characteristics curve to define the sensitivity and specificity of SUA as a discriminator of CAD prevalence in premenopausal women.

A meta-analysis of the hyperuricemia and CAD showed strong association between hyperuricemia and an increased risk of CAD prevalence, independently of traditional CHD risk factors [5]. Further analysis of the subgroups did not identify a significant association between hyperuricemia and CHD prevalence/mortality in men, but did show an increased risk for CHD mortality in women [5]. Another study showed that increased SUA levels were predictive of an increased risk of both cardiac and all-cause mortality, independent of traditional cardiovascular risk factors and that these associations followed a 'J-shaped' pattern [6]. Finally, this study also showed that the strongest association between SUA and mortality occurred in women and patients without arterial hypertension [6]. The well-recognized difference in cardiovascular risk profile of women, compared to men, may partly explain the stronger association between hyperuricemia and cardiovascular events in women.

Compared to their male counterparts, premenopausal women have lower SUA levels [12,13] and less cardiovascular risk factors. Hence, it is not clear why, in premenopausal patients with CAD, estrogen is not able to exert its cardiovascular protective function. One explanation suggests that the excessive inflammation, estrogen receptor deficit, and gene variation may be potential factors affecting the estrogen protective function [14,15]. Moreover, components associated with MS may modulate the platelet numbers, receptor-activated platelet secretory functions, and cellular activation of the vascular wall contributing to atherogenesis [16] while anti-atherogenic and anti-inflammatory properties of HDL may be diminished under certain inflammatory conditions [17–22]. The data from our current study showed a strong association between high level of SUA and development of multivessel disease and composite MACE. Findings from a previous study showed that the premenopausal CAD patients, more frequently presented with single vessel narrowing than their postmenopausal CAD counterparts (43.2% vs. 26.9%), had more severe lesions (≥90%) in the left main coronary artery (2.9% vs. 1.1%) and proximal left anterior descending artery (28.2% vs. 16.6%) [4]. These patients also had more triple vessel involvement (33.8% vs. 26.9%) [4]. Our study confirmed that in premenopausal women the rate of a single vessel attained was 53.4%. However, following the increase in SUA levels the rate of multivessel diseases was elevated. Moreover, ROC curve analysis

Table 3. Logistic regression analysis model of different CAD risk factors.

Variables	Univariate analysis	Multivariate analysis	
	OR (95% *CI*)	Full model	Final model
		OR (95% *CI*)	OR (95% *CI*)
Age (years)	1.08 (0.85–1.57)	1.10 (0.92–1.71)	
hs-CRP (mg/L)	1.57 (1.13–2.02)*	1.31 (1.03–2.84)*	1.29 (1.01–2.57)*
HDL-C (mg/dL)	0.81 (0.71–0.94)*	0.84 (0.66–1.07)	
LDL-C (mg/dL)	1.66 (1.31–2.21)*	1.49 (1.11–2.35)*	1.21 (1.04–2.15)*
Fasting blood sugar (mmol/L)	1.27 (1.08–2.11)*	1.17 (0.91–2.01)	
Hypercholesterolemia			
Yes	1.77 (1.22–2.56)*	1.64 (1.14–2.32)*	1.34 (1.07–2.12)*
No	1.00	1.00	
Hypertension			
Yes	1.05 (0.75–1.45)	0.89 (0.68–1.28)	
No	1.00	1.00	
Obesity			
Yes	1.09 (0.72–1.65)	1.01 (0.65–1.45)	
No			
Metabolic syndrome			
Yes	1.51 (1.05–2.19)*	1.27 (0.97–1.96)	
No	1.00	1.00	
Hyperuricemia			
Yes	1.60 (1.05–2.44)*	1.44 (1.01–2.12)*	1.51 (1.11–2.53)*
No	1.00	1.00	

Note: CAD, coronary artery disease; CI, confidence interval; HDL-C, high density lipoprotein cholesterol; hs-CRP, high-sensitivity C-reactive protein; LDL-C, low-density lipoprotein cholesterol; OR, odds ratio.
*$P<0.05$.

indicated that SUA may be developed as a clinical discriminator of CAD prevalence for use in screening premenopausal women.

For many years, SUA has been used in clinical practice as a marker of several metabolic disturbances. It has been generally agreed on that MS confers increased risk for CAD and poor long-term prognosis [23–24]. Due to its association with CAD, SUA could be used as a marker for a) cardiovascular risk factor burden, b) endothelial dysfunction, c) oxidative stress, d) diabetes, and e)

Table 4. Angiographical findings and follow-up results based on SUA levels in CAD patients.

	Q1 1.74–3.58 mg/dL (n = 92)	Q2 3.59–4.72 mg/dL (n = 93)	Q3 4.73–5.85 mg/dL (n = 92)	Q4 5.86–10.52 mg/dL (n = 92)	χ^2	*P*
Angiographical findings of vessel involvement						
Single vessel	59 (64.1)	52 (55.9)	46 (50.0)	40 (43.5)	8.560	0.036
Double vessel	16 (17.4)	20 (21.5)	22 (23.9)	25 (27.2)	2.688	0.442
Triple vessel	14 (15.2)	16 (17.2)	18 (19.6)	21 (22.8)	1.946	0.584
Main stem	3 (3.3)	5 (5.4)	6 (6.5)	6 (6.5)	1.273	0.736
Multivessel	32 (34.8)	39 (41.9)	45 (48.9)	52 (56.5)	9.676	0.022
Follow-up results						
Cardiac mortality	1 (1.1)	2 (2.3)	2 (2.3)	3 (3.4)	1.025	0.791
Angina	8 (8.9)	10 (11.2)	12 (13.6)	16 (18.0)	3.522	0.309
AMI	2 (2.2)	3 (3.4)	3 (3.4)	4 (4.5)	0.691	0.871
Repeated revascularization	5 (5.6)	7 (7.9)	8 (9.1)	9 (10.1)	1.320	0.710
Composite MACE	14 (15.6)	20 (22.5)	21 (23.9)	30 (33.7)	8.052	0.041

Data given as n (%). AMI, acute myocardial infarction; MACE, major adverse cardiac event.

hypertension [25,26], all of which are important predictors of CAD. In addition to hyperuricemia, our study results have shown that premenopausal women with CAD had higher incidents of hypercholesterolemia, MS, and increase in levels of hs-CRP, LDL-C and fasting blood sugar. Furthermore, levels of HDL-C were lower in these patients compared to non-CAD patients, potentially increasing their risk of MACE in during follow-up evaluations.

Our results further strengthen the notion that with high levels of SUA, premenopausal women have a greater chance of developing a composite MACE. However, currently available models used for the study of pathophysiological mechanisms of uric acid do not adequately explain the relationship between hyperuricemia and CAD. Soluble uric acid has been shown to act as a pro-oxidant, as well as facilitator of free radical production [27]. Uric acid can crystallize resulting in the formation of monosodium urate crystals (MSU), which precipitate in various tissues, triggering a local inflammatory response. The mechanistic actions involving MSU have been shown to be intimately involved in the pathology of CAD [27]. Moreover, SUA can stimulate oxidative stress, induce endothelial dysfunction, inflammation, and vasoconstriction [28]. These mechanisms may potentially contribute to the development of CAD observed in premenopausal patients with hyperuricemia.

SUA is associated with other risk factors. Therefore, decreasing SUA levels by administrating statin [29] in combination with other measures may reduce the risk of CAD. Further research is necessary to better understand the biological role of uric acid in CAD, potentially providing new therapeutic targets for the prevention and treatment of CAD in premenopausal women.

Study limitations

There are several limitations to this study. First, this was not a randomized trial, but a retrospective evaluation. Second, we had a relatively few premenopausal women who underwent coronary angiography. Third, estrogen levels were not measured in the study. Hence, the results of the present study should be interpreted with caution.

Conclusions

The prevalence of CAD in premenopausal women is significantly related to SUA levels. Hyperuricemia was identified as an independent risk factor for CAD after adjusting for potential confounding variables. SUA levels, measured at the time of positive angiographic CAD diagnosis, may represent a useful clinical predictor of incidence of major cardiovascular events in premenopausal women over a 3.5-year follow-up period.

Acknowledgments

Author Contributions

Conceived and designed the experiments: YJZ JWZ. Performed the experiments: JWZ. Analyzed the data: JWZ LJH. Contributed reagents/materials/analysis tools: SJC QY. Wrote the paper: JWZ SWY.

References

1. Ali NS (2002) Prediction of coronary heart disease preventive behaviors in women: a test of the health belief model. Women Health 35: 83–96.
2. King KB, Quinn JR, Delehanty JM, Rizzo S, Eldredge DH, et al. (2002) Perception of risk for coronary heart disease in women undergoing coronary angiography. Heart Lung 31: 246–252.
3. Oliver-Mcneil S, Artinian NT (2002) Women's perception of personal cardiovascular risk and their risk-reducing behaviors. Am J Crit Care 11: 221–227.
4. Dou KF, Xu B, Yang YJ, Lu R, Qiu H, et al. (2008) Clinical and angiographic characteristics of premenopausal women with coronary artery disease. Chin Med J 121: 2392–2396.
5. Kim SY, Guevara JP, Kim KM, Choi HK, Heitjan DF, et al. (2010) Hyperuricemia and coronary heart disease: a systematic review and meta-analysis. Arthritis Care Res (Hoboken) 62: 170–180.
6. Ndrepepa G, Braun S, King L, Fusaro M, Tada T, et al. (2013). Uric acid and prognosis in angiography-proven coronary artery disease. European journal of clinical investigation, 43(3), 256–266.
7. Ndrepepa G, Braun S, King L, Cassese S, Tada T, et al. (2013). Prognostic value of uric acid in patients with Type 2 diabetes mellitus and coronary artery disease. Clinical Science, 124(4), 259–268.
8. Calvo RY, Araneta MR, Kritz-Silverstein D, Laughlin GA, Barrett-Connor E (2014). Relation of Serum Uric Acid to Severity of and Progression of Coronary Artery Calcium in Postmenopausal White and Filipino Women (from The Rancho Bernardo Study). The American Journal of Cardiology. 113(7), 1153–1158.
9. Ndrepepa G, Cassese S, Braun S, Fusaro M, King L, et al. (2013). A gender-specific analysis of association between hyperuricaemia and cardiovascular events in patients with coronary artery disease. Nutrition, Metabolism and Cardiovascular Diseases, 23(12), 1195–1201.
10. Veeranna V, Zalawadiya S, Panaich S, Kottam A, Afonso L (2013). Uric acid and cardiovascular disease risk reclassification. Journal of the American College of Cardiology, 61(10_S).
11. Lin GM, Li YH, Zheng NC, Lai CP, Lin CL, et al. (2013). Serum uric acid as an independent predictor of mortality in high-risk patients with obstructive coronary artery disease: a prospective observational cohort study from the ET-CHD registry, 1997–2003. Journal of cardiology, 61(2), 122–127.
12. Katsiki N, Karagiannis A, Athyros VG, Mikhailidis DP (2013). Hyperuricaemia: more than just a cause of gout?. Journal of Cardiovascular Medicine, 14(6), 397–402.
13. Feig DI, Kang DH, Johnson RJ (2008) Uric acid and cardiovascular risk. N Engl J Med359: 1811–1821.
14. Pai JK, Kraft P, Cannuscio CC, Manson JE, Rexrode KM, Albert CM, et al. (2006) Polymorphisms in the CC-chemokine receptor-2 (CCR2) and -5 (CCR5) genes and risk of coronary heart disease among US women. Atherosclerosis186: 132–139.
15. Luster AD (1998) Chemokines-chemotactic cytokines that mediate inflammation. N Engl J Med 338: 436–445.
16. Jayachandran M, Litwiller RD, Lahr BD, Bailey KR, Owen WG, et al. (2011) Alterations in platelet function and cell-derived microvesicles in recently menopausal women: relationship to metabolic syndrome and atherogenic risk. J Cardiovasc Transl Res4: 811–822.
17. Navab M, Anantharamaiah GM, Reddy ST, Van Lenten BJ, Ansell BJ, et al. (2006) Mechanisms of disease: proatherogenic HDL–an evolving field. Nat Clin Pract Endocrinol Metab 2: 504–511.
18. Ansell BJ, Fonarow GC, Fogelman AM (2006) High-density lipoprotein: is it always atheroprotective? Curr Atheroscler Rep8: 405–411.
19. Keidar S, Bogner I, Gamliel-Lazarovich A, Leiba R, Fuhrman B, et al. (2009) High plasma high-density lipoprotein levels, very low cardiovascular risk profile, and subclinical carotid atherosclerosis in postmenopausal women. J of Clin Lipidol: 3345–350.
20. Corsetti JP, Ryan D, Rainwater DL, Moss AJ, Zareba W, et al. (2010) Cholesteryl Ester Transfer Protein Polymorphism (TaqIB) Associates With Risk in Postinfarction Patients With High CReactive Protein and High-Density Lipoprotein Cholesterol Levels. Arterioscler Thromb Vasc Biol 30: 1657–1664.
21. Ansell BJ, Fonarow GC, Fogelman AM (2007) The paradox of dysfunctional high-density lipoprotein. Curr Opin Lipidol18: 427–434.
22. Dullaart RP (2010) Increased Coronary Heart Disease Risk Determined by High High-Density Lipoprotein Cholesterol and C-Reactive Protein: Modulation by Variation in the CETP Gene. Arterioscler Thromb Vasc Biol30: 1502–1503.
23. Espinola-Klein C, Rupprecht HJ, Bickel C, Lackner K, Schnabel R, et al. (2007) Inflammation, atherosclerotic burden and cardiovascular prognosis. Atherosclerosis 195(2): e126–134.
24. Espinola-Klein C, Rupprecht HJ, Bickel C, Post F, Genth-Zotz S, et al. (2007) Impact of metabolic syndrome on atherosclerotic burden and cardiovascular prognosis. Am J Cardiol 99: 1623–1628.
25. Feig DI, Kang DH, Johnson RJ (2008). Uric acid and cardiovascular risk. N Engl J Med359: 1811–1821.
26. Heinig M, Johnson RJ (2006) Role of uric acid in hypertension, renal disease, and metabolic syndrome. Cleve Clin J Med 73: 1059–1064.
27. Jin M, Yang F, Yang I, Yin Y, Luo JJ, et al. (2012) Uric acid, hyperuricemia and vascular diseases. Front Biosci (Landmark Ed) 17: 656–669.

28. Kanbay M, Segal M, Afsar B, Kang DH, Rodriguez-Iturbe B, et al. (2013). The role of uric acid in the pathogenesis of human cardiovascular disease. Heart, 99(11): 759–766.
29. Athyros VG, Mikhailidis DP, Liberopoulos EN, Kakafika AI, Karagiannis A, et al. (2007) Effect of statin treatment on renal function and serum uric acid levels and their relation to vascular events in patients with coronary heart disease and metabolic syndrome A subgroup analysis of the GREek Atorvastatin and Coronary heart disease Evaluation (GREACE) Study. Nephrol Dial Transplant 22(1): 118–127.

CT-Angiography–Based Evaluation of the Aortic Annulus for Prosthesis Sizing in Transcatheter Aortic Valve Implantation (TAVI)–Predictive Value and Optimal Thresholds for Major Anatomic Parameters

Florian Schwarz[1]*, Philipp Lange[2], Dominik Zinsser[1], Martin Greif[2], Peter Boekstegers[3], Christoph Schmitz[4], Maximilian F. Reiser[1,5], Christian Kupatt[2,5], Hans C. Becker[1,5]

1 Institute for Clinical Radiology, Hospital of the Ludwig Maximilian University of Munich, Munich, Germany, **2** Medical Clinic I – Cardiology, Hospital of the Ludwig Maximilian University of Munich, Munich, Germany, **3** HELIOS Klinikum Siegburg, HELIOS Kliniken GmbH, Siegburg, Germany, **4** Department of Cardiac Surgery, Hospital of the Ludwig Maximilian University of Munich, Munich, Germany, **5** DZHK (German Centre for Cardiovascular Research), Partner Site Munich Heart Alliance, Munich, Germany

Abstract

Background/Objectives: To evaluate the predictive value of CT-derived measurements of the aortic annulus for prosthesis sizing in transcatheter aortic valve implantation (TAVI) and to calculate optimal cutoff values for the selection of various prosthesis sizes.

Methods: The local IRB waived approval for this single-center retrospective analysis. Of 441 consecutive TAVI-patients, 90 were excluded (death within 30 days: 13; more than mild aortic regurgitation: 10; other reasons: 67). In the remaining 351 patients, the CoreValve (Medtronic) and the Edwards Sapien XT valve (Edwards Lifesciences) were implanted in 235 and 116 patients. Optimal prosthesis size was determined during TAVI by inflation of a balloon catheter at the aortic annulus. All patients had undergone CT-angiography of the heart or body trunk prior to TAVI. Using these datasets, the diameter of the long and short axis as well as the circumference and the area of the aortic annulus were measured. Multi-Class Receiver-Operator-Curve analyses were used to determine the predictive value of all variables and to define optimal cutoff-values.

Results: Differences between patients who underwent implantation of the small, medium or large prosthesis were significant for all except the large vs. medium CoreValve (all p's<0.05). Furthermore, mean diameter, annulus area and circumference had equally high predictive value for prosthesis size for both manufacturers (multi-class AUC's: 0.80, 0.88, 0.91, 0.88, 0.88, 0.89). Using the calculated optimal cutoff-values, prosthesis size is predicted correctly in 85% of cases.

Conclusion: CT-based aortic root measurements permit excellent prediction of the prosthesis size considered optimal during TAVI.

Editor: Claudio Moretti, S. G. Battista Hospital, Italy

Funding: This work was supported by the DZHK (German Centre for Cardiovascular Research) and by the BMBF (German Ministry of Education and Research). The funders had no role in study design, data collection and analysis, decision to publish, or preparation of the manuscript.

Competing Interests: The authors have read the journal's policy and have the following conflicts: Professor Becker has received speaker honoraria from Siemens Healthcare. Professor Boekstegers is an employee of HELIOS Kliniken GmbH, yet his contribution to this study was made when he was an employee of the university hospital of the Ludwig-Maximilians-University of Munich.

* Email: Florian.Schwarz@med.uni-muenchen.de

Introduction

Aortic valve stenosis is the most common acquired valve disorder and symptomatic forms have dismal outcomes when treated medically [1,2]. For decades, surgical valve replacement has been the only curative treatment – however, due to comorbidities at the time of presentation up to one third of patients cannot undergo open heart surgery [3–5]. Transcatheter Aortic Valve Implantation (TAVI)/Transcatheter Aortic Valve Replacement (TAVR) is a novel, less invasive technique and is comparably safe even in patients with contraindications to surgery [6,7]. Results of the randomized controlled PARTNER-B-cohort comparing TAVI to best medical therapy have shown substantial survival benefits after 12 and 24 months [8,9]. In patients with a high surgical risk (PARTNER-A-cohort), TAVI was non-inferior to surgery after 12 months [10].

Unlike in surgical replacement, prosthesis sizing for TAVI significantly relies on imaging [11]. Imaging-derived measurements of the aortic root play the key role in patient and device selection. Transesophageal echocardiography and Multidetector

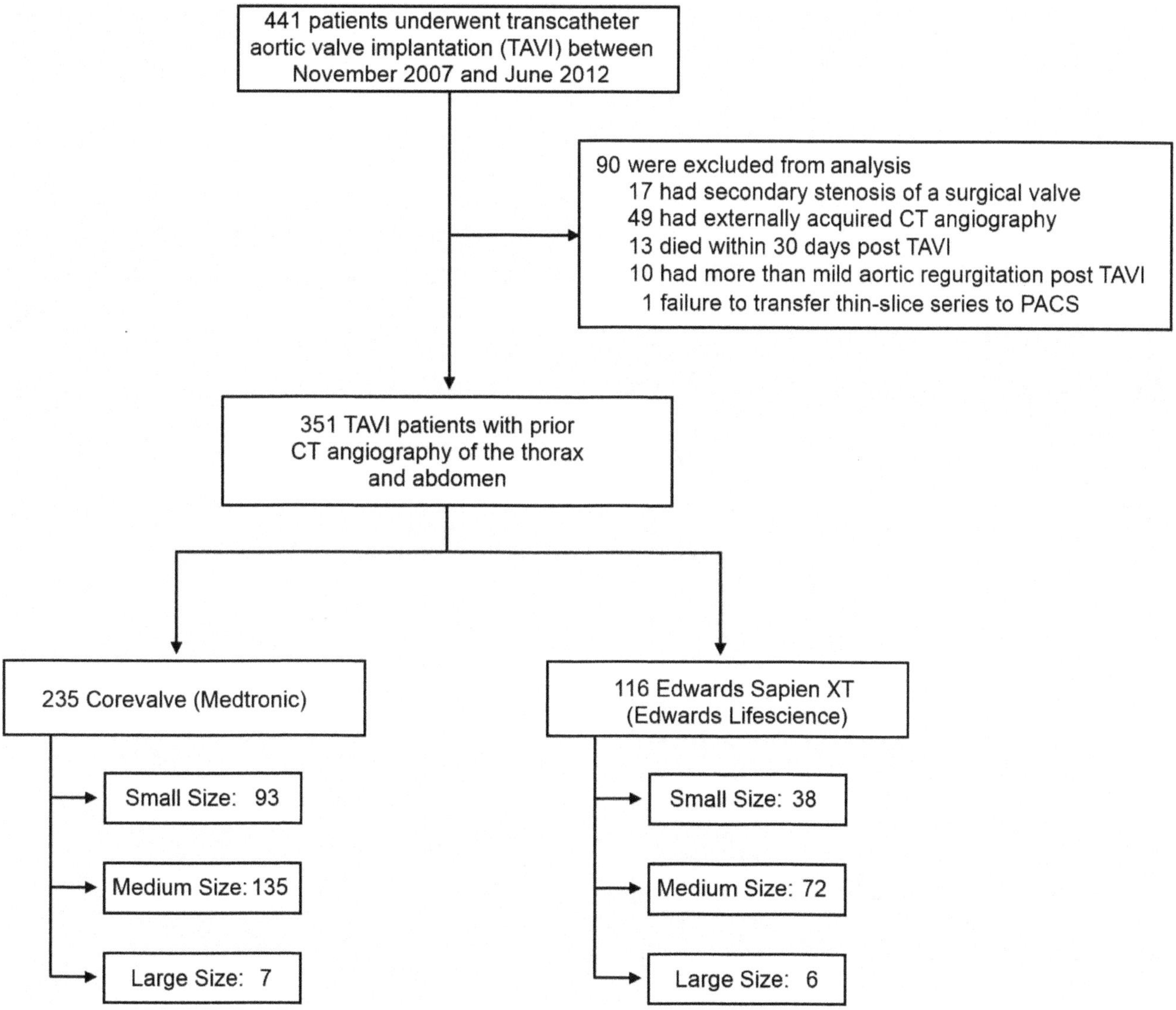

Figure 1. Inclusion chart for our analysis of 351 patients who underwent a successful TAVI procedure.

CT-angiography (CTA) have been applied extensively in this regard [12–14]. Several studies have consistently demonstrated that the aortic annulus has an elliptic shape described by a long and short axis with a wide range of reported eccentricities [15,16]. As a consequence, it is difficult to measure the true dimensions of the aortic annulus on the basis of a single plane obtained by 2D-echocardiography [17,18].

There is initial evidence favoring CTA over echocardiography for prosthesis selection. Recently, Jilaihawi et al had demonstrated for the SAPIEN XT valve (Edwards Lifesciences) that annular-sizing on the basis of CT resulted in lower rates of paravalvular regurgitation than sizing on the basis of 2D TEE [17]. Similar results had previously been reported by Hayashida et al for patients having undergone implantation of the Corevalve (Medtronic) or Sapien XT valve (Edwards Lifesciences) [19].

Several questions remain as to how select the optimal prosthesis size on the basis of CT-derived annulus parameters and most authors use a fixed algorithm suggesting certain annulus diameter ranges for distinct prosthesis sizes. Recently, Binder et al reported that the application of a CT-based annulus area sizing algorithm prior to TAVI resulted in the reduction of paravalvular regurgitation compared with simply providing quantitative results for anatomical parameters [20].

In this study, we analyzed all patients (n = 351) who had undergone dedicated CT-angiography prior to TAVI at our institution. We report descriptive statistics for the key anatomic parameters of the aortic root, determine interobserver reproducibility for CT-derived measurements and analyze various anatomic variables for their predictive value for the selection of optimal device size. Suggestions are provided for optimal cutoff values for CT-based measurements.

Methods

1. Patient Population

This analysis included patients with severe aortic valve stenosis who underwent a TAVI procedure at our institution between November 2007 and June 2012. Patients needed to have undergone CTA for the evaluation of aortic root anatomy within three months before TAVI. As all CT scans were performed as part of routine clinical workup and were analyzed anonymously,

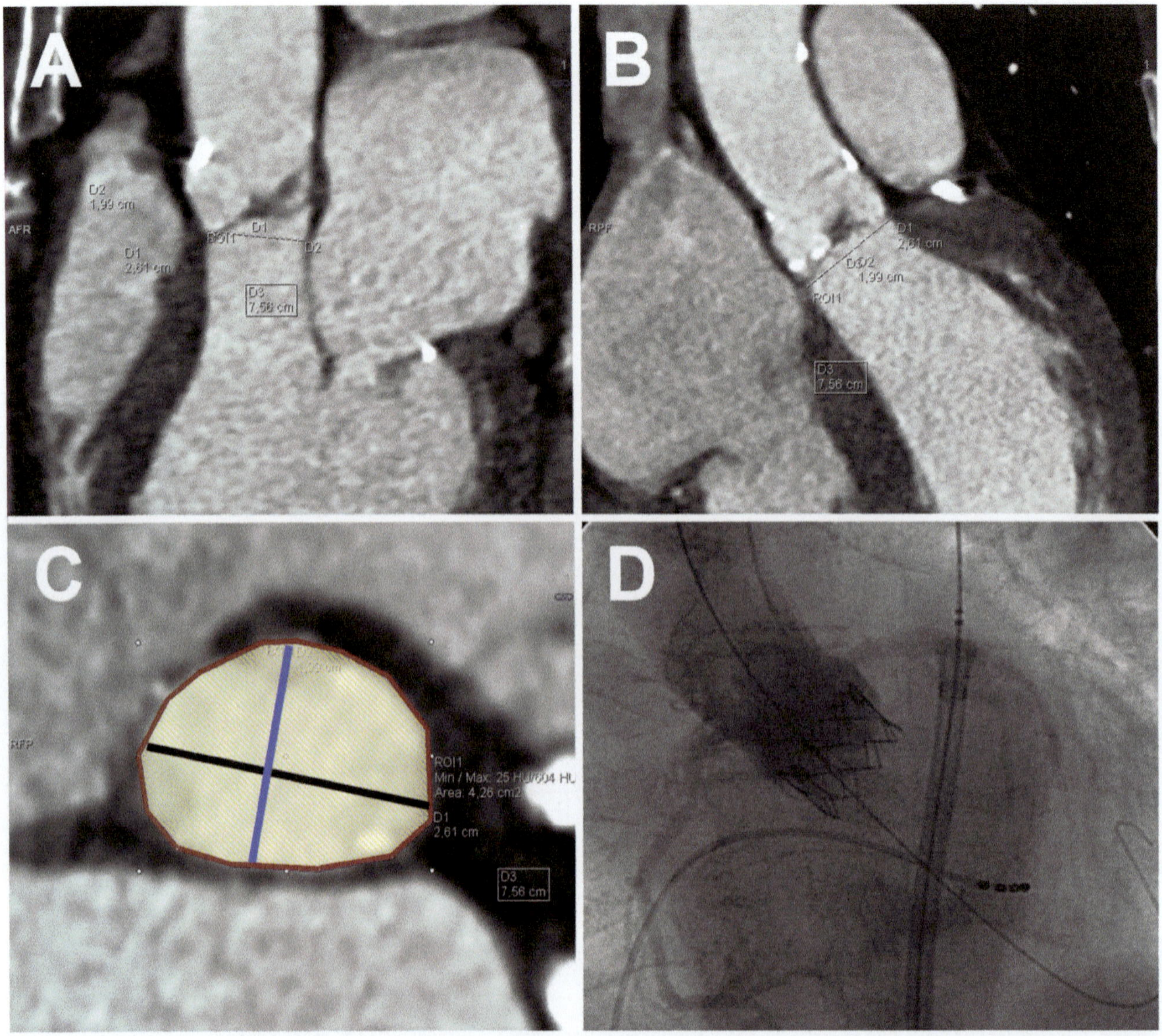

Figure 2. Examples of anatomic measurements at the aortic annulus performed for this study: isotropic small field-of-view CTA dataset of a 78 year old female patient with severe aortic stenosis, A) sagittal reformation and B) coronal reformation showing the orientation of the aortic annulus plane, C) double-oblique reformation of the aortic valve annulus, demonstrating the diameter of the long axis (black line), the diameter of the short axis (blue line), the annulus circumference (red polygonal), and annulus area (yellow shading). D) angiographic image after implantation of a 26 mm model of the Edward Sapien XT valve prosthesis demonstrates no paravalvular leakage.

the institutional review board of the Faculty of Medicine of the Ludwig Maximilian University of Munich waived the necessity to obtain consent beyond routine clinical requirements. All patients gave written consent to an anonymous analysis of the acquired data.

According to institutional policies patients with impaired renal function (glomerular filtration rate <30 ml/min), abnormal TSH-levels or a history of allergic reaction to iodine-containing contrast agents were excluded. After explicit education about the risks of iodinated contrast agents and exposure to x-rays, written informed consent was obtained (Figure 1).

2. CT Data Acquisition and Image Reconstruction

CT scans were performed either on a first-generation dual-source MDCT scanner (n = 49, Somatom Definition, Siemens Healthcare, Forchheim, Germany) or on a second-generation dual-source MDCT scanner (n = 302, Somatom Definition Flash, Siemens Healthcare) 3–90 days before TAVI. The ECG-signal was registered continuously throughout the scan. Images of the heart were acquired during diastole. Slice collimation was 2×64×0.6 mm (first generation) or 2×128×0.6 mm (second generation). Tube potential was 100 or 120 kV (depending on patient weight) and effective tube current-time product was 350–400 mAs/rotation. See Appendix S1 for detailed scan parameters.

In all patients, 90 ml of iomeprol 816.5 g/l (Imeron 400, Bracco Imaging, Milan, Italy) were administered via an ante-cubital vein at a flow-rate of 4 ml/s, followed by 100 ml of normal saline at the same flow rate. Contrast enhancement was controlled by bolus tracking within the ascending aorta.

Table 1. Patient parameters, N(%), mean ± SD or median [interquartile range] and summary of implanted valve sizes.

	All Patients	CoreValve Subgroup	Edward Sapien Subgroup	p
n	351 (100%)	235 (67%)	116 (33%)	
Female Patients	211 (58%)	132 (54%)	74 (62%)	0.18
Age at scan (yrs)	80.9±10.8	81.6±6.5	76.3±21.5	0.06
Height (cm)	165.7±8.9	165.5±13.9	163.2±18.2	0.125
Weight (kg)	72.9±14.7	72.6±15.0	72.1±17.0	0.83
BMI (kg/m^2)	26.5±4.8	26.3±4.5	26.8±5.4	0.62
Aortic Valve Area (cm^2)	0.70±0.15	0.69±0.16	0.72±0.13	0.21
Pressure gradient (mmHg)	66.9±22.4	67.3±23.8	66.0±19.6	0.65
Ejection fraction (%)	58.0±15.3	57.8±16.0	58.3±13.6	0.80
Logistic EuroSCORE	18.9 [13.4; 25.7]	19.6 [14.5; 26.7]	16.5 [11.0; 23.4]	<0.01
Valve Sizes:				
Small Size	131 (37%)	93 (40%)	38 (33%)	0.25
Medium Size	207 (59%)	135 (57%)	72 (62%)	0.44
Large Size	13 (4%)	7 (3%)	6 (5%)	0.52

Once intraluminal attenuation exceeded 150 HU, the table was repositioned for the desired scan range. Delay was 6 seconds (Somatom Definition) or 12 seconds (Somatom Definition Flash). Thereafter, the start of the scan was triggered by ECG automatically.

A medium-smooth convolution kernel was used to generate standard coronary CTA reconstructions (small field of view, slice thickness 0.75 mm, reconstruction increment 0.5 mm covering the entire heart). All series were pseudonymized and transferred to an external workstation.

3. CT Data Analysis

Two experienced readers analyzed all series independently using commercially available software (Syngo Via VA20, Siemens Healthcare, Germany). Readers determined subjective image quality and contrast enhancement on 4-point Likert scales (4: best image quality/contrast enhancement, 1: poor image quality/ contrast enhancement). Furthermore, both readers measured the size of the aortic annulus according to techniques suggested by various authors [12,21–23]. Using multiplanar reformations, readers independently established the double-oblique plane defined by the three 'hinge' points (i.e. the most apical points of the valvular cusps, see Figure 2). On this plane, both readers manually determined the lengths of the long axis (LA), short axis (SA), circumference (C) and area (A) of the elliptical shape of the the aortic valve annulus (Figure 2). Three virtual diameters (d_{mean}, d_C and d_A) were derived from these parameters according to the following formulae:

$$d_{mean} = \frac{LA + SA}{2};\ d_C = \frac{C}{\pi};\ d_A = 2 \times \sqrt{\frac{A}{\pi}}$$

4. Clinical and procedural data

In all patients, TAVI was performed at the department of cardiology of this institution as part of routine clinical care. Patients were admitted at least 1 day prior to TAVI and transferred to a high-level intensive care unit for at least 24 hours afterwards. All patients underwent a routine transthoracic echocardiography exam within 7 days prior to TAVI.

Selection of valve type (CoreValve by Medtronic, Minneapolis, USA vs. Edward Sapien XT by Edwards Lifesciences, Irvine, CA, USA) and size was performed by the heart team members before and during TAVI. According to the standard operating procedures of this institution, an initial estimation of annulus size was performed based on all available imaging information. During the procedure, a balloon catheter with the estimated size was inflated at the annulus position and snug fit was evaluated by fluoroscopy and balloon pressures [24–26]. Depending on the appearance of the balloon and the recorded pressures, valve size was either confirmed or changed. In the latter case, a different balloon catheter was used and the changed size tested. Once optimal size had been established, the respective valve was implanted using the techniques recommended by manufacturers. Thereafter, conventional angiography was performed to test for aortic regurgitation, which was rated on a three point Likert scale (1: no, minimal or first degree regurgitation, 2: second degree regurgitation, 3: severe regurgitation).

5. Statistical Analysis

The D'Agostino-Pearson test was used to test for normal distribution of continuous variables. Continuous variables are reported as mean ± standard deviation when normally distributed, otherwise as median (interquartile range).

For categorical variables, Cohen's kappa was used to address observer agreement and was reported with 95% confidence interval. For continuous variables, the intraclass correlation coefficient (ICC) was used [27].

Differences in proportions were assessed using the Chi-squared test. To test for differences in means of interval variables, the Student's t-test (for independent or paired samples) was applied if variables followed normal distribution. For comparison of means of three or more variables, a one-way analysis of variance (ANOVA) was performed. If significant differences were found, variables were compared using the Tukey-HSD post-hoc test with

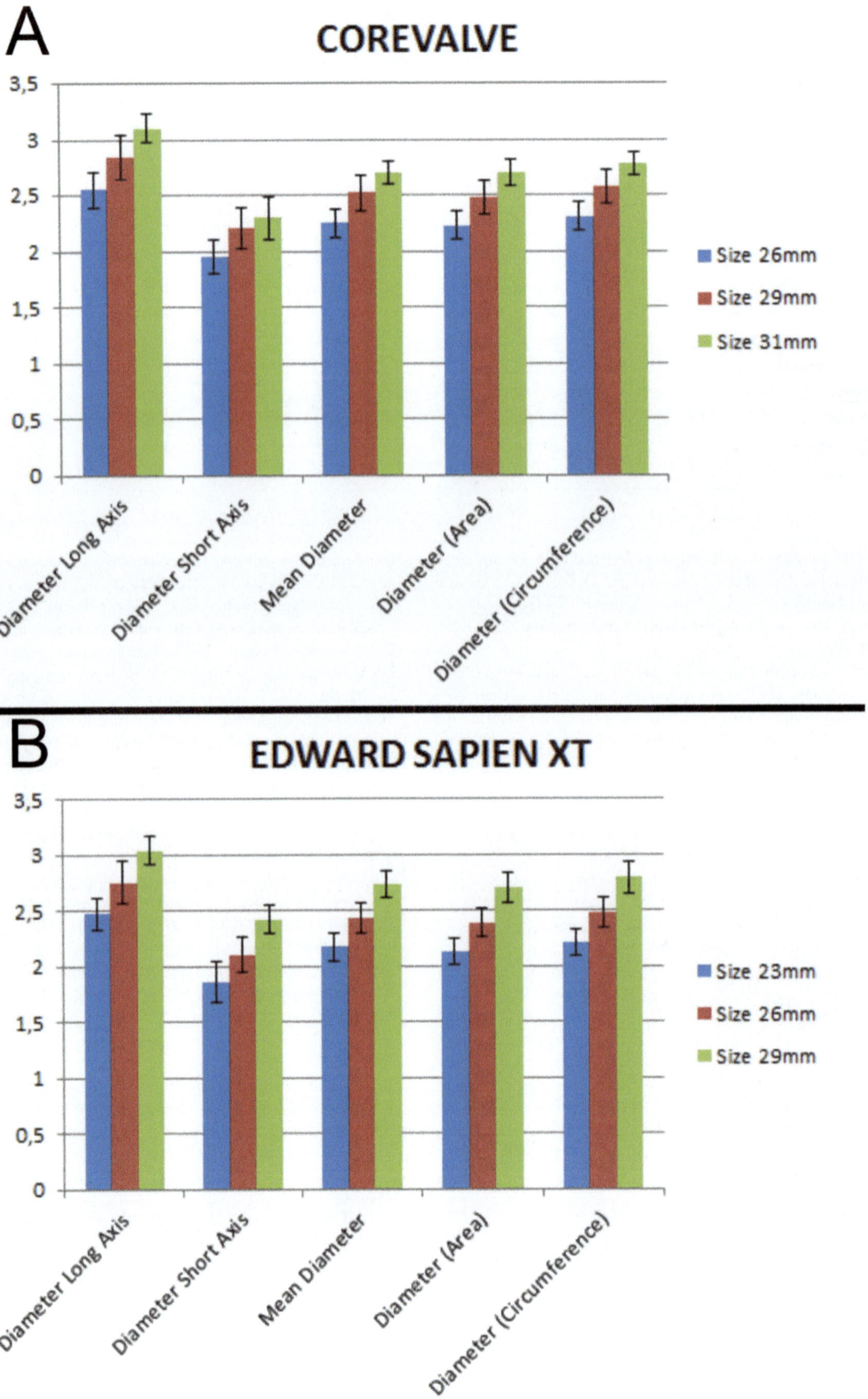
A
COREVALVE
3,5
3
2,5
2
1,5
1
0,5
0
Size 26mm
Size 29mm
Size 31mm
Diameter Long Axis
Diameter Short Axis
Mean Diameter
Diameter (Area)
Diameter (Circumference)
B
EDWARD SAPIEN XT
3,5
3
2,5
2
1,5
1
0,5
0
Size 23mm
Size 26mm
Size 29mm
Diameter Long Axis
Diameter Short Axis
Mean Diameter
Diameter (Area)
Diameter (Circumference)

Figure 3. Summary chart displaying major anatomic parameters (length of long and short axis; circumference-derived and area-derived virtual diameter) in patients in whom the small, medium or large size model was considered optimal for A) the CoreValve valve and the B) Edward Sapien XT valve. Except for the large vs. medium CoreValve size, all differences were statistically significant ($p<0.05$).

application of Bonferroni corrections to avoid errors due to multiple testing.

To compare means in variables not following normal distribution, a t-test was used if normal distribution was approximated after logarithmic transformation. In all other cases, non-parametric tests were used: the Mann-Whitney-test for independent variables and the Wilcoxon signed-rank test for paired variables.

To identify cut-off points that allow optimal prediction of implanted valve size on the basis of the particular anatomic parameter, and to estimate the associated generalization performance, we applied a 10-fold nested cross-validation approach. Details regarding this approach are included in Appendix S1.

P-values of 0.05 or less were considered statistically significant unless otherwise stated. Data were analyzed using MedCalc (Version 9.3.0.0, MedCalc Software, Mariakerke, Belgium), SPSS (21.0, IBM, Armonk, USA) and R [28].

Results

1. Patient Population

Between November 2007 and June 2012, 441 consecutive patients with high-grade aortic stenosis (mean AVA: 0.70 cm^2, SD: 0.15 cm^2) underwent a TAVI procedure at our institution. Of these, 17 patients were excluded as they presented with secondary stenosis of a surgical aortic valve prosthesis. Another 49 patients presented with externally acquired CT angiography datasets and were also excluded from this analysis. Of the remaining patients, 13 had died within 30 days after procedure and were not included into further analysis. 10 patients were excluded as they showed more than mild aortic regurgitation after valve implantation. Finally, one patient was excluded due to an error during archiving the small FOV (cardiac) series to PACS (Figure 1).

Of the remaining 351 patients, 235 had undergone implantation of a CoreValve prosthesis while in the remaining 116 patients the Edwards Sapien XT valve had been implanted. While differences in demographic parameters and preinterventional echocardiographic parameters between patients who underwent CoreValve vs. Edward Sapien XT valve implantation were not statistically significant, there was a difference in logarithmic Euro-Scores (19.6 [14.5; 26.7] vs. 16.5 [11.0; 23.4], $p<0.01$, see Table 1 for a summary of patient parameters) demonstrating a moderately less favorable risk profile in the CoreValve subgroup. In the entire cohort, no adverse events due to iv contrast administration during CT angiography were reported.

2. Subjective image quality and contrast enhancement of CTA datasets

There was substantial interobserver agreement for both subjective overall image quality (kappa = 0.76 [0.69–0.82]) and contrast enhancement (kappa = 0.72 [0.67–0.77]). Therefore, values from reader one were used for further analysis. Mean subjective image quality was 3.66 (SD: 0.58) and mean contrast enhancement was 3.88 (SD: 0.43).

3. CT-based anatomical measures of the aortic root

Interobserver agreement was excellent for all parameters with ICC-values consistently above 0.80. Bland-Altman-Analysis revealed no relevant systematic differences (Table 2 and Appendix S2). Therefore, arithmetic means between both observers were calculated for all variables.

Table 3 provides descriptive statistics on aortic valve measurements. Across all patients, length of the long axis and short axis were 2.70 [2.52; 2.90] and 2.05 [1.95; 2.25], respectively, and were slightly larger in the CoreValve subgroup than in the Edward Sapien subgroup (see Table 3). Median circumferences and median areas were 7.65 [7.28; 8.15] cm and 4.34 [3.90; 4.95] cm^2. There was a small but significant difference in average annulus diameters derived from circumference (2.44 [2.32; 2.60] cm) vs. those derived from annulus area (2.35 [2.23; 2.51] cm, $p<0.01$).

4. Annulus dimensions for different valve sizes

Of the 235 patients who underwent implantation of a CoreValve prosthesis, the 26 mm, 29 mm and 31 mm models were chosen in 93 (40%, 93/235), 135 (57%, 135/235) and 7 (3%, 7/235) cases. In 116 patients who received the Edward Sapien XT valve, the 23 mm, 26 mm and 29 mm were implanted in 38 (33%, 38/116), 72 (62%, 72/116) and 6 (5%, 6/118) cases.

Figure 3 provides details on long axis diameter, short axis diameter, circumference-derived and area-derived average annulus diameter measured for different sizes of CoreValve (Figure 3A) and Edward Sapien XT (Figure 3B). For all analyzed variables, one-way ANOVA showed significant differences between patients who underwent implantation of the small, middle or large valve (for the CoreValve: 26 mm, 29 mm, 31 mm; for the Edward Sapien XT: 23 mm, 26 mm, 29 mm, both p's<0.01). In Tukey-HSD post-hoc tests, differences between all size subgroups were statistically significant except for patients who underwent implantation of the CoreValve 31 mm vs. 29 mm ($p>0.05$), which was most likely due to the relatively small number of patients in the 31 mm CoreValve subgroup (n = 7).

Table 2. Interobserver Agreement for anatomical measurements of the aortic root reported as Intraclass Correlation Coefficient (ICC) and parameters of Bland-Altman-Analysis.

	Diameter long axis	Diameter short axis	$Diameter_{Mean}$	Annulus Circum-ference	Annulus Area
ICC [95% CI]	0.87 [0.84; 0.89]	0.86 [0.83; 0.88]	0.90 [0.88; 0.92]	0.92 [0.90; 0.93]	0.93 [0.92; 0.94]
Mean difference	0.00 cm	0.00 cm	0.00 cm	0.06 cm	0.03 cm^2
SD of differences	0.14 cm	0.12 cm	0.20 cm	0.54 cm	0.6 cm^2

Table 3. Primary anatomic parameters of the aortic annulus, N(%), mean ± SD or median [interquartile range] as well as "virtual diameters" derived from the mean of long axis and short axis, from annulus circumference and annulus area.

	All Patients	CoreValve Subgroup	Edward Sapien Subgroup	p
Diameter Long Axis [cm]	2.70 [2.52; 2.90]	2.75 [2.54; 2.90]	2.65 [2.50; 2.85]	0.049
Diameter Short Axis [cm]	2.05 [1.95; 2.25]	2.10 [1.95; 2.28]	2.05 [1.90; 2.20]	<0.01
Circumference [cm]	7.65 [7.28; 8.15]	7.73 [7.30; 8.25]	7.55 [7.05; 8.00]	<0.01
Area [cm^2]	4.34 [3.90; 4.95]	4.44 [3.98; 5.05]	4.19 [3.70; 4.75]	<0.01
Diameter$_{Mean}$ [cm]	2.40 [2.25; 2.55]	2.42 [2.27; 2.58]	2.35 [2.22; 2.52]	<0.01
Circumference- derived virtual diameter [cm]	2.44 [2.32; 2.60]	2.46 [2.32; 2.63]	2.40 [2.24; 2.55]	<0.01
Area-derived virtual diameter [cm]	2.35 [2.23; 2.51]	2.38 [2.25; 2.54]	2.31 [2.17; 2.46]	<0.01

5. Predictive value of different variables for device size selection and optimal cutoff values

Using multi-class ROC-analysis, the predictive value of all anatomic parameters for the size of prosthesis considered optimal was evaluated. For both valve types, all five analyzed parameters showed high predictive value for optimal prosthesis size (AUC: 0.75–0.91, Table 4). In particular, for the Medtronic CoreValve the short axis had a somewhat lower predictive value (multi-class AUC: 0.75) while there were no differences in predictive value between diameters of long axis, mean diameter, annulus area or annulus circumference (multi-class AUC's: 0.81, 0.80, 0.88, 0.9, $p>0.05$, Appendix S3). For the Edwards Sapien XT valve, differences in predictive value between the different parameters also did not reach statistical significance (multi-class AUC's: 0.83, 0.80, 0.88, 0.88, 0.89, $p>0.05$, Appendix S4). Application of the proposed cutoff-values in our sample of 351 patients results in the correct classification of 81.5% (286/351), 85.5% (300/351) and 82.9% (291/351) of cases if annulus circumference, annulus area or mean diameter are used.

Discussion

Transcatheter aortic valve implantation (TAVI) has been developed as a treatment strategy for patients with severe aortic stenosis who are at high risk or not eligible for heart surgery [29]. Several studies have demonstrated that MDCT is an ideal imaging modality prior to TAVI, providing isotropic datasets of the aortic root that can be reformatted in any spatial orientation [30–32]. There is some evidence favoring CT-derived annulus sizing over transthoracic echocardiography, particularly in regard to the incidence of postinterventional aortic regurgitation [17,19].

Several methods have been proposed to reduce the shape of the aortic annulus to a single measure for prosthesis sizing: calculation of the arithmetic mean between long and short axis [21], measurement of the length of the annulus circumference [12] or quantification of the annulus area [22,23]. To date, no consensus has been established on what the best technique is.

Binder et al have recently demonstrated for the Sapien XT valve that the recommendation of a particular prosthesis size on the basis of CT data results in more favorable outcomes than simply providing the annulus parameters [20]. In this regard

Table 4. Multi-Class AUC's as measures for the predictive value of the respective anatomic parameters for the valve size considered optimal by the implantation team.

	PARAMETER	OPTIMAL CUTOFF SMALL vs. MEDIUM	OPTIMAL CUTOFF MEDIUM vs. LARGE	MULTI-CLASS AUC
MEDTRONIC COREVALVE	Diameter Long Axis	2.70 cm	3.04 cm	0.8133
	Diameter Short Axis	2.05 cm	2.29 cm	0.7478
	Diameter$_{Mean}$	2.35 cm	2.70 cm	0.7974
	Annulus Area	4.30 cm^2	5.72 cm^2	0.8812
	Annulus Circumference	7.65 cm	8.60 cm	0.9146
EDWARDS SAPIEN XT	Diameter Long Axis	2.55 cm	3.05 cm	0.8347
	Diameter Short axis	1.95 cm	2.30 cm	0.7995
	Diameter$_{Mean}$	2.25 cm	2.55 cm	0.8793
	Annulus Area	3.85 cm^2	5.35 cm^2	0.8823
	Annulus Circumference	7.15 cm	8.20 cm	0.8884

Optimal cutoff values for the selection of the small, medium or large prosthesis size, defined as cutoff values that result in highest predictive accuracy.

however, uncertainty remains as to what the optimal size of prosthesis is for a given set of aortic annulus parameters.

In this analysis of over 350 patients who had undergone CT angiography prior to TAVI, we performed extensive anatomic measurements of the aortic root. Our results confirm previous analyses of Halpern et al [14], Gurvitch et al [12] and Delgado et al [33], since all relevant anatomic parameters can be measured in virtually all patients with excellent agreement between two experienced observers. Similar to the study by Gurvitch, observer agreement was highest for aortic annulus circumference and area (ICC's = 0.92, 0.93), even though in our study differences to observer agreement for long and short axis measurements were not significant.

In all patients included in this analysis, optimal prosthesis size was determined with the help of a sizing balloon catheter inflated during the implantation procedure [24–26]. Furthermore, all patients in whom this method might not have resulted in the selection of the correct prosthesis size – i.e. patients with more than mild regurgitation after TAVI (n = 10) and patients who died within 30 days after implantation (n = 13) – were deliberately excluded. No patient had to be excluded due to open heart surgery within 30 days. According to best professional judgment, prosthesis sizing was adequate in the remaining 351 patients. Thus, our data permit the unique opportunity to analyze the relation between different anatomic variables of the aortic root and the device size ultimately considered optimal. Even more importantly, the discriminatory power of different anatomic variables to predict prosthesis size as well as optimal cutoff values can be calculated.

Our results demonstrate that for all analyzed anatomic variables there are differences between patients who underwent implantation of the small, medium or large valve. Our results are both in line with but also extend those of Jilaihawi et al [17] and Delgado et al [34], demonstrating that on the basis of high-resolution MDCT datasets of the aortic root, the optimal valve size can be predicted. While in principle all evaluated anatomic parameters can be used for prosthesis sizing, the most favorable combination of high observer agreement and predictive value are observed for mean diameter, annulus area and annulus circumference (with multi-class AUC's of 0.88 and 0.91). Optimal thresholds for the selection of the small, medium or large size are given in Table 4. The use of these cutoff values in our cohort results in the correction prediction of valve size in 85% (300/351) of cases. In the remaining 15% (51/351), the application of a sizing balloon would result in a change of device size. Importantly, our 2-threshold-model does not take into account that a considerable number of patients will be suitable candidates for two valve sizes. Inclusion of the extent of aortic valve calcifications might further increase the predictive accuracy of our model.

Our single-center retrospective study has several limitations: first, the heart team members involved in valve implantation were not blinded towards the routine radiological reports derived from the CT dataset. While this would have been favorable from a scientific perspective, we feel that the information obtained from high-resolution CT angiography datasets prior to TAVI is of so essential a nature that withholding it would be clearly unethical. Furthermore, cardiologists integrated all available information regarding valve size, including transthoracic and transesophageal echocardiography and aortic angiography usually conducted before the TAVI procedure. In every single case, the presumed optimal valve size was simulated with a balloon catheter and changed if the size of the inflated balloon and the aortic annulus did not display the estimated ratio during aortography.

Second, we did not compare our measurements with a reference imaging modality such as 3D-echocardiography or MR angiography. However, our reference standard is the size of the implanted valve in those patients in whom – according to best professional judgment – prosthesis size turned out to be reasonably selected. For the purpose of this analysis we consider this outcome-oriented reference standard superior.

Third, we used only diastolic CT acquisitions to measure aortic annulus dimensions. However, it still is a matter of debate if systolic reconstructions are necessary for a reliable sizing of the aortic valve annulus: while some authors propose systolic reconstructions to avoid undersizing [35,36], others report no difference [37] or no substantial difference [38] between systolic and diastolic diameters. However, since we correlate our diastolic measures of annulus parameters with the prosthesis size considered optimal during implantation, a potential difference between systolic and diastolic dimensions is not a major concern; our results should rather be construed as a contribution to a prosthesis sizing algorithm from diastolic annulus parameters.

Fourth, we do not perform an analysis of the patients in whom valve implantation was not successful. However, the main intention of our manuscript is to perform a rigorous analysis of the dependencies between anatomical parameters of the aortic annulus and the implanted valve size for patients in whom the procedure was performed successfully. In that sense, we do not attempt to prove that an inadequate selection of prosthesis size increases the risk of a negative procedural outcome.

Finally, while our analysis suggests an ideal strategy to predict the appropriate valve size, we cannot answer the question how this strategy would perform in a prospective study context. However, the rate of excluded patients is comparatively small: only 23 patients had to be excluded due to either death within 30 days after the TAVI procedure (n = 13) or due to the development of more than mild aortic regurgitation (n = 10). Therefore, we are confident that our approach would permit a correct estimation of correct valve size in the vast majority of cases.

In conclusion, our analysis of 351 patients who successfully underwent TAVI shows that the valve size ultimately considered optimal can be predicted on the basis of CT-derived anatomic parameters of the aortic root. Mean diameter, annulus circumference and annulus area appear to have equally high reproducibility and predictive accuracy for both the Medtronic CoreValve and the Edwards Sapien XT prostheses. It remains to be shown that this approach holds up its predictive potential in a prospective study context.

Supporting Information

Appendix S1 Supplemental methods section including details on CT data acquisition, image reconstruction and statistical methods.

Appendix S2 Supplemental scatter plots and linear regression lines for the analysis of interobserver agreement.

Appendix S3 Extended results regarding the ANOVA analysis and post-hoc tests of differences in anatomic parameters of patients who underwent implantation of the large, middle or small version of either valve.

Appendix S4 Extended results regarding the analysis of differences in predictive values of the various anatomic

parameters for the valve size considered optimal by the TAVI team.

Author Contributions

Conceived and designed the experiments: FS PL DZ MG PB CS MFR CK HCB. Performed the experiments: FS PL DZ MG. Analyzed the data: FS PL DZ MG CK HCB. Contributed reagents/materials/analysis tools: MFR HCB. Wrote the paper: FS PL DZ MG PB CS MFR CK HCB.

References

1. Iung B, Baron G, Butchart EG, Delahaye F, Gohlke-Barwolf C, et al. (2003) A prospective survey of patients with valvular heart disease in Europe: The Euro Heart Survey on Valvular Heart Disease. Eur Hear J 24: 1231–1243. doi:S0195668X0300201X [pii].
2. Carabello BA, Paulus WJ (2009) Aortic stenosis. Lancet 373: 956–966. doi:S0140-6736(09)60211-7 [pii] 10.1016/S0140-6736(09)60211-7 [doi].
3. Bouma BJ, Van den Brink RBA, Van der Meulen JHP, Verheul HA, Cheriex EC, et al. (1999) To operate or not on elderly patients with aortic stenosis: the decision and its consequences. Heart 82: 143.
4. Iung B, Cachier A, Baron G, Messika-Zeitoun D, Delahaye F, et al. (2005) Decision-making in elderly patients with severe aortic stenosis: why are so many denied surgery? Eur Heart J 26: 2714.
5. Bach DS, Siao D, Girard SE, Duvernoy C, McCallister BD, et al. (2009) Evaluation of patients with severe symptomatic aortic stenosis who do not undergo aortic valve replacement. Circ Cardiovasc Qual Outcomes 2: 533.
6. Krishnaswamy A, Tuzcu EM, Kapadia SR (2010) Three-dimensional computed tomography in the cardiac catheterization laboratory. Catheter Cardiovasc Interv. doi:10.1002/ccd.22740.
7. Wood DA, Tops LF, Mayo JR, Pasupati S, Schalij MJ, et al. (2009) Role of multislice computed tomography in transcatheter aortic valve replacement. Am J Cardiol 103: 1295–1301. doi:S0002-9149(09)00110-6 [pii] 10.1016/j.amjcard.2009.01.034 [doi].
8. Leon M, Smith C, Mack M (2010) Transcatheter aortic-valve implantation for aortic stenosis in patients who cannot undergo surgery. N Engl J Med 363: 1597–1607. Available: http://www.nejm.org/doi/full/10.1056/nejmoa1008232. Accessed 2014 Jan 21.
9. Makkar RR, Fontana GP, Jilaihawi H, Kapadia S, Pichard AD, et al. (2012) Transcatheter aortic-valve replacement for inoperable severe aortic stenosis. N Engl J Med 366: 1696–1704. Available: http://www.ncbi.nlm.nih.gov/pubmed/23356420.
10. Smith CR, Leon MB, Mack MJ, Miller DC (2011) Transcatheter versus Surgical Aortic-Valve Replacement in High-Risk Patients. N Engl J Med 364: 2187–2198.
11. Achenbach S, Delgado V, Hausleiter J, Schoenhagen P, Min JK, et al. (2012) SCCT Expert Consensus Document on Computed Tomography Imaging Prior to Transcatheter Aortic Valve Implantation (TAVI)/Transcatheter Aortic Valve Replacement (TAVR). J Cardiovasc Comput Tomogr.
12. Gurvitch R, Webb JG, Yuan R, Johnson M, Hague C, et al. (2011) Aortic Annulus Diameter Determination by Multidetector Computed TomographyR-eproducibility, Applicability, and Implications for Transcatheter Aortic Valve Implantation. JACC Cardiovasc Interv 4: 1235–1245.
13. Wuest W, Anders K, Schuhbaeck A, May MS, Gauss S, et al. (2012) Dual source multidetector CT-angiography before transcatheter aortic valve implantation (TAVI) using a high-pitch spiral acquisition mode. Eur Radiol 22: 51–58.
14. Halpern EJ, Gupta S, Halpern DJ, Wiener DH, Owen AN (2012) Characterization and Normal Measurements of the Left Ventricular Outflow Tract by ECG-gated Cardiac CT: Implications for Disorders of the Outflow Tract and Aortic Valve. Acad Radiol.
15. Altiok E, Koos R, Schröder J, Brehmer K, Hamada S, et al. (2011) Comparison of two-dimensional and three-dimensional imaging techniques for measurement of aortic annulus diameters before transcatheter aortic valve implantation. Heart 97: 1578–1584.
16. Ng ACT, Delgado V, van der Kley F, Shanks M, van de Veire NRL, et al. (2010) Comparison of Aortic Root Dimensions and Geometries Before and After Transcatheter Aortic Valve Implantation by 2-and 3-Dimensional Transesophageal Echocardiography and Multislice Computed Tomography CLINICAL PERSPECTIVE. Circ Cardiovasc Imaging 3: 94–102.
17. Jilaihawi H, Kashif M, Fontana G, Furugen A, Shiota T, et al. (2012) Cross-sectional computed tomographic assessment improves accuracy of aortic annular sizing for transcatheter aortic valve replacement and reduces the incidence of paravalvular aortic regurgitation. J Am Coll Cardiol 59: 1275–1286.
18. Blanke P, Reinöhl J, Schlensak C, Siepe M, Pache G, et al. (2012) Prosthesis Oversizing in Balloon-Expandable Transcatheter Aortic Valve Implantation Is Associated With Contained Rupture of the Aortic Root. Circ Cardiovasc Interv 5: 540–548.
19. Hayashida K, Bouvier E, Lefevre T, Hovasse T, Morice M-C, et al. (2012) Impact of CT-guided valve sizing on post-procedural aortic regurgitation in transcatheter aortic valve implantation. J Am Coll Cardiol 59: E2142–E2142.
20. Binder RK, Webb JG, Willson AB, Urena M, Hansson NC, et al. (2013) The Impact of Integration of a Multidetector Computed Tomography Annulus Area Sizing Algorithm on Outcomes of Transcatheter Aortic Valve Replacement: A Prospective, Multicenter, Controlled Trial. J Am Coll Cardiol.
21. Leipsic J, Gurvitch R, LaBounty TM, Min JK, Wood D, et al. (2011) Multidetector Computed Tomography in Transcatheter Aortic Valve Implantation. JACC Cardiovasc Imaging 4: 416.
22. Schultz CJ, Moelker A, Piazza N, Tzikas A, Otten A, et al. (2010) Three dimensional evaluation of the aortic annulus using multislice computer tomography: are manufacturer's guidelines for sizing for percutaneous aortic valve replacement helpful? Eur Heart J 31: 849–856.
23. Blanke P, Siepe M, Reinöhl J, Zehender M, Beyersdorf F, et al. (2010) Assessment of aortic annulus dimensions for Edwards SAPIEN Transapical Heart Valve implantation by computed tomography: calculating average diameter using a virtual ring method. Eur J Cardio-Thoracic Surg 38: 750–758.
24. Babaliaros VC, Liff D, Chen EP, Rogers JH, Brown RA, et al. (2008) Can balloon aortic valvuloplasty help determine appropriate transcatheter aortic valve size? JACC Cardiovasc Interv 1: 580–586.
25. Babaliaros VC, Junagadhwalla Z, Lerakis S, Thourani V, Liff D, et al. (2010) Use of balloon aortic valvuloplasty to size the aortic annulus before implantation of a balloon-expandable transcatheter heart valve. JACC Cardiovasc Interv 3: 114–118.
26. Cerillo A, Mariani M, Berti S, Glauber M (2012) Sizing the aortic annulus. Ann Cardiothorac Surg 1: 245–256.
27. Bartko JJ (1966) The intraclass correlation coefficient as a measure of reliability. Psychol Rep 19: 3–11.
28. R Development Core Team (2010) R: A languae and environment for statistical computing. Available: http://www.r-project.org.
29. Cheung A, Soon JL (2011) Transcatheter aortic valve replacement: where will we be in 5 years? Curr Opin Cardiol 26: 106.
30. Schultz C, Moelker A, Tzikas A, Piazza N, De Feyter P, et al. (2010) The use of MSCT for the evaluation of the aortic root before transcutaneous aortic valve implantation: the Rotterdam approach. EuroIntervention 6: 505–511.
31. Del Valle-Fernandez R, Jelnin V, Panagopoulos G, Dudiy Y, Schneider L, et al. (2010) A method for standardized computed tomography angiography-based measurement of aortic valvar structures. Eur Hear J. doi:10.1093/eurheartj/ehq093.
32. Delgado V, Ng ACT, Shanks M, van der Kley F, Schuijf JD, et al. (2010) Transcatheter aortic valve implantation: role of multimodality cardiac imaging. Expert Rev Cardiovasc Ther 8: 113–123.
33. Delgado V, Ng ACT, Schuijf JD, van der Kley F, Shanks M, et al. (2011) Automated assessment of the aortic root dimensions with multidetector row computed tomography. Ann Thorac Surg 91: 716–723.
34. Delgado V, Ng ACT, Van De Veire NR, Van Der Kley F, Schuijf JD, et al. (2010) Transcatheter aortic valve implantation: role of multi-detector row computed tomography to evaluate prosthesis positioning and deployment in relation to valve function. Eur Heart J 31: 1114–1123.
35. Lehmkuhl L, Foldyna B, Von Aspern K, Lucke C, Grothoff M, et al. (2013) Inter-individual variance and cardiac cycle dependency of aortic root dimensions and shape as assessed by ECG-gated multi-slice computed tomography in patients with severe aortic stenosis prior to transcatheter aortic valve implantation: is it crucial for. Int J Cardiovasc Imaging 29: 693–703. doi:10.1007/s10554-012-0123-4.
36. Blanke P, Russe M, Leipsic J, Reinohl J, Ebersberger U, et al. (2012) Conformational pulsatile changes of the aortic annulus: impact on prosthesis sizing by computed tomography for transcatheter aortic valve replacement. JACC Cardiovasc Interv 5: 984–994. doi:10.1016/j.jcin.2012.05.014.
37. Bolen MA, Popovic ZB, Dahiya A, Kapadia SR, Tuzcu EM, et al. (2012) Prospective ECG-triggered, axial 4-D imaging of the aortic root, valvular, and left ventricular structures: a lower radiation dose option for preprocedural TAVR imaging. J Cardiovasc Comput Tomogr 6: 393–398. doi:10.1016/j.jcct.2012.10.006.
38. Bertaso AG, Wong DTL, Liew GYH, Cunnington MS, Richardson JD, et al. (2012) Aortic annulus dimension assessment by computed tomography for transcatheter aortic valve implantation: differences between systole and diastole. Int J Cardiovasc Imaging 28: 2091–2098.

20

Chronic Total Occlusions in Sweden – A Report from the Swedish Coronary Angiography and Angioplasty Registry (SCAAR)

Truls Råmunddal[1]*[9], Loes Hoebers[2][9], Jose P. S. Henriques[2], Christian Dworeck[1], Oskar Angerås[1], Jacob Odenstedt[1], Dan Ioanes[1], Göran Olivecrona[3], Jan Harnek[3], Ulf Jensen[4], Mikael Aasa[4], Risto Jussila[4], Stefan James[5], Bo Lagerqvist[5], Göran Matejka[1], Per Albertsson[1], Elmir Omerovic[1]

1 Department of Cardiology, Sahlgrenska University Hospital, Gothenburg, Sweden, **2** Department of Cardiology, Academic Medical Center, Amsterdam, The Netherlands, **3** Department of Coronary Heart Disease, Skåne University Hospital, Scania, Sweden, **4** Department of Cardiology, Stockholm South General Hospital, Stockholm, Sweden, **5** Department of Medical Sciences, Uppsala University, Uppsala, Sweden

Abstract

Introduction: Evidence for the current guidelines for the treatment of patients with chronic total occlusions (CTO) in coronary arteries is limited. In this study we identified all CTO patients registered in the Swedish Coronary Angiography and Angioplasty Registry (SCAAR) and studied the prevalence, patient characteristics and treatment decisions for CTO in Sweden.

Methods and Results: Between January 2005 and January 2012, 276,931 procedures (coronary angiography or percutaneous coronary intervention) were performed in 215,836 patients registered in SCAAR. We identified all patients who had 100% luminal diameter stenosis known or assumed to be ≥3 months old. After exclusion of patients with previous coronary artery bypass graft (CABG) surgery or coronary occlusions due to acute coronary syndrome, we identified 16,818 CTO patients. A CTO was present in 10.9% of all coronary angiographies and in 16.0% of patients with coronary artery disease. The majority of CTO patients were treated conservatively and PCI of CTO accounted for only 5.8% of all PCI procedures. CTO patients with diabetes and multivessel disease were more likely to be referred to CABG.

Conclusion: CTO is a common finding in Swedish patients undergoing coronary angiography but the number of CTO procedures in Sweden is low. Patients with CTO are a high-risk subgroup of patients with coronary artery disease. SCAAR has the largest register of CTO patients and therefore may be valuable for studies of clinical importance of CTO and optimal treatment for CTO patients.

Editor: Ingo Ahrens, University Hospital Medical Centre, Germany

Funding: The SCAAR registry is sponsored by the Swedish Health Authorities only and is independent of commercial funding. No current funding sources for this study. The funders had no role in study design, data collection and analysis, decision to publish, or preparation of the manuscript.

Competing Interests: Dr Stefan James has during the last 3 years received institutional research grants from Medtronic, Terumo Inc,Vascular Solutions and served as an advisory board member for Medtronic. Dr Jose P.S. Henriques has received unrestricted research grant from Abbott Vascular. Dr Elmir Omerovic serves as an advisory board member for Astra Zeneca and has received lecturing fees from Medtronic and Astra Zeneca. All other co-authors have no disclosures or potential conflicts of interest.

* Email: truls@wlab.gu.se

[9] These authors contributed equally to this work.

Introduction

Chronic total occlusions (CTO) are difficult to treat with percutaneous coronary intervention (PCI) [1]. Revascularization of CTO demands expert skills, longer procedural time and is associated with higher procedural risks such as coronary perforation, contrast nephropathy, radiation exposure, and loss of collateral circulation [1,2]. According to the European and American guidelines, PCI of CTO has class-IIa recommendation (weight of evidence in favour of the treatments usefulness/efficacy) [3,4] but this recommendation is based on small retrospective studies and on expert consensus.

The true prevalence of a CTO in the general population is unknown and few studies have addressed this question. In observational studies, a CTO was found in approximately one third of the patients referred for coronary angiography [5–7]. However, these studies were based on low number of patients and participating hospitals, and may therefore be prone to selection bias. To date, no epidemiological study has investigated the prevalence and clinical characteristics of CTO patients at the nationwide level.

The Swedish Coronary Angiography and Angioplasty Registry (SCAAR) is a prospective national registry that collects data about all patient undergoing coronary angiography and PCI in Sweden [8]. Therefore, we identified all CTO patients registered in SCAAR and studied prevalence, patient characteristics and treatment decision for CTO in Sweden.

Methods

Swedish Coronary Angiography and Angioplasty Registry (SCAAR)

The SCAAR registry was established in 1999 after the unification of Swedish Coronary Angiography registry (Acta Coronaria) and the Swedish Coronary Angioplasty registry (SCAP). SCAAR, which is a part of the national SWEDEHEART registry, holds data on all consecutive patients from all centres that perform coronary angiography and PCI in Sweden. The registry is independent of commercial funding and is sponsored by the Swedish Health Authorities only. The technology has been developed and administered by the Uppsala Clinical Research Center. Since 2001, SCAAR has been Internet-based, with recording of data online through an Internet interface in the catheterization laboratory; data are transferred in an encrypted format to a central server at the Uppsala Clinical Research Center.

In total, there are 30 hospitals with cardiac catheterization facilities in Sweden of which 9 are university hospitals. In SCAAR, a coronary angiography procedure is described by approximately 50 variables while a PCI procedure allows for is described by approximately 200 variables. The information about clinical characteristics and procedural details is entered into the registry immediately after the procedure by the PCI physician after the review of clinical information.

Ethics statement

The study was approved by the regional ethical review board of Gothenburg University, Gothenburg,Sweden. The regional ethical review board waived the need for written informed consent from the participants according to Swedish legislation and because data were de-identified and anonymized before analysis.

Definitions

We defined CTO as 100% luminal diameter stenosis and the absence of antegrade flow known or assumed to be ≥3 months duration [6,9,10]. Coronary artery disease was defined as a luminal narrowing ≥50% on angiography. Procedural success after PCI treatment of the coronary lesion is defined as residual stenosis <50%, decreased grade of stenosis after intervention by at least 20%, normal blood flow and no serious complications.

Study cohort

We used two different methods to identify CTO patients in SCAAR between January 2005 and January 2012.

The first method is based on the information about %-luminal stenosis at the level of coronary segments that was introduced in 2005. From this date onwards, the information derived from a diagnostic coronary angiogram can also be used to determine if a coronary segment was totally occluded. In order to differentiate between acute and chronic occlusions, we excluded patients who underwent a procedure for acute coronary syndrome in whom the occlusion was located in the same coronary artery as the culprit vessel. Furthermore, we excluded patients who underwent a procedure in the same vessel within the previous 3 months. The CTO patients identified by this method constitute the *coronary segment subcohort*.

The second method is based on the separate variable by which PCI operators classify a treated occlusion either as a chronic occlusion ≥3 months duration or as an acute/subacute occlusion ≤3 months duration.

The patients with previous coronary artery bypass graft (CABG) surgery were excluded from analysis as the patency of the graft could not be determined. The study was scrutinised and approved by the ethics board according to the Swedish law and regulations.

Total CTO cohort

The total CTO cohort contains all CTO patients identified by either of the two methods (**Figure 1**). Patients and procedures in which the same CTO lesion was registered through both methods or at multiple occasions were identified and duplicate observations were excluded from the analysis. For each patient, the procedure where the CTO was observed first was selected.

Coronary segment subcohort

We also present data from the subcohort of patients who were identified according to whether they had a 100% luminal stenosis and considered to be a CTO based on the above mentioned inclusion criteria. We compared patient characteristics and treatment decisions between patients with significant coronary artery disease in whom a CTO was observed or not. Prevalence of a CTO was calculated only from the coronary segment subcohort and in relation to three different denominators: the number of unique procedures, the number of unique patients and the number of unique patients with significant coronary artery disease.

Validation of CTO

Validation of the CTO definition was performed in a subgroup of 955 patients from one university hospital (Sahlgrenska University Hospital) and from three county hospitals (Norra Älvsborgs Hospital, Borås Hospital, Skövde Hospital). This subgroup represents 5.7% of all identified CTO patients in SCAAR in the study period. The patients were randomly selected by means of random number generator using Stata software (Version 12.1, StataCorp, College Station, Texas, USA). The validation procedure was conducted by a panel consisting of five experienced interventional cardiologists. The panellists examined individual coronary angiograms according to a monitoring plan defined in advance. Each angiogram was evaluated in regard to whether the patient had previous CABG, whether the treated occlusion was ≥3 months old and whether 100% segmental stenosis on angiogram was an occlusion ≥3 months old. The results from the validation procedure were then compared to the data entered in SCAAR.

Statistical analysis

Differences in baseline characteristics between the groups were tested by the χ^2 test for categorical variables while Mann–Whitney U test and Kruskal-Wallis test were used for comparison of continuous non-normally distributed variables. We used Shapiro-Wilks test to test for normal distribution. Tests for trends were made using linear contrasts of means in a one-way analysis of variance model for numerical data and the Armitage-Cohrane trend test for categorical data. We used logistic regression with test for linear trend to evaluate whether annual incidence of CTO and success rate for PCI of CTO changed during the study period. Statistical significance was defined as a P-value<0.05. All analyses were performed using Stata software (Version 13.1, StataCorp, College Station, Texas, USA).

Results

Prevalence of CTO in Sweden

As of January 2012, 497,572 procedures (coronary angiographies and PCIs) performed in 348,863 patients were registered in SCAAR. The numbers of PCIs and coronary angiographies

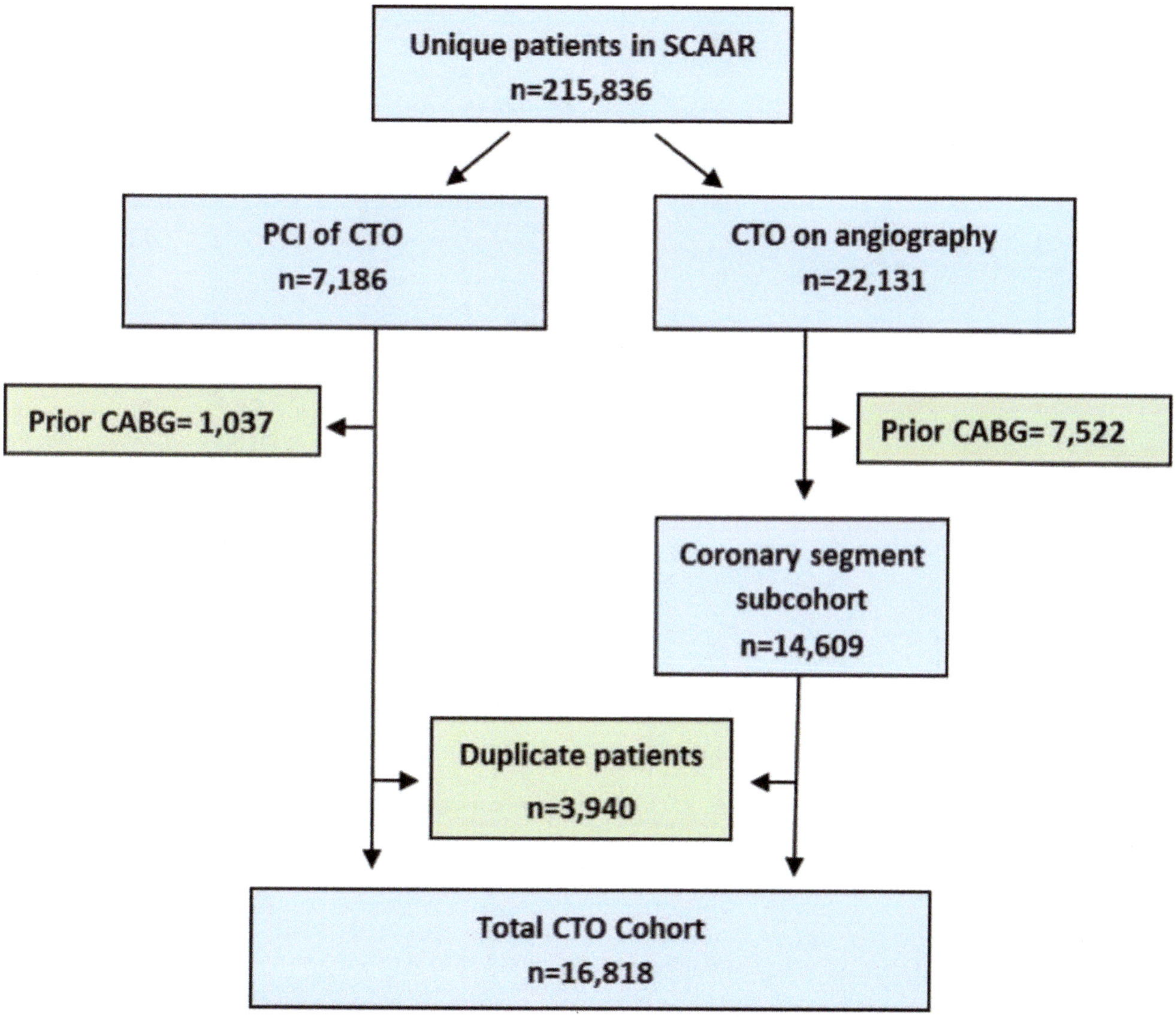

Figure 1. Flow chart for identification and selection of CTO patients in SCAAR. Based on the selection methods we have defined two CTO groups. The first group - *the total CTO cohort-* contains all CTO patients recognized by one or both methods during the period. The second group is the subcohort that contains the patients in whom a CTO was identified through the %-luminal stenosis on the coronary segments – *the coronary segment subcohort.*

increased since 1999 (**Figure 2**). The annual rate of PCIs for CTO remained low (~1200 in 2011).

Between January 2005 and January 2012, Swedish interventionalists completed 276,931 procedures in 215,836 patients. The total number of CTO patients without previous CABG during the same period was 16,818 and these patients constitute the total CTO cohort (**Figure 1**).

Information about age of the treated CTO was missing in 0.8% (n = 1077) of all procedures. Of the 134,087 reported PCIs, 7,816 (5.8%) involved the treatment of a CTO. These procedures were performed in 29 different hospitals on 7,186 unique patients of whom 6,149 without prior CABG. Almost half (43%) of all CTO procedures were performed at university hospitals. Data on procedural success was missing in 12 procedures (0.2%). The overall success rate was 53.1%. The annual success rate did not change significantly during the study period with 54.4% in 2005 and 56.6% in 2012 (OR 1.02, 95% CI 0.99–1.06; P = 0.15 test for linear trend).

Complete information about luminal %-stenosis was available in 160,159 (57.8%) angiographies of which 144,744 were from in patients without previous CABG. A CTO was observed in 10.6% of angiographies from 126,745 patients. Of these patients, 14,609 had at least one CTO resulting in a prevalence of 11.5%. Coronary artery disease was diagnosed in 91,154 patients of which 16.0% had a CTO. In patients who underwent multiple procedures, the CTO was diagnosed on the first diagnostic angiogram in 90% of the cases. The annual number of diagnosed CTO in patients undergoing coronary angiography decreased gradually by 25% from 11.5% in 2005 to 8.6% in 2012 (OR 0.97; 95% CI 0.96–0.98; P<0.001 test for linear trend). In patients with significant coronary artery disease, CTO decreased by 12% from 17.2 in 2005 to 15.1 in 2012 (OR 0.95; 95% CI 0.94–0.96; P< 0.001 test for linear trend).

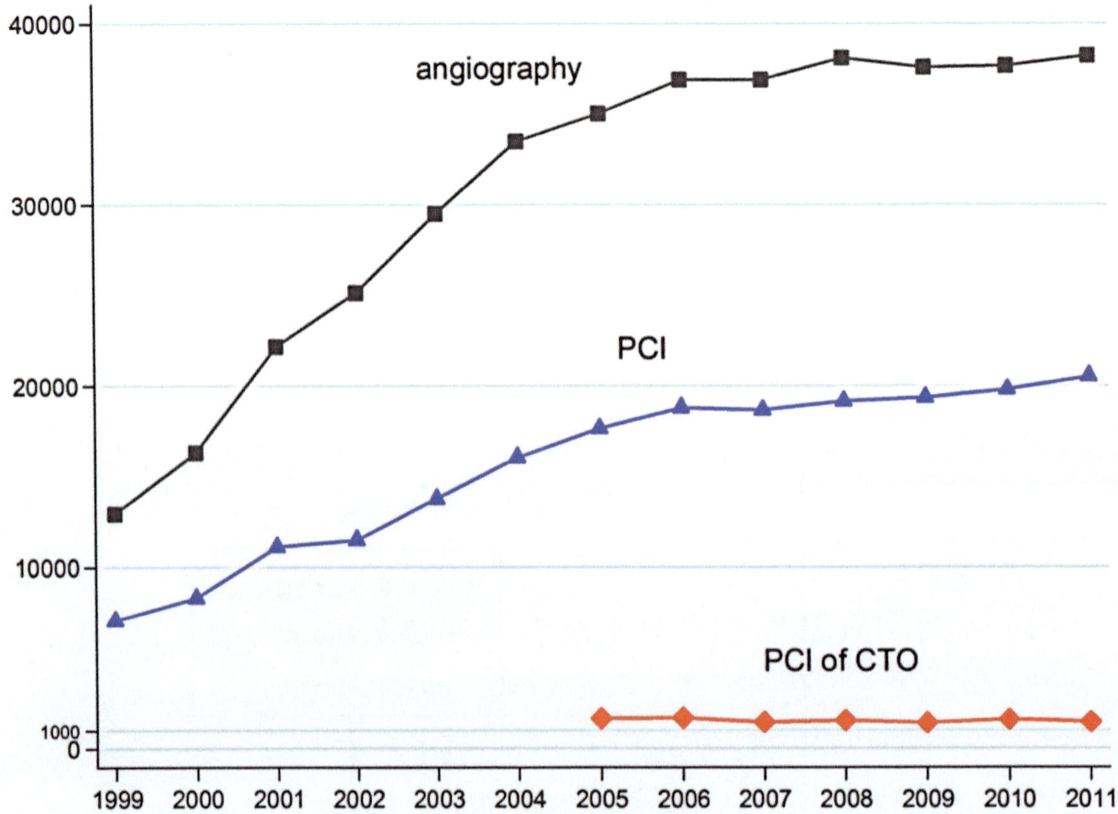

Figure 2. Annual number of coronary angiographies, PCI's, and PCI's performed in CTO patients in Sweden reported in SCAAR since 1999.

Patient characteristics

The clinical characteristics of all CTO patients - the total CTO cohort - registered in SCAAR since 2005 are summarized in **Table 1**. The majority of CTO patients were male. The high occurrence of previous MI (37%) and the presence of traditional cardiovascular risk factors make CTO patients a high-risk population.

Table 2 shows the baseline demographic and angiographic characteristics of patients with coronary artery disease stratified for the presence of a CTO on angiography (coronary segment subcohort). CTO patients were more often males and were more likely to have risk factors including previous MI. In addition, the extent of coronary artery disease was more severe in CTO patients with more multivessel and left main disease. Although CTO was diagnosed in the majority of cases during a coronary angiography for stable angina, a substantial proportion was diagnosed in patients with acute coronary syndrome. Furthermore, patients with a CTO more often presented in cardiogenic shock at presentation for STEMI compared to patients without a CTO. The CTO was more frequently located in the right coronary artery (RCA) followed by the left anterior descending artery (LAD) and left circumflex artery (LCx) (**Figure 3**). In approximately 14%, CTOs were observed in more than one vessel of which only 0.1% included the left main.

Treatment of CTO patients

Table 3 shows the differences in baseline demographic and angiographic characteristics of CTO patients identified through the coronary segment stenosis, according to the received treatment at baseline. After diagnosis, the majority of the CTO patients (56%) received medical treatment only. The CTO patients who received invasive treatment were evenly distributed between PCI (22.3%) and referral for CABG (21.7%). CTO patients, who received medical treatment only, had more often previous MI, presented more often with STEMI, had a lower creatinine clearance and had less severe angina symptoms in comparison to the patients who were treated invasively for a CTO. Patients who were referred for CABG were more often male with a higher prevalence of cardiovascular risk factors including diabetes, had less often previous MI or PCI, presented more often with stable angina and suffered more frequently from extensive coronary artery disease than CTO patients treated with PCI. CTO patients treated for stable angina received medical treatment in 41.6%, PCI in 20.6% and CABG in 37.8%. CTO patients who were treated for acute coronary syndrome received medical treatment in 28.6%, PCI in 71.2%, and were referred to CABG in 0.2%. Procedure-related complications were reported in 5.4% CTO patients treated with PCI. The following complications were reported: death (0%), major bleeding (1.3%), stroke (0.3%), pericardial tamponade (0.4%) renal insufficiency (0.7%), emergency PCI (0.1%), emergency CABG (0%), procedure-related MI (1.1%), anaphylactic reaction (0.1%), other (1.4%)

Validation of CTO

The validation analysis revealed 36 (3.8%) erroneously classified patients. Of these, 18 patients did not have a 100% occluded coronary artery on the coronary angiogram. Another 5 patients

Table 1. Baseline characteristics of the total CTO cohort in SCAAR at the time of diagnosis based on data collected during the period 2005–2012.

	All CTO patients (n = 16,818)	Missing %
Male (%)	77.5	0.0
Age (median, IQR)	68 (60–76)	0.2
Diabetes (%)	23.9	1.0
Hypertension (%)	61.9	2.5
Hyperlipidemia (%)	62.7	2.9
Smoking status (%)		6.2
Current smoker	19.9	
Previous smoker	40.2	
Previous MI (%)	37.2	3.8
Previous PCI (%)	18.4	0.1
Cardiogenic shock (%)*	10.2	1.2
Creatinine Clearance (ml/min)	81 (61–104)	28.2
CCS class (%)**		7.0
I	9.0	
II	52.2	
III	37.4	
IV	1.4	
Indication (%)		0.0
Stable CAD	45.5	
Unstable CAD/NSTEMI	27.5	
STEMI	14.3	
Other	12.7	
Extent of CAD (%)		1.1
1 vessel	20.4	
2 vessel	35.1	
3 vessel	36.1	
Left main disease***	8.4	

CAD: coronary artery disease, CCS: Canadian cardiovascular society, CTO: chronic total occlusion, IQR: inter quartile range, MI: myocardial infarction, (N)STEMI: (non-)ST-elevation myocardial infarction, PCI: percutaneous coronary intervention.
* Cardiogenic shock only displayed for the indication STEMI.
**CCS class only displayed for the indication stable CAD.
*** Left main (LM) disease includes: LM+1 vessel, LM+2 vessel and LM+3 vessel.

had prior CABG and 13 patients had acute or subacute coronary occlusions.

Discussion

In this study, we identified and studied 16,818 CTO patients in SCAAR. We found CTO in every tenth patient undergoing coronary angiography, and that the prevalence of CTO in Sweden decreased by one quarter in these patients between January 2005 and January 2012.

The true prevalence of a CTO in the general population is unknown and not well studied. In a few older studies based on small populations, CTO prevalence was 35% [7] and 52% [5] in patients with significant coronary artery disease. In a recent study from Canada based on 1697 patients, CTO prevalence was 14.7% in all patients undergoing angiography [6]. However, our study shows that the prevalence of CTO was 11.5% in Sweden. The reason for the difference in CTO prevalence between Sweden and other countries may be due to selection bias. While all previous studies were based on selected and relatively small populations, SCAAR holds information from all hospitals that perform coronary angiography and PCI in Sweden which reduces selection bias. Another explanation may be that prevalence of CTO differs between the countries due to variance in severity of coronary artery disease, treatment algorithms for acute coronary syndromes and organization of health care system [11].

Our study shows that CTO patients are a high-risk population with more traditional cardiovascular risk factors, multivessel disease, history of MI and PCI, which is in accordance with previous reports [1,6,9]. Furthermore, a substantial number (14%) of patients had multiple CTO's in separate vessels.

Majority of CTO patients had stable angina but approximately 40% had acute coronary syndrome at the time when CTO was diagnosed. Overall, 56% of the CTO patients were treated with medical treatment initially. The remaining patients were evenly distributed between percutaneous and surgical revascularization similar to the Canadian study [9]. The success rate for CTO procedures in all Swedish hospitals was 53% which is lower than 70% and 80% reported by others [2,6,12]. However, the success

Table 2. Baseline characteristics of patients from coronary segment subcohort with coronary artery disease, stratified for the presence of a CTO observed on angiography.

	CTO observed (n = 14,609)	Missing %	CTO not observed (n = 76,545)	Missing %	P-value
Male gender (%)	77.7	0	70.6	0.0	<0.01
Age (median, IQR)	68 (61–76)	0.2	68 (60–75)	0.2	<0.01
Diabetes (%)	24.0	1.0	18.6	0.8	<0.01
Hypertension (%)	62.0	2.4	52.5	2.0	<0.01
Hyperlipidemia (%)	61.9	2.8	44.4	2.5	<0.01
Smoking status (%)		5.8		5.5	<0.01
Current smoker	20.0		21.6		
Previous smoker	40.0		35.0		
Previous MI (%)	37.0	3.8	16.5	2.3	<0.01
Previous PCI (%)	17.5	0.1	10.7	0.05	<0.01
Cardiogenic shock(%)*	10.1	1.0	3.5	1.3	<0.01
Creatinine Clearance	80	28.2	81	34.2	<0.01
(ml/min)	(60–103)		(62–103)		
CCS class (%)**		6.9		5.5	0.19
I	9.3		9.6		
II	53.4		54.7		
III	36.0		34.5		
IV	1.3		1.2		
Indication (%)		0		0	<0.01
Stable CAD	44.5		17.1		
Unstable CAD/NSTEMI	26.3		49.6		
STEMI	15.1		26.0		
Other	14.0		7.3		
Extent of CAD (%)		1.5		1.2	<0.01
1 vessel	17.4		48.7		
2 vessel	35.1		25.9		
3 vessel	38.3		17.2		
Left main disease***	9.2		8.2		

CAD: coronary artery disease, CCS: Canadian cardiovascular society, CTO: chronic total occlusion, IQR: inter quartile range, MI: myocardial infarction, (N)STEMI: (non-)ST-elevation myocardial infarction, PCI: percutaneous coronary intervention.
* Cardiogenic shock only displayed for the indication STEMI.
**CCS class only displayed for the indication stable CAD.
*** Left main (LM) disease includes: LM+1 vessel, LM+2 vessel and LM+3 vessel.

rate in this study is based on all CTO procedures performed in our country rather than in a single hospital or smaller registries in other studies. The average success of 53% in SCAAR is unlikely to be representative for low- versus high-volume CTO centers [2,10]. Among the 30 hospitals reporting to SCAAR there are only a few high-volume centres with a dedicated CTO program and less than half of the CTO procedures in Sweden were performed at university hospitals. Some evidence suggest that procedural success is closely related to operator experience [13]. However, the recommendation that CTO procedures should be concentrated to dedicated high-volume hospitals needs stronger evidence.

Although CTO patients are common in clinical work, the evidence for the current guidelines and clinical practice is limited. The need for randomized clinical trials in this patient population is pressing; however, only a few such trials are initiated and on-going [12,14]. Until evidence from randomized trials becomes available we will need to identify and utilize the information available from

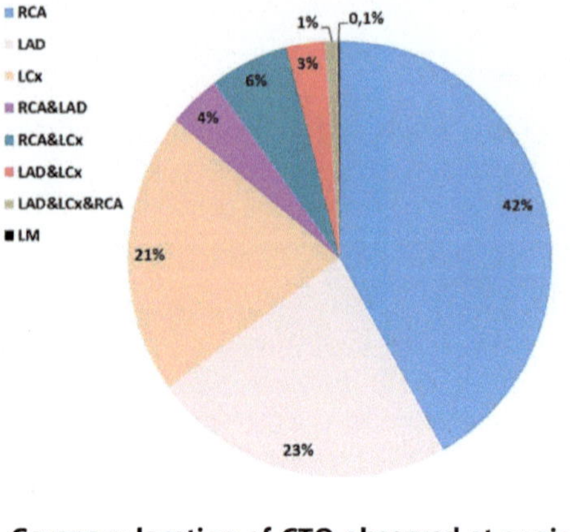

Figure 3. Coronary location of CTO observed at angiography. RCA = right coronary artery, LAD = left descending coronary artery, LCx = left circumflex coronary artery, LM = left main.

Table 3. Baseline characteristics of CTO patients from coronary segment subcohort according to the treatment strategy.

	No PCI of CTO (n = 8,182)		PCI of CTO (n = 3,251)		Referral for CABG (n = 3,172)		
	(%)	Missing (%)	(%)	Missing (%)	(%)	Missing (%)	P-value
Male gender	76.2	0	76.5	0	82.9	0	<0.01
Age (median, IQR)	69 (61–77)	0.2	66 (59–74)	0.2	68 (61–74)	0.2	<0.01
Diabetes	24.0	1.1	21.0	1.2	26.9	0.4	<0.01
Hypertension	61.6	3.0	59.8	2.3	65.2	1.5	<0.01
Hyperlipidemia	58.6	3.4	60.2	2.7	71.2	1.3	<0.01
Smoking status		7.0		5.0		3.6	<0.01
Current smoker	21.4		20.7		15.5		
Previous smoker	39.4		39.5		42.1		
Previous MI	41.3	4.1	33.4	3.5	29.4	3.2	<0.01
Previous PCI	19.9	0.1	20.3	0.2	8.3	0.03	<0.01
Cardiogenic Shock**	10.0	1.0	10.4	0.9	0	0	0.84
Creatinine Clearance (ml/min)	77 (57–101)	31.6	85 (65–109)	26.1	82 (64–102)	21.8	<0.01
CCS class*		7.1		4.6		7.8	<0.01
I	13.2		8.6		5.3		
II	55.2		56.3		49.8		
III	30.3		34.3		43.3		
IV	1.4		0.8		1.6		
Indication		0		0		0	<0.01
Stable CAD	33.1		41.3		77.4		
Unstable CAD/NSTEMI CAD/NSTEMI	31.1		39.8		0.4		
STEMI	21.7		13.5		0		
Other	14.2		5.5		22.2		
Extent of CAD (%)		1.2		1.3		1.3	<0.01
1 vessel	14.9		36.5		4.2		
2 vessel	40.9		39.6		15.8		
3 vessel	37.9		21.1		56.8		
Left main disease***	6.3		2.8		23.2		

CAD: coronary artery disease, CCS: Canadian cardiovascular society, CTO: chronic total occlusion, IQR: inter quartile range, MI: myocardial infarction, (N)STEMI: (non-)ST-elevation myocardial infarction, PCI: percutaneous coronary intervention.
* Cardiogenic shock only displayed for the indication STEMI.
**CCS class only displayed for the indication stable CAD.
*** Left main (LM) disease includes: LM+1 vessel, LM+2 vessel and LM+3 vessel.
Data about initial treatment strategy were missing in four CTO patients.

contemporary databases and quality registries. The SCAAR registry with its distinctive structure covering the whole Swedish nation provides unique possibility to study several important features of CTO's including epidemiology, patients characteristic as well as health outcomes. It contains information about both past and current treatment strategies of these complex patients not only from specialized centers, but also from all hospitals that preforms PCI. Given these circumstances, the SCAAR registry can be an important instrument to address many key questions in CTO.

The prevalence of CTO in Sweden decreased by one quarter during the study period. We hypothesize that this primarily reflects the increasing rate of timely revascularisation with PCI of patients with acute coronary syndrome – STEMI and non-STEMI. Because the prevalence decreased by 25% while the number of procedures remained unchanged, the proportion of CTO procedures increased by the same percentage. Besides the decreased prevalence, the relatively low annual rate of CTO procedures in Sweden may be related to improved treatment of symptoms, better quality of life, fear of complications, technical complexity, and low evidence-level.

There are some important limitations that need to be addressed. First, this is an observational study and as such it provides only associative evidence, not causative. Second, we cannot rule out the possibility of selection bias, as only hospitalized patients are included in the registry. Substantial proportion of missing data in the coronary segment subcohort may have resulted in biased estimate on CTO prevalence. Third, patients with missing data tend to have higher risk and their exclusion from the analysis might have produced biased results. Fourth, we cannot exclude the possibility that some occlusions had duration of less than three months, however the validation of CTO diagnosis and procedures in SCAAR have shown that only 3.8% were erroneously classified.

Conclusions

SCAAR is the largest database of CTO patients to date. CTO is a frequent finding in Swedish population and is diagnosed in every 10th patient undergoing coronary angiography. The prevalence of CTO has decreased by one quarter. Patients with a CTO represent a high risk subgroup of CAD patients. SCAAR may be a valuable source of data in the process of evidence-building in the CTO field.

Acknowledgments

We would like to acknowledge Rosie Perkins for excellent support and scientific editing.

Author Contributions

Conceived and designed the experiments: TR EO LH JPSH CD DI JO OA UJ MA RJ SJ BL GO JH PA GM. Analyzed the data: TR EO LH JPSH CD DI JO OA UJ MA RJ SJ BL GO JH PA GM. Wrote the paper: TR EO LH JPSH CD DI JO OA UJ MA RJ SJ BL GO JH PA GM.

References

1. Grantham JA, Marso SP, Spertus J, House J, Holmes DR Jr, et al. (2009) Chronic total occlusion angioplasty in the United States. JACC Cardiovascular Interventions 2: 479–486.
2. Galassi AR, Tomasello SD, Reifart N, Werner GS, Sianos G, et al. (2011) In-hospital outcomes of percutaneous coronary intervention in patients with chronic total occlusion: insights from the ERCTO (European Registry of Chronic Total Occlusion) registry. EuroIntervention 7: 472–479.
3. Task Force on Myocardial Revascularization of the European Society of C, the European Association for Cardio-Thoracic S, European Association for Percutaneous Cardiovascular I, Kolh P, Wijns W, et al. (2010) Guidelines on myocardial revascularization. Eur J Cardiothorac Surg 38 Suppl: S1–S52.
4. Members WC, Levine GN, Bates ER, Blankenship JC, Bailey SR, et al. (2011) 2011 ACCF/AHA/SCAI Guideline for Percutaneous Coronary Intervention: A Report of the American College of Cardiology Foundation/American Heart Association Task Force on Practice Guidelines and the Society for Cardiovascular Angiography and Interventions. Circulation 124: e574–e651.
5. Christofferson RD, Lehmann KG, Martin GV, Every N, Caldwell JH, et al. (2005) Effect of chronic total coronary occlusion on treatment strategy. AmJCardiol 95: 1088–1091.
6. Fefer P, Knudtson ML, Cheema AN, Galbraith PD, Osherov AB, et al. (2012) Current perspectives on coronary chronic total occlusions: the Canadian Multicenter Chronic Total Occlusions Registry. JAmCollCardiol 59: 991–997.
7. Kahn JK (1993) Angiographic suitability for catheter revascularization of total coronary occlusions in patients from a community hospital setting. AmHeart J 126: 561–564.
8. Angeras O, Albertsson P, Karason K, Ramunddal T, Matejka G, et al. (2013) Evidence for obesity paradox in patients with acute coronary syndromes: a report from the Swedish Coronary Angiography and Angioplasty Registry. Eur Heart J 34: 345–353.
9. Prasad A, Rihal CS, Lennon RJ, Wiste HJ, Singh M, et al. (2007) Trends in outcomes after percutaneous coronary intervention for chronic total occlusions: a 25-year experience from the Mayo Clinic. J Am Coll Cardiol 49: 1611–1618.
10. Mehran R, Claessen BE, Godino C, Dangas GD, Obunai K, et al. (2011) Long-term outcome of percutaneous coronary intervention for chronic total occlusions. JACC Cardiovasc Interv 4: 952–961.
11. Fox KA, Goodman SG, Klein W, Brieger D, Steg PG, et al. (2002) Management of acute coronary syndromes. Variations in practice and outcome; findings from the Global Registry of Acute Coronary Events (GRACE). Eur Heart J 23: 1177–1189.
12. Joyal D, Afilalo J, Rinfret S (2010) Effectiveness of recanalization of chronic total occlusions: a systematic review and meta-analysis. Am Heart J 160: 179–187.
13. Thompson CA, Jayne JE, Robb JF, Friedman BJ, Kaplan AV, et al. (2009) Retrograde techniques and the impact of operator volume on percutaneous intervention for coronary chronic total occlusions an early US experience. JACC Cardiovasc Interv 2: 834–842.
14. van der Schaaf RJ, Claessen BE, Hoebers LP, Verouden NJ, Koolen JJ, et al. (2010) Rationale and design of EXPLORE: a randomized, prospective, multicenter trial investigating the impact of recanalization of a chronic total occlusion on left ventricular function in patients after primary percutaneous coronary intervention for acute ST-elevation myocardial infarction. Trials 11: 89.

21

Self-Navigation with Compressed Sensing for 2D Translational Motion Correction in Free-Breathing Coronary MRI

Gabriele Bonanno[1,2], Gilles Puy[3¤], Yves Wiaux[1,2,3,4,5], Ruud B. van Heeswijk[1,2], Davide Piccini[1,2,6], Matthias Stuber[1,2]*

1 Department of Radiology, University Hospital (CHUV) and University of Lausanne (UNIL), Lausanne, VD, Switzerland, **2** Center for Biomedical Imaging (CIBM), Lausanne, VD, Switzerland, **3** Institute of Electrical Engineering, École Polytechnique Fédérale de Lausanne (EPFL), Lausanne, VD, Switzerland, **4** Department of Radiology and Medical Informatics, University of Geneva (UniGE), Genève, GE, Switzerland, **5** Institute of Sensors, Signals & Systems, Heriot Watt University, Edinburgh, United Kingdom, **6** Advanced Clinical Imaging Technology, Siemens Healthcare IM BM PI, Lausanne, Switzerland

Abstract

Purpose: Respiratory motion correction remains a challenge in coronary magnetic resonance imaging (MRI) and current techniques, such as navigator gating, suffer from sub-optimal scan efficiency and ease-of-use. To overcome these limitations, an image-based self-navigation technique is proposed that uses "sub-images" and compressed sensing (CS) to obtain translational motion correction in 2D. The method was preliminarily implemented as a 2D technique and tested for feasibility for targeted coronary imaging.

Methods: During a 2D segmented radial k-space data acquisition, heavily undersampled sub-images were reconstructed from the readouts collected during each cardiac cycle. These sub-images may then be used for respiratory self-navigation. Alternatively, a CS reconstruction may be used to create these sub-images, so as to partially compensate for the heavy undersampling. Both approaches were quantitatively assessed using simulations and in vivo studies, and the resulting self-navigation strategies were then compared to conventional navigator gating.

Results: Sub-images reconstructed using CS showed a lower artifact level than sub-images reconstructed without CS. As a result, the final image quality was significantly better when using CS-assisted self-navigation as opposed to the non-CS approach. Moreover, while both self-navigation techniques led to a 69% scan time reduction (as compared to navigator gating), there was no significant difference in image quality between the CS-assisted self-navigation technique and conventional navigator gating, despite the significant decrease in scan time.

Conclusions: CS-assisted self-navigation using 2D translational motion correction demonstrated feasibility of producing coronary MRA data with image quality comparable to that obtained with conventional navigator gating, and does so without the use of additional acquisitions or motion modeling, while still allowing for 100% scan efficiency and an improved ease-of-use. In conclusion, compressed sensing may become a critical adjunct for 2D translational motion correction in free-breathing cardiac imaging with high spatial resolution. An expansion to modern 3D approaches is now warranted.

Editor: Xiaoming Yang, University of Washington School of Medicine, United States of America

Funding: This work is supported by the grant #320030_143923 of the Swiss National Science Foundation (www.snf.ch) and by the Centre d'Imagerie BioMédicale (CIBM) of the UNIL, UNIGE, HUG, CHUV, EPFL and the Leenaards and Jeantet Foundations. The funders had no role in study design, data collection and analysis, decision to publish, or preparation of the manuscript.

Competing Interests: The authors have read the journal's policy and have the following conflicts: D. Piccini is an employee of Siemens Healthcare.

* Email: matthias.stuber@chuv.ch

¤ Current address: INRIA, Centre Inria Rennes - Bretagne Atlantique, Rennes, France

Introduction

One of the major challenges in free-breathing coronary magnetic resonance imaging (MRI) is the compensation of respiratory motion. If uncorrected, respiratory motion leads to blurring or ghosting and results in decreased diagnostic value of the acquired images. To account for respiratory-induced motion, most commonly used strategies involve navigator (NAV) echoes obtained from the dome of the right hemi-diaphragm [1,2,3,4]. Nevertheless, navigator techniques suffer from several limitations, including limited scan efficiency and ease-of-use problems. Respiratory self-navigation (Self-Nav) has been proposed [5,6] as an alternative approach for respiratory motion compensation in coronary MRI. Using Self-Nav, respiratory motion parameters are extracted directly from the readouts used for imaging of the heart. These motion parameters are then used to correct for motion during image reconstruction, after scan completion. This allows for 100% scan efficiency and an improved ease-of-use, as laborious scout scanning and navigator placement are no longer required. One category of self-navigated approaches consists of methods that initially acquire a central k-space line in superior-inferior (SI) direction at the beginning of each data segment acquisition, followed by a 3D radial acquisition. From the SI projection, the position of the heart can be estimated and a one-dimensional respiratory motion correction [6,7,8] may be performed. With this approach, average scanning time of 3D radial coronary techniques decreased from ~16 min (for NAV) to ~6 min (for Self-Nav) [8]. However, similarly to the conventional NAV, the displacement of the heart in non-SI directions cannot easily be determined. Thus, to account for 2D respiratory displacement of the heart, image-based self-navigation techniques have been proposed. These 2D techniques make use of additional low-resolution Cartesian images to extract motion in multiple directions [9]. Alternatively, by using a 2D radial acquisition strategy, ghosting artifacts are no longer an issue for undersampled acquisitions and the very same projections used in the final image reconstruction may also be exploited to extract respiratory motion parameters. However, while two-dimensional motion information may be extracted from the radial k-space readouts that are acquired in each cardiac cycle, the limited amount of radial readouts per data segment provide a rather sparse representation in the Fourier domain with aliasing, or streaking, in the image domain. Therefore, simply extracting two-dimensional motion parameters from such radial data segments with the goal to augment self-navigation may not be straightforward [10,11,12]. Recently, compressed sensing (CS) has been widely studied to accelerate MR acquisitions [13,14,15,16]. CS theory shows that it is possible to accurately reconstruct sparse MR images from only a few number of k-space measurements. Images are then reconstructed from these measurements with the use of non-linear techniques. In dynamic cine cardiac MRI, CS has recently not only been applied to accelerate image acquisition but also to support motion compensation with Cartesian [17] and non-Cartesian trajectories [17,18,19]. Similarly, parallel imaging [20] and a combination of CS with parallel imaging [21,22] has been employed for respiratory motion compensation. In coronary MR angiography (MRA), CS has been used to assist final image reconstruction [23], to abbreviate scanning time for navigator gated [24] and multiple breath-hold [25] approaches, and, preliminarily, to support motion correction and final image reconstruction in a self-navigated 3D Cartesian trajectory [26]. In the present study, we hypothesized that image quality in self-navigated, volume targeted free-breathing radial coronary MRA can be improved by exploiting CS to extract accurate 2D respiratory motion parameters. Here, CS is used to reconstruct heavily undersampled images (henceforth referred to as sub-images) from the radial k-space readouts acquired during each cardiac cycle. To test this hypothesis, an image-based self-navigation technique that incorporates CS reconstruction, and allows for two-dimensional motion correction, was first implemented as a 2D imaging technique. It was then tested in healthy volunteers by acquiring images of, and then analyzing, the proximal segments of the right coronary artery. Specifically, for testing the feasibility of such an approach, targeted free-breathing in vivo coronary MRA scans were acquired with an interleaved 2D radial sampling scheme where undersampled sub-images were reconstructed either with or without CS from each data segment (interleave). In these sub-images, in-plane translational motion parameters were extracted for each cardiac cycle and motion correction was then performed in k-space for each individual sub-image. All motion corrected sub-images were then combined to create the final coronary MRA dataset. The image quality from both the CS-assisted and the non-CS assisted self-navigation techniques was quantitatively assessed and compared to that from conventional navigator gating.

Methods

Upon written request to the authors, the data used and produced in this study can be made available under the condition that local Ethics Committee approval to share said data is obtained. Some of the algorithms utilized are already available in the public domain, which is clearly indicated below.

Self-navigation incorporating compressed sensing

In the proposed image-based self-navigation method, sub-images are generated using CS reconstruction to suppress artifacts due to undersampling. Motion is measured by co-registering all sub-images to a reference sub-image. In the present implementation, only in-plane translational displacement is corrected. A diagram that illustrates the pipeline of the technique is shown in Fig. 1. An interleaved 2D radial acquisition strategy is used for imaging, since aliasing in undersampled radial sub-images leads to incoherent noise-like artifacts that may be reduced with a non-linear iterative reconstruction [15].

Sub-image reconstruction. To estimate the respiratory motion parameters of the heart with self-navigation, undersampled sub-images were reconstructed from each interleave (resulting in 2.89% of Nyquist equivalent undersampling) with a) a non-linear reconstruction algorithm (Self-Nav CS method) based on a Total Variation prior [27] and with b) a conventional linear reconstruction (Self-Nav LN method) that consisted of density compensation and convolution-based gridding [28] of the radial profiles and fast Fourier transform (FFT) for comparison purposes. Because of the undersampling, the reconstruction becomes an ill-posed inverse problem and, for the Self-Nav CS method, the image is estimated through a non-linear iterative process in order to find the best match with the given data by minimizing the following functional:

$$\arg\min_{x} \frac{1}{2}\|Fx-y\|_2^2+\lambda R_{TV}(x), \tag{1}$$

On the right hand side of Eq. 1, the first functional is a squared L_2-norm of the residual between the measured noisy data $\boldsymbol{y}$ and $\boldsymbol{Fx}$. The matrix $\boldsymbol{F}$ models the acquisition and denotes the subsampled Fourier operator, implemented using the non-uniform FFT [29,30,31], that computes the k-space coefficients of the estimated image $\boldsymbol{x}$. The second term $R_{TV}(\boldsymbol{x})$ is a prior term used to regularize the ill-posed inverse problem. Its effect is weighted by $\lambda>0$, which was experimentally found to be optimal at 10^{-5}. In this coronary imaging scenario, the following Total Variation prior was chosen to search for an image estimate with sparse gradient:

$$R_{TV}(x)=\sum_{i}\sqrt{|D_x(x_i)|^2+|D_y(x_i)|^2}, \tag{2}$$

where D_x and D_y represent the spatial derivatives of the image $\boldsymbol{x}$ at pixel $\boldsymbol{i}$, computed as the finite difference between neighboring pixels in x and y direction respectively. The underlying idea is that by minimizing the derivatives, regions with homogenous and constant intensities are recovered and streaking artifacts and noise are removed. The magnitude of the derivatives was used in order to preserve the edges on the image and to simultaneously help suppress Gibbs ringing artifacts and noise, as suggested by Block et

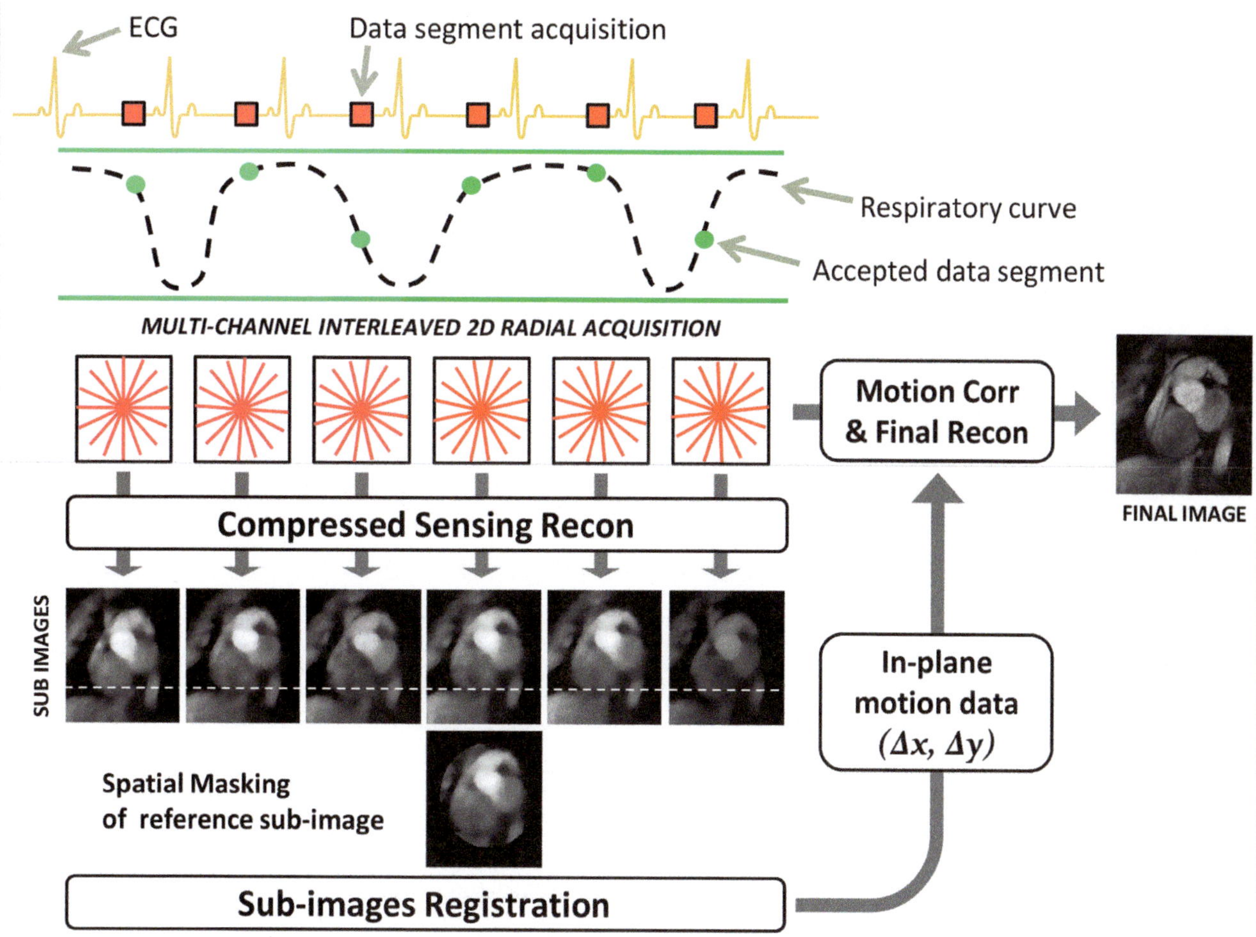

Figure 1. Schematic of the self-navigation method using compressed sensing (Self-Nav CS). An interleaved two-dimensional radial acquisition is performed with ECG triggering and during free-breathing. Undersampled sub-images are reconstructed from k-space data acquired during each heart-beat (interleaved red stars) using a compressed sensing algorithm based on a Total Variation prior. Motion detection is performed by registering all the sub-images to extract in-plane translation data. A binary mask is generated by the user on the reference sub-image and is used for the similarity measure computation during registration. Motion parameters are then extracted as displacements in two dimensions (Δx, Δy) and used to correct k-space data on a beat-to-beat basis prior to conventional, final image reconstruction.

al. [15]. The problem in Eq. 1 was solved using the method described by Beck et al. [32,33].

Motion detection. Each of the sub-images obtained with the Self-Nav CS and Self-Nav LN methods, as described above, represents the heart at the position in the respiratory cycle during which the corresponding interleave was acquired. Once all sub-images were acquired, they were co-registered to extract in-plane motion parameters of each interleave. The image registration framework was developed with the open source toolkit ITK ("The Insight Segmentation and Registration Toolkit" [34]), as an iterative process where a sub-image is modified iteratively by a given transform to match a randomly chosen reference sub-image. A rigid translation transformation was used to obtain relative in-plane displacements (Δx, Δy) that were subsequently used for motion correction. For each iteration, the transformed sub-image was linearly interpolated onto a Cartesian grid and compared with its reference counterpart by computing the mean square error. This similarity measure represents the cost function of the iterative process, which used a gradient descent optimizer to search for a local minimum in the transform space (corresponding to the smallest difference between the two sub-images).

For an accurate image registration, a binary ROI mask with an ellipsoidal shape was applied onto the heart and used for the computation of the similarity measure only. The ROI was manually selected in order to encompass the heart only and the mask assumed values of 1 inside the ROI while 0 elsewhere. This was implemented to avoid errors in the displacement calculation step caused by both static tissues (e. g. posterior chest wall, spinal cord), and tissues that move asynchronously with the sought cardiac motion (e. g. anterior chest wall, liver).

Motion correction. The estimated motion parameters of each sub-image were then used to correct the radial readouts in k-space. According to the Fourier shift theorem, a radial profile in k-space can be corrected for a rigid displacement by means of a linear phase modulation $\Delta\beta$ (Eq. 3):

$$\Delta\beta(k) = 2\pi\frac{k}{N}(\Delta x\cos\theta + \Delta y\sin\theta), \qquad (3)$$

where the pair (Δx, Δy) denotes the in-plane displacements that are projected onto the radial line with the azimuthal angle θ. N is the total number of data points sampled during signal-readout and k refers to the index of the sampling point along the readout line. Subsequently, all corrected subsets of k-space data were combined and an image was reconstructed with the conventional linear method (gridding [28] followed by FFT) for each channel individually. The final magnitude image was obtained as the square root of the sum-of-squares of all channel images.

MR experiments – simulations

As a first validation step, in order to investigate the performance of the proposed reconstruction algorithm, volume-targeted electrocardiogram (ECG) triggered *breath-hold* images (see protocol parameters below) of the right coronary artery (RCA) were acquired in vivo in one healthy adult subject. Breath-holding was used to obtain a dataset that is free of respiratory motion [35]. Then, to quantitatively ascertain the accuracy of the sub-image reconstruction strategies used for self-navigation, the interleaved k-space data were artificially corrupted with known in-plane displacement values that were extracted from one of the free-breathing volunteer scans (see below). These in-plane displacement values were within a range of 0 to 7 mm. The corrupted image was then retrospectively corrected with the proposed self-navigation method with both linear and non-linear reconstructions. The motion detection error relative to the known respiratory displacement values (ground truth) was then evaluated for both reconstruction methods. Specifically, the Euclidean distance between the ground truth displacements and those obtained from the Self-Nav LN and Self-Nav CS methods were computed.

MR experiments – volunteer study

In vivo experiments were performed in 12 healthy adult volunteers (3 women, 26.9±5.1 years) on a 3T clinical scanner (MAGNETOM Trio, Siemens AG, Healthcare Sector, Erlangen, Germany) with a 32-channel cardiac radiofrequency (RF) coil (Invivo, Gainesville, FL). All in vivo MR acquisitions were approved by the Institutional Review Board of the University Hospital of Lausanne (CHUV, Lausanne, Switzerland), and written informed consent was obtained from all study subjects. All clinical investigations were conducted according to the principles expressed in the Declaration of Helsinki. After survey imaging, three 2D ECG gated cine-scans with axial slice orientation were acquired at the base, mid-ventricular level and the apex of the heart. These cine images were used to visually identify the onset of the minimal coronary motion period (= trigger delay) that was then used for the subsequent targeted coronary MRA acquisition. Using the cine frames acquired at the trigger delay time and from all 3 anatomical levels, the RCA was visually identified and the double-oblique plane of the RCA was defined as previously reported [36]. ECG-triggered images of the RCA were then acquired using either navigator gating (NAV, 4 mm gating window, no slice tracking) or free breathing without NAV. The coronary MRA imaging sequence consisted of an interleaved 2D radial gradient-echo acquisition with T_2-preparation, fat saturation, and the following sequence parameters: 360 radial projections in k-space, 320 samples per projection, 24 interleaves, 15 projections per interleave, 320×320 matrix, 320×320 mm field-of-view (FoV), 1×1×8 mm spatial resolution, repetition time (TR) =8.9 ms, echo time (TE) =4.2 ms, TE_{T2prep} = 50 ms, RF excitation angle $\alpha = 15^{\circ}$, receiver bandwidth = 200 Hz/pixel. Reconstruction of all NAV and free-breathing images was performed off-line, on a stand-alone PC in MATLAB (Mathworks, Natick, MA), with C and C++ subroutines called for gridding and ITK registration. Free-breathing images were reconstructed both without any motion compensation as a post processing step (No Resp Gating) and with the reconstructions used by the Self-Nav LN and Self-Nav CS methods. During these Self-Nav data acquisitions, the navigator signal from the dome of the right hemi-diaphragm was still recorded, but was not actually used for gating or tracking.

Data analysis. For each subject, four different targeted images of the RCA were available for analysis (No Resp Gating, Self-Nav LN, Self-Nav CS, NAV). Since there is no ground-truth for the measurement of respiratory-induced heart motion, the four imaging strategies were compared for acquisition time, scan efficiency and image quality. Quantitative image quality assessment was performed with the Soap-Bubble software [37]. The SNR of the blood pool and the blood pool-to-myocardium contrast to noise ratio (CNR) were computed according to the formulas:

$$SNR = \frac{S_{aorta}}{\sigma_{noise}}, \; CNR = \frac{S_{aorta} - S_{myo}}{\sigma_{noise}}, \tag{4}$$

where S_{aorta} and S_{myo} represent the mean signal value of a region of interest (ROI) manually traced inside the aorta and the myocardium of the left ventricle respectively, while σ_{noise} is the standard deviation of the signal measured in an ROI outside the thorax. In all images, the average vessel diameter and the percent vessel sharpness (%VS) were computed for the proximal 2 cm of the RCA.

For further validation of the proposed techniques, the SI components of the in-plane displacements of the Self-Nav LN and Self-Nav CS methods were compared to the displacements measured by the diaphragmatic navigator for each subject. In particular, to obtain these self-navigated SI components, first the in-plane displacements were expressed as a function of the patient coordinate system after multiplication by the inverse of the slice rotation matrix. The projection of the thus-obtained absolute displacements onto the z-axis was then considered as the SI component.

Statistical analysis

For the in vivo simulations, the motion detection error with respect to the known displacement values was obtained with both the Self-Nav LN and Self-Nav CS methods, for each of the 24 simulated interleaves. A paired two-tailed Student's t-test was used to compare two methods, with $P<0.05$ considered statistically significant.

For the volunteer study, acquisition time, scan efficiency and image quality parameters (SNR, CNR, lumen diameter and %VS) of each acquisition strategy were measured and compared. A paired two-tailed Student's t-test was used, with $P\leq 0.008$ considered statistically significant after Bonferroni correction for multiple comparisons. The correlation coefficient (CC) was then computed between the SI displacements detected by the Self-Nav methods and NAV, as a measure of synchronicity between the motion detected at the level of the heart by self-navigation and the motion of the diaphragm [38]. Hence, high CC values indicate that the motion detected by self-navigation is correlated with the respiratory cycle. Linear regression analysis was also performed to compute the regression coefficients. This measure relates to a subject-specific correction factor between respiration-induced cardiac and diaphragmatic motion. Statistical comparisons were then made using a paired two-tailed Student's t-test with $P<0.05$ considered statistically significant.

Results

Sub-image reconstruction

In Fig. 2, a fully sampled image (360 acquired radial profiles) from a NAV acquisition (Fig. 2-a) is shown as a reference adjacent to two sub-image reconstructions shown in Fig. 2-b and Fig. 2-c. Both of these images were reconstructed using one interleave consisting of 15 radial profiles. The sub-image in Fig. 2-b was reconstructed with the conventional Self-Nav LN method and streaking artifacts, noise, and regional signal loss are clearly visible at the level of the heart. However, when the same k-space data were reconstructed with the Self-Nav CS method (Fig. 2-c), streaking artifacts and noise appear reduced and smoothed out at the level of the heart, while the signal appears increased and the anatomy better defined when compared to the conventional reconstruction.

MR experiments – simulations

As expected, the breath-held targeted acquisition displayed in Fig 3-a does not present streaking or blurring and the RCA appears well depicted (arrows). After artificial motion corruption of the same k-space data, the reconstructed image appears blurred (Fig. 3-b) and segments of the RCA can no longer be identified. In the images reconstructed with either self-navigation technique, the coronary becomes visible again and improved quality can be appreciated. With linear reconstruction of the sub-images, much of the blurring is suppressed and the anatomy is partially restored when compared to the motion corrupted image in Fig 3-b. However, streaking artifacts originating from the surrounding structures can still be identified at the level of the mid RCA, and residual blurring at the borders of the left ventricle (LV) can be identified (Fig. 3-c). When using non-linear CS reconstruction of the sub-images, streaking artifacts are reduced and the borders of the RCA and the LV visually appear more clearly defined (Fig. 3-d). Consistent with these findings, the average error of the motion detection among all 24 sub-images was 0.38 ± 0.29 mm when using non-linear reconstruction and 1.58 ± 1.11 mm with linear reconstruction ($P<0.001$). Expressed as relative average error (divided by the displacement), this was $16.9 \pm 16.7\%$ and $76.3 \pm 97.6\%$ respectively ($P<0.003$).

MR experiments – volunteer study

When the acquisition was performed without respiratory gating or motion correction, the anatomy in the reconstructed images appeared blurred as shown in Fig. 4-a. The same data can be corrected for respiratory motion using the proposed self-navigation method with linear reconstruction of the sub-images. As expected, this leads to an overall sharper image where the anatomy is restored (Fig. 4-b). When using non-linear reconstruction of the sub-images, however, a further improvement in the visual delineation of the RCAs is obtained (Fig. 4-c) and the image quality approaches that of the navigator-gated images (Fig. 4-d). Consistent with these findings, the proposed Self-Nav CS method led to significantly improved vessel sharpness ($36.2 \pm 10.7\%$) as compared to the No Resp Gating acquisition ($27.9 \pm 10.4\%$, $P=0.0027$) and to the Self-Nav LN approach ($33.3 \pm 10.2\%$, $P=0.005$). Superior vessel sharpness ($38.54 \pm 10.6\%$) was still obtained with the NAV acquisition. However, this did not reach statistical significance when compared to Self-Nav CS ($P=0.22$, Table 1). Simultaneously, no statistically significant difference in SNR, CNR or average vessel diameter was found among the images obtained with the three motion compensation strategies and the corrupted data. Acquisition time, scan efficiency and image quality parameters are reported in Table 1 for both gated and non-gated techniques. Relative to the duration of the NAV acquisition, the scan efficiency increased 2.8 times by using the proposed Self-Nav techniques, which led to an acquisition time reduction of 69% ($P<0.001$).

When comparing the respiratory displacement regression measurements between the navigator and self-navigation, the average CC value was higher for Self-Nav CS than for Self-Nav LN (0.97 ± 0.01 vs 0.93 ± 0.07 respectively, $P=0.04$). Accordingly, linear regression plots of SI shifts from all subjects show a narrower distribution of data points around the regression line when using Self-Nav CS (Fig. 5-a) and when compared to Self-Nav LN (Fig. 5-b). As a representative example, SI motion measured in a healthy adult subject with both Self-Nav CS and NAV shows high synchronicity in Fig.5-c. Averaged over all subjects, the subject-specific correction factor that relates respiration induced diaphragmatic and heart displacement was 0.36 ± 0.14 for Self-Nav LN and 0.37 ± 0.13 for Self-Nav CS, with the amplitude of respiratory displacement measured at the level of the heart being

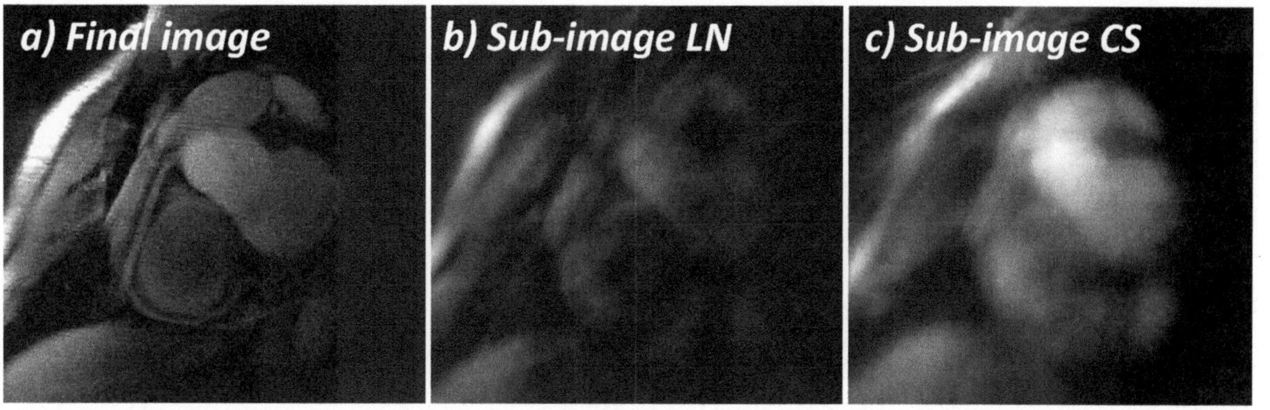

Figure 2. Reconstruction of in vivo sub-images. a) Representative targeted RCA from a conventional NAV acquisition. b) Sub-image obtained in the same subject from one interleave (15 radial spokes out of a total of 360) reconstructed with the linear approach (gridding followed by FFT). c) Sub-image obtained from the same interleave as in (b), however, reconstructed with the compressed sensing method based on Total-Variation.

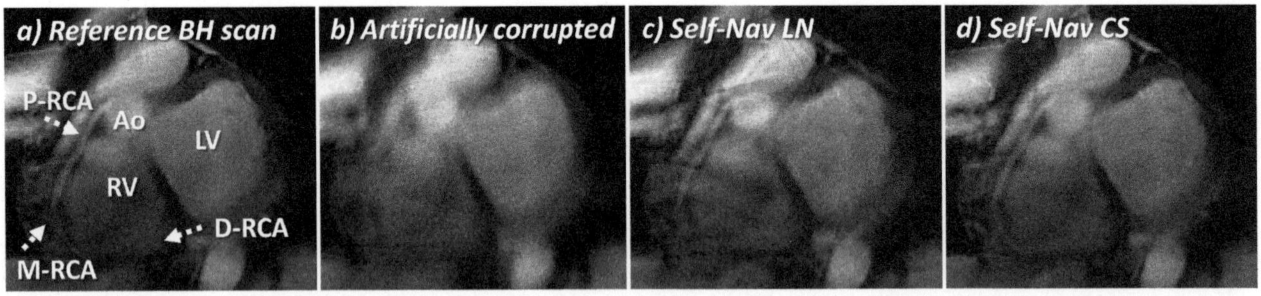

Figure 3. In vivo motion correction simulation. On the targeted acquisition of the right coronary artery (RCA), the following anatomical structures are visible: left ventricle (LV), right ventricle (RV), aorta (Ao), proximal (P), mid (M) and distal (D) segments of the RCA (dotted arrows). To test the performance of the self-navigation (Self-Nav) techniques, an RCA image was acquired during a breath-hold (BH) and serves as the reference standard of optimal respiratory motion suppression (a). In vivo respiratory displacement parameters were extracted at the level of a heart from a free-breathing acquisition in a healthy volunteer. These data were then used to corrupt each interleave of the standard of reference BH data simulating respiratory motion (b). These artificially corrupted data were then retrospectively corrected with the Self-Nav techniques using linear (c) and compressed sensing (CS) (d) reconstruction of the sub-images. While much of the blurring is suppressed with the Self-Nav LN method (c), residual streaking artifacts remain visible. Improved image quality and anatomy depiction were instead obtained with the Self-Nav CS method (d). This also provided more accurate motion detection, as evidenced by a 76% decrease of the error between the estimated displacements and the ground truth.

smaller than that measured at the level of the right hemi diaphragm.

Discussion

A novel image-based self-navigation approach was developed for coronary MRI and preliminarily tested for feasibility with a 2D acquisition sequence. The method takes advantage of compressed sensing for improved 2D translation respiratory motion correction. While CS has primarily been exploited for reducing scanning time by undersampling and, in some applications, to simultaneously support motion compensation, in the proposed self-navigation approach, the final image is fully sampled and reconstructed with conventional linear methods and CS is solely used to reduce streaking artifacts on the aliased sub-images that are used for improved motion estimation. These sub-images are intrinsically undersampled since they are extrapolated from the individual interleaves that are a sub-set of the fully sampled acquisition. Simultaneously, in comparison to a recently described image-based navigator approach [9], no additional image acquisition is required and, as such, temporal delays no longer occur between the extraction of motion information and the actual imaging.

Several implementations that combine CS and motion estimation/correction for the purpose of enhancing reconstruction have recently been proposed for dynamic cardiac MRI [17,18]. In coronary MRI, Akçakaya et al. [23] achieved 6-fold accelerated scanning time without significant change in image quality for targeted 3D Cartesian acquisitions. In a first attempt to support motion correction, Moghari et al. [24] proposed a combined scheme where NAV-rejected data were not reacquired to create variable density sampling for the final CS reconstruction, thus achieving gating efficiency as high of ~80%. Recently, Prieto et al. [39] extracted undersampled sub-images from a 3D golden-step Cartesian acquisition with an iterative SENSE algorithm [40] to resolve and correct for respiratory motion. While the information from a diaphragmatic navigator was employed to populate the 3D sub-images, average acquisition times were in the order of ~9 min.

All these studies proposed cardiac MRI techniques that exploit iterative methods to reconstruct the final images from 3D undersampled data with increased image quality, while simultaneously correcting for motion. In this contribution, we propose a modified version of a known image-based self-navigation approach [11], which incorporates non-linear reconstruction [32] to improve accuracy of motion detection and still uses linear algorithms to reconstruct a final image of the coronaries. The performance of this method as part of a 2D radial self-navigation technique was then investigated. In particular, the above-mentioned accuracy of beat-to-beat respiratory motion measurements and final image quality were measured. As a surrogate for

Table 1. In vivo results: quantitative analyses.

	No Resp Gating	*Self-Nav LN*	*Self-Nav CS*	*NAV*
SNR [-]	40.78±5.85	40.04±6.97	40.16±6.77	40.63±10.02
CNR [-]	26.11±4.38	25.02±6.97	25.98±5.62	27.48±5.47
Average Diameter [mm]	3.02±0.54	2.85±0.35	2.90±0.40	2.81±0.37
Vessel Sharpness [%]	27.86±10.38†	33.34±10.25†	36.20±10.66	38.54±10.59
Acquisition Time [s]	22.77±2.72	22.77±2.72	22.77±2.72	73.58±33.57†
Scan efficiency [%]	100±0	100±0	100±0	35.60±10.55†

Mean values ± one standard deviation from 12 healthy adult subjects are shown.
†indicates a significant difference when compared to the proposed Self-Nav CS technique, (Student's t-test with Bonferroni correction for multiple comparisons, $P< 0.008$). SNR = signal-to-noise ratio of the blood pool; CNR = contrast-to-noise ratio between blood pool and myocardium.

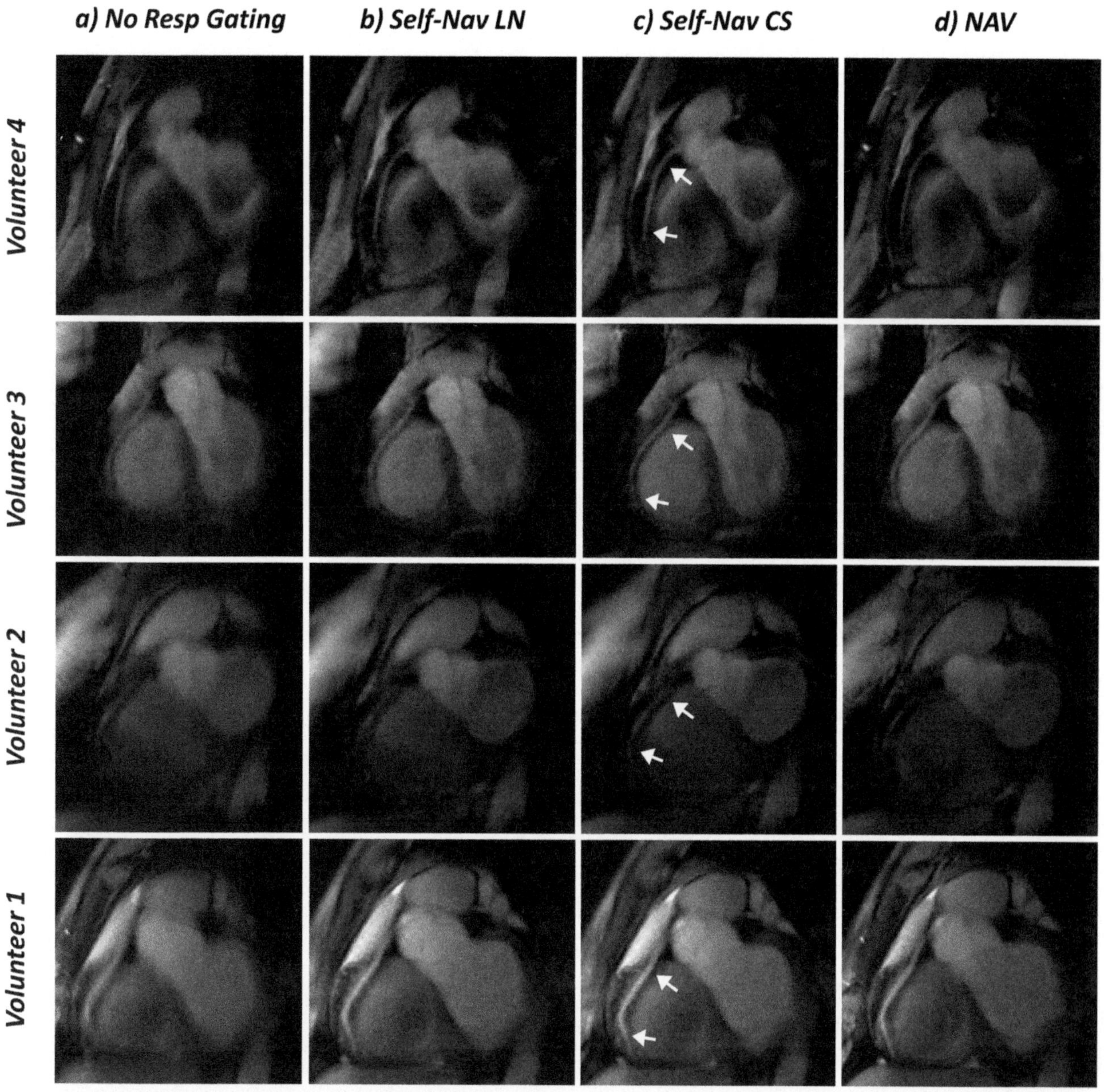

Figure 4. In vivo results from four healthy volunteers. a) Respiratory motion corrupted images from targeted acquisitions of the right coronary artery (RCA) without any respiratory gating. The images appear blurred and the RCAs not well depicted. When the same image data are retrospectively motion compensated using self-navigation with linear reconstruction (Self-Nav LN) of the sub-images (b), motion artifacts are suppressed and the anatomy is restored in the image with improved visibility of the RCA. c) Self-navigation with non linear reconstruction of the sub-images (Self-Nav CS) provides an improved image quality with better coronary delineation (arrows) when compared to the images obtained with the No Resp Gating and Self-Nav LN methods. The overall image quality approaches that of the standard of reference NAV acquisition in (d), albeit with a 2.8-fold reduction in scanning time.

image quality, vessel definition or vessel sharpness was quantified as previously reported [23,39,41,42,43].

As a result, this study showed that in respiratory motion simulation, based on in vivo data, CS was been shown to reduce the motion detection error of self-navigation by 76%, when compared to a purely linear reconstruction of the sub-images. This may be due to the fact that the abrupt intensity variations of the streaking artifacts that are generated due to undersampling may impair the search for the best image match during sub-image registration. In line with what was hypothesized, the use of CS reduces these artifacts and may therefore provide for a better sub-image "match", resulting in more accurate motion detection. With the non-linear reconstruction, the error range is constrained to half of the pixel size or even lower. Accordingly, a higher image quality was found for Self-Nav CS when compared to Self-Nav LN. However, in the above-described CS framework only first order derivatives of the sub-images were used to exploit sparsity. While a sufficient image quality was achieved for the estimation of motion parameters, the reconstruction of the sub-images may still appear "patchy" because of the high degree of undersampling (4% of the full dataset). To minimize this effect, it might be useful to investigate a recently proposed CS technique that uses a weighted

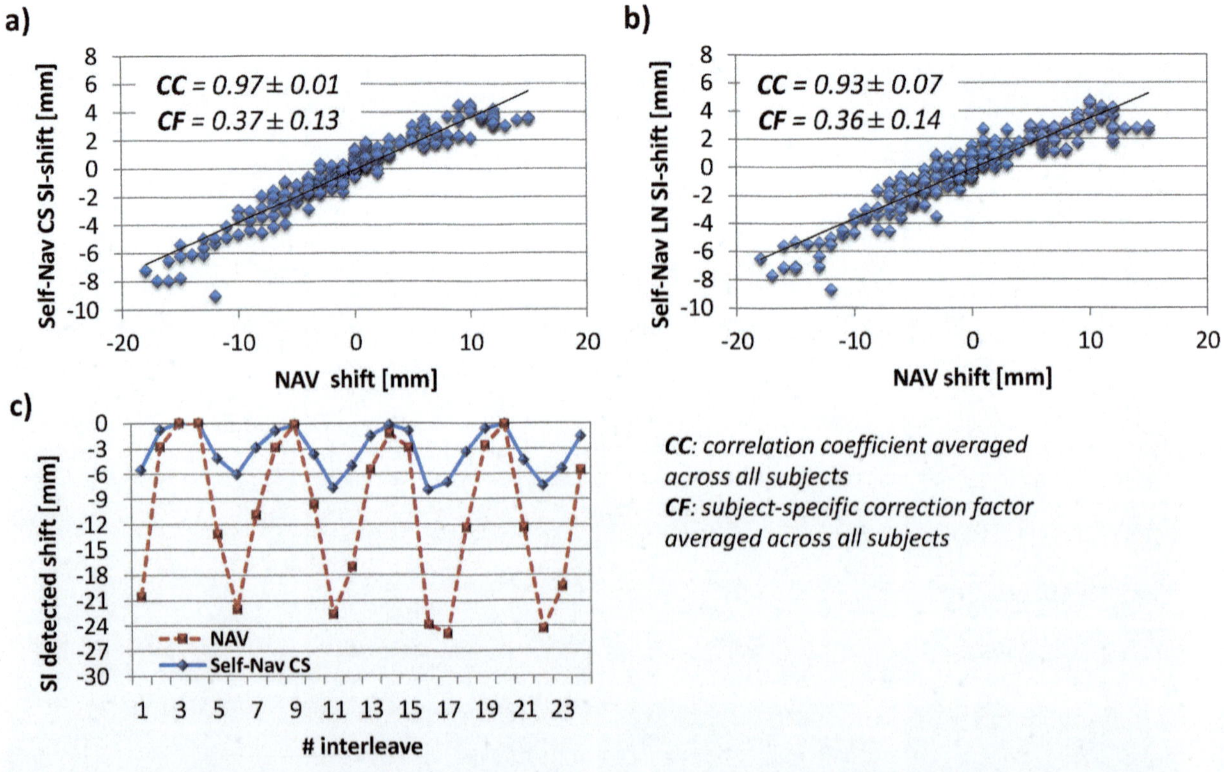

Figure 5. Detected motion in SI direction. Linear regression plot of the SI shifts detected in all subjects show a good correlation between NAV and Self-Nav methods: average correlation coefficient (CC) for Self-Nav CS (a) was significantly higher than that from Self-Nav LN (b) (0.97±0.01 vs 0.93±0.07, P=0.04), indicating higher synchronicity between Self-Nav CS and NAV. Average subject-specific correction factor (CF) between diaphragmatic and respiratory-induced motion were 0.37±0.13 and 0.36±0.14 for Self-Nav CS (a) and Self-Nav LN (b), respectively. An example of the SI-component of the in-plane displacement detected with the Self-Nav CS technique (solid blue line) together with the signal detected by the diaphragmatic navigator (NAV – red dashed line) is shown in (c). In this healthy subject, the motion detected with the proposed method and the reference standard NAV show strong synchronicity, also confirmed by CC=0.98.

average of different wavelet transforms as regularization prior in order to achieve higher levels of sparsity and improved reconstruction as a result [44]. In addition, a method that takes coil sensitivities into account, as presented before [15], may also lead to a further improvements for non-linear reconstruction of the sub-images. In vivo MR experiments in 12 healthy adult volunteers suggest that the use of CS for motion detection significantly improves vessel sharpness relative to motion corrupted images and, albeit to a lesser extent, also relative to Self-Nav LN. When comparing Self-Nav CS to the reference standard NAV, acquisition time was reduced by 69% and scan efficiency increased 2.8 times, while vessel sharpness was not significantly different than in images obtained with NAV. One might expect that an image-based Self-Nav correction would be superior to any conventional NAV correction, since the respiratory-induced motion is detected in multiple dimensions and directly at the level of the heart. However, in our study, NAV vessel sharpness was still found to be superior - a result consistent with the findings of Henningsson et al. [9]. This can be attributed to the fact that both linear and non-linear Self-Nav correct for the whole range of respiratory induced cardiac displacement, while this range was significantly constrained using NAV with a gating window of 4 mm only. As a result, Self-Nav acquisitions may also be subject to trough-plane motion, whereas the narrow range of NAV acceptance may automatically prevent such displacements from adversely affecting image quality. Some combination of the two - such as using NAV to discard data from extreme respiratory positions and reconstructing the rest with Self-Nav - may prove superior. This combined approach may also be a solution for compensation of irregular respiration, which was not tested in this study. In fact, irregular breathing is expected to be characterized by a non-periodic pattern and extreme respiratory positions: while the former is taken into account by the beat-to-beat motion detection, the latter may lead to adverse effects related to amplified through-plane motion and non-rigid deformation.

Despite the substantial gain in acquisition time using self-navigation, SNR and CNR did not show significant differences among the investigated acquisition- and reconstruction strategies. In the NAV acquisitions the increase in acquisition time is not linked with an increase in SNR since many of the acquired data segments do not contribute to the final image. However, with the proposed approach this inefficiency can be avoided, while scanning time is significantly reduced. Simultaneously, image quality was shown to be comparable to that obtained with the conventional NAV acquisitions, which may be attributable to the documented and improved accuracy of the CS-assisted motion detection.

The spatial masking of the reference sub-image employed in the image registration process was used to facilitate the motion estimation task. This method ensures that the alignment is obtained at the level of the heart, minimizing adverse effects originating from signal of surrounding anatomical structures. In the current implementation, the masking is performed manually during offline reconstruction. While this allows a precise placement and adjustment of the ellipsoidal ROI around the heart only, it remains operator–dependent and may adversely affect the robustness of the method. Moreover, manual ROI placement represents a limitation for inline processing in a clinical workflow. Nevertheless, a template- and atlas based segmentation of the heart might be used as an automatic manner to define an ROI of the heart [45].

However, regardless of the accuracy of motion detection, static structures can adversely affect the quality of the final corrected image. Since the motion-correction is performed in k-space, this results in translation of the entire image. Therefore, static structures are also shifted by the same amount leading to blurring and streaking artifacts. Selective radiofrequency excitations [46] might reduce this effect and, simultaneously, improve the motion detection by only exciting the targeted moving structures. Alternatively, a region-specific image registration of the sub-images might be used to correct locally for motion, such that static structures that surround the heart undergo minimal correction and, consequently, will produce much less streaking artifacts on the heart. Methods using local-affine [47] or non-rigid [48] transformation have been adopted for this purpose and remain to be investigated. The high correlation between the SI-component of the respiratory-induced motion of the heart as detected by Self-Nav CS and the diaphragmatic navigator suggests high synchronicity between these two measurements. Simultaneously, we found an average correction factor between respiratory-induced cardiac and diaphragmatic motion of 0.37 for Self-Nav CS and 0.36 for Self-Nav LN. While this corroborates the findings by Nagel et al. [49], where a correction factor of 30% yielded improved image quality for the proximal coronary arteries, it also suggests that the respiratory displacement of the heart is attenuated when compared to that of the diaphragm. This is also consistent with other reports [38,42]. Just as a 2D extension of self-navigation provides a theoretical improvement over a traditional one-dimensional navigation, a 3D correction may ultimately prove best, as it should better account for the three-dimensional nature of the respiratory-induced motion of the heart. This remains to be investigated, though. Wang et al. [38] have demonstrated that the SI displacement is much more significant than that in the anterior-posterior or left-right direction. Still, the slice orientation for targeted imaging of the RCA is double-oblique with the imaging plane being oriented predominantly in the foot-head direction. This slice orientation, in combination with an 8 mm slice thickness, encompasses most of the respiratory-induced motion of the heart in-plane, but through-plane motion remains unaccounted for in our current implementation. Together with the relatively large range of correction, this may contribute to an image quality that still does not surpass that of the conventional NAV technique, given that the latter accepts only a small range of respiratory motion, minimizing the effects of through-plane displacement.

One of the major limitations of our technique includes the need of the imaging plane to be in parallel with the principal direction of respiratory motion. Therefore, the utility of the proposed approach for RCA imaging was investigated as a first step. However, off-sagittal or off-coronal image plane orientations still fulfill this requirement and may enable the motion compensated acquisition of LAD and LCX as well, but this remains to be studied. Nevertheless, out of plane motion may lead to partial coverage of a coronary artery, which, in turn, may appear as a regional narrowing and a false positive result. While false positives may be preferred over false negatives, this still is a limitation, which mandates appropriate planning of both slice orientation and thickness, and which makes the approach more operator dependent. This limitation can be avoided by increasing the volumetric coverage. Therefore, an extension of this CS technique with a 3D radial imaging sequence is currently planned. Alternatively, multiple 2D image navigators may be exploited as recently reported [41] but the time delay between navigator and imaging still needs to be considered [50] as the respiratory displacement parameters are not directly extracted from the imaging data themselves. Nevertheless, while this study represents a proof of concept of this methodology, it allowed testing the motion detection strategy with breath-hold acquisitions that were used to simulate motion on in vivo data. This demonstrated improved accuracy for the proposed motion correction strategy in our 2D setting. In contrast, with a 3D acquisition scheme, a comparison with a dataset acquired during a breath-hold would not have been possible because of the required breath-hold duration. Hence, future efforts will be directed towards an extension of Self-Nav CS with a 3D acquisition, for which a CS-assisted motion detection algorithm will likely be critical to minimize motion artifacts in 3D and to maximize the diagnostic yield. A technique that makes use of CS-reconstructed sub-images to extract more accurate 3D motion parameters is currently being investigated. With the extension of this methodology to 3D, several challenges will be encountered. Specifically, with a volumetric FoV, several data segments have to be combined to reconstruct a sub-image with an adequate amount of signal and information about motion. To this end, a respiratory signal that can be obtained from diaphragmatic navigators [12] or 1D self-navigators [51] will be needed to bin different data segments into a common respiratory phase. It would also be beneficial if the binned raw data of an individual respiratory phase were uniformly distributed in k-space in order to limit streaking artifacts on the relative undersampled reconstructed sub-image. This could be obtained by using an hybrid 3D radial stack-of-star acquisition [52] or 3D radial trajectories [8,53] that are interleaved with golden-angle steps. Simultaneously, extension with affine or non-rigid deformation [47] may also need to be integrated, as a further improvement. In conclusion, a novel image-based self-navigation approach that incorporates compressed sensing reconstruction for 2D translation motion correction in free-breathing coronary MRI has been demonstrated to provide images with an image quality similar to that obtained with conventional diaphragmatic navigators, albeit with the advantage of a 69% reduction in scanning time. Based on the above observations, the extension of the CS methodology with a 3D imaging strategy is now justified.

Author Contributions

Conceived and designed the experiments: GB BP YW RBvH DP MS. Performed the experiments: GB. Analyzed the data: GB. Contributed reagents/materials/analysis tools: GB GP YW RBvH DP MS. Wrote the paper: GB. Critically revised the article for important intellectual content: GB BP YW RBvH DP MS. Approved final version of manuscript: GB BP YW RBvH DP MS.

References

1. Ehman RL, Felmlee JP (1989) Adaptive technique for high-definition MR imaging of moving structures. Radiology 173: 255–263.
2. Li D, Kaushikkar S, Haacke EM, Woodard PK, Dhawale PJ, et al. (1996) Coronary arteries: three-dimensional MR imaging with retrospective respiratory gating. Radiology 201: 857–863.

3. Oshinski JN, Hofland L, Mukundan S Jr, Dixon WT, Parks WJ, et al. (1996) Two-dimensional coronary MR angiography without breath holding. Radiology 201: 737–743.
4. McConnell MV, Khasgiwala VC, Savord BJ, Chen MH, Chuang ML, et al. (1997) Prospective adaptive navigator correction for breath-hold MR coronary angiography. Magn Reson Med 37: 148–152.
5. Larson AC, White RD, Laub G, McVeigh ER, Li D, et al. (2004) Self-gated cardiac cine MRI. Magn Reson Med 51: 93–102.
6. Stehning C, Bornert P, Nehrke K, Eggers H, Stuber M (2005) Free-breathing whole-heart coronary MRA with 3D radial SSFP and self-navigated image reconstruction. Magn Reson Med 54: 476–480.
7. Lai P, Larson AC, Park J, Carr JC, Li D (2008) Respiratory self-gated four-dimensional coronary MR angiography: a feasibility study. Magn Reson Med 59: 1378–1385.
8. Piccini D, Littmann A, Nielles-Vallespin S, Zenge MO (2012) Respiratory self-navigation for whole-heart bright-blood coronary MRI: Methods for robust isolation and automatic segmentation of the blood pool. Magn Reson Med 68: 571–579.
9. Henningsson M, Koken P, Stehning C, Razavi R, Prieto C, et al. (2012) Whole-heart coronary MR angiography with 2D self-navigated image reconstruction. Magn Reson Med 67: 437–445.
10. Hardy CJ, Zhao L, Zong X, Saranathan M, Yucel EK (2003) Coronary MR angiography: respiratory motion correction with BACSPIN. J Magn Reson Imaging 17: 170–176.
11. McLeish K, Kozerke S, Crum WR, Hill DL (2004) Free-breathing radial acquisitions of the heart. Magn Reson Med 52: 1127–1135.
12. Bhat H, Ge L, Nielles-Vallespin S, Zuehlsdorff S, Li D (2011) 3D radial sampling and 3D affine transform-based respiratory motion correction technique for free-breathing whole-heart coronary MRA with 100% imaging efficiency. Magn Reson Med 65: 1269–1277.
13. Tsai CM, Nishimura DG (2000) Reduced aliasing artifacts using variable-density k-space sampling trajectories. Magn Reson Med 43: 452–458.
14. Santos JM, Cunningham CH, Lustig M, Hargreaves BA, Hu BS, et al. (2006) Single breath-hold whole-heart MRA using variable-density spirals at 3T. Magn Reson Med 55: 371–379.
15. Block KT, Uecker M, Frahm J (2007) Undersampled radial MRI with multiple coils. Iterative image reconstruction using a total variation constraint. Magn Reson Med 57: 1086–1098.
16. Lustig M, Donoho D, Pauly JM (2007) Sparse MRI: The application of compressed sensing for rapid MR imaging. Magn Reson Med 58: 1182–1195.
17. Jung H, Sung K, Nayak KS, Kim EY, Ye JC (2009) k-t FOCUSS: a general compressed sensing framework for high resolution dynamic MRI. Magn Reson Med 61: 103–116.
18. Usman M, Atkinson D, Odille F, Kolbitsch C, Vaillant G, et al. (2013) Motion corrected compressed sensing for free-breathing dynamic cardiac MRI. Magn Reson Med 70: 504–516.
19. Jung H, Park J, Yoo J, Ye JC (2010) Radial k-t FOCUSS for high-resolution cardiac cine MRI. Magn Reson Med 63: 68–78.
20. Hansen MS, Sorensen TS, Arai AE, Kellman P (2012) Retrospective reconstruction of high temporal resolution cine images from real-time MRI using iterative motion correction. Magn Reson Med 68: 741–750.
21. Otazo R, Kim D, Axel L, Sodickson DK (2010) Combination of compressed sensing and parallel imaging for highly accelerated first-pass cardiac perfusion MRI. Magn Reson Med 64: 767–776.
22. Otazo R, Kim D, Axel L, Sodickson DK (2011) Combination of compressed sensing and parallel imaging with respiratory motion correction for highly-accelerated cardiac perfusion MRI. Journal of Cardiovascular Magnetic Resonance 13: O98.
23. Akcakaya M, Nam S, Hu P, Moghari MH, Ngo LH, et al. (2011) Compressed sensing with wavelet domain dependencies for coronary MRI: a retrospective study. IEEE Trans Med Imaging 30: 1090–1099.
24. Moghari MH, Akcakaya M, O'Connor A, Basha TA, Casanova M, et al. (2011) Compressed-sensing motion compensation (CosMo): a joint prospective-retrospective respiratory navigator for coronary MRI. Magn Reson Med 66: 1674–1681.
25. Forman C, Piccini D, Grimm R, Hutter J, Hornegger J, et al. (2014) High-resolution 3D whole-heart coronary MRA: a study on the combination of data acquisition in multiple breath-holds and 1D residual respiratory motion compensation. MAGMA.
26. Doneva M, Stehning S, Nehrke K, Börnert P (2011) Improving Scan Efficiency of Respiratory Gated Imaging Using Compressed Sensing with 3D Cartesian Golden Angle Sampling. Proc Intl Soc Mag Reson Med 19, Montreal, Canada, 23 April 2011.
27. Rudin LI, Osher S, Fatemi E (1992) NONLINEAR TOTAL VARIATION BASED NOISE REMOVAL ALGORITHMS. Physica D 60: 259–268.
28. Jackson JI, Meyer CH, Nishimura DG, Macovski A (1991) Selection of a convolution function for Fourier inversion using gridding [computerised tomography application]. IEEE Trans Med Imaging 10: 473–478.
29. Greengard L, Lee J-Y (2004) Accelerating the Nonuniform Fast Fourier Transform. Society for Industrial and Applied Mathematics REVIEW 46: 443–454.
30. Liu QH, Nguyen N (1998) An accurate algorithm for nonuniform fast Fourier transforms (NUFFT's). Ieee Microwave and Guided Wave Letters 8: 18–20.
31. NUFFT Non-Uniform FFT Toolbox. Available: http://www.cims.nyu.edu/cmcl/nufft/nufft.html. Accessed 2014 Jul 29.
32. Beck A, Teboulle M (2009) Fast gradient-based algorithms for constrained total variation image denoising and deblurring problems. IEEE Trans Image Process 18: 2419–2434.
33. Perraudin N, Shuman D, Puy G, Vandergheynst P (2014) UNLocBoX A matlab convex optimization toolbox using proximal splitting methods. arXiv:14020779 Available: http://unlocbox.sourceforge.net. Accessed 2014 Jul 29.
34. ITK The Insight Segmentation and Registration Toolkit. Available: www.itk.org. Accessed 2014 Jul 29.
35. Fischer RW, Botnar RM, Nehrke K, Boesiger P, Manning WJ, et al. (2006) Analysis of residual coronary artery motion for breath hold and navigator approaches using real-time coronary MRI. Magn Reson Med 55: 612–618.
36. Stuber M, Botnar RM, Danias PG, Sodickson DK, Kissinger KV, et al. (1999) Double-oblique free-breathing high resolution three-dimensional coronary magnetic resonance angiography. J Am Coll Cardiol 34: 524–531.
37. Etienne A, Botnar RM, Van Muiswinkel AM, Boesiger P, Manning WJ, et al. (2002) "Soap-Bubble" visualization and quantitative analysis of 3D coronary magnetic resonance angiograms. Magn Reson Med 48: 658–666.
38. Wang Y, Riederer SJ, Ehman RL (1995) Respiratory motion of the heart: kinematics and the implications for the spatial resolution in coronary imaging. Magn Reson Med 33: 713–719.
39. Prieto C, Doneva M, Usman M, Henningsson M, Greil G, et al. (2014) Highly efficient respiratory motion compensated free-breathing coronary mra using golden-step Cartesian acquisition. J Magn Reson Imaging.
40. Pruessmann KP, Weiger M, Bornert P, Boesiger P (2001) Advances in sensitivity encoding with arbitrary k-space trajectories. Magn Reson Med 46: 638–651.
41. Henningsson M, Smink J, Razavi R, Botnar RM (2012) Prospective respiratory motion correction for coronary MR angiography using a 2D image navigator. Magn Reson Med.
42. Kawaji K, Spincemaille P, Nguyen TD, Thimmappa N, Cooper MA, et al. (2013) Direct coronary motion extraction from a 2D fat image navigator for prospectively gated coronary MR angiography. Magn Reson Med DOI 10.1002/mrm.24698.
43. Botnar RM, Stuber M, Danias PG, Kissinger KV, Manning WJ (1999) Improved coronary artery definition with T2-weighted, free-breathing, three-dimensional coronary MRA. Circulation 99: 3139–3148.
44. Carrillo R, McEwen J, Van De Ville D, Thiran JP, Wiaux Y (2013) Sparsity Averaging for Compressive Imaging. IEEE Signal Processing Letters 20: 591–594.
45. Piccini D, Maréchal B, Coppo S, Chaptinel J, Bonanno G, et al. (2014) Automated and Subject-Specific Coil Selection for Respiratory Self-Navigation in Coronary MRA. Proc Intl Soc Magn Reson Med 23, pp 2503, Milan, Italy, 2014 April 26.
46. Abd-Elmoniem KZ, Barmet C, Stuber M (2012) Free-breathing inner-volume black-blood imaging of the human heart using two-dimensionally selective local excitation at 3 T. Magn Reson Med 68: 822–829.
47. Buerger C, Schaeffter T, King AP (2011) Hierarchical adaptive local affine registration for fast and robust respiratory motion estimation. Med Image Anal 15: 551–564.
48. Chefd'Hotel C, Hermosillo G, Faugeras O (2002) Flows of diffeomorphisms for multimodal image registration. Proc IEEE ISBI, pp 753–756, 10 July 2002.
49. Nagel E, Bornstedt A, Schnackenburg B, Hug J, Oswald H, et al. (1999) Optimization of realtime adaptive navigator correction for 3D magnetic resonance coronary angiography. Magn Reson Med 42: 408–411.
50. Spuentrup E, Stuber M, Botnar RM, Manning WJ (2001) The impact of navigator timing parameters and navigator spatial resolution on 3D coronary magnetic resonance angiography. J Magn Reson Imaging 14: 311–318.
51. Pang J, Bhat H, Sharif B, Fan Z, Thomson LE, et al. (2013) Whole-heart coronary MRA with 100% respiratory gating efficiency: Self-navigated three-dimensional retrospective image-based motion correction (TRIM). Magn Reson Med.
52. Adluru G, Chen L, Kim SE, Burgon N, Kholmovski EG, et al. (2011) Three-dimensional late gadolinium enhancement imaging of the left atrium with a hybrid radial acquisition and compressed sensing. J Magn Reson Imaging 34: 1465–1471.
53. Piccini D, Littmann A, Nielles-Vallespin S, Zenge MO (2011) Spiral phyllotaxis: the natural way to construct a 3D radial trajectory in MRI. Magn Reson Med 66: 1049–1056.

22

The Cost-Utility of CT Angiography and Conventional Angiography for People Presenting with Intracerebral Hemorrhage

Richard I. Aviv[1]*, Adam G. Kelly[2], Babak S. Jahromi[3,4¤], Curtis G. Benesch[2,3], Kate C. Young[2,3,4¤]

1 Department of medical Imaging, University of Toronto, Division of Neuroradiology Sunnybrook Health Sciences Centre, Toronto, Ontario, Canada, **2** Department of Neurology, University of Rochester, Rochester, New York, United States of America, **3** Department of Neurosurgery, University of Rochester, Rochester, New York, United States of America, **4** Department of Imaging Sciences, University of Rochester, Rochester, New York, United States of America

Abstract

Objective: To determine the optimal imaging strategy for ICH incorporating CTA or DSA with and without a NCCT risk stratification algorithm.

Methods: A Markov model included costs, outcomes, prevalence of a vascular lesion, and the sensitivity and specificity of a risk stratification algorithm from the literature. The four imaging strategies were: (a) CTA screening of the entire cohort; (b) CTA only in those where NCCT suggested a high or indeterminate likelihood of a lesion; (c) DSA screening of the entire cohort and (d) DSA only for those with a high or indeterminate suspicion of a lesion following NCCT. Branch d was the comparator.

Results: Age of the cohort and the probability of an underlying lesion influenced the choice of optimal imaging strategy. With a low suspicion for a lesion (<12%), branch (a) was the optimal strategy for a willingness-to-pay of $100,000/QALY. Branch (a) remained the optimal strategy in younger people (<35 years) with a risk below 15%. If the probability of a lesion was >15%, branch (b) became preferred strategy. The probabilistic sensitivity analysis showed that branch (b) was the optimal choice 70–72% of the time over varying willingness-to-pay values.

Conclusions: CTA has a clear role in the evaluation of people presenting with ICH, though the choice of CTA everyone or CTA using risk stratification depends on age and likelihood of finding a lesion.

Editor: Michael Lim, Johns Hopkins Hospital, United States of America

Funding: The authors have no support or funding to report.

Competing Interests: The authors have declared that no competing interests exist.

* E-mail: Richard.Aviv@sunnybrook.ca

¤ Current address: Oxford PharmaGenesis, Inc., Newtown, Pennsylvania, United States of America

Introduction

Following the diagnosis of intracranial hemorrhage (ICH) on non contrast CT (NCCT), the American Heart Association guidelines recommend the use of non-invasive vascular imaging such as CT angiography (CTA) to evaluate for the presence of underlying vascular lesions.[1] The guidelines, however, limit this recommendation to ICH where a clinical or radiological (based on non-contrast CT - NCCT) suspicion of an underlying lesion exists.

Traditionally, the role of NCCT has been confined to ICH diagnosis and facilitation of management decisions pertaining to ICH-related complications. Additionally, radiological and clinical features have been described that suggest the possibility of an underlying structural lesion.[2–5] Only one prospective study has quantified NCCT performance for the detection of an underlying secondary vascular lesion and demonstrated a modest sensitivity and specificity of 77% and 84% respectively. A recent retrospective study, stratified NCCT scan appearances into low, indeterminate and high risk and reported the performance of NCCT for predicting an underlying vascular lesions. Acknowledging that both indeterminate and high risk NCCT scans require further vascular workup, the study demonstrated a sensitivity and specificity of 96% and 33% respectively.[2]

Pure reliance on clinical and NCCT features to determine the risk of an underlying lesion is an historic approach stemming from prior practice where only digital subtraction angiography (DSA) was available to confirm clinical or NCCT suspicion.[6] Fear of DSA- associated morbidity and mortality led to the procedure being performed only in a limited and highly selected population where the procedural risks were outweighed by the perceived benefit of the confirmatory diagnosis. These fears, however, likely contributed to a selection and verification bias that has distorted the true prevalence of secondary vascular lesions. Although safety and accuracy of CTA is well established for aneurysm, its performance in non-subarachnoid ICH is only more recently established. There are now numerous publications demonstrating sensitivities and specificities of CTA for secondary vascular causes ranging from 92–100%.[2–5,7] We have previously proposed that

CTA screening should be implemented in all ICH patients irrespective of NCCT risk stratification or perceived clinical risk.[6] However, acknowledging the widespread reliance on NCCT to risk stratify ICH presentations, we sought to determine the optimal angiographic strategy for ICH work-up by exploring the future costs and outcomes related to CTA and DSA use without and with a NCCT risk stratification algorithm.

Methods

Model Description

We developed a Markov model to predict the future costs and health-related outcomes of different imaging strategies (Figure 1). Markov modeling allowed for future estimation of outcomes based on several potential health states after the initial event. The Markov cycle length was one year. The time horizon was the lifetime of the cohort.

There were four branches at the decision node: (a) immediate CTA screening of the entire cohort; (b) A stratified CTA approach - CTA performed only in those where the NCCT suggested a high or indeterminate (medium) likelihood of an underlying lesion. Patients with a low suspicion of an underlying lesion on NCCT do not undergo CTA vascular imaging [8]; (c) DSA screening of the entire cohort and (d) A stratified DSA approach - DSA performed where the NCCT suggested a high or indeterminate likelihood of an underlying lesion. As above, patients with a low suspicion of an underlying lesion on NCCT would not undergo DSA vascular imaging. Branch (d) was the comparator or the strategy against which the other three were compared. The sensitivity and specificity of CTA and NCCT to identify a lesion were derived from prior studies (Table 1).[2,3,5,7,8].

The hypothetical cohort presented with ICH on the NCCT. The etiology could be either primary (e.g. hypertensive) or secondary ICH relating to an underlying vascular lesion. Hemorrhage as a result of tumor was not included for model simplicity. Any lesion identified by DSA or CTA was considered successfully treated. If a recurrent primary or secondary hemorrhage occurred, we assumed that all subjects underwent DSA and any previously missed lesions would then be successfully treated. Adverse outcomes following DSA in which there was no successful diagnostic treatment were limited to permanent disabling neurological deficits for model simplicity. We assumed that permanent disabling deficits due to the DSA were not separated from permanent disabling deficits due to treatment and were thus captured sufficiently in the mRS distribution following treatment.

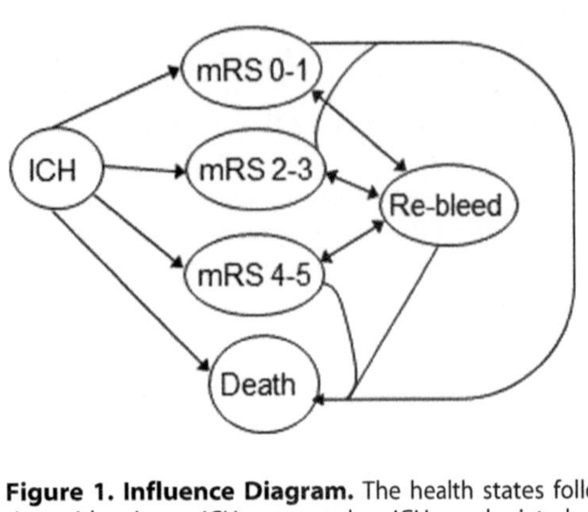

Figure 1. Influence Diagram. The health states following presentation with primary ICH or secondary ICH are depicted.

Probabilities

There is a paucity of large randomized trial data for outcomes estimates, thus a combination of sources were used (Table 1). The probability of a vascular anomaly was taken from prior studies and varied with age.[9] Bayes revision was then used with the sensitivity and specificity of NCCT (and/or CTA as appropriate) to determine the post-test probability of a lesion. The distribution of modified Rankin Scale scores after primary ICH was modeled according to the FAST trial.[10] Sample weighted outcomes after secondary ICH were used.[11,12]

We assumed one rate of recurrent secondary ICH and used a relative risk term to change the likelihood of recurrent hemorrhage with treatment. The relative risk was calculated as the incidence of hemorrhage after treatment based on a meta-analysis divided by the incidence of hemorrhage for the natural history of known vascular lesions.[13,14]

Costs and Health Care Utilization

We used a payer perspective. Direct medical costs included the costs of hospitalization, rehabilitation or long-term care, CTA and DSA.[15–19] Charges for the hospitalization were converted to costs using data and cost-to-charge ratios from 2009 Nationwide Inpatient Sample (NIS), Healthcare Cost and Utilization Project (HCUP), Agency for Healthcare Research and Quality.[20] The cost of a hospitalization was based on whether or not a lesion was repaired. Repair was identified using ICD-9 procedure codes: 39.72, 39.51, 39.53 with ICD-9 diagnosis code 431. All prices were adjusted to 2011 USD using the Consumer's Price Index for medical care.

A positive CTA implies a readily visible, unequivocal abnormality with lesions proceeding to neurosurgical or endovascular therapy as arbitrated by the physician. We assumed that if endovascular therapy is decided upon, selective DSA of the vessel(s) of interest is undertaken limiting exposure to other vessels. Therefore a separate DSA for diagnosis of the CTA-confirmed abnormality is not performed prior to the planned therapy. Similarly, if a surgical treatment is considered appropriate following diagnostic CTA we assume the patient goes to the operating room without a pre-procedural diagnostic DSA.

If CTA correctly identified a vascular anomaly, the subject underwent successfully treatment without a confirmatory DSA, reflecting widespread clinical practice. The cost structure was:

CTA identified vascular anomaly (true positive):

$$\text{Cost}_{\text{CTA}} + \text{Cost}_{\text{HOSPITALIZATION SECONDARY ICH}}.$$

False negative CTA results were assumed to have the cost structure of primary ICH with their treatment plan based on the primary ICH assumption. This cost structures was:

CTA does not detect a vascular anomaly (false negative):

$$\text{Cost}_{\text{CTA}} + \text{Cost}_{\text{HOSPITALIZATION PRIMARY ICH}}$$

The remaining cost structures were:

CTA identified vascular anomaly (false positive):

$$\text{Cost}_{\text{CTA}} + \text{Cost}_{\text{DSA}} + \text{Cost}_{\text{HOSPITALIZATION PRIMARY ICH}}$$

Table 1. Model inputs.

Parameter	Base Case	Range	Distribution for PSA	References
Initial Age	40	10–80	Normal (SD = 12.5)	Author estimate
Sensitivity of CTA	0.96	0.8–1.0	Beta	[2,3,5,7]
Specificity of CTA	0.99	0.8–1.0	Beta	[2,3,5,7]
Sensitivity of NCCT high/indeterminate risk	0.95	0.7–1.0	Beta	[45]
Specificity of NCCT high/indeterminate risk	0.35	0–0.6	Beta	[45]
Probabilities, %				
mRS after Primary ICH			Dirichlet	
mRS 0–1	8	0–18		[10]
mRS 2–3	23	0–50		[10]
mRS 4–5	40	30–50		[10]
mRS 6	29	15–45		[10]
mRS after Secondary ICH			Dirichlet	
mRS 0–1	69.4	30–100		[11,12]
mRS 2–3	22.4	0–50		[11,12]
mRS 4–5	3.5	0–20		[11,12]
mRS 6	4.7	0–20		[11,12]
Vascular anomaly, %	45	0–70		[9]
Primary ICH re-bleed, % per cycle	2.08	0–6	Beta	[46]
Secondary ICH re-bleed, % per cycle	3.92	0–10	Beta	[13]
Relative Risk of re-bleed after repair of vascular anomaly	0.35	0–2	Log	[13,14]
Costs (2011 USD)				
CTA	425	100–1500	Normal	[47]
DSA	1100	450–2000	Normal	[48]
Hospitalization, Secondary ICH	85,400	10,000–300,000	LogNormal	[20]
Hospitalization, Primary ICH & missed lesion	25,300	3,000–120,000	LogNormal	[20]
			LogNormal	
Long-term care, mRS 2–3	8,438	0–20,000	LogNormal	[15–19,49]
Long-term care, mRS 4–5, 1st year	71,428	30,000–150,000	LogNormal	[15–19,49]
Long-term care, mRS 4–5, 2nd year	37,140	10,000–90,000	LogNormal	[15–19,49]
Utility values				
mRS 0–1	0.9	0.2–1.0	Beta	[21]
mRS 2–3	0.75	0–1.0	Beta	[21]
mRS 4–5	0.25	−0.1–1.0	Beta	[21]
mRS 6	0			
Discount Rate (%)	3	0–8	Not included	[22]

The range presented is for the one-way sensitivity analysis. The relative risk is for re-bleed after the lesion is fixed. CTA = CT Angiography; DSA = digital subtraction angiogram; ICH = intracerebral hemorrhage; mRS = modified Rankin Scale score; NCCT = non-contract head CT; PSA = probabilistic sensitivity analysis; RR = relative risk; USD = United States Dollars.

CTA does not detect a vascular anomaly (true negative):

$$\mathrm{Cost}_{\mathrm{CTA}} + \mathrm{Cost}_{\mathrm{HOSPITALIZATION\ PRIMARY\ ICH}}$$

For the cohort in branch (d): high or indeterminate suspicion of a vascular anomaly based on NCCT, we assumed that the DSA cohort incurred the cost of DSA in addition to their hospitalization cost.

Utility

Utility is the desirability or preference for one health state over another. Perfect health has a utility of one while death is zero. Negative values are allowed representing a state worse than death. Quality adjusted life years (QALYs) are the utility of a health state multiplied by the duration of the health state summed over a lifetime. Utility values were adapted from the *Factor Seven for Acute Hemorrhagic Stroke* trial which measured quality of life at 90 days.[21]

Analysis

Future costs and outcomes were discounted at 3%.[22] The incremental cost-effectiveness ratio (ICER) is the average net costs of branches a, b or c divided by the net QALYs from branch d of a Markov cohort. For example [($\$_{CTA\ ALL}$ - $\$_{DSA\ high/indeterminate}$) per ($QALY_{CTA\ ALL}$ − $QALY_{DSA\ high/indeterminate}$)]. Assumptions about each individual model variable were tested by a one-way sensitivity analysis. A probabilistic sensitivity analysis was used to estimate second order uncertainty about cost, probability and utility data (n = 1000 samples).

Results

Case Vignettes

Since the probability of identifying a vascular lesion varies with age, we conducted a two-way sensitivity analysis varying these inputs to discern the optimal imaging strategy for different combinations of these two inputs (Figure 2).[9] Three case vignettes are presented to demonstrate which imaging pathway is the optimal choice. Optimal choice balanced the lifetime costs of care with lifetime outcomes for a willingness-to-pay of $100,000/QALY.

(1) *A 40-year old presented with ICH on NCCT and a 20% probability of an underlying lesion.*

Using 40 years on the x-axis and 20% on the y-axis of Figure 2, the optimal pathway was NCCT with CTA for a high or indeterminate suspicion of a lesion.

(2) *A 25-year old presented with ICH on NCCT and a 40% probability of an underlying lesion*

With a high index of suspicion for a lesion, the optimal pathway was NCCT with CTA for a high or indeterminate suspicion of a lesion.

(3) *A 60-year old presented with ICH on NCCT and a 2% probability of an underlying lesion.*

With a low index of suspicion for a lesion, the optimal pathway was NCCT with CTA for all persons.

Broadly speaking, when the probability of an underlying lesion is ≥15%, stratified CTA for high or indeterminate NCCT is the optimal strategy regardless of age using net monetary benefits with a willingness-to-pay of $100,000 per QALY. When probability of an underlying lesion was below 15% the dominant strategy was NCCT and CTA in all patients below 60 years of age. Above 60 years, stratified CTA for high or indeterminate NCCT became cost effective for a lesion probability of 13–14%.

Several factors contribute to the value of the ICER beyond the costs of the initial screening strategies accounting for cost-effectiveness of CTA screening in all older patients (scenario 3) but selectively applying CTA in the younger cohort. ICERs and net benefit models used in these analyses reflect the contribution of many factors including total lifetime costs, health related outcomes, the balance of the proportion of primary and secondary ICH as well as the age of the cohort. The numerator of an ICER is the incremental net costs of a strategy accumulated over a lifetime following hospitalization, long-term care and adverse events, thus the numerator reflects more than just the incremental cost of DSA

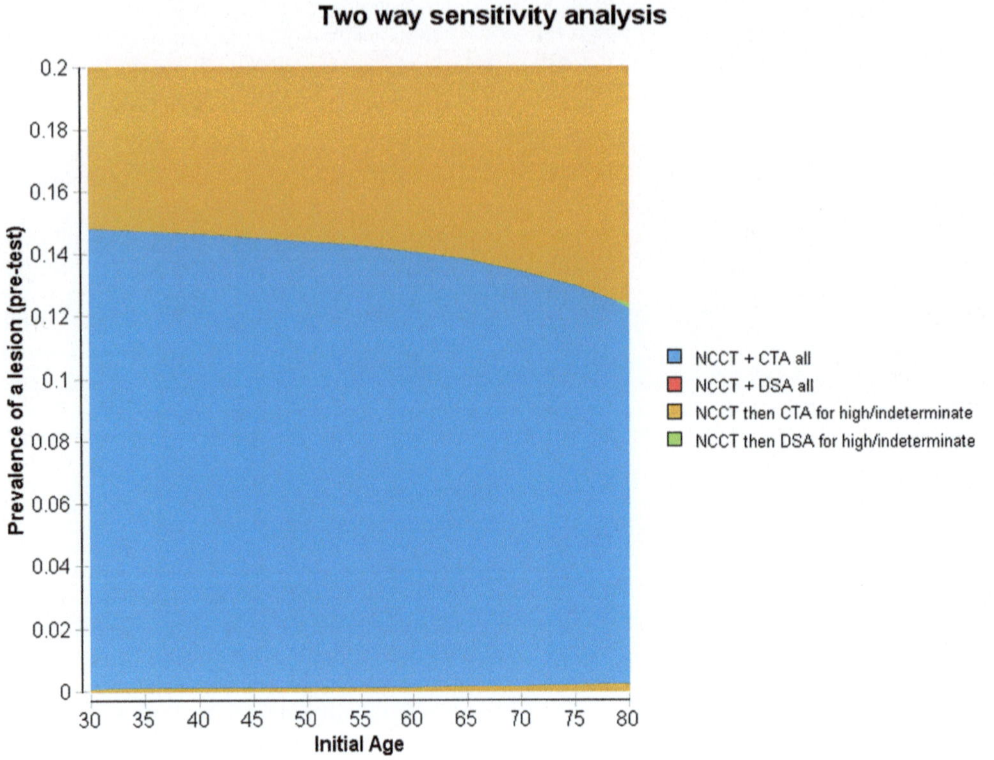

Figure 2. Two-way sensitivity analysis. The prevalence of a lesion and cohort age were tested in a two-way deterministic sensitivity analysis with a willingness-to-pay of $100,000/QALY. The optimal imaging strategy - CTA of the entire cohort (blue), CTA for high or indeterminate suspicion of a lesion on NCCT (orange) and DSA for a high or indeterminate suspicion of a lesion on NCCT (green) – depends on the age and probability of a lesion.

or CTA. Compared to secondary hemorrhage primary hemorrhage has, relatively speaking, (a) a worse distribution of mRS scores for outcomes, (b) lower hospitalization costs but higher long-term care costs experienced due to greater disability, (c) and lower overall utility. There is also additional burden (higher probability of re-bleed if a lesion is not fixed, cost and outcomes) for missed lesions on the CTA. The individual influence of each of these factors is explored by using sensitivity analyses.

One-way Sensitivity Analyses

One-way sensitivity analyses were conducted to identify which individual model inputs influenced the ICER. To complete these analyses, we specified a base case analysis with a 40-year old cohort the prevalence of vascular anomaly reported for this age.[9] The strategy of using stratified CTA for a 40-year old cohort with a high or indeterminate NCCT had lower net costs (-$2,100) and greater QALYs (0.133) than stratified DSA for those with a high or indeterminate NCCT making it the dominant screening strategy (Figure 3 and Table S1 in File S1). DSA screening of the entire cohort had an ICER of $70,000 per QALY while the ICER for CTA screening of the entire cohort was $600,000 per QALY.

To address the uncertainty around the likelihood of finding a vascular anomaly, we tested our model by varying this probability in a 40-year old cohort. The choice of optimal imaging strategy was sensitive to the probability of a vascular lesion (Table 2). When the probability of a lesion was ≤6%, CTA screening of the entire 40-year old cohort became the dominant option with the lowest costs and greatest QALYs (dark green) compared to all other imaging strategies. CTA screening of the entire cohort was a reasonable option, for up to a 15% probability of a lesion (light green). Stratified CTA following high or indeterminate NCCT was the optimal strategy compared to all others tested when the probability of an underlying lesion was 16–60%.

Changing the initial age of the cohort also influenced the optimal imaging strategy for a 45% probability of a lesion. Stratified CTA following high or indeterminate NCCT was the dominant strategy compared to all other strategies tested for ages 10–40 and 51–80 (Tables S2 in File S1 and S3 in File S1). DSA screening of the entire cohort became cost-ineffective (ICER > $100,000 per QALY) at age ≥41 years; CTA screening of the entire cohort became cost-effective (ICER <$100,000 per QALY) only for ages 41–50. However, this change is likely due to the 8% probability of a lesion, rather than age itself (see Two-way Sensitivity Analysis).[9]

Changes in the assumptions of two model inputs increased ICER of DSA screening of the entire cohort beyond $100,000 per QALY. DSA screening of the entire cohort became cost-ineffective if either the re-bleed for secondary ICH was <3% per cycle or the relative risk of re-bleed after treatment of the vascular anomaly was >0.42. The results of other one-way sensitivity analyses were presented in Table S2 in File S1.

The relative risk of a re-bleed was tested with the re-bleed rate as another two-way sensitivity analysis. Stratified CTA for high or indeterminate suspicion of lesion following NCCT was the optimal strategy across all combinations using a net monetary benefit model with a willingness-to-pay of either $50,000 or $100,000 per QALY (data not shown).

Probabilistic Sensitivity Analysis

Monte Carlo simulations showed that stratified CTA for high or indeterminate suspicion of a lesion on NCCT was the optimal screening strategy 70–72% of the time varying slightly with the willingness-to-pay (Figure 4).

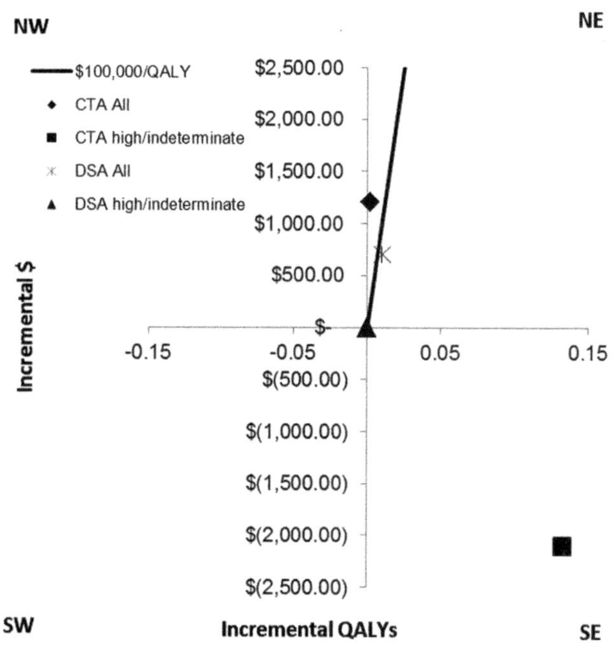

Figure 3. Base Case graphs. The base case analyses are presented on a two-dimensional graph showing the net costs and net QALYs for CTA of the entire cohort (diamond), CTA for high or indeterminate suspicion of a lesion on NCCT (square), DSA for the entire cohort (asterisk) and DSA for those with a high or indeterminate suspicion of a lesion on NCCT (triangle).

Discussion

The most cost effective strategy for screening of ICH patients is dependent on both age and underlying vascular lesion prevalence. However, a CTA strategy for all patients was the optimal imaging strategy regardless of age when the risk of an underlying vascular lesion was below 12%. This strategy remained optimal in younger patients (<~35 years) with a risk below 15%. When the risk exceeds 15%, a strategy first stratifying patients into high and indeterminate risk categories by NCCT prior to CTA is the preferred strategy regardless of age. Furthermore, the results of the probabilistic sensitivity analysis which showed stratified CTA is an optimal screening strategy in ~70% of the simulations.

In a large recent retrospective study 623 patients were divided according to their NCCT scan appearances into low, indeterminate and high risk for underlying vascular lesions. High risk scans constituted only a minority of ICH presentations (19/623; 3%). The large majority of patients demonstrated indeterminate (421; 68%) scans, while low risk scans constituted the remaining 29%. More recent studies confirm frequencies of high, intermediate and low risk scans of 2–11%, 42–61% and 32–36% respectively.[23–25] Acknowledging the need to further investigate patients with indeterminate risk and confirm NCCT suspicion in the high risk group, up to 90% of the ICH population would still require further angiographic imaging with this stratification approach. NCCT stratification would spare only the 11–30% defined as low risk from angiographic imaging but yield a 1.6–8%% false negative rate.[2,24,26] An external validation of attempts to combine NCCT risk stratification with clinical variables including age, gender, hypertensive/anticoagulation status to define 'low risk' [1,2,7,9,24,26] yielded an AUCs of 0.82 for predicting underlying

Table 2. One way sensitivity analysis for the probability of a lesion in a 40-year old cohort.

Probability of a Lesion	NCCT + CTA All	NCCT + CTA high/indeterminate	NCCT + DSA All	NCCT + DSA high/indeterminate
1–15%	**Dominant**	*Not optimal*	*Not optimal*	Comparator
16–17%	**Dominant**	**Dominant**	*Not optimal*	Comparator
18–20%	<$100,000/QALY	**Dominant**	*Not optimal*	Comparator
21–33%	*Not optimal*	**Dominant**	*Not optimal*	Comparator
34–60%	*Not optimal*	**Dominant**	<$100,000/QALY	Comparator
vs all other strategies				
1–6%	**Dominant**			
16–60%		**Dominant**		

Bold: The strategy is dominant (less costly and more QALYs than the comparator). Normal: The ICER falls in an acceptable range. Italics: Not optimal - the strategy is dominated, in the southwest quadrant, or in the northwest quadrant above the $100,000 per QALY line.

vascular lesion presence with NCCT stratification faring as well as a combined imaging/radiological score.[27] The average performance of NCCT therefore provides a compelling argument for consideration of a CTA base screening algorithm given its sensitivity and specificity ranging from 92–100% for secondary vascular lesion detection.[2–5,7]

The notion of negligible risk in 'typical hypertensive' locations is largely derived from a prospective study of 206 patients examined by DSA reporting a 0% prevalence of secondary vascular lesions for basal ganglia ICH in older (>45 yrs) hypertensive patients.[9] A reappraisal of the study, however suggests that this group remains worthy of further angiographic study as the caudate head was erroneously omitted from the study's basal ganglia definition. The authors actually demonstrated 1 caudate hemorrhage secondary to an aneurysm in an old hypertensive patient. Rightful inclusion of the caudate head into the basal ganglia definition results in a secondary vascular lesion in 1/29 or 2.4% of older patients with 'typical hypertensive' locations. Similarly, older hypertensive patients with any ICH location demonstrated an angiographic yield of 11% (age >50 yrs) in a prospective and 9.5% (age >46 yrs) in a retrospective study.[2,8] Finally a recent study from a center adopting a more liberal DSA approach demonstrated a 15% incidence of vascular lesions in a patient subgroup that was hypertensive (or impaired coagulation; 72%), older and more likely to present with a low probability scan (56%). In this study 7% of deep location ICH was associated with a secondary vascular lesion. According to our results the combination of age >40 and low vascular lesion prevalence suggests that this specific patient group would be best served with a combined

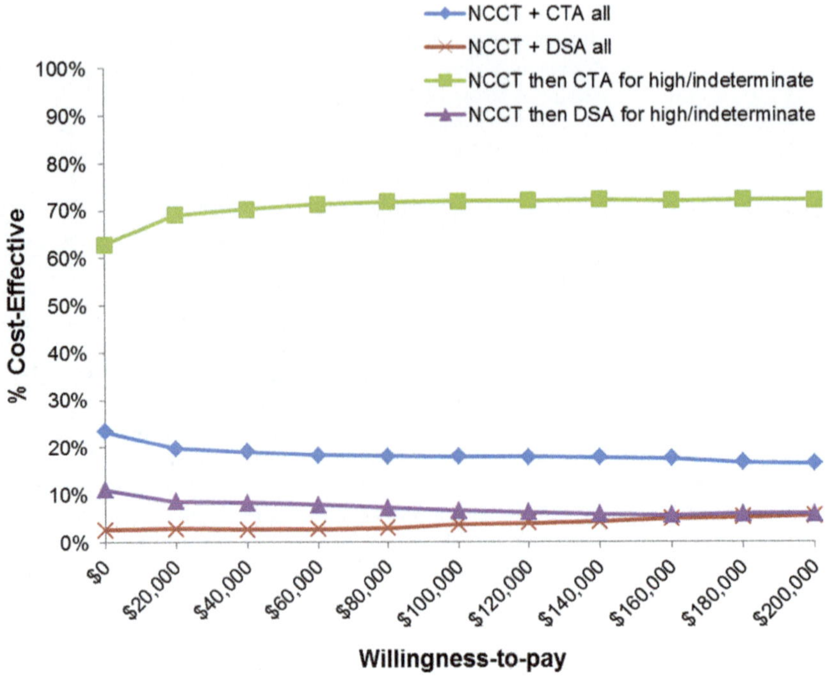

Figure 4. Probabilistic sensitivity analysis. Variables in the model were sampled simultaneously to show the probability that a given strategy was optimal strategy in relation to the willingness-to-pay (x-axis) using net monetary benefits calculations.

NCCT and CTA strategy. Indeed a CTA–all-patients strategy was recommended by the same group.[28]

The reliance on DSA as a reference standard to exclude vascular lesions in ICH before the maturation of CTA as an accepted technique undoubtedly resulted in both a selection and verification bias. It is noteworthy that prospective angiographic studies show a higher (34–53%) prevalence of secondary ICH than the 20% commonly cited.[7–9,29] CTA is associated with a lower overall patient risk than DSA and can be performed safely with limited morbidity and mortality. Several studies report the safety of contrast use in the stroke population with the incidence of contrast induced nephropathy (CIN) below 5%.[30–36] The American college of radiology states that the concern for the development of CIN is a relative but not absolute contraindication to the administration of intravascular contrast.[37] The role of contrast in the development of nephropathy is overstated with only 1 of 8 studies that included a control group showing a link between contrast and CIN. [30,32,38–43]

Limitations of this study relate to the paucity of prospective data available on which to base the incidence of secondary vascular lesions. Additionally, new information about outcomes by age, volume and etiology, primary vs secondary, would help strengthen the model. While the included study is the only prospective study available that utilizes the reference standard procedure DSA, the single center nature and non-North American demographic studied could limit its application to other population. Models of cost effectiveness rely on underlying assumptions that, while tested, remain assumptions. However the purpose of any cost-effectiveness model is to help frame questions and inform medical decision making.[44]

In summary a strategy imaging all patients with NCCT and CTA is optimal when the risk of an underlying lesion is below 10% whereas an NCCT stratification strategy is dominant where risk exceeds this threshold.

Supporting Information

File S1 Tables S1–S3. Table S1. Base Case Analysis. The cohort was 40 years and had a 45% probability of a vascular anomaly. Table S2. One way sensitivity analyses (except age and probability of a lesion). *Initial age 41–50 has to do with the probability of an underlying lesion. The look-up table used for the analysis had a lower probability for this decade. Bold: The strategy is dominant (less costly and more QALYs than the comparator). Table S3. One-way sensitivity analysis for age. Normal: The ICER falls in an acceptable range. Italics: Not optimal - the strategy is dominated, in the southwest quadrant, or in the northwest quadrant above the $100,000 per QALY line.

Author Contributions

Conceived and designed the experiments: RA AK BJ CB KY. Performed the experiments: KY. Analyzed the data: KY. Wrote the paper: RA KY. Critical revision of manuscript: AK BJ CB.

References

1. Morgenstern LB, Hemphill JC III, Anderson C, Becker K, Broderick JP, et al. (2010) Guidelines for the management of spontaneous intracerebral hemorrhage: a guideline for healthcare professionals from the American Heart Association/American Stroke Association. Stroke 41: 2108–2129.
2. Delgado Almandoz JE, Schaefer PW, Forero NP, Falla JR, Gonzalez RG, et al. (2009) Diagnostic accuracy and yield of multidetector CT angiography in the evaluation of spontaneous intraparenchymal cerebral hemorrhage. AJNR Am J Neuroradiol 30: 1213–1221.
3. Yeung R, Ahmad T, Aviv RI, de Tilly LN, Fox AJ, et al. (2009) Comparison of CTA to DSA in determining the etiology of spontaneous ICH. Can J Neurol Sci 36: 176–180.
4. Romero JM, Artunduaga M, Forero NP, Delgado J, Sarfaraz K, et al. (2009) Accuracy of CT angiography for the diagnosis of vascular abnormalities causing intraparenchymal hemorrhage in young patients. Emerg Radiol 16: 195–201.
5. Yoon DY, Chang SK, Choi CS, Kim WK, Lee JH (2009) Multidetector row CT angiography in spontaneous lobar intracerebral hemorrhage: a prospective comparison with conventional angiography. AJNR Am J Neuroradiol 30: 962–967.
6. Khosravani H, Mayer SA, Demchuk AM, Jahromi BS, Gladstone DJ, et al. (In Press) Emergency Noninvasive Angiography for Acute Intracerebral Hemorrhage. AJNR Am J Neuroratiol.
7. Wong GK, Siu DY, Abrigo JM, Poon WS, Tsang FC, et al. (2011) Computed tomographic angiography and venography for young or nonhypertensive patients with acute spontaneous intracerebral hemorrhage. Stroke 42: 211–213.
8. Halpin SF, Britton JA, Byrne JV, Clifton A, Hart G, et al. (1994) Prospective evaluation of cerebral angiography and computed tomography in cerebral haematoma. J Neurol Neurosurg Psychiatry 57: 1180–1186.
9. Zhu XL, Chan MS, Poon WS (1997) Spontaneous intracranial hemorrhage: which patients need diagnostic cerebral angiography? A prospective study of 206 cases and review of the literature. Stroke 28: 1406–1409.
10. Mayer SA, Brun NC, Begtrup K, Broderick J, Davis S, et al. (2005) Recombinant activated factor VII for acute intracerebral hemorrhage. N Engl J Med 352: 777–785.
11. Hartmann A, Mast H, Mohr JP, Koennecke HC, Osipov A, et al. (1998) Morbidity of intracranial hemorrhage in patients with cerebral arteriovenous malformation. Stroke 29: 931–934.
12. van BJ, Lovelock CE, Cordonnier C, Rothwell PM, Klijn CJ, et al. (2009) Outcome after spontaneous and arteriovenous malformation-related intracerebral haemorrhage: population-based studies. Brain 132: 537–543.
13. Ondra SL, Troupp H, George ED, Schwab K (1990) The natural history of symptomatic arteriovenous malformations of the brain: a 24-year follow-up assessment. J Neurosurg 73: 387–391.
14. van BJ, van der Worp HB, Buis DR, Al-Shahi SR, Kappelle LJ, et al. (2011) Treatment of brain arteriovenous malformations: a systematic review and meta-analysis. JAMA 306: 2011–2019.
15. Oster G, Huse DM, Lacey MJ, Epstein AM (1994) Cost-effectiveness of ticlopidine in preventing stroke in high-risk patients. Stroke 25: 1149–1156.
16. Kuntz KM, Kent KC (1996) Is carotid endarterectomy cost-effective? An analysis of symptomatic and asymptomatic patients. Circulation 94: II194–II198.
17. Cronenwett JL, Birkmeyer JD, Nackman GB, Fillinger MF, Bech FR, et al. (1997) Cost-effectiveness of carotid endarterectomy in asymptomatic patients. J Vasc Surg 25: 298–309; discussion 310–291.
18. Yin D, Carpenter JP (1998) Cost-effectiveness of screening for asymptomatic carotid stenosis. J Vasc Surg 27: 245–255.
19. Post PN, Kievit J, van Baalen JM, van den Hout WB, van Bockel JH (2002) Routine duplex surveillance does not improve the outcome after carotid endarterectomy: a decision and cost utility analysis. Stroke 33: 749–755.
20. HCUP Nationwide Inpatient Sample (NIS). Healthcare cost and Utilization Project (HCUP). 2009.Agency for Healthcare Research and Quality, Rockville, MD.
21. Christensen MC, Mayer S, Ferran JM (2009) Quality of life after intracerebral hemorrhage: results of the Factor Seven for Acute Hemorrhagic Stroke (FAST) trial. Stroke 40: 1677–1682.
22. (1996) Cost-effectiveness in health and medicine. Gold MB, Siegel JE, Rusell LB, Weinstein MC, eds. New York: Oxford University Press.
23. Kadkhodayan Y, Cross DT III, Derdeyn CP, Moran CJ (2007) Carotid angioplasty and stenting in the elderly. Neuroradiology 49: 933–938.
24. Delgado Almandoz JE, Jagadeesan BD, Moran CJ, Cross DT III, Zipfel GJ, et al. (2012) Independent validation of the secondary intracerebral hemorrhage score with catheter angiography and findings of emergent hematoma evacuation. Neurosurgery 70: 131–140; discussion 140.
25. van Asch CJ, Velthuis BK, Greving JP, van Laar PJ, Rinkel GJ, et al. (2013) External validation of the secondary intracerebral hemorrhage score in The Netherlands. Stroke 44: 2904–2906.
26. Kadkhodayan Y, Delgado Almandoz JE, Kelly JE, Kale SP, Jagadeesan BD, et al. (2012) Yield of catheter angiography in patients with intracerebral hemorrhage with and without intraventricular extension. J Neurointerv Surg 4: 358–363.
27. Gerlach UA, Pascher A (2012) Technical advances for abdominal wall closure after intestinal and multivisceral transplantation. Current Opinion in Organ Transplantation 17: 258–267.
28. Kadkhodayan Y, Delgado Almandoz JE, Kelly JE, Kale SP, Jagadeesan BD, et al. (2012) Yield of catheter angiography in patients with intracerebral hemorrhage with and without intraventricular extension. J Neurointervent Surg 4: 358–363.
29. Toffol GJ, Biller J, Adams HP Jr, Smoker WR (1986) The predicted value of arteriography in nontraumatic intracerebral hemorrhage. Stroke 17: 881–883.

30. Oleinik A, Romero JM, Schwab K, Lev MH, Jhawar N, et al. (2009) CT angiography for intracerebral hemorrhage does not increase risk of acute nephropathy. Stroke 40: 2393–2397.
31. Tippins RB, Torres WE, Baumgartner BR, Baumgarten DA (2000) Are screening serum creatinine levels necessary prior to outpatient CT examinations? Radiology 216: 481–484.
32. Lima FO, Lev MH, Levy RA, Silva GS, Ebril M, et al. (2010) Functional contrast-enhanced CT for evaluation of acute ischemic stroke does not increase the risk of contrast-induced nephropathy. AJNR Am J Neuroradiol 31: 817–821.
33. Olsen JC, Salomon B (1996) Utility of the creatinine prior to intravenous contrast studies in the emergency department. J Emerg Med 14: 543–546.
34. Aulicky P, Mikulik R, Goldemund D, Reif M, Dufek M, et al. (2010) Safety of performing CT angiography in stroke patients treated with intravenous thrombolysis. J Neurol Neurosurg Psychiatry 81: 783–787.
35. Hopyan JJ, Gladstone DJ, Mallia G, Schiff J, Fox AJ, et al. (2008) Renal safety of CT angiography and perfusion imaging in the emergency evaluation of acute stroke. AJNR Am J Neuroradiol 29: 1826–1830.
36. Krol AL, Dzialowski I, Roy J, Puetz V, Subramaniam S, et al. (2007) Incidence of radiocontrast nephropathy in patients undergoing acute stroke computed tomography angiography. Stroke 38: 2364–2366.
37. ACR Committee on Drugs and Contrast Medoa (2013) ACR Manual on Contrast Media. Version 9. American College of Radiology.
38. Bruce RJ, Djamali A, Shinki K, Michel SJ, Fine JP, et al. (2009) Background fluctuation of kidney function versus contrast-induced nephrotoxicity. AJR Am J Roentgenol 192: 711–718.
39. Cramer BC, Parfrey PS, Hutchinson TA, Baran D, Melanson DM, et al. (1985) Renal function following infusion of radiologic contrast material. A prospective controlled study. Arch Intern Med 145: 87–89.
40. Heller CA, Knapp J, Halliday J, O'Connell D, Heller RF (1991) Failure to demonstrate contrast nephrotoxicity. Med J Aust 155: 329–332.
41. Langner S, Stumpe S, Kirsch M, Petrik M, Hosten N (2008) No increased risk for contrast-induced nephropathy after multiple CT perfusion studies of the brain with a nonionic, dimeric, iso-osmolal contrast medium. AJNR Am J Neuroradiol 29: 1525–1529.
42. McGillicuddy EA, Schuster KM, Kaplan LJ, Maung AA, Lui FY, et al. (2010) Contrast-induced nephropathy in elderly trauma patients. J Trauma 68: 294–297.
43. Tremblay LN, Tien H, Hamilton P, Brenneman FD, Rizoli SB, et al. (2005) Risk and benefit of intravenous contrast in trauma patients with an elevated serum creatinine. J Trauma 59: 1162–1166; discussion 1166–1167.
44. Young KC, Kelly AG, Holloway RG (In Press) Reading a Cost-effectiveness or Decision Analysis Study: 5 Things to Consider. Neurology: Clinical Practice 3: 413–420.
45. Delgado Almandoz JE, Schaefer PW, Goldstein JN, Rosand J, Lev MH, et al. (2010) Practical scoring system for the identification of patients with intracerebral hemorrhage at highest risk of harboring an underlying vascular etiology: the Secondary Intracerebral Hemorrhage Score. AJNR AmJNeuroradiol 31: 1653–1660.
46. Vermeer SE, Algra A, Franke CL, Koudstaal PJ, Rinkel GJ (2002) Long-term prognosis after recovery from primary intracerebral hemorrhage. Neurology 59: 205–209.
47. (2012) Reimbursement Information for CT Perfusion in the Diagnosis of Acute Stroke. Available: http://www3.gehealthcare.com/en/Products/~/media/Downloads/us/Product/Reimbursement/Customer-Advisories/GEHealthcare-Customer-Advisory_CT-Perfusion-Diagnosis-Acute-Stroke-Reimbursement-Info-2012.pdf. Accessed March 21, 2013.
48. (2011) 2011 Medicare Physician Fee Schedule Payment Rates: Angiography/Vascular Procedures. Available: http://www.medical.siemens.com/siemens/en_US/rg_marcom_FBAs/files/Reimbursement/Angio_2011_Final_MPFS_Payment_Rates.pdf. Accessed March 21, 2013.
49. Kilaru S, Korn P, Kasirajan K, Lee TY, Beavers FP, et al. (2003) Is carotid angioplasty and stenting more cost effective than carotid endarterectomy? J Vasc Surg 37: 331–339.

23

Characterization of a Spontaneous Retinal Neovascular Mouse Model

Eiichi Hasegawa[1,2], Harry Sweigard[1,2], Deeba Husain[1,2], Ana M. Olivares[3], Bo Chang[4], Kaylee E. Smith[1], Amy E. Birsner[5], Robert J. D'Amato[2,5], Norman A. Michaud[1], Yinan Han[3], Demetrios G. Vavvas[1,2], Joan W. Miller[1,2], Neena B. Haider[2,3], Kip M. Connor[1,2]*

1 Angiogenesis Laboratory, Department of Ophthalmology, Massachusetts Eye & Ear Infirmary, Boston, Massachusetts, United States of America, **2** Department of Ophthalmology, Harvard Medical School, Boston, Massachusetts, United States of America, **3** Schepens Eye Research Institute, Massachusetts Eye & Ear Infirmary, Boston, Massachusetts, United States of America, **4** The Jackson Laboratory, Bar Harbor, Maine, United States of America, **5** Vascular Biology Program, Department of Surgery, Boston Children's Hospital, Harvard Medical School, Boston, Massachusetts, United States of America

Abstract

Background: Vision loss due to vascular disease of the retina is a leading cause of blindness in the world. Retinal angiomatous proliferation (RAP) is a subgroup of neovascular age-related macular degeneration (AMD), whereby abnormal blood vessels develop in the retina leading to debilitating vision loss and eventual blindness. The novel mouse strain, neoretinal vascularization 2 (NRV2), shows spontaneous fundus changes associated with abnormal neovascularization. The purpose of this study is to characterize the induction of pathologic angiogenesis in this mouse model.

Methods: The NRV2 mice were examined from postnatal day 12 (p12) to 3 months. The phenotypic changes within the retina were evaluated by fundus photography, fluorescein angiography, optical coherence tomography, and immunohistochemical and electron microscopic analysis. The pathological neovascularization was imaged by confocal microscopy and reconstructed using three-dimensional image analysis software.

Results: We found that NRV2 mice develop multifocal retinal depigmentation in the posterior fundus. Depigmented lesions developed vascular leakage observed by fluorescein angiography. The spontaneous angiogenesis arose from the retinal vascular plexus at postnatal day (p)15 and extended toward retinal pigment epithelium (RPE). By three months of age, histological analysis revealed encapsulation of the neovascular lesion by the RPE in the photoreceptor cell layer and subretinal space.

Conclusions: The NRV2 mouse strain develops early neovascular lesions within the retina, which grow downward towards the RPE beginning at p15. This retinal neovascularization model mimics early stages of human retinal angiomatous proliferation (RAP) and will likely be a useful in elucidating targeted therapeutics for patients with ocular neovascular disease.

Editor: Michael E. Boulton, Indiana University College of Medicine, United States of America

Funding: Research reported in this publication was supported by a Special Scholar Award (to KMC) and unrestricted grant (to JM) from Research to Prevent Blindness, as well as a Bright Focus Foundation grant (to KMC and NH). Additionally, research reported in this publication was supported by National Eye Institute of the National Institutes of Health under award numbers R01EY022084/S1 (to KMC) and P30EY014104. The content is solely the responsibility of the authors and does not necessarily represent the official views of the National Institutes of Health. The funders had no role in study design, data collection and analysis, decision to publish, or preparation of the manuscript.

* Email: kip_connor@meei.harvard.edu

Introduction

Vision loss due to vascular disease of the retina is a leading cause of blindness in the world and affects all age groups. Neovascularization is a hallmark of complex, polygenic diseases, such as retinopathy of prematurity, proliferative diabetic retinopathy, and age-related macular degeneration (AMD). AMD, affects 1 in 3 individuals over age 65, occurs in two forms: exudative ("wet") and nonexudative ("dry"). Advanced exudative AMD is defined by the formation of abnormal blood vessels that grow from the choroidal vasculature, through breaks in Bruch's membrane, into the outer retina [1]. Less commonly, the abnormal vessels originate from retinal vasculature and can form a retinal–choroidal anastomosis (RCA) with the choroidal vascular bed [1–4]. These blood vessels are immature and leaky, resulting in subretinal and intraretinal edema and hemorrhage, which leads to vision loss [1,5]. Neovascular AMD accounts for 10–15% of AMD cases, and if left untreated, rapidly leads to substantial vision loss [1,6]. In recent years, a subgroup of neovascular AMD coined as retinal angiomatous proliferation (RAP) has been described where the disease starts as neovessels originating from the retinal vascular bed and grow towards the outer retina, ultimately forming choroidal neovascularization [7–9]. RAP [9], has been classified into three stages: stage I, when intraretinal neovascularization (IRN) arises from the deep capillary vascular plexus within the retina; stage II, is determined by growth of these abnormal retinal vessels into the subretinal space to form subretinal neovascularization (SRN); and Stage III occurs when choroidal neovascularization is observed, retinal–choroidal anastomosis (RCA) is a persistent feature of this stage. While it is well known that RAP follows a different natural course and response to treatment from typical neovascular AMD [10], there are few established models that allow us to fully understand the disease pathophysiology or to test new treatments for RAP [11,12].

There are several animal models of retinal neovascularization [13–17], however, the precise molecular mechanism of RAP remains to be elucidated. The neoretinal vascularization (NRV) 2 mouse line, also called JR5558 mice, was discovered through The Jackson Laboratory Eye Mutant Screening program, which has identified a large number of new mouse models that exhibit unique eye phenotypes [18]. In this study, we characterize a novel mutant mouse model, NRV2, which appear to have a recessive mode of inheritance characterized by multiple areas of retinal depigmentation and vascular leakage in the posterior fundus. In this study, we focused on the characterization of the early ocular phenotype and etiology of angiogenesis in NRV2 mice. We discovered that depigmentation and neovascularization occur spontaneously and are concurrent with the presence of the abnormal blood vessels in the photoreceptor cell layer of the retina. Furthermore, NRV2 neovascularization originates from the retinal vascular plexus and grows outwards to the subretinal space, forming neovascularization structures at the RPE Bruch's membrane interface and mimicking the early clinical presentation of RAP in humans. This genetic model of retinal neovascularization will provide a significant tool that will aid in our understanding of the molecular causes of retinal neovascular disease as well as in developing preclinical therapeutics.

Materials and Methods

Animals

JR5558 mice were obtained from The Jackson Laboratory (Bar Harbor, ME) and named neoretinal vascularization 2 (NRV2) mice. As far as we have observed, there is close to 100% penetrance of the ocular phenotype in this strain and we have not found any other gross abnormalities in other organ systems to date. All animal procedures adhered to the Association for Research in Vision and Ophthalmology Statement for the Use of Animals in Ophthalmic and Vision Research. The Animal Care and Use Committee of Massachusetts Eye and Ear Infirmary approved the protocol for experiments outlined herein. The n's expressed are reflective of an individual mouse, not an individual eye.

Fundus photography

Fundus images were taken using the Micron III Retinal Imaging Microscope (Phoenix Research Laboratories, Pleasanton, CA). Mice were anesthetized with Avertin (Sigma, St. Louis, MO) and placed on the 37°C heating pad to keep body temperature. The pupils were dilated with 5% phenylephrine and 0.5% tropicamide. Images were taken by attaching cornea covered with 2.5% Goniovisc (HUB Pharmaceuticals, Rancho Cucamonga, CA) to the Micron camera lens using the StreamPix software (Phoenix Research Laboratories, Pleasanton, CA).

Fluorescein angiography

Fluorescein angiography (FA) was performed using a Micron III Retinal Imaging system directly following imaging of the fundus. Fluorescein images were captured at 3–5 minutes after i.p. injection of 0.1 ml of 2% fluorescein sodium (Akorn, Lake Forest, IL) and used to quantify the number of the vascular leakage areas. The images were captured at 1, 3–5 and 10 minutes after injection to define the time course of vascular leakage over time.

Spectral Domain Optical Coherence Tomography (SD-OCT)

OCT images were taken using the Micron III Retinal Imaging Microscope. OCT images were taken by line scan under the guide of bright or Fluorescein field. The line scan is made up of a series of 1024 single point A-scans.

Histology

Eyes were enucleated and fixed with Methanol/Acetic acid (3:1) overnight at 4°C. Tissues were paraffin embedded. Serial 5 μm thick sections were cut and stained with hematoxylin and eosin (H&E), examined under bright field light microscopy.

Immunohistochemical Staining and 3D reconstruction of retinal vascular structure

Eyes were enucleated and fixed in 4% paraformaldehyde for 1 hour at room temperature. Retinas were isolated and blocked in PBS with 0.5% Triton X-100 and 5% goat serum. Retinas were rinsed in PBS, permeabilized overnight at 4°C with 0.5% Triton X-100 in PBS, and stained overnight with FITC-conjugated G. simplicifolia isolectin B4 (Alexa Fluor 488-I21411, 1:100 dilution; Life Technologies, Carlsbad, CA) in 1 mM $CaCl_2$ in PBS. After 2 hours of washes, retinas were whole-mounted onto microscope slides (Superfrost/Plus; Fisher Scientific, Pittsburgh, PA) with the photoreceptor side down and embedded in reagent (PermaFluor; Thermo Scientific, Fremont, CA). Retinal wholemounts were visualized with a confocal microscope (SP5; Leica, Wetzlar, Germany). Retinal vascular structures were reconstructed with Amira 5.2 software (Visualization Sciences Group, Burlington, MA) from the pictures taken by the confocal microscope.

Electron microscopy

Eyes were enucleated and cleaned of all extraneous tissue then rinsed with saline. Eyes were immediately placed into fixative consisting of 2.5% gluteraldehyde and 2% formaldehyde in 0.1 M cacodylate buffer with 0.08 M $CaCl_2$ at 4°C. After a short 10 to 15 minute fixation, eyes were bisected at the limbus and the anterior segment was separated from the posterior segment and the parts to be examined were placed back in the fixative. Within 24 hours of enucleation, the tissues were washed in 0.1 M cacodylate buffer and stored at 4°C. The tissues were post-fixed for 1.5 hours in 2% aqueous OsO_4. The tissues were dehydrated in graded ethanols, transitioned in propylene oxide, infiltrated with propylene oxide and epon mixtures (tEpon, Tousimis) embedded in epon and cured for 24–48 hours at 60°C. One-micron sections were cut on a Leica Ultracut UCT and stained with 1% toluidine blue in 1% borate buffer. Areas selected from the 1 micron thick sections were further sectioned at 70–90 nm, stained with saturated Uranyl Acetate and Sato's lead stain and examined with a Philips CM-10 electron microscope.

ELISAs for VEGF and sFLT-1

The retina tissue was homogenized with a lysis buffer (Roche Diagnostics) containing protease inhibitors (Roche Diagnostics), and the homogenates were centrifuged at 16,200×*g* for 10 min at 4°C. The amounts of VEGF and sFLT-1 protein were assayed using ELISA systems (R&D Systems).

Statistical analysis

Data are presented as means ± SEM and were analyzed with Student t test for comparisons between two groups. P value of < 0.05 was considered statistically significant.

Results

Depigmentation and vascular leakage observed in retinas of NRV2 mice

A longitudinal study was conducted to determine the onset and progression of clinical manifestations of neovascular disease in NRV2 mice. Fundus exams were performed using a fundus imaging microscope at postnatal day p17 through postnatal day p35. Diffuse areas of depigmentation were observed in the retina beginning at p17 (Fig. 1A, Fig. S1A, B). Depigmented areas begin to become more focal in nature and increase in number at p21 (Fig. 1B). The lesions become well demarcated and larger in size at p25 (Fig. 1C). After p25, these areas become more diffuse in nature (Fig. 1D, E, Fig. S1E, F). Vascular leakage was detected by fluorescein angiography (FA). No leakage is observed at p17 (Fig. 1F, Fig. S1C, D). The vascular leakage pattern follows the appearance of retinal depigmentation becoming evident at p21 (Fig. 1G) and peaks at p25, corresponding with the height of focal depigmentation in these animals (Fig. 1H). The areas of depigmentation correlated with the development of vascular leakage, indicating a vascular component to this disease phenotype. As with the focal depigmentation, fluorescein leakage gradually decreased after p25 (Fig. 1I, J, Fig. S1G, H). Early, moderate and late phase fluorescein angiograms were performed to determine the degree of vascular leakage in NRV2 mice. At p25, early leakage was observed that became both brighter and larger in size as time progressed to the late phase of the angiogram, indicating active neovascularization (Fig. 2A–C). At p31, minimal leakage was observed from the onset of the angiogram, which persisted through the late phase without any further increase in leakage (Fig. 2D–F), indicating that vascular leakage develops fairly early in these mice at p25 and begins to resolve by p31. Longitudinal fundus analysis from p21 through 16 weeks revealed both the number of depigmentation areas (Fig. 3A) and FA leakage areas (Fig. 3B) peaked at p25. By day 31 the areas of depigmentation became more diffuse and enlarged, but the vascular leakage largely subsided (Fig. 3A, B).

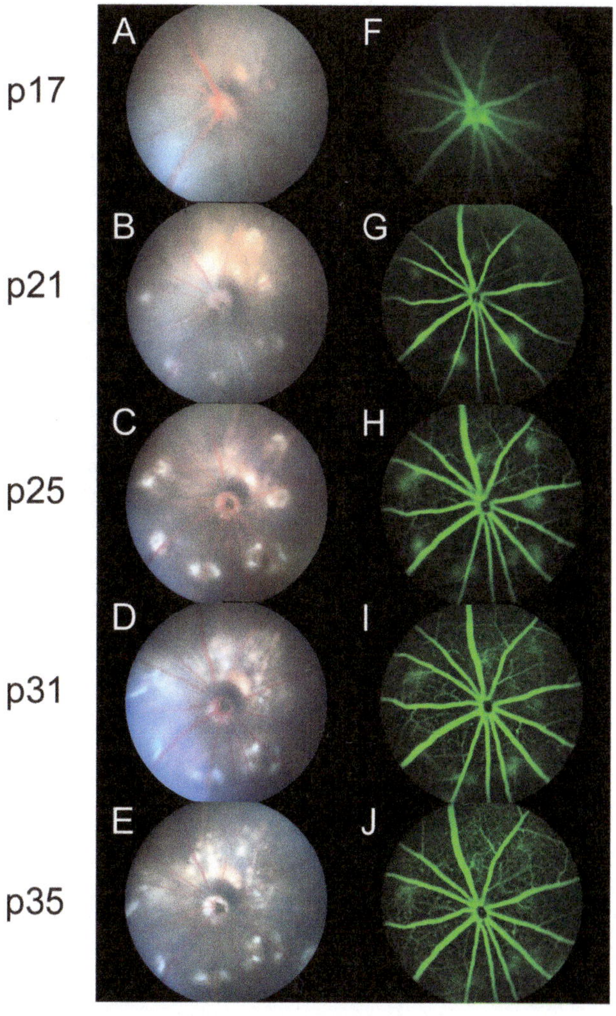

Figure 1. Time course representing the morphological changes found in the fundus of NRV2 mice. Fundus photographs and fluorescein angiography of NRV2 mice from p17 to p35. *(A–E)* Fundus images show the emergence of depigmented regions at p17 that increase in size and number through p35. *(F–J)* Fluorescein angiography indicates vascular leakage corresponding to the areas of depigmentation, peaking at p25 and subsiding by p35. n = 10, Representative images are shown. p = postnatal day.

Spectral domain optical coherence tomography reveals dysmorphic outer and inner retinal layers

Spectral domain optical coherence tomography (SD-OCT) allows for a detailed, noninvasive evaluation of the retinal architecture *in vivo*, and has been found to accurately reflect retinal morphological changes that occur during retinal disease progression. We followed lesion development in the NRV2 mouse by SD-OCT at p17, p21, and p25. Depigmentation areas first appear at p17, however, no vascular leakage is evident on FA (Fig. 4A, B). In the SD-OCT, a disruption is apparent in the outer plexiform layer (OPL) and a highly reflective lesion is present in the inner segment/outer segment (IS/OS) (Fig. 4C). As the lesion develops from p21–p25, the depigmentation area becomes more prominent (Fig. 4D, G) and is associated with increased vascular leakage (Fig. 4E, H) The SD-OCT assessment reveals enlargement of the subretinal and inner segment/outer segment (IS/OS) zone along with a highly reflective area and persistent irregularity of the ONL and OPL (arrows, Fig. 4C, F, I).

Retinal neovascular development in the NRV2 mouse originates in the inner retina and extends outwards to the RPE

Fundus characterization of the NRV2 eye strongly indicates the presence of neovascular structures within retina. Retinal histology was performed on NRV2 ocular tissue to determine the origin of the neovascularization. Normal retina (Fig. 5A, B and Fig. S2) was compared to retinal areas with lesions in the NRV2 mouse. Retinal cross-sections revealed the presence of lesions containing a lumenal structure near photoreceptor outer segments (Fig. 5C, D). The abnormal vascular structure appears to originate from the deep layer of the retinal vascular plexus, at the outer edge of the inner nuclear layer (INL). Neovessels descend into the outer nuclear layer (ONL), which is typically an avascular area, and then

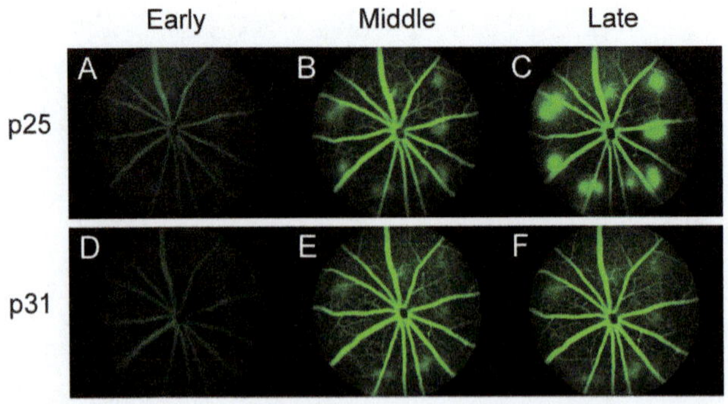

Figure 2. Vascular leakage in retinal lesions of NRV2 mice during postnatal development. Fluorescein angiography images taken of NRV2 mice at the early through late phases after fluorescein injection for p25 and p31. (*A–C*) At p25 NRV2 mice have increased vascular leakage through the late phase of fluorescein angiography, compare B and C. (*D–F*) By p31, there is reduced vascular leakage relative to p25, that does not increase from the middle to late phase of fluorescein angiography, compare E and F. Early = 1 minute after fluorescein injection, middle = 3–5 minutes after fluorescein injection, late = 10 minutes after fluorescein injection. n = 10, Representative images are shown. p = postnatal day.

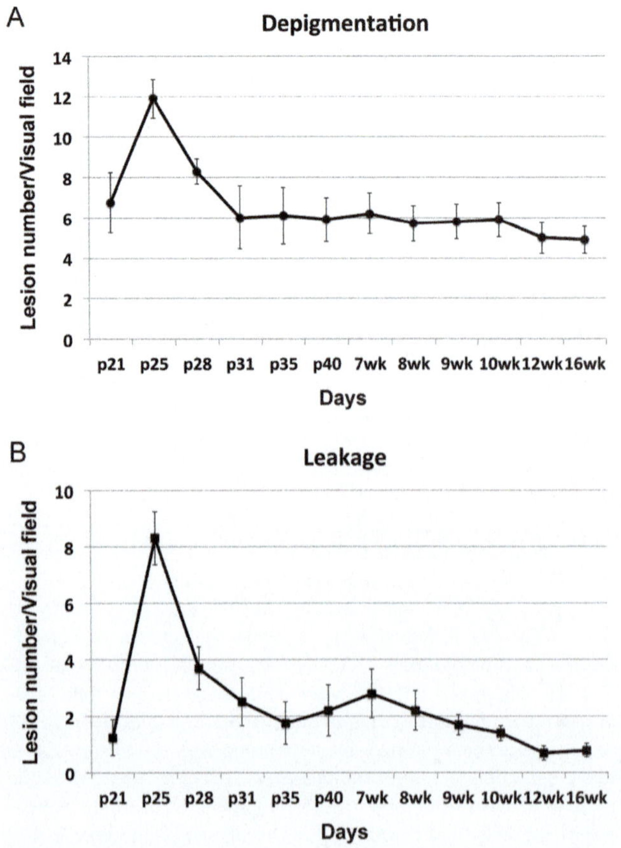

Figure 3. The peak time for depigmentation and vascular leakage in NRV2 mice is at p25. Developmental time course of depigmentation and vascular leakage assessed by funduscopy and fluorescein angiography in NRV2 mice. (*A*) Quantitation of the number of depigmented regions observed by fundus imaging. The peak number of depigmented regions occurs at p25, followed by a relative stabilization. (*B*) Quantitation of the number of fluorescein angiography leakage, measured by the number of leakage regions, also peaks at p25. Each plot on the graph is an average of 10 eyes, p = postnatal day.

reach the RPE and spread, initially, above the RPE (Fig. 5E, F). The RPE and choriocapillaris appear normal in these sections. These findings are supported by our SD-OCT images, which show abnormal structures originating from the OPL and extending into the subretinal space (Fig. 4C, D). However, it still remained unclear if these vessels originated from the retinal vasculature or if they were of choroidal origin, which subsequently anastamosed to the outer retinal plexus. We assessed the formation of the subretinal neovascular lesions in retinal flatmounts stained with isolectin to gain a more complete understanding of the origin of these vessels. A confocal z-stack was taken through the retina and the vasculature was reconstructed into three-dimensional models using Amira software. We assessed eyes at p12, p15, p17, p21 and p25 in order to capture the development of these lesions. At p12, normal reticulated retinal vasculature was present in the INL and no abnormal vessels were observed in the ONL (Fig. 6B). In contrast, beginning at p15, neovessels begin to grow and extend into the ONL from the INL (Fig. 6C, movie S1). These vessels continued to extend downward until they reach the RPE, where they balloon above the RPE from p17 through p25 (Fig. 6C–E, movie S2, S3).

Transmission electron microscopy (TEM) of NRV2 reveals lesion architecture and development

Morphological features at the RPE-Bruch's interface were assessed using electron microscopy to further delineate ultrastructural characteristics of NRV2 neovascular lesions. The outer segments, RPE, Bruch's membrane, and choriocapillaris are well organized in C57BL/6 mice (Fig. 7A). In contrast, new vessels are evident at the photoreceptor outer segment-RPE interface at p21 in NRV2 mice (Fig. 7B). Here the outer segments appear disorganized (damaged and or missing) and are lacking their typical morphologic structure (Fig. 7B). Two new vessels are observed among the outer segments above the RPE and choriocapillaris, which appear normal at p21 (Fig. 7B). Higher magnification of the lesion identifies pericytes that are clearly evident around the new vessels in these lesions (Fig. 7C). These new vessel structures are also observed in 3 months old NRV2 mice. However, by 3 months of age, the RPE layer is disrupted and proliferating RPE cells have enveloped the neovascular lesion (Fig. 7D).

Interestingly, there are infoldings of the RPE at the surface of the cell in contact with the new vessels (Fig. 7E). The new vessels in turn show fenestrations along this contact area, mimicking the usual RPE- choriocapillaris interaction (Fig. 7F). Some of these new vessels are located directly over the Bruch's membrane without an intervening RPE layer (Fig. 7G). Bruch's membrane appeared intact and the choriocapillaris seemed normal at all time points as seen by Fig. 1C, by light microscopy and TEM using step sections.

It is well known that vascular endothelial growth factor (VEGF) is a potent inducer of intraocular neovascularization [19]. Several clinical studies have demonstrated that Anti-VEGF monotherapy has a certain inhibitory effect to RAP progression [20–22]. On the other hand, soluble FLT-1 (also known as soluble VEGF receptor-1) is a natural inhibitor of VEGF, which is produced in the photoreceptor layer [23]. It binds VEGF and regulates VEGF-mediated angiogenesis [24–26]. Both suppression of sFLT-1 by neutralizing antibodies and conditional knockdown of sFLT-1 in photoreceptor cells increased VEGF levels and caused vessels to enter the normally avascular photoreceptor layer [23]. We assessed the levels of VEGF and sFLT-1 in the retina of NRV2

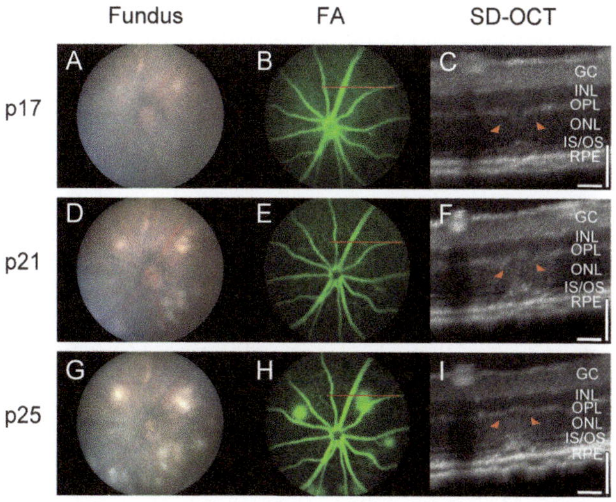

Figure 4. Vascular leakage corresponds to disturbances in the outer plexiform and outer nuclear layers of the retina. Images showing the representative time course of lesion development in a NRV2 mouse. (*A–C*) Fundus image taken at p17, showing areas that have slight depigmentation, at the 1 o'clock position of the image (*A*, left panel). In the same area, vascular leakage can be seen by fluorescein angiography (*B*, middle panel). Examination by SD-OCT at the region of vascular leakage (red bar in *B*) reveals a disturbance in the ONL and OPL of the retina (*C*, right panel). Arrowheads point to the retinal disturbance. (*D–F*) Fundus image taken at p21, of the same mouse, shows increased depigmentation at the 1 o'clock position of the image (*D*, left panel). In the same area vascular leakage can be seen by fluorescein angiography (*E*, middle panel). Examination by SD-OCT at the region of vascular leakage (red bar in *E*) reveals a disturbance in the ONL and OPL of the retina (*F*, right panel). Arrowheads point to the retinal disturbance. (*G–I*) Fundus image of the same mouse taken at p25, the height of leakage in NRV2 mice, shows depigmentation, at the 1 o'clock position of the image (*G*, left panel). In the same area, vascular leakage is pronounced compared to the earlier time points as seen by fluorescein angiography (*H*, middle panel). Examination by SD-OCT at the region of vascular leakage (red bar in *H*) reveals a disturbance in the ONL and OPL of the retina (*I*, right panel). Arrowheads point to the retinal disturbance. p = postnatal day, GC: ganglion cells; INL: inner nuclear layer; OPL: outer plexiform layer; ONL: outer nuclear layer; IS/OS: photoreceptor inner segment/outer segments. n = 10, Representative images are shown. Scale bars: 50 μm.

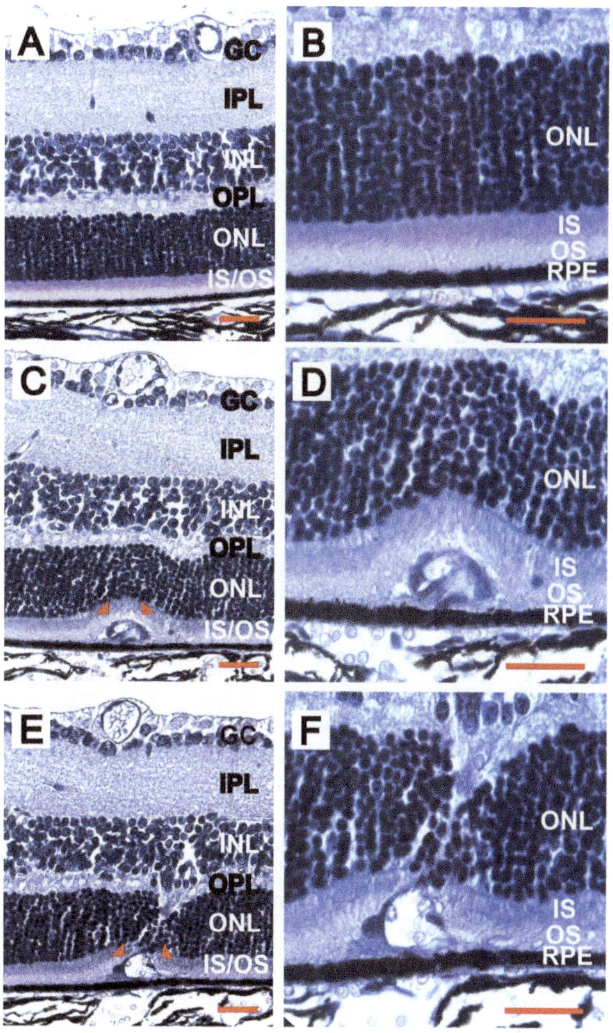

Figure 5. Neovessels extend from the INL to the RPE in NRV2 mice. Retinal cross-sections stained by H&E through a neovascular lesion. (*A*) Cross-section from a C57Bl6 mouse showing the normal architecture of the retinal layers. (*B*) Higher magnification of (*A*) focusing on the normal architecture between the ONL and RPE interface. (*C*) Cross section from an NRV2 mouse at p25, showing a disturbance in the outer retina. (*D*) Higher magnification of (*C*) to show that the lesion is at the interface of the ONL and RPE, in the outer segments of the photoreceptors. (*E*) Retinal cross-section from another NRV2 mouse at p25, capturing the track of a neovessel spanning from the INL to the RPE. (*F*) Higher magnification of (*E*) showing the vessel extending through the ONL. Arrowheads in (*C*) and (*E*) indicate the lesion areas that are magnified in (*D*) and (*F*). GC: ganglion cells; IPL: inner plexiform layer; INL: inner nuclear layer; OPL: outer plexiform layer; ONL: outer nuclear layer; IS/OS: photoreceptor inner segment/outer segments. n = 3, Representative images are shown. Scale bars: 25 μm.

mice during disease progression. VEGF levels of NRV2 mice were significantly higher than those of C57BL/6 control mice (Fig. S3A). However, there was no significant difference between the sFLT-1 levels in the retina of NRV2 mice and those of C57BL/6 mice (Fig. S3B), suggesting that overexpression of VEGF in the retina is involved in the cause of retinal angiogenesis in NRV2 mice.

Discussion

In the present study, we characterized a novel mouse model of ocular neovascular disease, NRV2, by fundus, histological, and ultrastructural analysis. As shown in Figure 1–3, NRV2 mice spontaneously develop retinal depigmentation and vascular leakage in the fundus during early postnatal days. The NRV2 phenotype is bilateral with no bias for gender observed. Additionally, gross observation revealed no differences in other organs. Histological analysis revealed abnormal vessel structures present from the outer plexiform layer to the retinal pigment epithelium (Fig. 5C–F). Moreover, three-dimensional reconstruction of the retinal vasculature at p15 clearly demonstrates that these neovessels originate from the deep retinal vascular plexus in the outer plexiform layer, which grow through the outer retina towards the subretinal space between p17–p25 (Fig. 6). SD-OCT examination captured balloon-like neovessel structures in the photoreceptor cell layer (Fig. 4C, F, I). We could not identify any vascular structures of choroidal origin and three-dimensional reconstruction images of vasculature did not show vessels growing up from the choroidal vascular bed into the retina's ONL layer. Our findings indicate that the retinal origin of angiogenesis in NRV2 mice is consistent with stage 1 and stage 2 of human RAP

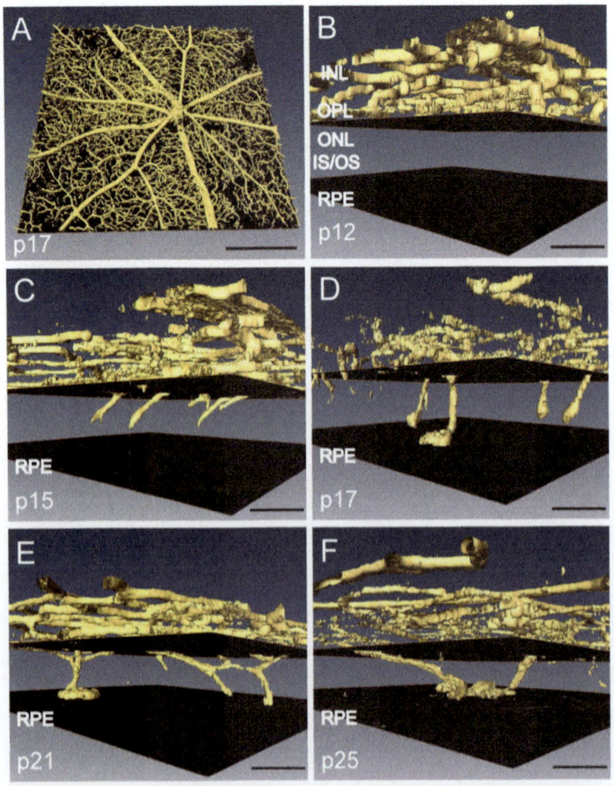

Figure 6. Neovessels originate from the INL and grow towards the RPE in NRV2 mice. Retinal cross-sections stained with isolectin B4 that have been reconstructed into 3D images (Amira software) using confocal Z stacks to show the development of retinal blood vessels in NRV2 mice. (*A*) Low magnification overview of the 3D reconstruction of a retinal flatmount stained with isolectin B4 for blood vessels. (*B–F*) High magnification images of retinal cross-sections from NRV2 mice stained with isolectin B4 that have been reconstructed into a 3D montage. (*B*) At p12, there are only vessels in the INL with no apparent irregular vessel development. (*C*) At p15, vessels are found extending from the INL towards the RPE cell layer. (*D*) At p17, the vessels have reached the RPE interface. (*E*) At p21, vessels have mostly interfaced with the RPE cell layer and have begun to expand across the surface of the RPE. (*F*) At p25, the vessels have fully interacted with the RPE and formed balloon like structures. p = postnatal day, INL: inner nuclear layer; OPL: outer plexiform layer; ONL: outer nuclear layer; IS/OS: photoreceptor inner segment/outer segments. The upper black square shows the border of the OPL and ONL. The lower black square shows the interface of the RPE layer. n = 3/timepoint, Representative images are shown. Scale bars: (*A*): 500 μm, (*B–F*): 50 μm.

as defined by Yannuzzi et al [9]. Contrary to our findings, Nagai N et al. concluded that the neovessels in this mouse model originate from choriocapillaris [27]. They identify vascular structures in the subretinal space by immunohistochemical and histological analysis. Our ultrastrucutural analysis revealed that NRV2 neovessels proliferate into the subretinal space, located between the RPE and photoreceptor cell layer (Fig. 7B). As the neovascular lesions age, the neovessels become encapsulated by RPE (Fig. 7D) and likely blocks the fluorescein leakage initially seen from p21 to p25 (Fig. 1). Moreover, it was also observed that the neovessels can descend to the border of Bruch's membrane at three months with no RPE cells or processes between the vessels and Bruch's membrane (Fig. 7G). However, no breaks in Bruch's membrane were ever identified in serial light or electron microscopic sections and the choriocapillaris morphology was normal. These findings further suggest that neovessels in NRV2 mice are of retinal origin and the growth of the neovessels into the subretinal space corresponds to the stage 2 of human RAP. Müller cells play an important role for retinal homeostasis [28]. Recently, it has been shown that ablation of Müller cells results in intraretinal neovascularization and vascular leakage [29]. However, in NRV2 mice, GFAP positive glial cells accumulated close to the neovascular area in the retina [27]. They might have pro-angiogenic effects in this mouse strain because Müller cells are also known to be a source of VEGF and TNF in hypoxic or inflammatory conditions [30]. The role of Müller cells in NRV2 mice remains to be elucidated.

Interestingly, the NRV2 neovessels were found to have fenestrations similar to the choriocapillaris (Fig. 7E, F). Previous reports show that RPE cells play an essential role in the development and maintenance of fenestrated choroidal vasculature [31]. RPE cells are also reported to have the ability to induce fenestrations in endothelial cells of retinal vessels by encapsulating them [32]. Given these prior findings, we propose that these retinal neovessels originate from the deep retinal vascular plexus and extend downward through the retina until they reach the RPE where they proliferate until RPE cells encapsulate the lesions, isolating them from the retinal microenvironment.

Yannuzzi et al. proposed three-stages of retinal angiomatous proliferation in AMD [9]. They considered the origin of the neovascularization in RAP to be derived from the inner retina. In the early stage of RAP, angiomatous proliferation arises spontaneously from intraretinal capillaries. During the second stage, the intraretinal neovessels extends outwards into the subretinal space. Finally, choroidal neovascularization occurs and forms retinal-choroidal anastomoses. In contrast, Gass et al. [33] suggested that focal atrophy of the RPE and type 1 occult choroidal neovascularization under the RPE are the initial lesions of RAP. These lesions permit the retinal neovasculature to infiltrate into the outer retina and form chorioretinal anastomoses with the original type 1 occult choroidal vessel. Using immunohistochemistry, Shimada et al. demonstrated the existence of intraretinal neovascularization, but not choroidal neovascularization, in excised RAP specimens from patients with stage 2 RAP [34]. They also showed that both choroidal neovascularization and chorioretinal anastomosis existed in the stage 3 RAP specimens. Their histopahological findings supported Yannuzzi's original hypothesis, in which RAP originates from the inner retina [9].

Several mouse models have been reported to show RCA, which is seen in stage 3 of RAP [35–37]. Very low-density lipoprotein receptor (VLDLR) knock out mice begin to show abnormal retinal blood vessels originating from the outer plexiform layer and grow into the subretinal space around p14 [35], which is similar to the process of NRV2 mice. In the VLDLR knock out mouse model, RCA occurs approximately at 10 months of age and RPE cells surround the vessels [36]. Additionally, photoreceptor degeneration and the loss of the ONL were also observed [36]. In contrast, the neovascularization in mice lacking CYP27A1, which is the principal cholesterol hydroxylase in the retina, occurred in both retina and choroid [37]. This angiogenesis process was detected around 1.5 months. The major abnormalities included dilated blood vessels in the OPL and thickened fibrovascular structures between the RPE and Bruch's membrane. The RCA formation was observed at 11 months, which is later than VLDLR knock out mice. This angiogenesis process might be more representative of Gass's original hypothesis [33]. Electron microscopy of NRV2 mice revealed significant RPE disturbances in the lesion of these animals (Fig. 7D). The changes of RPE morphology would be consistent with decreased oxygen supply to the outer retina due to

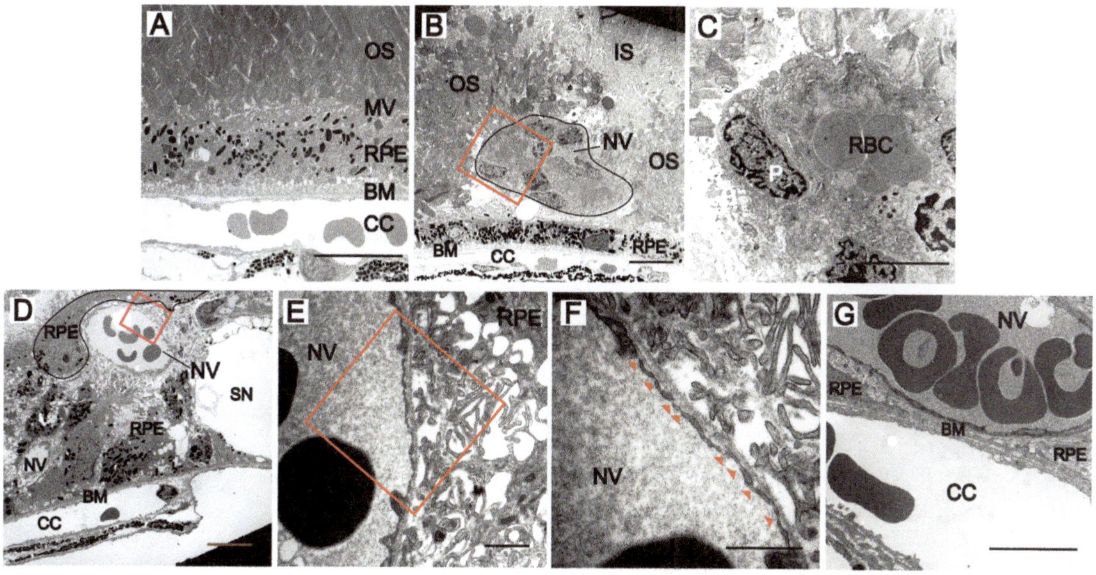

Figure 7. Neovessels that interface with the RPE form characteristic morphological features of more mature vessels. Electron micrographs taken of NRV2 mice illustrate commonly observed morphological findings of neovessels when they come in contact with the RPE/Bruch's membrane. (*A*) Electron micrograph of a C57BL/6 mouse at 3 months of age shows the normal architecture of the outer retina. (*B*) Neovessels (outlined in black) from an NRV2 mouse at p21, surrounded by disorganized outer photoreceptor segments. (*C*) High magnification image (red box in *B*) that shows the presence of pericytes in the neovessels. (*D*) A 3 months old, NRV2 mouse with an RPE cell (outlined in black) surrounding the neovessel. (*E*) High magnification (red box in *D*) that shows a contact point between the neovessel and RPE cell. (*F*) Higher magnification (red box in *E*) of the contact point reveals fenestrations (arrowheads). (*G*) A 3 months old, NRV2 mouse where the neovessel has come in direct contact with the Bruch's membrane. IS: inner segment; OS: outer segment; MV: microvilli; BM: Bruch's membrane; CC: choriocapillaris; NV: new vessels; P: pericyte; n = 3/timepoint, Representative images are shown. Scale bars: (*A–D, G*): 5 μm, (*E, F*): 1 μm.

reduced diffusion from the choroidal capillaries, subsequently leading to a rise in the ischemic factors, inflammatory factors, and retinal angiogenesis in this mouse strain. However, we did not observe any features of choroidal involvement, as seen in RCA, at any of the time points examined in NRV2 mice. Further observation is needed to elucidate the progression of RCA in this mouse model.

In conclusion, the origin and progression of angiogenesis observed in the NRV2 mouse strain closely resembles human RAP. The underlying etiopathogenesis, including genetic etiology and mode of disease progression in patients with RAP, is not well defined, in spite of several mouse models of RCA. Therefore, future studies using the NRV2 mouse could include genetic analysis that defines the specific genes and pathways involved in the angiogenic process, along with the role of potential growth factors that guide the neovessels to extend from the inner retina towards the choroid. This study begins to define a novel mouse model of ocular neovascularization that could become an important tool in developing future anti-angiogenic therapies.

Supporting Information

Figure S1 The fundus morphological changes found in NRV2 mice. Fundus photographs and fluorescein angiography of NRV2 mice at p17 (*A–D*), 2 M (*E, G*) and 3 M (*F, H*). (*A, B*) Fundus images showed the emergence of depigmented regions at p17. (*C, D*) Fluorescein angiography did not show any vascular leakage corresponding to the areas of depigmentation at p17. (*E, F*) The depigmentation areas become faint at 2 M (*E*) and faded away at 3 M (*F*). (*G, H*) Fluorescein leakage almost disappeared after 2 M. Fluorescein angiography images were taken 3 minutes after fluorescein intraperitoneal injection; n = 5–10, Representative images are shown. p = postnatal day.

Figure S2 H&E section of normal C57BL/6 mouse retina. Retinal cross-sections of normal C57BL/6 mouse at p30 stained by H&E. (*A*) Cross-section from a C57BL/6 mouse showing the normal architecture of the retinal layers. (*B*) Higher magnification of (*A*) focusing on the normal architecture between the ONL and RPE interface. n = 3. Scale bars: 25 μm.

Figure S3 VEGF and sFLT-1 protein expression in the retina of NRV2 mice. (A) VEGF and (B) sFLT-1 protein concentration in the retina of NRV2 mice were quantified by ELISA and compared to age-matched C57BL/6 mice at several time points. (A) VEGF expression in NRV2 mice was significantly higher than C57BL/6 mice at p12, p17, p21, and p30. (B) sFLT-1 didn't show any significant differences between NRV2 and C57BL/6. n = 3/timepoint *$P<0.05$, **$P<0.01$.

Movie S1 The rotation image of 3D retinal vascular structure of NRV2 mouse at p15 from Figure 6C.

Movie S2 Confocal images were taken every 1 micron in the p25 retinal flat mount stained with isolectin B4. Images were compiled sequentially, from superficial layers to deep layers, into video format. These images were used for making the 3D images of Fig. 6F and Movie S3.

Movie S3 The rotation image of 3D retinal vascular structure of NRV2 mouse at p25 from Figure 6F.

Acknowledgments

Research reported in this publication was supported by a Special Scholar Award (to K.M.C.) and unrestricted grant (to J.W.M.) from Research to Prevent Blindness as well as a Bright Focus Foundation grant (K.M.C. and N.H.). Additionally, research reported in this publication was supported by *National Eye Institute* of the National Institutes of Health under award numbers: R01EY022084/S1 (K.M.C.) and P30EY014104. The content is solely the responsibility of the authors and does not necessarily represent the official views of the National Institutes of Health.

Author Contributions

Conceived and designed the experiments: EH DH NH KMC JM. Performed the experiments: EH NAM AMO HS KS YH KMC. Analyzed the data: EH AMO NAM KMC DH HS. Contributed reagents/materials/analysis tools: BC AEB RJD DGV. Contributed to the writing of the manuscript: EH HS DH NH KMC JM.

References

1. Lim LS, Mitchell P, Seddon JM, Holz FG, Wong TY (2012) Age-related macular degeneration. Lancet 379: 1728–1738.
2. Jager RD, Mieler WF, Miller JW (2008) Age-related macular degeneration. N Engl J Med 358: 2606–2617.
3. Zhang K, Zhang L, Weinreb RN (2012) Ophthalmic drug discovery: novel targets and mechanisms for retinal diseases and glaucoma. Nature reviews Drug discovery 11: 541–559.
4. Liakopoulos S, Ongchin S, Bansal A, Msutta S, Walsh AC, et al. (2008) Quantitative optical coherence tomography findings in various subtypes of neovascular age-related macular degeneration. Invest Ophthalmol Vis Sci 49: 5048–5054.
5. Gragoudas ES, Adamis AP, Cunningham ET, Jr., Feinsod M, Guyer DR (2004) Pegaptanib for neovascular age-related macular degeneration. The New England journal of medicine 351: 2805–2816.
6. Miller JW (2013) Age-related macular degeneration revisited–piecing the puzzle: the LXIX Edward Jackson memorial lecture. Am J Ophthalmol 155: 1–35 e13.
7. Hartnett ME, Weiter JJ, Garsd A, Jalkh AE (1992) Classification of retinal pigment epithelial detachments associated with drusen. Graefes Arch Clin Exp Ophthalmol 230: 11–19.
8. Hartnett ME, Weiter JJ, Staurenghi G, Elsner AE (1996) Deep retinal vascular anomalous complexes in advanced age-related macular degeneration. Ophthalmology 103: 2042–2053.
9. Yannuzzi LA, Negrao S, Iida T, Carvalho C, Rodriguez-Coleman H, et al. (2001) Retinal angiomatous proliferation in age-related macular degeneration. Retina 21: 416–434.
10. Viola F, Massacesi A, Orzalesi N, Ratiglia R, Staurenghi G (2009) Retinal angiomatous proliferation: natural history and progression of visual loss. Retina 29: 732–739.
11. Bottoni F, Massacesi A, Cigada M, Viola F, Musicco I, et al. (2005) Treatment of retinal angiomatous proliferation in age-related macular degeneration: a series of 104 cases of retinal angiomatous proliferation. Arch Ophthalmol 123: 1644–1650.
12. Silva RM, Cachulo ML, Figueira J, de Abreu JR, Cunha-Vaz JG (2007) Chorioretinal anastomosis and photodynamic therapy: a two-year follow-up study. Graefes Arch Clin Exp Ophthalmol 245: 1131–1139.
13. Okamoto N, Tobe T, Hackett SF, Ozaki H, Vinores MA, et al. (1997) Transgenic mice with increased expression of vascular endothelial growth factor in the retina: a new model of intraretinal and subretinal neovascularization. Am J Pathol 151: 281–291.
14. Tobe T, Okamoto N, Vinores MA, Derevjanik NL, Vinores SA, et al. (1998) Evolution of neovascularization in mice with overexpression of vascular endothelial growth factor in photoreceptors. Invest Ophthalmol Vis Sci 39: 180–188.
15. Ohno-Matsui K, Hirose A, Yamamoto S, Saikia J, Okamoto N, et al. (2002) Inducible expression of vascular endothelial growth factor in adult mice causes severe proliferative retinopathy and retinal detachment. Am J Pathol 160: 711–719.
16. Lai CM, Dunlop SA, May LA, Gorbatov M, Brankov M, et al. (2005) Generation of transgenic mice with mild and severe retinal neovascularisation. Br J Ophthalmol 89: 911–916.
17. Yetemian RM, Brown BM, Craft CM (2010) Neovascularization, enhanced inflammatory response, and age-related cone dystrophy in the Nrl−/− Grk1−/− mouse retina. Invest Ophthalmol Vis Sci 51: 6196–6206.
18. Won J, Shi LY, Hicks W, Wang J, Hurd R, et al. (2011) Mouse model resources for vision research. J Ophthalmol 2011: 391384.
19. Miller JW, Le Couter J, Strauss EC, Ferrara N (2013) Vascular endothelial growth factor a in intraocular vascular disease. Ophthalmology 120: 106–114.
20. Saito M, Iida T, Kano M (2013) Two-year results of combined intravitreal anti-VEGF agents and photodynamic therapy for retinal angiomatous proliferation. Jpn J Ophthalmol 57: 211–220.
21. Engelbert M, Zweifel SA, Freund KB (2009) "Treat and extend" dosing of intravitreal antivascular endothelial growth factor therapy for type 3 neovascularization/retinal angiomatous proliferation. Retina 29: 1424–1431.
22. Hemeida TS, Keane PA, Dustin L, Sadda SR, Fawzi AA (2010) Long-term visual and anatomical outcomes following anti-VEGF monotherapy for retinal angiomatous proliferation. Br J Ophthalmol 94: 701–705.
23. Luo L, Uehara H, Zhang X, Das SK, Olsen T, et al. (2013) Photoreceptor avascular privilege is shielded by soluble VEGF receptor-1. Elife 2: e00324.
24. Kendall RL, Thomas KA (1993) Inhibition of vascular endothelial cell growth factor activity by an endogenously encoded soluble receptor. Proc Natl Acad Sci U S A 90: 10705–10709.
25. Lai CM, Shen WY, Brankov M, Lai YK, Barnett NL, et al. (2005) Long-term evaluation of AAV-mediated sFlt-1 gene therapy for ocular neovascularization in mice and monkeys. Mol Ther 12: 659–668.
26. Lukason M, DuFresne E, Rubin H, Pechan P, Li Q, et al. (2011) Inhibition of choroidal neovascularization in a nonhuman primate model by intravitreal administration of an AAV2 vector expressing a novel anti-VEGF molecule. Mol Ther 19: 260–265.
27. Nagai N, Lundh von Leithner P, Izumi-Nagai K, Hosking B, Chang B, et al. (2014) Spontaneous CNV in a novel mutant mouse is associated with early VEGF-A-driven angiogenesis and late-stage focal edema, neural cell loss, and dysfunction. Invest Ophthalmol Vis Sci 55: 3709–3719.
28. Reichenbach A, Bringmann A (2013) New functions of Muller cells. Glia 61: 651–678.
29. Shen W, Fruttiger M, Zhu L, Chung SH, Barnett NL, et al. (2012) Conditional Mullercell ablation causes independent neuronal and vascular pathologies in a novel transgenic model. J Neurosci 32: 15715–15727.
30. Eichler W, Yafai Y, Wiedemann P, Reichenbach A (2004) Angiogenesis-related factors derived from retinal glial (Muller) cells in hypoxia. Neuroreport 15: 1633–1637.
31. Marneros AG, Fan J, Yokoyama Y, Gerber HP, Ferrara N, et al. (2005) Vascular endothelial growth factor expression in the retinal pigment epithelium is essential for choriocapillaris development and visual function. Am J Pathol 167: 1451–1459.
32. Burns MS, Hartz MJ (1992) The retinal pigment epithelium induces fenestration of endothelial cells in vivo. Curr Eye Res 11: 863–873.
33. Gass JD, Agarwal A, Lavina AM, Tawansy KA (2003) Focal inner retinal hemorrhages in patients with drusen: an early sign of occult choroidal neovascularization and chorioretinal anastomosis. Retina 23: 741–751.
34. Shimada H, Kawamura A, Mori R, Yuzawa M (2007) Clinicopathological findings of retinal angiomatous proliferation. Graefes Arch Clin Exp Ophthalmol 245: 295–300.
35. Heckenlively JR, Hawes NL, Friedlander M, Nusinowitz S, Hurd R, et al. (2003) Mouse model of subretinal neovascularization with choroidal anastomosis. Retina 23: 518–522.
36. Hu W, Jiang A, Liang J, Meng H, Chang B, et al. (2008) Expression of VLDLR in the retina and evolution of subretinal neovascularization in the knockout mouse model's retinal angiomatous proliferation. Invest Ophthalmol Vis Sci 49: 407–415.
37. Omarova S, Charvet CD, Reem RE, Mast N, Zheng W, et al. (2012) Abnormal vascularization in mouse retina with dysregulated retinal cholesterol homeostasis. J Clin Invest 122: 3012–3023.

24

Assessment of the Coronary Venous System Using 256-Slice Computed Tomography

Chunjuan Sun[1,2], Yinghua Pan[2], Hongbo Wang[2], Jian Li[2], Pei Nie[1], Ximing Wang[1]*, Heng Ma[2]*, Futao Huo[2]

1 Shandong Provincial Key Laboratory of Diagnosis and Treatment of Cardio-Cerebral Vascular Diseases, Shandong Medical Imaging Research Institute, Shandong University, Jinan, Shandong, China, **2** Department of Radiology, Yuhuangding Hospital, Yantai, Shandong, China

Abstract

Purpose: To investigate the coronary venous system and its relation to adjacent structures using 256-slice computed tomography (CT).

Materials and Methods: The study consisted of 102 patients who underwent coronary CT angiography (CTA) using 256-slice CT. For each patient, the coronary venous system and its relation to adjacent structures were evaluated. The appropriate locations and diameters of the posterior interventricular vein (PIV), posterior vein of the left ventricle (PVLV) and the left marginal vein (LMV) were detected. The paired student's *t* test was used to evaluate the difference between the diameter of the coronary sinus (CS) ostium in anteroposterior direction and that in superoinferior direction.

Results: The CS, great cardiac vein (GCV), PIV, and anterior interventricular vein (AIV) were visualized in all cases. It was possible to evaluate at least one main vein with adequate caliber and regular course for cardiac resynchronization therapy (CRT) in 96.1% of these cases. The diameter of the CS ostium in superoinferior direction (11.7±2.1 mm) was larger than that in anteroposterior direction (9.0±2.0 mm) ($t = 13.511$, $P < 0.05$). For the majority of the cases, the CS-GCV was located above the level of the mitral valve annulus (MVA), while the left circumflex coronary artery (LCX) was coursed between the CS-GCV and the MVA. LMV had more intersection with the circumflex or circumflex marginal than PVLV.

Conclusion: 256-slice CT provides superior noninvasive evaluation of the coronary venous system which has important clinical implications.

Editor: Denice Hodgson-Zingman, University of Iowa Carver College of Medicine, United States of America

Funding: Funding was received from the Shandong Province Natural Science Foundation (ZR2012HM013) and Yantai City Science and Technology Development Plan (2012090). The funders had no role in study design, data collection and analysis, decision to publish, or preparation of the manuscript.

Competing Interests: The authors have declared that no competing interests exist.

* Email: wangximing369@126.com (XW); mahengyhd@163.com (HM)

Introduction

Investigations of the coronary venous system are overshadowed by numerous studies of the coronary arteries. In contrast to that for coronary arteries, the literature for coronary veins is scarce. The clinical importance of the coronary venous system, nevertheless, should not be underestimated [1].

The coronary venous system is being used increasingly for various electrophysiological purposes, such as radiofrequency catheter ablation (RFA), mapping, defibrillation, local drug delivery, gene delivery, percutaneous mitral annuloplasty (PMA) and cardiac resynchronization therapy (CRT) [2,3]. A thorough knowledge of the coronary venous anatomy prior to the procedure will not only ease the intervention process but also increase the success rate. Catheter-based venous angiography is an invasive method with the possibilities for serious complications. In recent years, ECG-gated multi-slice spiral computed tomography (MSCT) has become an important noninvasive tool to evaluate coronary venous system. Up to now, a number of previous studies have used 4-, 16-, 64-, and128-slice MSCT to describe the coronary venous tree [4–10]. Compared with the older generation MSCT, the 256-slice MSCT with the reduction of scanning time, breath-holding duration, motion artifacts, contrast medium and radiation dose can provide superior noninvasive visualization of coronary artery and venous anatomy [11]. However, to our best knowledge, there are no published papers regarding coronary venous system depiction using the latest generation 256-slice CT.

The aim of our study was to assess coronary venous system and its relation to adjacent structures using 256-slice CT.

Materials and Methods

Our study received the approval from Shandong Medical Imaging Research Institute Ethics Board. Our institutional review board waived the need for written informed consent from the participants, because it was a retrospective review of coronary CT angiography performed for clinical reasons.

Patients

The study population was composed of 102 consecutive patients (55 females and 47 males; mean age: 58.8±8.8 years, range: 28–79years) who had undergone coronary CTA between July 2013 and November 2013 for suspected coronary artery disease. Patients with a creatinine level above 2 mg/dL, pregnancy and any known allergy to non-ionic contrast agents were excluded from the study.

CT protocol

Imaging was performed with a retrospectively ECG-gated CT coronary angiogram using 256-slice CT (Brilliance iCT, Philips, Cleveland,Ohio,USA). The scan coverage was planned from the tracheal bifurcation to the diaphragm. The coronary CTA scan parameters were as follows: tube voltage, 100 kVp; effective tube current–time product, 700 mAs; pitch, 0.18; detector configuration, 128×0.625 mm; rotation time, 270 ms. The heart rate was controlled under 90 beats per minute (bpm) by β-blocker prior to CTA. On average, 75 ml of non-ionic contrast agent (Ultravist 370, Bayer Schering Pharma AG, Berlin, Germany) was injected into the antecubital vein at a rate of 5 ml/s using a dual-head injector. The contrast agent was given in 3 phases: 60 ml of contrast agent (average), then 15 ml of contrast agent and 15 ml of saline (50%/50%) and finally 30 ml of saline flush. Automatic bolus tracking (Bolus Pro, Philips Healthcare, Cleveland, OH, USA) was used by defining a region of interest (ROI) in the ascending aorta at the level of aorto-pulmonary fenestration, with the scans initiated 6 s after the signal attenuation reached a pre-determined threshold of 180 Hounsfield Units (HU).

Data reconstruction was performed on a dedicated workstation (IntelliSpace Portal, Cleveland,Ohio,USA). Transverse images were reconstructed at 45% of the RR interval with 0.9 mm slice thickness and 0.6 mm intervals using a medium smooth-tissue convolution kernel (B26f). Multiplanar reformation (MPR), maximum intensity projection (MIP) and volume rendering (VR) were used for image interpretation. All images were interpreted by two independent radiologists with more than 6-year cardiac CT experience. Consensus agreement was achieved between the two observers if disagreement existed.

Anatomic observations

The tributaries of the coronary venous system and its relation to adjacent structures were identified on volume-rendered images (Figure 1). The presence of the following coronary veins was evaluated: CS, GCV, AIV, PIV, PVLV, LMV, small cardiac vein (SCV) and the vein of Marshall. The number of side branches of these tributaries was also recorded.

Quantitative data

The ostium of the CS is defined as the site where the CS makes an angle with the right atrium in the crux cordis area. Multi-planar reformatting was used to determine the size of the ostium in 2 directions (Figure 2). The diameters of the proximal parts of the PIV, PVLV, and LMV were measured. The distance from the ostium to tributaries and the angle between the tributaries and CS were measured on volume-rendered images (Figure 3).

Statistical analysis

The statistical SPSS 17.0 software (SPSS, Chicago, IL, USA) was used for statistical analysis. Continuous variables were expressed as mean ± standard deviation. Categorical variables were expressed as absolute number (percentage). The paired student's t test was used to evaluate the difference between the diameter of the CS ostium in anteroposterior direction and that in superoinferior direction. Statistical tests were 2-tailed, and a P value<0.05 was considered significant.

Results

The Anatomy of coronary venous system

The coronary sinus (CS) is the most prominent feature of the coronary venous system running along the posterior coronary groove to the right atrium. It was visualized in all cases (100%).

The great cardiac vein (GCV) terminates in the coronary sinus, a junction defined by the presence of the Marshall vein. It was visualized in all cases (100%).

The anterior interventricular vein (AIV) originates at the apex of the heart, returns back along the anterior inter-ventricular groove, and ends in the great cardiac vein. It was visualized in all cases (100%).

The posterior interventricular vein (PIV) originates close to the apex of the heart and follows the posterior inter-ventricular groove toward the base where, in most cases, flows into the CS. It was visualized in all cases (100%).

The posterior vein of the left ventricle (PVLV) runs through the diaphrag-matic aspect of the left ventricle and ends in the GCV. It was visualized in 79 cases (77.5%). There were 2 PVLVs in 10 cases (12.7%).

The left marginal vein (LMV) runs along the lateral border of the heart ending in the GCV. It was visualized in 68 cases (66.7%). There were 2 or 3 LMVs in 8cases (11.8%).

The small cardiac vein (SCV) originates on the front side of the heart and runs on the diaphragmatic portion of the right coronary groove. It was observed as a very small vein in 28 cases (27.5%), and 57.1% of which directly drained into PIV.

The Marshall vein descends obliquely along the back surface of the left atrium up to the confluence of the CS and GCV. It was present in 7 cases (6.9%).

Table 1 lists the quantitative data of the PIV, PVLV, and LMV. It was possible to evaluate at least one main vein with adequate caliber and regular course for CRT in 96.1% (98/102) of the cases. The diameter of the CS ostium in superoinferior direction (11.7±2.1 mm) was larger than that in anteroposterior direction (9.0±2.0 mm). (t = 13.511, P<0.05).

Relationship between CS-GCV, MVA and LCX (Figures 4–5)

The CS-GCV was located above the level of the MVA in 93.1% (95/102) of cases, and only 6.9% (7/102) of cases was located along the MVA. The relationship between LCX and CS-GCV was defined by the medial/lateral orientation with respect to determination of the vessel closer to epicardium in overlapping segments. The CS-GCV was lateral to the LCX in 68.6% (70/102) of cases and medial to the LCX in 29.4% (30/102) of cases. The CS-GCV was medial in one segment and lateral in another segment in 2 cases.

Relationship between AIV and the left anterior descending artery (LAD) (Figure 6)

In 29.4% (30/102) of cases, AIV crossed LAD. In these 30 cases, the vein was lateral to and therefore overlying the LAD in 53.3% (16/30), and medial to the LAD in 46.7% (14/30). In the remaining cases (70.6%), AIV was concomitant with LAD. AIV crossed a diagonal with the vein lateral and therefore overlying the artery in 33.3% (34/102) of cases, and the vein medial to the diagonal (between epicardium and artery) in 66.7% (68/102) of cases.

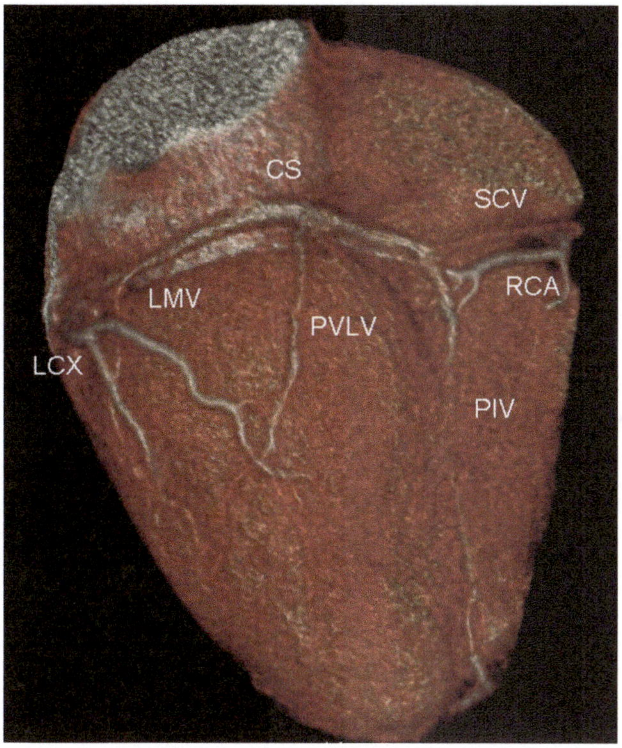

Figure 1. Volume-rendered image provides an overview of coronary venous anatomy. It clearly depicts the coronary sinus (CS), posterior interventricular vein (PIV), posterior vein of the left ventricle (PVLV), left marginal vein (LMV), and small cardiac vein (SCV). Also notes the right coronary artery (RCA) and the left circumflex coronary artery (LCX).

Relationship between PVLV, LMV and circumflex or circumflex marginal (Figure 7)

The LMV crossed the circumflex or circumflex marginal in 82.4% (56/68) of cases. The LMV was lateral to the circumflex or circumflex marginal in 67.9% (38/56) of cases, and medial to the circumflex or circumflex marginal in 32.1% (18/56) of cases. The LMV was concomitant with circumflex or circumflex marginal in 7.4% (5/68) of cases. Because of the decrease in size of the circumflex, there was an intersection point between the PVLV and circumflex marginal branches only in 32.9% (26/79) of cases.

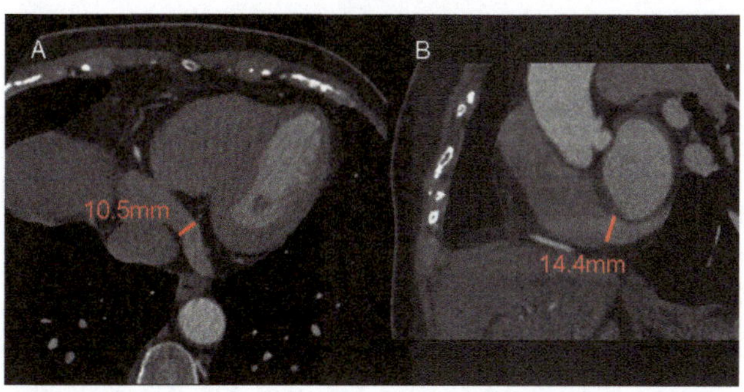

Figure 2. Measurement of the diameter of the coronary sinus (CS). Multiplanar reformatting is used to determine the diameter of the ostium in the anteroposterior(A) and supero-inferior (B)position.

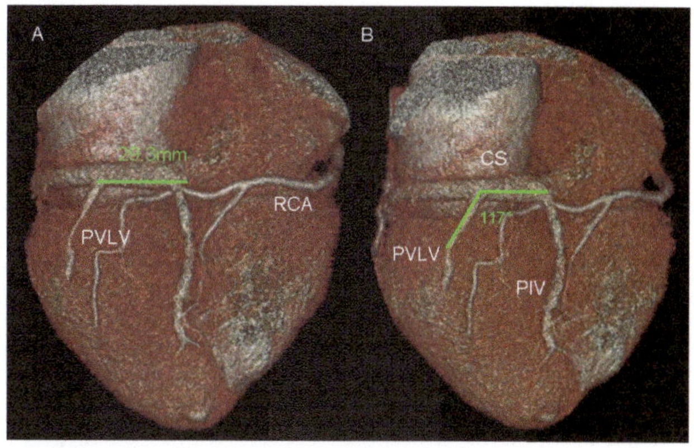

Figure 3. Measurement of the distance and angle between the tributaries and coronary sinus (CS). A. the distance from the ostium to tributaries B, the angle between the tributaries and CS.

Relationship between PIV and posterior descending artery (PDA) (Figure 8)

PIV was concomitant with PDA in 35 cases and intersected with PDA in 63 cases. Of these intersected cases, the vein was lateral to the PDA in 92.1% (58/63) of cases, and medial to the PDA in 7.9% (5/63) of cases.

Discussion

Imaging methods for coronary venous system

There are several imaging methods to assess coronary venous system. Each of these methods has its own advantages and disadvantages [12–17].

Retrograde cardiac venography is currently the gold standard technique for defining coronary venous anatomy; however, it is invasive, technically challenging, and unable to define the relationship between the coronary veins and coronary arteries. It also has a lot of disadvantages such as coronary sinus trauma due to balloon occlusion, a longer imaging time, and a high dose of contrast material. Compared to retrograde cardiac venography, electron-beam CT is a better option, as it is noninvasive and has a higher imaging success rate. However, a considerable number of patients may not be adequately assessed by this modality because not all parts of the heart are examined, and the image quality is suboptimal. Compared with other techniques for imaging the cardiac venous system, MRA is noninvasive and does not require injection of iodinated contrast medium or expose patients to ionizing radiation. However, the major challenges for MRA are the long scan time, image artifacts caused by motion instability during the long scan time and a relatively low spatial resolution.

In recent years, MSCT has become the preferred noninvasive method to assess the coronary venous system. Unlike retrograde venography, MSCT angiography allows both simultaneous imaging of the coronary veins and assessment of arteriovenous relationships. There is no vessel overlap. The newer-generation MSCT scanner, especially the 256-slice CT with faster gantry rotation time and larger detector coverage can provide better visualization of the coronary veins with a lower radiation dose.

Main findings

The followings are our main findings in this study. First, to the best of our knowledge, this is the first report to assess the coronary venous system using 256-slice CT. Second, the 256-slice CT

Table 1. Quantitative measurement of cardiac veins.

	Ostial diameter (mm)	Distance from the ostium of CS (mm)	Angle between the identified veins and CS/GCV
PIV (n=102)	4.8±1.0	10.6±4.0	71°±17°
PVLV (n=79)	3.1±1.0	27.8±9.3	109°±18°
LMV (n=68)	2.7±0.7	57.3±15.1	116°±29°

CS, coronary sinus; PIV, posterior interventricular vein; PVLV, posterior vein of the left ventricle; LMV, left marginal vein; GCV, great cardiac vein.

coronary angiography, in addition to coronary artery imaging, can provide important information of the coronary venous system, as well as its relation to adjacent structures. The latter has important clinical implications. Third, this kind of study can provide guidance for patients who need device implantation.

Clinical implications

Cardiac resynchronization therapy (CRT) is an attractive treatment for selected heart failure patients. Left ventricular (LV) pacing is established by a pacemaker lead in a tributary of the CS during CRT. The LV lead is the most challenging part of CRT implantation. Because the postero-lateral left ventricular wall is usually the optimal location for pacing [18]. Common target veins are the LMV or PVLV [19]. Vessel size is an important criterion for selecting the target vein for LV pacemaker lead insertion. A too-small coronary sinus diameter and a too-small or too-big target vein may cause CRT to be unsuccessful [20]. The diameter of target vein for the smallest LV lead must be greater than 1.5 mm [19]. Before CRT implantation, the following question has to be answered: which cardiac vein is suitable for LV lead placement? 256-slice CT is a reliable technique to depict the coronary venous system, which can not only confirm the presence of a target vein but also provide information on the course of the vessel, the side branches, the diameter, the distance from the ostium to tributaries, the angle between the tributaries and CS and the relation to adjacent artery. In our study, the PVLV was visualized in 77.5% of all cases, and the LMV was visualized in 66.7% of all cases. The mean diameter of PVLV and LMV was 3.1±1.0 mm, and 2.7±0.7 mm, respectively. It was possible to evaluate at least one main vein with adequate caliber and regular course running on the postero-lateral wall of left ventricle in 96.1% of the cases, only 4 cases had no target veins (Figure 9). The CS is the most constant component of the coronary venous system and was detected in all patients. The diameter of the CS ostium in superoinferior direction(11.7±2.1 mm) was larger than that in anteroposterior direction (9.0±2.0 mm), indicating an oval shape of the ostium, which is confirmed by the 16-slice MSCT observations of Jongbloed et al [5] and magnetic resonance imaging observations of Ma H et al [17]. In addition, LMV had more intersection with the circumflex or circumflex marginal than PVLV and the LMV was lateral to the circumflex or circumflex marginal in most cases. Circumflex artery compression may be caused as a serious complication with such a close relation between LMV and circumflex artery during CRT. A thorough knowledge of the coronary venous system anatomy prior to the procedure will ease the intervention process and increase the success rate.

Percutaneous mitral annuloplasty (PMA) has been proposed as an alternative to surgical annuloplasty [21]. With this technique, a double-anchor PMA device is implanted in the CS-GCV at the level of the superior and inferior commissures of the mitral valve. Evaluation of the CS anatomy and its relation to the MVA and the coronary arteries may be of great value in patients who are considered for PMA. In the present study, the CS is located above the level of the MVA in 93.1% of cases. Sometimes, the CS can lie on the left atrial wall for almost its entire course (Figure 10). In 68.6% of the patients, the LCX courses between the CS and the MVA, with a potential risk of compression of the LCX by PMA devices when percutaneous mitral annuloplasty is applied. The close relationship between the CS, coronary arteries, and MVA may result the limits to use PMA, particularly when the artery is

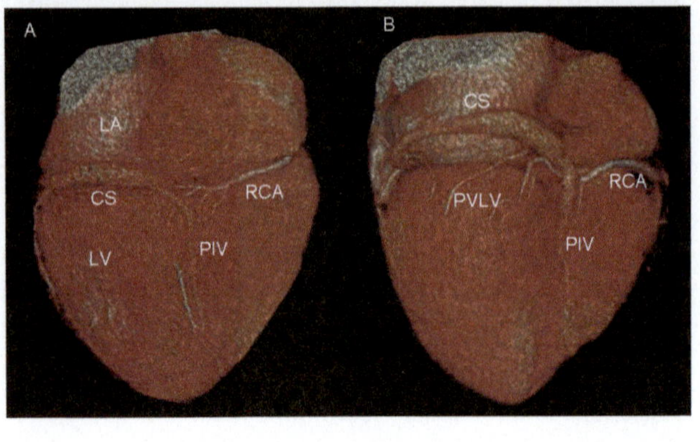

Figure 4. Volume-rendered images show the relationship between the coronary sinus (CS) and mitral valve annulus (MVA). A. the CS is located along the MVA. B. the CS is located above the level of the MVA.; LA=left atrium; LV=left ventricle.

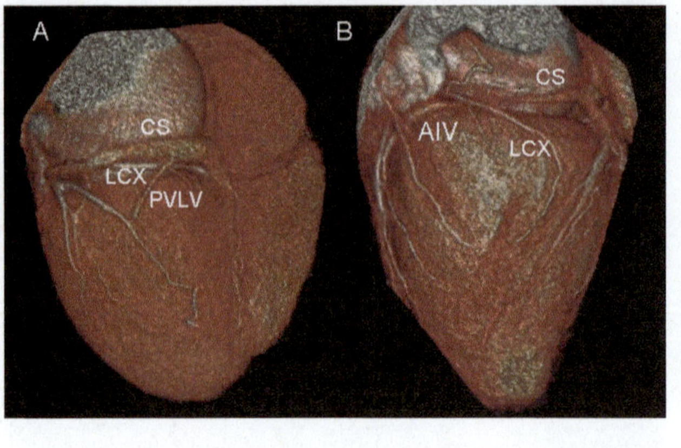

Figure 5. Volume-rendered images show the relationship between the coronary sinus (CS) and the left circumflex coronary artery (LCX). A. LCX courses between the CS and the mitral valve annulus (MVA), with a potential risk of compression of the LCX when percutaneous mitral annuloplasty (PMA) is applied. B. LCX courses superiorly to the CS.

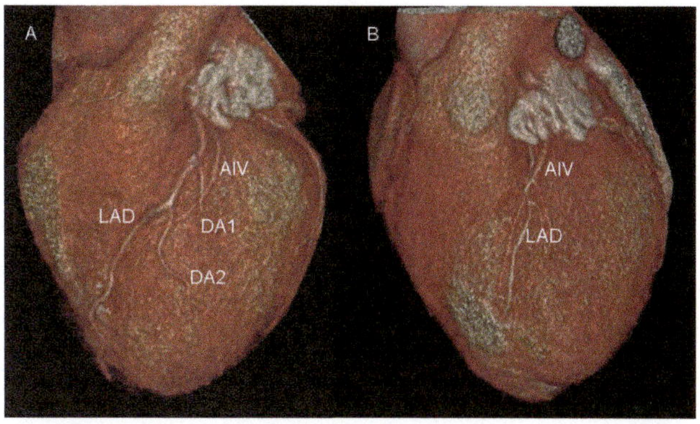

Figure 6. Volume-rendered images show the relationship between anterior interventricular vein (AIV) and left anterior descending artery (LAD). A. AIV is concomitant with LAD, and AIV crosses two diagonals with the vein medial to the diagonals (between epicardium and arteries). B. AIV crosses LAD, and the vein is lateral to and therefore overlying the LAD.

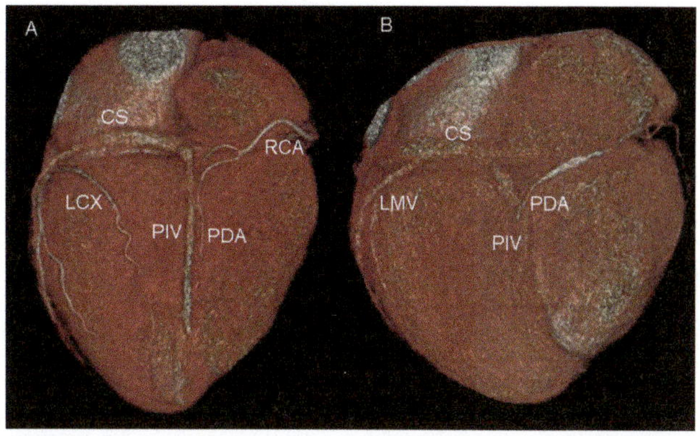

Figure 8. Volume-rendered images show the relationship between posterior interventricular vein (PIV) and posterior descending artery (PDA). A. PIV is concomitant with PDA. B. PIV crosses PDA with the vein medial to the PDA.

interlaced with the CS over a long distance (Figure 11). A surgical approach may be preferred over a percutaneous approach. Knowledge of a detailed anatomic relationship between the CS, coronary arteries, and MVA in humans is essential to define the safety and efficacy of PMA [22].

Radiofrequency catheter ablation (RFA) is a procedure to correct a disturbance in heart rhythm. As a less invasive option to the surgical incisions used in the procedure, such ablation may be performed either by within the chambers of the heart (endocardial ablation) or by outside the heart (epicardial ablation). Epicardial arrhythmias originating from the coronary venous system are usually performed through instrumentation of the CS and its branches. For example, in some idiopathic ventricular tachychardia, coronary veins provide endovascular access to the epicardial regions of the ventricles, especially the crucial area between the junction of the great cardiac vein and the anterior interventricular vein [23]. Ablation can be performed safely from within the

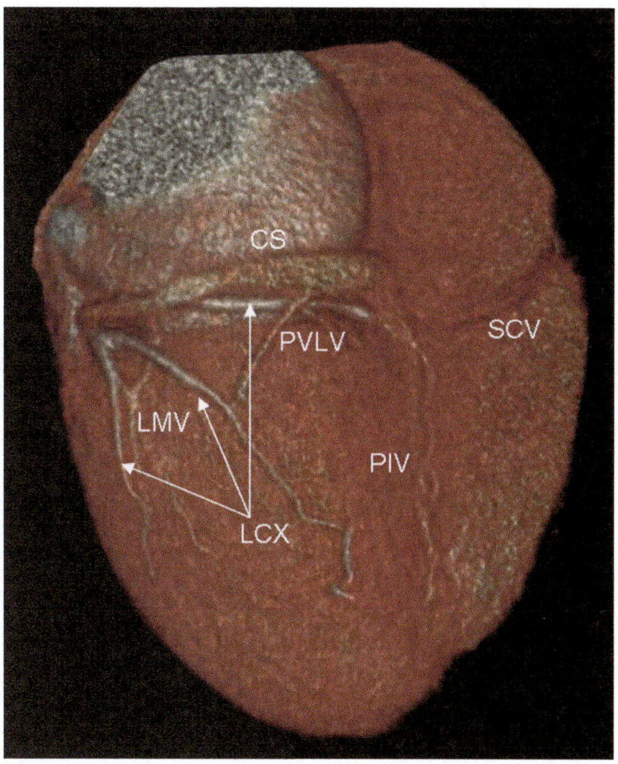

Figure 7. Volume-rendered image shows the relationship between posterior vein of the left ventricle (PVLV), left marginal vein (LMV) and circumflex or circumflex marginal. The LMV and PVLV cross the circumflex or circumflex marginal.

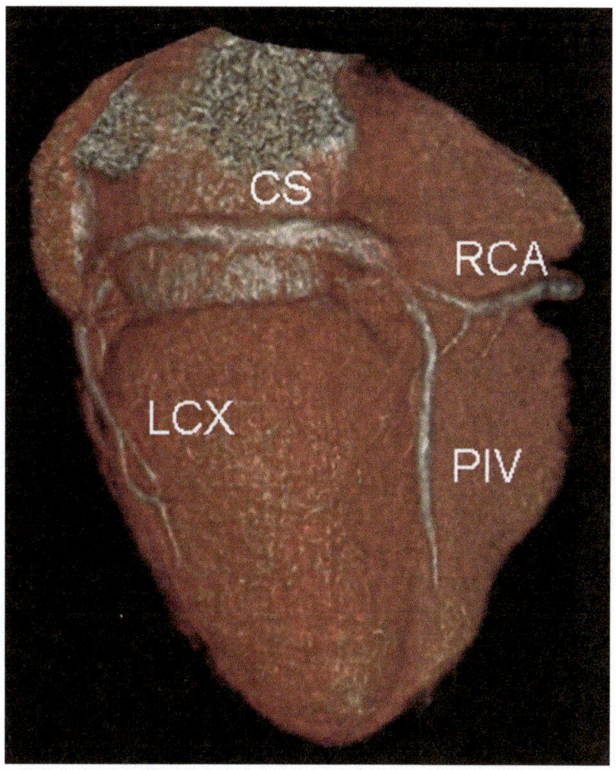

Figure 9. A case with no target veins for Cardiac resynchronization therapy (CRT). Volume-rendered image shows the presence of multiple thin and short posterior cardiac veins representing a contraindicated site for CRT leads placement.

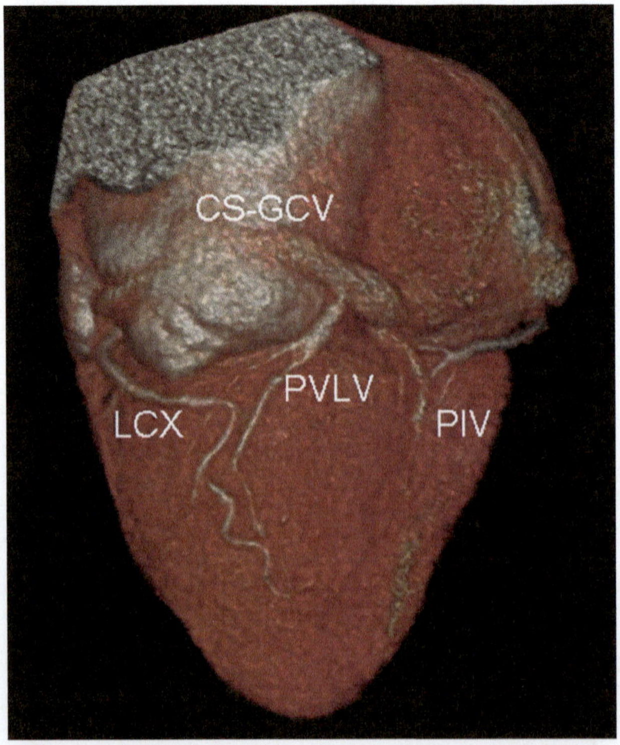

Figure 10. Volume-rendered image shows the spatial relationship of the coronary sinus (CS) and left atrial wall. In this patient, the CS lies on the left atrial wall for almost its entire course and part of the CS is not visualized because of the compression of left atrial wall, which may limit the use of Percutaneous mitral annuloplasty (PMA).

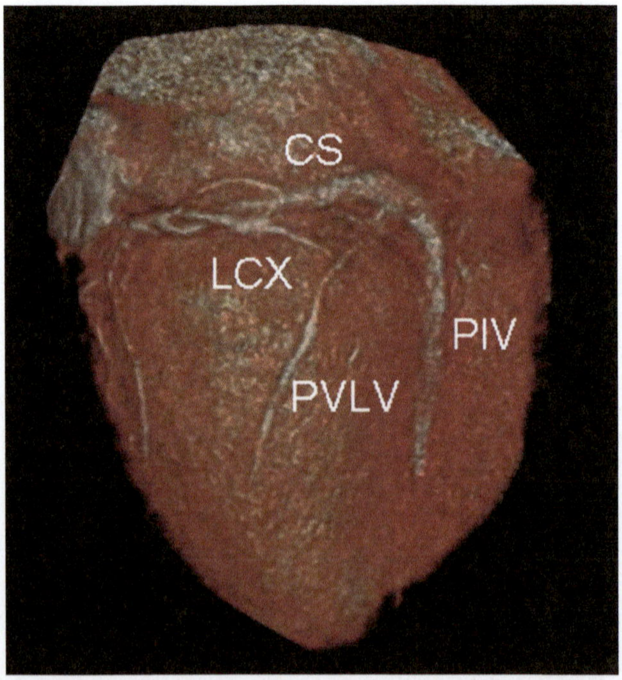

Figure 11. Volume-rendered image shows the spatial relationship of the coronary sinus (CS) and left circumflex artery (LCX). The LCX is interlaced with the CS over a long distance. This close relationship may limit the use of Percutaneous mitral annuloplasty (PMA).

coronary venous system. However, coronary artery injury is an ever-present risk, especially near the proximal part of the AIV. A thorough knowledge of the anatomy of veins and arteries prior to the procedure will increase the success rate and will reduce complications.

In addition, the coronary venous system as a route for administering pharmacologic therapy, gene therapy, growth factors, and stem cells to the myocardium has shown higher success rate than intra-arterial or systemic delivery.

Study limitations

We also acknowledged some limitations in our study. First, the 256-slice CT scans were tailored for optimal visualization of the coronary arteries, which may also be limited in showing the side branches with a small diameter of the coronary veins. Van de Veire et al. [24] reported that an additional 2-second delay was applied after the contrast bolus reached the descending aorta before triggering the scan and the use of saline chasing was omitted for optimal visualization of the coronary venous system. Second, the radiation dose in CT is a limitation that can be modified using dose reduction techniques, for instance, the use of prospective ECG-gating for coronary CTA [25]. Finally, there were no patients with advanced heart failure, atrial fibrillation or mitral valve disease in our study. Most of patients were examined because of a suspicion of CAD, so we did not have the possibility to compare our 256-slice CT technique with the current invasive gold standard, retrograde cardiac venography.

Conclusion

256-slice CT is a feasible tool for non-invasive evaluation of the coronary venous system and can provide accurate information of the coronary venous system which has important clinical implications.

Author Contributions

Conceived and designed the experiments: CS XW HM FH. Performed the experiments: CS YP JL. Analyzed the data: CS PN HW. Contributed reagents/materials/analysis tools: HW. Contributed to the writing of the manuscript: CS.

References

1. Loukas M, Bilinsky S, Bilinsky E, el-Sedfy A, Anderson RH (2009) Cardiac veins: a review of the literature. Clin Anat 22: 129–145.
2. Tada H, Kurosaki K, Naito S, Koyama K, Itoi K, et al. (2005) Three-dimensional visualization of the coronary venous system using multidetector row computed tomography. Circ J 69:165–170.
3. Echeverri D, Cabrales J, Jimenez A (2013) Myocardial Venous Drainage: From Anatomy to Clinical Use. J Invasive Cardiol 25:98–105.
4. Mühlenbruch G, Koos R, Wildberger JE, Günther RW, Mahnken AH (2005) Imaging of the cardiac venous system: comparison of MDCT and conventional angiography. AJR Am J Roentgenol 185:1252–1257.
5. Jongbloed MR, Lamb HJ, Bax JJ, Schuijf JD, de Roos A, et al. (2005) Noninvasive visualization of the cardiac venous system using multi-slice computed tomography. J Am Coll Cardiol 45:749–753.
6. Abbara S, Cury RC, Nieman K, Reddy V, Moselewski F, et al. (2005) Noninvasive evaluation of cardiac veins with 16-MDCT angiography. AJR Am J Roentgenol 185:1001–1006.
7. Van de Veire NR, Schuijf JD, De Sutter J, Devos D, Bleeker GB, et al. (2006) Non-invasive visualization of the cardiac venous system in coronary artery disease patients using 64-slice computed tomography. J Am Coll Cardiol 48: 1832–1838.

8. Mlynarski R, Mlynarska A, Sosnowski M (2011) Anatomical variants of coronary venous system on cardiac computed tomography. Circ J 75: 613–618.
9. Malagò R, Pezzato A, Barbiani C, Sala G, Zamboni GA, et al. (2012) Non invasive cardiac vein mapping: role of multi-slice CT coronary angiography. Eur J Radiol 81: 3262–3269.
10. Genc B, Solak A, Sahin N, Gur S, Kalaycioglu S, et al. (2013) Assessment of the coronary venous system by using cardiac CT. Diagn Interv Radiol 19:286–293.
11. Klass O, Walker M, Siebach A, Stuber T, Feuerlein S, et al. (2010) Prospectively gated axial CT coronary angiography: comparison of image quality and effective radiation dose between 64- and 256-slice CT. Eur Radiol 20: 1124–1131.
12. Blendea D, Shah RV, Auricchio A, Nandigam V, Orencole M, et al. (2007) Variability of coronary venous anatomy in patients undergoing cardiac resynchronization therapy: a high-speed rotational venography study. Heart Rhythm 4:1155–1162.
13. Arbelo E, García-Quintana A, Caballero E, Hernández E, Caballero-Hidalgo A, et al. (2008) Usefulness of hyperemic venous return angiography for studying coronary venous anatomy prior to cardiac resynchronization device implantation. Rev Esp Cardiol 61:936–944.
14. Mao S, Shinbane JS, Girsky MJ, Child J, Carson S, et al. (2005) Coronary venous imaging with electron beam computed tomographic angiography: three-dimensional mapping and relationship with coronary arteries. Am Heart J 150:315–322.
15. Knackstedt C, Mühlenbruch G, Mischke K, Schimpf T, Spüntrup E, et al. (2008) Imaging of the coronary venous system in patients with congestive heart failure: comparison of 16 slice MSCT and retrograde coronary sinus venography: comparative imaging of coronary venous system. Int J Cardiovasc Imaging 24:783–791.
16. Chiribiri A, Kelle S, Götze S, Kriatselis C, Thouet T, et al. (2008) Visualization of the cardiac venous system using cardiac magnetic resonance. Am J Cardiol 101:407–412.
17. Ma H, Tang Q, Yang Q, Bi X, Li H, et al. (2011) Contrast-enhanced whole-heart coronary MRA at 3.0T for the evaluation of cardiac venous anatomy. Int J Cardiovasc Imaging 27:1003–1009.
18. Koos R, Sinha AM, Markus K, Breithardt OA, Mischke K, et al. (2004) Comparison of left ventricular lead placement via the coronary venous approach versus lateral thoracotomy in patients receiving cardiac resynchronization therapy. Am J Cardiol 94:59–63.
19. Saremi F, Muresian H, Sánchez-Quintana D (2012) Coronary Veins: Comprehensive CT-Anatomic Classification and Review of Variants and Clinical Implications. Radiographics 32:E1–32.
20. Hasdemir C (2007) Cardiac resynchronizationtherapy: implantation tips and tricks. Anadolu Kardiyol Derg 7:53–56.
21. Tops LF, Van de Veire NR, Schuijf JD, de Roos A, van der Wall EE, et al. (2007) Noninvasive evaluation of coronary sinus anatomy and its relation to the mitral valve annulus: implications for percutaneous mitral annuloplasty. Circulation 115: 1426–1432.
22. Maselli D, Guarracino F, Chiaramonti F, Mangia F, Borelli G, et al. (2006) Percutaneous Mitral Annuloplasty: An Anatomic Study of Human Coronary Sinus and Its Relation With Mitral Valve Annulus and Coronary Arteries. Circulation 114:377–380.
23. Vaseghi M, Shivkumar K (2010) Catheter Ablation of Idiopathic Ventricular Tachycardia. Circ Arrhythm Electrophysiol 3:219–221.
24. Van de Veire NR, Marsan NA, Schuijf JD, Bleeker GB, Wijffels MC, et al. (2006) Noninvasive Imaging of Cardiac Venous Anatomy With 64-Slice Multi-Slice Computed Tomography and Noninvasive Assessment of Left Ventricular Dyssynchrony by 3-Dimensional Tissue Synchronization Imaging in Patients With Heart Failure Scheduled for Cardiac Resynchronization Therapy. Am J Cardiol 101:1023–1029.
25. Hosch W, Heye T, Schulz F, Lehrke S, Schlieter M, et al. (2011) Image quality and radiation dose in 256-slice cardiac computed tomography:Comparison of prospective versus retrospective image acquisition protocols. Eur J Radiol 80:127–135.

25

Improved Cerebral Time-of-Flight Magnetic Resonance Angiography at 7 Tesla – Feasibility Study and Preliminary Results Using Optimized Venous Saturation Pulses

Karsten H. Wrede[1,2]*, Sören Johst[1,3], Philipp Dammann[1,2], Neriman Özkan[2], Christoph Mönninghoff[3], Markus Kraemer[4], Stefan Maderwald[1,3], Mark E. Ladd[1,3,5], Ulrich Sure[2], Lale Umutlu[1,3], Marc Schlamann[3]

1 Erwin L. Hahn Institute for Magnetic Resonance Imaging, University Duisburg-Essen, Essen, Germany, **2** Department of Neurosurgery, University Hospital Essen, Essen, Germany, **3** Department of Diagnostic and Interventional Radiology and Neuroradiology, University Hospital Essen, Essen, Germany, **4** Department of Neurology, Alfried Krupp von Bohlen und Halbach Hospital, Essen, Germany, **5** Division of Medical Physics in Radiology (E020), German Cancer Research Center (DKFZ), Heidelberg, Germany

Abstract

Purpose: Conventional saturation pulses cannot be used for 7 Tesla ultra-high-resolution time-of-flight magnetic resonance angiography (TOF MRA) due to specific absorption rate (SAR) limitations. We overcome these limitations by utilizing low flip angle, variable rate selective excitation (VERSE) algorithm saturation pulses.

Material and Methods: Twenty-five neurosurgical patients (male n = 8, female n = 17; average age 49.64 years; range 26–70 years) with different intracranial vascular pathologies were enrolled in this trial. All patients were examined with a 7 Tesla (Magnetom 7 T, Siemens) whole body scanner system utilizing a dedicated 32-channel head coil. For venous saturation pulses a 35° flip angle was applied. Two neuroradiologists evaluated the delineation of arterial vessels in the Circle of Willis, delineation of vascular pathologies, presence of artifacts, vessel-tissue contrast and overall image quality of TOF MRA scans in consensus on a five-point scale. Normalized signal intensities in the confluence of venous sinuses, M1 segment of left middle cerebral artery and adjacent gray matter were measured and vessel-tissue contrasts were calculated.

Results: Ratings for the majority of patients ranged between good and excellent for most of the evaluated features. Venous saturation was sufficient for all cases with minor artifacts in arteriovenous malformations and arteriovenous fistulas. Quantitative signal intensity measurements showed high vessel-tissue contrast for confluence of venous sinuses, M1 segment of left middle cerebral artery and adjacent gray matter.

Conclusion: The use of novel low flip angle VERSE algorithm pulses for saturation of venous vessels can overcome SAR limitations in 7 Tesla ultra-high-resolution TOF MRA. Our protocol is suitable for clinical application with excellent image quality for delineation of various intracranial vascular pathologies.

Editor: Xiaoming Yang, University of Washington School of Medicine, United States of America

Funding: An IFORES grant to KHW from the University Duisburg-Essen supported the research [http://www.uni-due.de/med/forschung/forschungsfoerderung/ifores.shtml]. The funders had no role in study design, data collection and analysis, decision to publish, or preparation of the manuscript.

Competing Interests: The authors have declared that no competing interests exist.

* Email: karsten.wrede@uk-essen.de

Introduction

In recent years, time-of-flight magnetic resonance angiography (TOF MRA) [1] has become an important diagnostic tool to depict cerebral vasculature [2–4]. This non-invasive technique is now widely considered equivalent to the gold standard, digital subtraction angiography for some applications such as follow-up of coiled cerebral aneurysms [3–7]. One important factor for the increasing relevance of TOF MRA has been the availability of higher magnetic field strengths. Better signal-to-noise ratio at 3 Tesla has already significantly improved the spatial resolution compared to 1.5 Tesla [8–13], and 7 Tesla has pushed spatial resolution to the sub-millimeter scale [8,9,14–18] while maintaining reasonable acquisition times.

Ultra-high-field magnetic resonance imaging (MRI) at 7 Tesla is currently being introduced in clinical application [19–22]. Many technical difficulties have been overcome already, but several restricting issues have still to be resolved. One major limitation is imposed by specific absorption rate (SAR) restriction. To unleash the full potential of 7 Tesla MRI, modified pulse sequences have to be employed. Such sequences with special spatial presaturation pulses were first described by Felmlee [23], and their implementation, application, and clinical relevance have been demonstrated in several subsequent publications [1–3,24,25]. SAR limitations restrict conventional saturation pulses at 7 Tesla, due to the fact

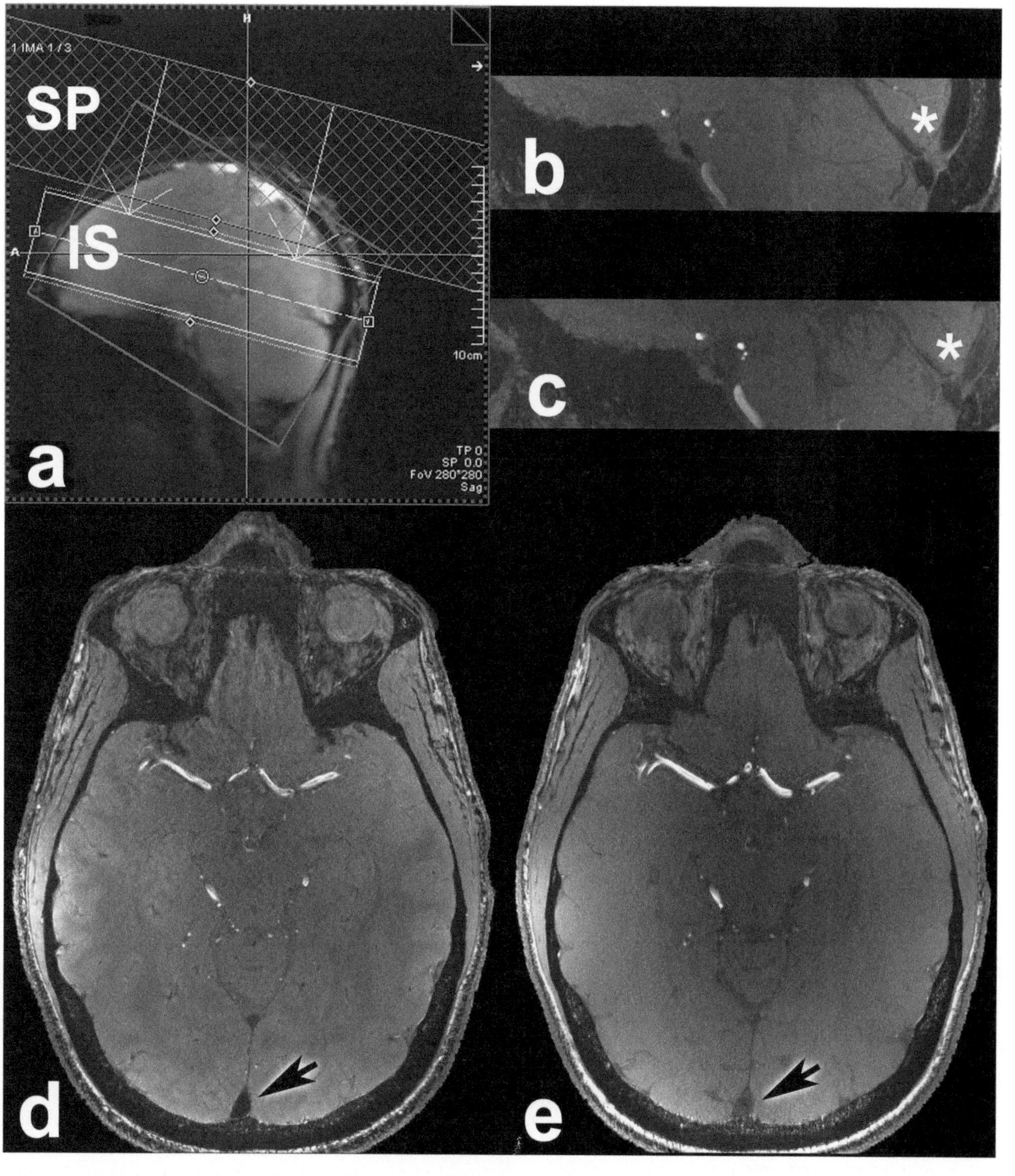

Figure 1. Shown is the localizer scan (a) of a 51-year-old male patient (subject 24) with a large arteriovenous malformation in the left hemisphere with thickness of TOF MRA imaging slab (IS) and saturation pulse (SP) illustrated. In a 29-year-old healthy subject a TOF MRA slab with identical coverage and spatial resolution was acquired with the non-optimized sequence in 17:48 min (**b**: sagittal view, **d**: transverse view). With the optimized sequence the identical slab was acquired in 6:22 min (**c**: sagittal view, **e**: transverse view). The same representative slice is shown for both sequences for direct comparison. In the optimized sequence TE could be reduced from 6.62 ms to 4.34 ms (due to a different asymmetric echo factor) and TR could be reduced from 56 ms to 20 ms (mainly due to reduced SAR) leading to better image contrast.

Table 1. Basic demographic data for all patients and average SAR for TOF MRA sequence.

Subject	Sex	Age in Years	SAR	Pathology
1	female	52	9.988	aneurysm
2	female	26	9.116	aneurysm
3	female	56	9.088	aneurysm
5	female	56	8.166	aneurysm
7	male	70	9.47	aneurysm
9	male	45	9.035	aneurysm
12	female	66	9.351	aneurysm
13	female	52	8.666	aneurysm
14	female	54	6.657	aneurysm
15	female	69	6.264	aneurysm
16	female	51	6.077	aneurysm
17	female	60	6.684	aneurysm
21	female	53	9.7	aneurysm
4	male	40	9.955	AVM
22	male	49	9.363	AVM
23	male	40	7.701	AVM
24	male	51	8.031	AVM
11	male	58	7.306	AVF
25	male	61	7.228	AVF
6	female	35	9.658	Moyamoya
8	female	34	9.13	Moyamoya
10	female	29	7.911	Moyamoya
18	female	58	9.004	Moyamoya
19	female	34	9.088	Moyamoya
20	female	42	9.677	Moyamoya

TOF MRA: time-of-flight magnetic resonance angiography.
SAR: time-averaged local specific absorption rate; 10 Watts/kg allowed maximum.

that these limits lead to unreasonable extension of acquisition time or suboptimal image contrast based on lowered flip angles of imaging excitation pulses. This study presents a protocol for ultra-high-resolution TOF MRA suitable for clinical application.

Materials and Methods

Ethics Statement

The study was conducted according to the principles expressed in the Declaration of Helsinki and was approved by the local university institutional review board (Ethik-Kommission der medizinischen Fakultät der Universität Duisburg-Essen). Written informed consent was obtained before each examination.

Study Design and Population

This prospective study evaluated the diagnostic ability of high-resolution 7 Tesla TOF MRA for various intracranial vascular pathologies (aneurysms, AVM, AVF, Moya-Moya). The study group comprised of 25 neurosurgical patients (male n = 8, female n = 17; average age 49.64 years; range 26–70 years). Inclusion criteria were: 1) single or multiple intracranial vascular pathologies, 2) age 18–80 years, 3) ability to give informed consent and 4) legal competence. Exclusion criteria were: 1) monitoring on intensive care or intermediate care unit 2) cardiac pacemakers or any other electronic implants, 3) metallic implants, 4) pregnancy or breast feeding period, 5) claustrophobia and 6) chronic or episodic vertigo.

Scanner and Coil System

All images were acquired on a 7 Tesla whole-body MRI system (Magnetom 7 T, Siemens Healthcare, Erlangen, Germany) equipped with a 32-channel Rx/Tx head coil (Nova Medical, Wilmington, MA, USA). The scanner has a gradient system of 45 mT/m maximum amplitude and a slew rate of 200 mT/m/ms.

Examination at 7 Tesla

Prior to sequence acquisition, B_0 shimming was performed using a vendor-provided gradient echo sequence and an algorithm based on the work of Schar [26]. A vendor-provided spin-echo sequence was used for B_1 field mapping and local flip angle optimization. Following slice-selective excitation, two refocusing pulses sequentially generate a spin-echo and a stimulated echo. Transmitter adjustment volume was placed in the center of the brain leading to an average flip angle variation of less than 20% in the superior sagittal sinus. Spatial coverage of the TOF MRA slab and the saturation pulse is demonstrated on a sagittal localizer scan of a 40-year-old male patient suffering from a large right parietal AVM (Figure 1). Time-averaged local SAR in Watts/kg was assessed for every scan. The values were measured by the SAR

Table 2. Consensus ratings for arterial vessel and pathology delineation, vessel-tissue contrast, artifacts and overall image quality.

Subject	Delineation of Circle of Willis	Delineation of vascular pathologies	Vessel-tissue contrast	artifacts	image quality	Pathology
1	5	5	5	5	5	aneurysm
2	5	5	5	4	4	aneurysm
3	5	5	5	4	5	aneurysm
5	5	5	5	4	5	aneurysm
7	5	5	5	5	5	aneurysm
9	5	5	5	5	5	aneurysm
12	5	5	5	5	5	aneurysm
13	5	5	5	4	5	aneurysm
14	5	5	5	5	5	aneurysm
15	5	5	5	4	5	aneurysm
16	5	5	5	5	5	aneurysm
17	5	5	5	5	5	aneurysm
21	5	5	5	5	5	aneurysm
4	5	5	2	4	5	AVM
22	5	5	4	4	5	AVM
23	5	5	5	5	5	AVM
24	5	5	5	4	5	AVM
11	5	3	3	4	4	AVF
25	5	4	3	4	4	AVF
6	3	5	5	4	4	Moyamoya
8	3	5	5	4	4	Moyamoya
10	3	5	5	4	4	Moyamoya
18	4	5	5	4	4	Moyamoya
19	3	5	5	4	4	Moyamoya
20	3	5	5	4	4	Moyamoya

For qualitative analysis images were evaluated, utilizing a five-point scale:
5 = excellent, 4 = good, 3 = moderate, 2 = poor, and 1 = non-diagnostic.
AVM: arteriovenous malformation AVF: dural arteriovenous fistula.

supervision system of the MR scanner and read out from the DICOM header of the acquired imaging data.

TOF MRA Sequence

The TOF MRA sequence is based on a 3D FLASH sequence with flow compensation and tilt-optimized non-saturated excitation (TONE) across the slab [27]. Datasets were acquired with an excitation flip angle of $\alpha = 18°$, TE = 4.34 ms, TR = 20 ms, FOV 200 mm × 169 mm × 46 mm, 112 slices per slab (oversampling 14%), GRAPPA acceleration factor R = 4 (phase direction), partial Fourier 6/8 in both slice and phase directions, matrix of 896 × 756 (non-interpolated), and a voxel size of 0.22 × 0.22 × 0.41 mm^3 in a total acquisition time of 6 min 22 s. For a shorter echo time, compared to the standard protocol, a different factor for the asymmetric echo was implemented in the modified protocol: 0.2 instead of 0.3 (ratio of columns acquired before and after echo). The variable-rate selective excitation (VERSE) algorithm [28] was used to reduce SAR contribution of excitation and venous saturation RF pulses [29]. Cutoff thresholds (percentage of maximum amplitude of the original pulse at which the pulse is cropped by the VERSE algorithm) of 50%/30% were chosen for excitation/saturation. The resulting duration was 0.6 ms/2 ms for excitation/saturation RF pulse (compared to 1 ms/3.8 ms in the unmodified standard protocol). A lower VERSE cutoff threshold for the saturation pulses than for the excitation pulses can be chosen because an exact saturation slice profile is not important as long as the saturation area is not overlapping with the imaging slice. The flip angle of the saturation RF pulses was additionally reduced ($\alpha_{SAT} = 35°$ instead of 90° which is normally used) to face SAR constraints [27].

Venous Saturation Pulse

Modified saturation pulses were used to suppress the venous system within the slab and above including the superior sagittal sinus. To reduce total measurement time, the RF pulse and the following spoiler gradient were made shorter (2.3 ms [chosen duration before VERSE was applied]/4 ms instead of 4 ms/ 11 ms). To reduce SAR of the RF pulses, the VERSE algorithm was used on the saturation pulses with a 30% cut-off threshold. The flip angle, α_{SAT}, of the saturation pulses was set to nominally 35° (variation of less than 20% in the superior sagittal sinus due to B_1 inhomogeneity) as suggested in our previously published paper [27] to allow high saturation without exceeding the SAR limitations.

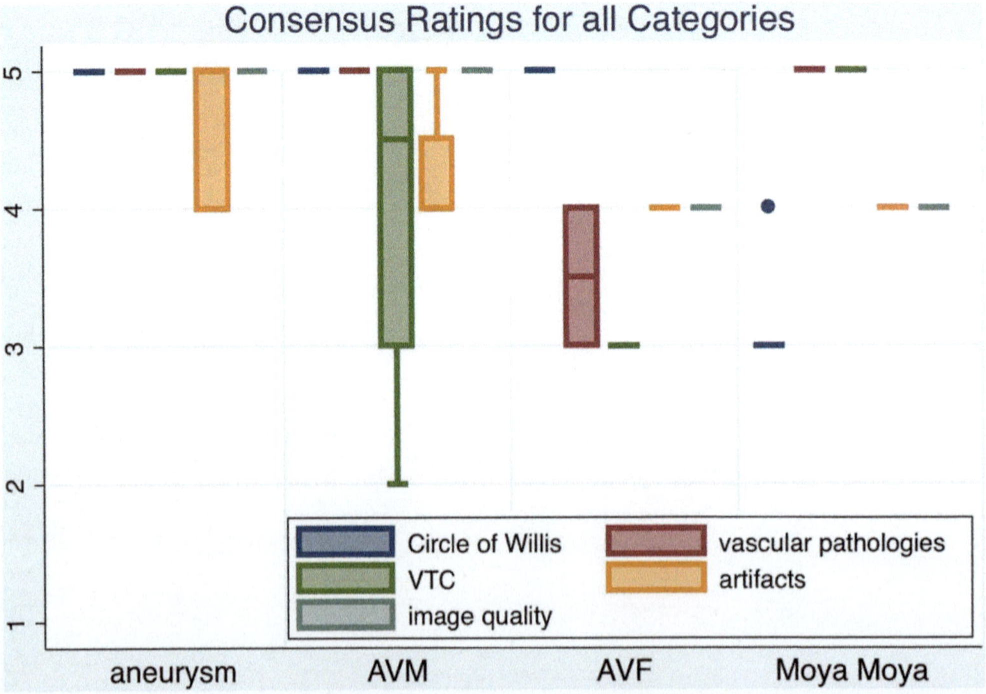

Figure 2. This figure shows the boxplots for all pathologies (aneurysms, AVM, AVF and Moyamoya angiopathy) and all rated categories. Delineation of Circle of Willis was rated excellent except for Moyamoya angiopathy, mainly due to the disease specific early ramifications of the middle cerebral artery branches. Delineation of vascular pathologies was rated excellent except for AVF. The complex angioarchitecture and close relationship to the skull bone complicate depiction in this pathology. Vessel tissue contrast was excellent in aneurysms and Moyamoya angiopathy, but poor to excellent in AVM and AVF. Arterialized hyperintense venous blood alters vessel tissue contrast in these patients. Presence of artifacts was rated mainly good to excellent for all pathologies and only pulsation artifacts led to lower ratings. VERSE specific artifacts did not significantly alter the images. Overall image quality was good to excellent for all pathologies.

Image Evaluation

Image evaluation was performed in consensus by two experienced neuroradiologists on standard post-processing Picture Archiving and Communcation system workstations (Centricity RIS 4.0i, GE Healthcare, USA). Visual evaluation was performed on 3D image reconstructions and on the source images in axial orientation.

For qualitative analysis the following features were evaluated, utilizing a five-point scale (5 = excellent, 4 = good, 3 = moderate, 2 = poor, and 1 = non-diagnostic):

1. Delineation arterial vessels in Circle of Willis
2. Delineation of vascular pathologies
4. Presence of artifacts
5. Vessel tissue contrast
6. Overall image quality

Prior to quantitative measurements, signal intensities of all scans were normalized. The image histogram of each subject was stretched, and shifted to match the baseline histogram of subject 1. Although this method does not correct for intra-subject B_1 inhomogeneities, inter-scan variability of signal intensities caused by e.g. different transmitter voltage, head size and other factors is successfully minimized [30]. The histogram normalization was performed using the inormalize tool by Zijdenbos (version 1.5.1 for OS X as part of Medical Imaging NetCDF toolbox - MINC). MINC is a medical imaging data format and associated set of tools and libraries developed at the Montreal Neurological Institute and freely available online (http://www.bic.mni.mcgill.ca/ServicesSoftware). After preprocessing quantitative signal intensity measurements were then performed by region-of-interest (ROI) analysis using the interactive display tool "fslview" (version 3.1.8 for OS X, http://www.fmrib.ox.ac.uk/fsl/fslview). Vessel-tissue contrast ratio $\left(VTCR\_CoS = \frac{Signal_{GM} - Signal_{CoS}}{Signal_{GM} + Signal_{CoS}} \right)$ of the confluence of sinuses (CoS) and $(VTCR\_MCA = \frac{Signal_{MCA} - Signal_{GM}}{Signal_{MCA} + Signal_{GM}})$ middle cerebral artery (MCA) were assessed in correlation to surrounding gray matter (GM). Therefore, ROIs were placed in the largest diameter of the CoS ($Signal_{CoS}$) and proximal left M1 segments ($Signal_{MCA}$) as well as adjacent gray matter ($Signal_{GM}$). Diameters for ROIs slightly varied between subjects to account for anatomical variations and to maximize ROI size without including voxels from other tissue classes. The average diameter for the ROI of the CoS was 8–12 mm; the ROI for MCA was 3–5 mm in diameter; the ROI for brain parenchyma amounted to approximately 10 mm. In surgically treated Moyamoya patients ROIs were placed in the superficial temporal artery to middle cerebral artery bypass instead of the proximal M1 segment. Sufficient venous saturation in the confluence of sinuses was achieved by definition, if signal intensities in CoS were lower than in GM (VTCR_CoS>0). Arterial vessel tissue contrast was rated subjectively by both raters with focus on local angioarchitecture (VTCR_MCA>0.2 was defined as sufficient).

Differences of continuous scaled variables were tested by Student's t-test. For every mean value the standard error of mean (SE, $\sigma/\sqrt{n}$) was calculated as an estimate of the population mean. Statistical analysis was carried out with the STATA software

Table 3. Quantitative normalized signal intensity measurements.

Subject	CoS	GM	VTC_CoS	MCA	GM	VTC_MCA	Pathology
1	203	482	0.407	1270	244	0.678	aneurysm
2	217	470	0.368	1130	237	0.653	aneurysm
3	179	440	0.422	1082	228	0.652	aneurysm
5	150	479	0.523	1105	266	0.612	aneurysm
7	137	415	0.504	968	225	0.623	aneurysm
9	204	443	0.369	1195	225	0.683	aneurysm
12	168	430	0.438	1072	227	0.651	aneurysm
13	160	373	0.400	1221	212	0.704	aneurysm
14	107	416	0.591	1157	202	0.703	aneurysm
15	113	348	0.510	1117	196	0.701	aneurysm
16	158	479	0.504	1147	257	0.634	aneurysm
17	159	399	0.430	1084	221	0.661	aneurysm
21	110	274	0.427	862	154	0.697	aneurysm
4	429	533	0.108	1112	280	0.598	AVM
22	147	301	0.344	1080	152	0.753	AVM
23	90	251	0.472	1108	122	0.802	AVM
24	126	366	0.488	1074	211	0.672	AVM
11	347	461	0.141	1032	236	0.628	AVF
25	259	330	0.121	1168	184	0.728	AVF
6	162	336	0.349	1027	174	0.710	Moyamoya
8	108	261	0.415	1053	133	0.776	Moyamoya
10	147	449	0.507	986	245	0.602	Moyamoya
18	187	460	0.422	1004	220	0.641	Moyamoya
19	117	234	0.333	1007	117	0.792	Moyamoya
20	161	407	0.433	973	215	0.638	Moyamoya

Quantitative normalized signal intensity measurements were performed by region-of-interest (ROI) analysis.

Vessel-tissue contrast ratio $\left(VTCR\_CoS = \frac{Signal_{GM} - Signal_{CoS}}{Signal_{GM} + Signal_{CoS}}\right)$ of the confluence of sinuses (CoS) and $\left(VTCR\_MCA = \frac{Signal_{MCA} - Signal_{GM}}{Signal_{MCA} + Signal_{GM}}\right)$.
middle cerebral artery (MCA) were assessed in correlation to surrounding gray matter (GM). Therefore, ROI were placed in the largest diameter of the CoS $(Signal_{CoS})$ and proximal left M1 segments $(Signal_{MCA})$ as well as adjacent gray matter $(Signal_{GM})$.

The average diameter for the ROI of the CoS was 8–12 mm; the ROI for MCA was 3–5 mm in diameter; the ROI for brain parenchyma amounted to approximately 10 mm. In surgically treated Moyamoya patients ROI were placed in the superficial temporal artery to middle cerebral artery bypass instead of the proximal M1 segment.

AVM: arteriovenous malformation AVF: dural arteriovenous fistula.

CoS: confluence of sinuses SSS: superior sagittal sinus.

GM: gray matter MCA: middle cerebral artery M1 segment.

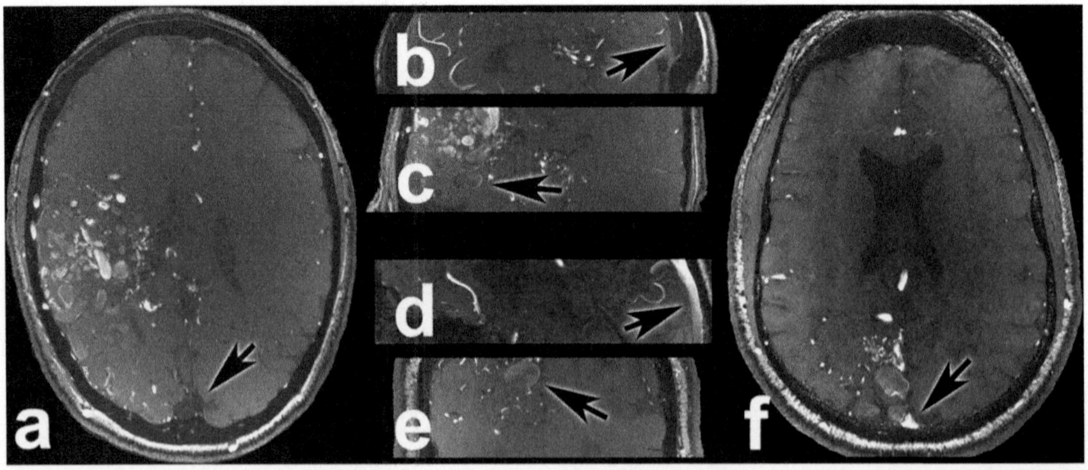

Figure 3. This 40-year-old male patient (a–c) (subject 23) suffered from a right hemispherical AVM (Spetzler-Martin [31] grade IV). Arrows are in transversal (**a**) and sagittal (**b**) views are indicating the saturated superior sagittal sinus. Arrow in coronal view (**c**) is marking a partially saturated draining vein. This 40-year-old male patient (**d–f**) (subject 4) suffered of a right parietal parasagittal fistulous AVM. Signal intensity in the upper part of the sagittal sinus next to the outlet of the draining vein was equal to signal intensity of left middle cerebral artery M1 segment (**f**): arrow in this transverse view is marking unsaturated superior sagittal sinus). In the further distal part of the superior sagittal sinus close to the confluence of sinuses, signal intensity is gradually decreasing until it is lower than in the neighboring occipital gray matter (**d**: arrow in this sagittal view is marking gradually saturated superior sagittal sinus). Arrow marks a partially saturated draining vein in coronal view (**e**). Depending on the individual cerebrovascular anatomy and venous drainage of the AVM, venous saturation can be altered significantly in parts of the TOF MRA imaging slab. Regardless of lower venous saturation in some cases overall image quality was nevertheless rated good to excellent.

package (Stata/SE 12.1 for Mac (64-bit Intel), StataCorp, 4905 Lakeway Drive, College Station, Texas 77845 USA).

Results

All 25 neurosurgical patients tolerated the examination well and were successfully examined without exceeding SAR limitations (time averaged applied RF power in Watts/kg 8.493, range 6.077–9.988, SE 0.241) using 35° flip angles for saturation pulses. Table 1 gives an overview of basic demographic data and time-averaged local SAR in Watts/kg for every scan. Table 2 lists detailed information about consensus ratings for vessel and pathology delineation, vessel-tissue contrast, artifacts and overall image quality. A lower rating for presence of artifacts in some of the patients was solely due to pulsation artifacts. Slight aliasing artifacts were observable only in the uppermost/lowermost 2–3 slices in the axial images, which did not impair evaluation by the raters. Further VERSE specific artifacts (e.g. slice profile distortions or slice shifts especially for off-resonant spins) were not observed. Ratings were good to excellent for the majority of patients and pathologies. Figure 2 presents the ratings in boxplots for all pathologies and all rated categories. Table 3 shows detailed information on ROI mean signal intensity in confluence of sinuses, middle cerebral artery M1 segment (superficial temporal artery to middle cerebral artery bypass in surgically treated patients) and adjacent gray matter. Calculations of vessel-tissue contrast ratios show sufficient vessel-tissue contrast for venous vessels, arterial vessels and adjacent gray matter for the majority of patients and pathologies. The applied venous saturation pulses resulted in vessel-tissue contrast ratios for all patients as follows: mean VTCR_CoS = 0.401 (range 0.108–0.591, SE 0.024); VTCR_MCA = 0.68 (range 0.598–0.802, SE 0.011). The applied venous saturation pulses resulted in vessel-tissue contrast ratios for the patient subgroup with aneurysms and Moyamoya angiopathy as follows: mean VTCR_CoS = 0.44 (range 0.333–0.591, SE 0.015); VTCR_MCA = 0.674 (range 0.602–0.792, SE 0.012). The applied venous saturation pulses resulted in vessel-tissue contrast ratios for the patient subgroup with AVM and AVF as follows: mean VTCR_CoS = 0.279 (range 0.108–0.488, SE 0.073); VTCR_MCA = 0.697 (range 0.598–0.802, SE 0.032). Student's t-test showed significantly higher VTCR_CoS ($p = 0.003$) for the patient subgroup with aneurysms and Moyamoya angiopathy compared to the subgroup of patients suffering of AVM or AVF.

Aneurysms

Thirteen patients with a total of 19 intra-cranial unruptured aneurysms were enrolled in the study (male n = 2, female n = 11; average age 54.61 years; range 26–70 years). Consensus ratings were excellent for delineation of Circle of Willis (mean 5.0, range 5–5, SE 0.0), excellent for vascular pathology delineation (mean 5.0, range 5–5, SE 0.0), excellent for vessel-tissue contrast (mean 5.0, range 5–5, SE 0.0), good for presence of artifacts (mean 4.69, range 4–5, SE 0.133) and excellent for overall image quality (mean 5.0, range 5–5, SE 0.0). The applied venous saturation pulses resulted in vessel-tissue contrast ratios as follows: mean VTCR_CoS = 0.45 (range 0.368–0.591, SE 0.019); VTCR_MCA = 0.667 (range 0.612–0.704, SE 0.009).

Arteriovenous malformations

Four patients with intracranial AVM were enrolled in the study (male n = 4, female n = 0; average age 45 years; range 40–51 years). Consensus ratings were excellent for delineation of Circle of Willis (mean 5.0, range 5–5, SE 0.0), excellent for vascular pathology delineation (mean 5.0, range 5–5, SE 0.0), good for vessel-tissue contrast (mean 4.0, range 2–5, SE 0.707), good for presence of artifacts (mean 4.25, range 4–5, SE 0.25) and excellent for overall image quality (mean 5.0, range 5–5, SE 0.0). The applied venous saturation pulses resulted in vessel-tissue contrast ratios as follows: mean VTCR_CoS = 0.353 (range 0.108–0.488, SE 0.088); VTCR_MCA = 0.706 (range 0.578–0.802, SE 0.045). Venous saturation was lower compared to other pathologies due to inherent features of AVMs, in particular the arterialized venous

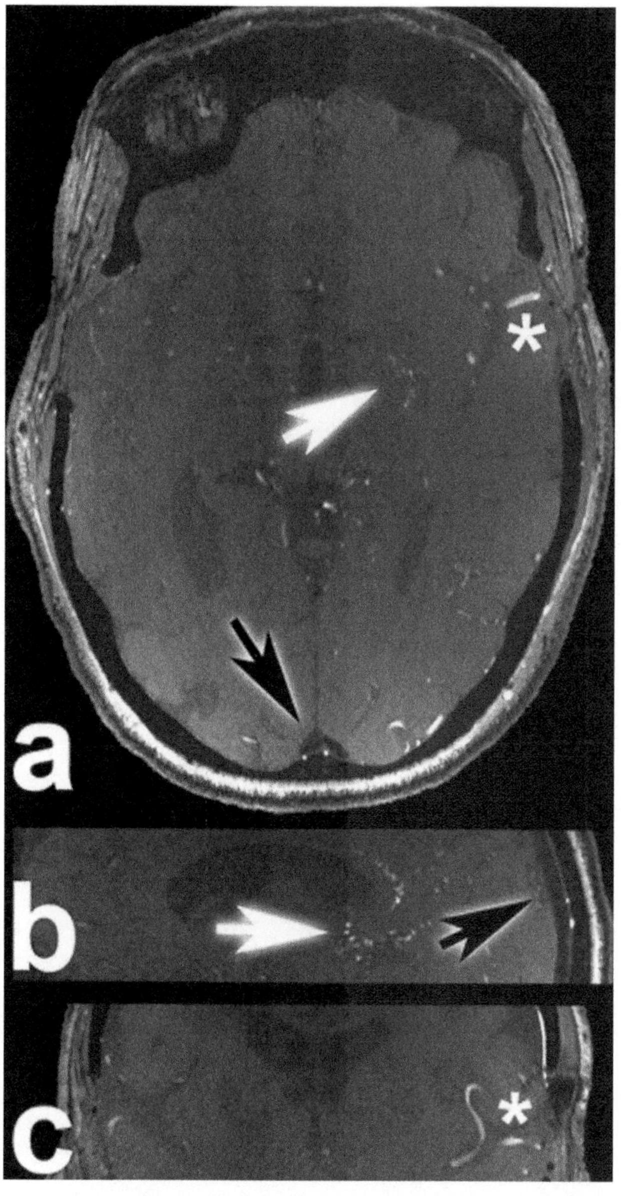

Figure 4. These are the transversal (a), sagittal (b) and coronal (c) views of a 42-year-old female Moyamoya patient (subject 20) after bilateral superficial temporal artery to middle cerebral artery bypass surgery (asterisks next to bypass, black arrows pointing on saturated superior sagittal sinus). The Moyamoya typical anomalously early ramification of middle cerebral artery branches are best depicted in axial and coronal views (white arrows in **a** and **b**).

drainage. Decreasing volume of arterialized draining blood flowing through the saturation slab increases signal intensity. Patient 4 suffered of a right parietal parasagittal fistulous AVM. Signal intensity in the upper part of the sagittal sinus next to the outlet of the draining vein was equal to signal intensity of left middle cerebral artery M1 segment. In the confluence of venous sinuses signal intensity was lower than in the neighboring occipital gray matter (Figure 3 d, gradually decreasing signal intensity in sagittal view). Figure 3 b depicts a partially saturated draining vein in a 40-year-old male patient (subject 23) who suffered from a right hemispherical AVM (Spetzler-Martin [31] grade IV). Depending on the individual cerebrovascular anatomy and venous drainage of the AVM, venous saturation can be altered significantly in parts of the TOF MRA imaging slab. The specific features of AVM delineation in 7 Tesla TOF MRA scans are presented in transversal, sagittal and coronal views for subject 4 and 23.

Moyamoya angiopathy

Six patients suffering from Moyamoya angiopathy were enrolled in the study (male n = 0, female n = 6; average age 38.67 years; range 29–58 years). Consensus ratings were moderate for delineation of Circle of Willis (mean 3.167, range 3–4, SE 0.167), excellent for vascular pathology delineation (mean 5.0, range 5–5, SE 0.0), excellent for vessel-tissue contrast (mean 5.0, range 5–5, SE 0.0), good for presence of artifacts (mean 4.0, range 4–4, SE 0.0) and good for overall image quality (mean 4.0, range 4–4, SE 0.0). The inherent features of Moyamoya angiopathy with slim and sometimes completely blocked arteries in the Circle of Willis and complex collateral circulation especially in surgically treated patients resulted in only moderate ratings for delineation of the Circle of Willis. The applied venous saturation pulses resulted in vessel-tissue contrast ratios as follows: mean VTCR_CoS = 0.41 (range 0.333–0.507, SE 0.026); VTCR_MCA = 0.693 (range 0.602–0.792, SE 0.032). Figure 4 shows a scan of a 42 years-old female patient (subject 20) after bilateral superficial temporal artery to middle cerebral artery bypass surgery.

Dural arteriovenous fistula (AVF)

Two patients with arteriovenous fistulas were enrolled in the study (male n = 2, female n = 0; average age 59.5 years; range 58–61 years). Consensus ratings were excellent for delineation of Circle of Willis (mean 5.0, range 5–5, SE 0.0), moderate and good for vascular pathology delineation (mean 3.5, range 3–4, SE 0.5), moderate for vessel-tissue contrast (mean 3.0, range 3–3, SE 0.0), good for presence of artifacts (mean 4.0, range 4–4, SE 0.0) and good for overall image quality (mean 4.0, range 4–4, SE 0.0). The applied venous saturation pulses resulted in vessel-tissue contrast ratios as follows: mean VTCR_CoS = 0.131 (range 0.121–0.141, SE 0.01); VTCR_MCA = 0.678 (range 0.628–0.728, SE 0.05). As in AVM patients venous saturation was lower compared to other pathologies due to inherent features of dural AVFs, in particular direct shunting of arterialized blood into the venous sinuses. High signal intensity of arterialized blood is similar to signal intensity of the left middle cerebral artery M1 segment. Signal intensity of venous sinuses decays the further away from the fistula point it is measured. The special features of dural AVF in 7 Tesla TOF MRA scans are exemplarily illustrated (Figure 5) in a 58-year-old male patient (subject 11) with a complex occipital dural AVF (Cognard [32] type IIb) fed by branches of both external carotid and vertebral arteries.

Discussion

Time-of-flight MRA is a non-invasive imaging technique using FLASH gradient-echo magnetic resonance sequences to visualize the contrast between the high signal intensity of inflowing blood and saturated stationary tissue. TOF MRA utilizing 1.5 Tesla has been established as an excellent clinical diagnostic method for pre-operative and pre-interventional planning as well as for follow-up controls in cerebro-vascular pathologies, and has gained ground on the accepted gold standard, invasive digital subtraction angiography.

The increase of the magnetic field strength from 1.5 Tesla to 3 Tesla has been proven beneficial for clinical neuroimaging and

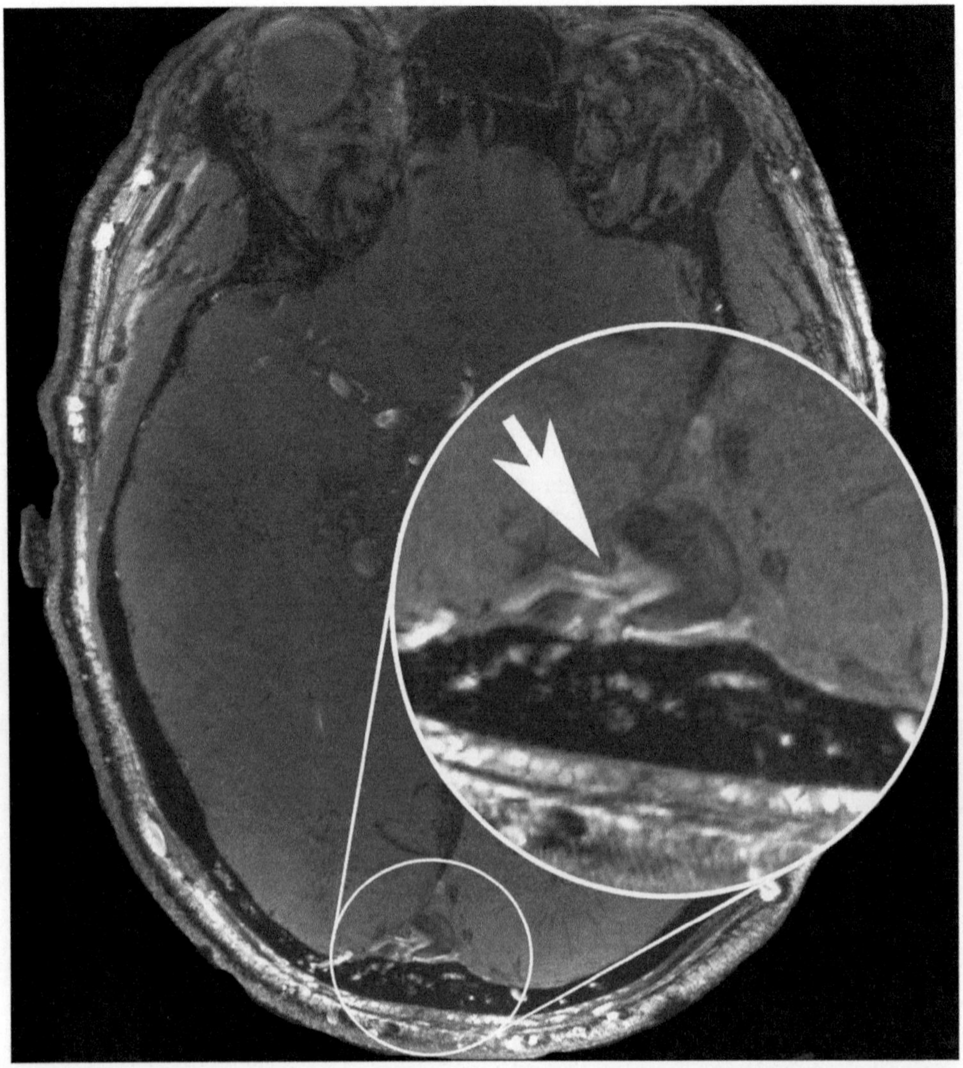

Figure 5. This figure shows the scan of a 58-year-old male patient (subject 11) with a complex occipital dural AVF (Cognard type IIb) fed by branches of both external carotid and vertebral arteries. It highlights the advantages of venous saturation pulses in 7 Tesla TOF MRA. The exact location of the fistulous point (arrow in magnified image section) is depicted by mixing hyperintense unsaturated arterial blood with hypointense saturated venous blood in the superior sagittal sinus.

feasible for ultra-high-field 7 Tesla MRI, facilitating a significant increase in spatial resolution [4,8,9,15–17,33,34]. Moenninghoff et al. presented a high-resolution 7 Tesla TOF MRA protocol for clinical application including venous saturation pulses. To maintain SAR limitations, time-of-repetition (TR) had to be increased up to 57 ms, resulting in an increase in acquisition time to almost 15 minutes for comparable spatial coverage as the presented protocol. The previously suggested solution [27] to overcome SAR limitations within a patient tolerable scanning time has not yet been applied in a clinical setting for various intracerebral vascular pathologies.

The impairment of venous saturation at ultra-high field strength is mainly due to SAR limitations that prohibit the usage of venous saturation pulses within reasonable acquisition times.

One proposed solution to overcome SAR limitations is to play out a regular 90° saturation pulse only every n-th readout of the k-space [8]. The drawback of this approach would be that either measurement time is not used efficiently or excitation RF pulses experience different effective TRs which could lead to an artifact appearing similar to aliasing [35] caused by periodic signal variation in k-space lines. The exact effect of different effective TRs would have to be assessed prior to routine clinical application. It is also difficult to achieve a good balance between venous saturation and optimal SAR utilization, as this method is more rigid than mere flip angle variations. Our approach to overcome SAR limitations uses customized low flip angle VERSE algorithm [28,29] saturation pulses to significantly reduce the SAR of each individual saturation pulse rather than reducing the number of saturation pulses. The VERSE algorithm was used to decrease SAR contribution of excitation and saturation RF pulses. Based on this reduction, flip angles of saturation pulses were optimized for adequate venous saturation while remaining within SAR restrictions. Without optimization of flip angles and VERSE algorithm acquisition time was almost 3 times longer (6:22 min versus 17:48 min) in a 29-year-old healthy volunteer and TE had to be increased from 4.34 ms to 6.62 ms. Also the TR had to be increased from 20 ms to 56 ms to stay within SAR limits. Especially the prolonged TR leads to lower image contrast. A detailed description of the applied pulse sequence and considerations on ideal flip angles for saturation pulses have previously been published [27]. Differences in image contrast between non-optimized and optimized TOF MRA sequences are illustrated in Figure 1.

Only in patients with AVMs and AVF, venous saturation was reduced compared to other pathologies. This was presumably due to the inherent features of both pathologies, specifically the fast blood flow of venous drainage. In addition, only part of the AVMs were within the field of saturation pulses and consequently unsaturated blood was drained over the veins. Even though the venous saturation was reduced in these patients, the application of saturation pulses could still partially suppress the signal of draining veins with an overall good image quality.

The high diagnostic relevance of saturation pulses in combination with ultra-high-resolution TOF MRA is exemplarily shown in the case of Subject 12 (Figure 5). The complex dural AVF (Cognard [32] type IIb) could be clearly visualized and the fistulous point with the hyperintense artery entering the hypointense venous sinus was clearly depicted by mixed unsaturated arterial and saturated venous blood. This effect can presumably only be visualized with effective venous saturation, and might not be clearly visible in TOF MRA imaging without venous saturation pulses or in contrast-enhanced T_1-weighted images. Future patients suffering of AVF will be examined with and without venous saturation pulses to further investigate the diagnostic potential of this effect.

Consensus ratings of two experienced readers ranged between good and excellent for the majority of patients and most of the evaluated features. In combination with short acquisition time and possibility to visualize the complete intracranial arterial vasculature with ultra-high resolution the presented TOF MRA protocol is suitable for clinical application.

Clearly, this study is not free of limitations. The study group comprised of patients suffering from various intracranial vascular pathologies and therefore patient numbers for individual pathologies are small. Nevertheless, to the authors knowledge this is one of the largest neurosurgical patients cohorts scanned with TOF MRA at 7 Tesla, published in literature. Further investigations with larger patient cohorts of single pathologies should be the focus of future studies. Ultra-high-field imaging in patients who underwent treatment has been restricted so far, as Guglielmi detachable coils, aneurysm clips, most cranial fixation plates and other metallic implants are not certified for 7 Tesla MR imaging. Although preliminary results on implant safety in cerebral 7 Tesla MRI have been recently demonstrated [36–38], up to now avoiding metallic implants during surgery is the only feasible way for postoperative scans. The excellent image quality is exemplarily shown in a 42-year-old female patient (subject 25) after bilateral superficial temporal artery to middle cerebral artery bypass surgery (Figure 4). Future studies on the diagnostic potential of 7 Tesla MRI for follow-up of treated aneurysms, AVM, AVF and patients with Moyamoya angiopathy would be of high scientific and clinical interest. Another limitation is posed by the lack of a comparison to digital subtraction angiography, the diagnostic gold standard. However, with MRA offering equivalent non-invasive vessel diagnostics to DSA, the main focus of this trial was set on testing the feasibility and diagnostic potential of high-resolution TOF MRA at 7 Tesla utilizing novel low flip angle venous saturation pulses in a variety of intracranial vascular pathologies.

In summary, this study presents the clinical application of the previously reported practical solution for saturation pulses in 7 Tesla ultra-high-resolution TOF MRA that maintains SAR levels within the accepted safety standards combined with short acquisition times [27]. Excellent imaging quality was shown for the majority of patients in a larger cohort suffering from diverse cerebro-vascular pathologies.

Acknowledgments

The authors thank Lena C. Schäfer (RT) for performing all in vivo examinations.

Author Contributions

Conceived and designed the experiments: KHW SJ PD NÖ CM MK SM MEL US LU MS. Performed the experiments: KHW SJ PD NÖ CM MK SM MEL US LU MS. Analyzed the data: KHW SJ PD NÖ CM MK SM MEL US LU MS. Contributed reagents/materials/analysis tools: KHW SJ LU MS. Wrote the paper: KHW SJ PD NÖ CM MK SM MEL US LU MS.

References

1. Keller PJ, Drayer BP, Fram EK, Williams KD, Dumoulin CL, et al. (1989) MR angiography with two-dimensional acquisition and three-dimensional display. Work in progress. Radiology 173: 527–532.
2. Brugieres P, Ricolfi F, Revel MP, Combes C, Gaston A (1993) Functional exploration of brain vessels by MRI. Usefulness of presaturation techniques. Journal of Neuroradiology 20: 239–251.
3. Brugières P, Blustajn J, Le Guérinel C, Méder JF, Thomas P, et al. (1998) Magnetic resonance angiography of giant intracranial aneurysms. Neuroradiology 40: 96–102.
4. Monninghoff C, Maderwald S, Theysohn JM, Kraff O, Ladd SC, et al. (2009) Evaluation of intracranial aneurysms with 7 T versus 1.5 T time-of-flight MR angiography - initial experience. RoFo: Fortschritte auf dem Gebiete der Rontgenstrahlen und der Nuklearmedizin 181: 16–23.
5. Chung TS, Joo JY, Lee SK, Chien D, Laub G (1999) Evaluation of cerebral aneurysms with high-resolution MR angiography using a section-interpolation technique: correlation with digital subtraction angiography. Am J Neuroradiol 20: 229–235.
6. Majoie CBLM, Sprengers ME, Van Rooij WJJ, Lavini C, Sluzewski M, et al. (2005) MR angiography at 3 T versus digital subtraction angiography in the follow-up of intracranial aneurysms treated with detachable coils. American Journal of Neuroradiology 26: 1349–1356.
7. Papke K, Brassel F (2006) Modern cross-sectional imaging in the diagnosis and follow-up of intracranial aneurysms. Eur Radiol 16: 2051–2066.
8. Hendrikse J, Zwanenburg JJ, Visser F, Takahara T, Luijten P (2008) Noninvasive Depiction of the Lenticulostriate Arteries with Time-of-Flight MR Angiography at 7.0 T. Cerebrovascular diseases 26: 624–629.
9. Heverhagen JT, Bourekas E, Sammet S, Knopp MV, Schmalbrock P (2008) Time-of-flight magnetic resonance angiography at 7 Tesla. Invest Radiol 43: 568–573.
10. Willinek WA, Born M, Simon B, Tschampa HJ, Krautmacher C, et al. (2003) Time-of-Flight MR Angiography: Comparison of 3.0-T Imaging and 1.5-T Imaging-Initial Experience. Radiology 229: 913–920.
11. Gaa J, Weidauer S, Requardt M, Kiefer B, Lanfermann H, et al. (2004) Comparison of intracranial 3D–ToF-MRA with and without parallel acquisition techniques at 1.5 T and 3.0 T: Preliminary results. Acta radiologica 45: 327–332.
12. Nowinski WL, Puspitasaari F, Volkau I, Marchenko Y, Knopp MV (2013) Comparison of Magnetic Resonance Angiography Scans on 1.5, 3, and 7 Tesla Units: A Quantitative Study of 3-Dimensional Cerebrovasculature. J Neuroimaging: 86–95.
13. Gibbs GF, Huston J 3rd, Bernstein MA, Riederer SJ, Brown RD Jr (2005) 3.0-Tesla MR angiography of intracranial aneurysms: comparison of time-of-flight and contrast-enhanced techniques. J Magn Reson Imaging 21: 97–102.
14. Cho ZH, Kang CK, Han JY, Kim SH, Kim KN, et al. (2008) Observation of the lenticulostriate arteries in the human brain in vivo using 7.0 T MR angiography. Stroke 39: 1604–1606.
15. von Morze C, Xu D, Purcell DD, Hess CP, Mukherjee P, et al. (2007) Intracranial time-of-flight MR angiography at 7 T with comparison to 3 T. J Magn Reson Imaging 26: 900–904.
16. Kang CK, Park CW, Han JY, Kim SH, Park CA, et al. (2009) Imaging and analysis of lenticulostriate arteries using 7.0-Tesla magnetic resonance angiography. Magn Reson Med 61: 136–144.

17. Martin-Vaquero P, Da Costa RC, Echandi RL, Tosti CL, Knopp MV, et al. (2011) Time-of-flight magnetic resonance angiography of the canine brain at 3.0 Tesla and 7.0 Tesla. American Journal of Veterinary Research 72: 350–356.
18. Zwanenburg JJ, Hendrikse J, Takahara T, Visser F, Luijten PR (2008) MR angiography of the cerebral perforating arteries with magnetization prepared anatomical reference at 7 T: comparison with time-of-flight. J Magn Reson Imaging 28: 1519–1526.
19. Ladd ME (2007) High-field-strength magnetic resonance: potential and limits. Top Magn Reson Imaging 18: 139–152.
20. Fujii Y, Uzuka T, Matsuzawa H, Igarashi H, Nakada T (2010) Neuroscientific application of ultra high-field (7 tesla) MRI. Neurological Surgery 38: 107–116.
21. Kollia K, Maderwald S, Putzki N, Schlamann M, Theysohn JM, et al. (2009) First clinical study on ultra-high-field MR imaging in patients with multiple sclerosis: comparison of 1.5 T and 7 T. Am J Neuroradiol 30: 699–702.
22. Wrede KH, Dammann P, Mönninghoff C, Johst S, Maderwald S, et al. (2014) Non-Enhanced MR Imaging of Cerebral Aneurysms: 7 Tesla versus 1.5 Tesla. PLoS ONE 9: e84562.
23. Felmlee JP, Ehman RL (1987) Spatial presaturation: A method for suppressing flow artifacts and improving depiction of vascular anatomy in MR imaging. Radiology 164: 559–564.
24. King KF (2004) Spatial Saturation Pulses. In: Bernstein MA, King KF, Zhou ZJ, editors. Handbook of MRI pulse sequences. Amsterdam; Boston: Academic Press. 148–152.
25. Tkach JA, Ruggieri PM, Ross JS, Modic MT, Dillinger JJ, et al. (1993) Pulse sequence strategies for vascular contrast in time-of-flight carotid MR angiography. J Magn Reson Imaging 3: 811–820.
26. Schar M, Kozerke S, Fischer SE, Boesiger P (2004) Cardiac SSFP imaging at 3 Tesla. Magn Reson Med 51: 799–806.
27. Johst S, Wrede KH, Ladd ME, Maderwald S (2012) Time-of-Flight Magnetic Resonance Angiography at 7 T Using Venous Saturation Pulses With Reduced Flip Angles. Invest Radiol 47: 445–450.
28. Conolly S, Nishimura D, Macovski A, Glover G (1988) Variable-rate selective excitation. J Magn Reson Imaging 78: 440–458.
29. Schmitter S, Bock M, Johst S, Auerbach EJ, Ugurbil K, et al. (2012) Contrast enhancement in TOF cerebral angiography at 7 T using saturation and MT pulses under SAR constraints: impact of VERSE and sparse pulses. Magn Reson Med 68: 188–197.
30. Loizou CP, Pantziaris M, Pattichis CS, Seimenis I (2012) Brain MR image normalization in texture analysis of multiple sclerosis. Journal of Biomedical Graphics and Computing 3.
31. Spetzler RF, Martin NA (1986) A proposed grading system for arteriovenous malformations. J Neurosurg 65: 476–483.
32. Cognard C, Gobin YP, Pierot L, Bailly AL, Houdart E, et al. (1995) Cerebral dural arteriovenous fistulas: clinical and angiographic correlation with a revised classification of venous drainage. Radiology 194: 671–680.
33. Conijn MM, Hendrikse J, Zwanenburg JJ, Takahara T, Geerlings MI, et al. (2009) Perforating arteries originating from the posterior communicating artery: a 7.0-Tesla MRI study. Eur Radiol 19: 2986–2992.
34. Kang CK, Hong SM, Han JY, Kim KN, Kim SH, et al. (2008) Evaluation of MR angiography at 7.0 Tesla MRI using birdcage radio frequency coils with end caps. Magn Reson Med 60: 330–338.
35. Johst S, Orzada S, Fischer A, Schafer LC, Nassenstein K, et al. (2014) Sequence Comparison for Non-Enhanced MRA of the Lower Extremity Arteries at 7 Tesla. PLoS One 9: e86274.
36. Kraff O, Wrede KH, Schoemberg T, Dammann P, Noureddine Y, et al. (2013) MR safety assessment of potential RF heating from cranial fixation plates at 7 T. Med Phys 40: 042302.
37. Noureddine Y, Kraff O, Ladd ME, Schaefers G, Wrede KH, et al. (2012) RF Safety of Aneurysm Clips at 7 Tesla: Effect of Field Polarization. Proc. Intl. Soc. Mag. Reson. Med. (ISMRM) 20: 2767.
38. Noureddine Y, Kraff O, Ladd ME, Schaefers G, Wrede KH, et al. (2013) In Silico and in Vitro Investigation of Temperature Elevation Close to an Aneurysm Clip at 7T. In: ISMRM 21st Annual Meeting & Exhibition 20–26 April 2013, Salt Lake City, USA. pp. 4416.

Right Ventricular Function Quantification in Takotsubo Cardiomyopathy Using Two-Dimensional Strain Echocardiography

Felix Heggemann[1*], Karsten Hamm[2], Joachim Brade[3], Florian Streitner[1], Christina Doesch[1], Theano Papavassiliu[1], Martin Borggrefe[1], Dariusch Haghi[1]

1 First Medical Department, University Medical Center Mannheim, University of Heidelberg, Mannheim, Germany, **2** Department of Cardiology, Center of Cardiovascular Medicine, Bad Neustadt, Germany, **3** Department of Biometrics and Statistics, University Medical Center Mannheim, University of Heidelberg, Mannheim, Germany

Abstract

Aims: This study sought to characterize global and regional right ventricular (RV) myocardial function in patients with Takotsubo cardiomyopathy (TC) using 2D strain imaging.

Methods: We compared various parameters of RV and left ventricular (LV) systolic function between 2 groups of consecutive patients with TC at initial presentation and upon follow-up. Group 1 had RV involvement and group 2 did not have RV involvement.

Results: At initial presentation, RV peak systolic longitudinal strain (RVPSS) and RV fractional area change (RVFAC) were significantly lower in group 1 (−13.2±8.6% vs. −21.8±5.4%, p = 0.001; 30.7±9.3% vs. 43.5±6.3%, p = 0.001) and improved significantly upon follow-up. Tricuspid annular plane systolic excursion (TAPSE) did not differ significantly at initial presentation between both groups (14.8±4.1 mm vs. 17.9±3.5 mm, p = 0.050). Differences in regional systolic RV strain were only observed in the mid and apical segments. LV ejection fraction (LVEF) and LV global strain were significantly lower in group 1 (36±8% vs. 46±10%, p = 0.006 and −5.5±4.8% vs. −10.2±6.2%, p = 0.040) at initial presentation. None of the parameters were significantly different between the 2 groups upon follow-up. A RVPSS cut-off value of >−19.1% had a sensitivity of 85% and a specificity of 71% to discriminate between the 2 groups.

Conclusion: In TC, RVFAC, RVPSS, LVEF and LV global strain differed significantly between patients with and without RV dysfunction, whereas TAPSE did not. 2 D strain imaging was feasible for the assessment of RV dysfunction in TC and could discriminate between patients with and without RV involvement in a clinically meaningful way.

Editor: M. Faadiel Essop, Stellenbosch University, South Africa

Funding: The authors have no funding or support to report.

Competing Interests: The authors have declared that no competing interests exist.

* Email: felixheggemann@gmx.de

These authors contributed equally to this work.

Introduction

In 1991 Dote et al. [1] described a novel syndrome named Takotsubo Cardiomyopathy (TC) consisting of transient left ventricular apical dysfunction ("apical ballooning"), minimal elevation of myocardial enzymes in the absence of coronary artery disease and electrocardiographic ST-T segment changes [2].

In a previous work we characterized global and regional LV function in patients with TC using 2D strain echocardiography [2]. RV involvement is another known feature of TC, occurring roughly in one-quarter of patients [3–7]. Right ventricular involvement in patients with TC is correlated with more severe complications and longer hospitalisation and is an important prognostic factor of the clinical course [6]. Therefore, it is desirable to accurately assess RV function in this disease entity.

Estimation of RV function is challenging due to the complex RV geometry [8,9]. Usage of TAPSE (tricuspid annular systolic excursion) for the diagnosis of RV dysfunction is limited, because hyperkinetic basal segments may compensate for hypokinetic midventricular- and apical parts. RVFAC (right ventricular fractional area change) measures RV function in a single plane and therefore may not be a reliable measure of global RV function. 2D strain is a novel method that allows for a segment-based measurement of myocardial deformation and may therefore have the potential to quantify RV dysfunction more precisely than conventional parameters of RV function.

To the best of our knowledge, detailed echocardiographic quantification of RV function in TC using 2D strain echocardiography has not been performed so far. Therefore, in this study we sought to analyse RV function by using this novel technique in addition to conventional parameters of RV function.

Table 1. Baseline clinical and echocardiographic characteristics for patients with TC with biventricular involvement (group 1) and only left ventricular involvement (group 2).

Parameters	group 1	group 2	p-value
Age (years)	68±8	70±12	0.265
Female, n (%)	12 (86)	14 (100)	0.541
Hypertension, n (%)	6 (43)	10 (71)	0.21
Diabetes, n (%)	2 (14)	4 (29)	0.541
Current smoker, n (%)	4 (29)	3 (21)	0.769
Hypercholesterolemia, n (%)	3 (30)	1 (8)	0.376
Pleural effusion (%)	5 (36)	0 (0)	0.003
Presenting symptom, n (%)			
Angina	6 (43)	11 (49)	0.114
Dyspnoea	6 (43)	2 (14)	0.210
Other	2 (14)	1 (8)	0.769
ECG upon presentation			
ST elevation	4 (29)	4 (29)	1.000
T wave inversion	12 (86)	11 (79)	0.769
Type TC, n (%)			
Classical	11 (79)	9 (64)	0.541
Variant	3 (21)	5 (36)	0.541
Peak troponin I (μg/l) [normal range: 0–0.4]	2.4±1.8	2.4±2.2	0.402
Triggering factor, n (%)			
Physical stress	7 (50)	2 (14)	0.114
Emotional stress	7 (50)	5 (36)	0.541
Strain obtainable in % of segments of the RV free wall (acute/follow-up)	81/76	83/71	

TC: Takotsubo cardiomyopathy, ECG: electrocardiogram, RV: right ventricular

Methods

Study population

Twenty-eight patients with the clinical diagnosis of TC undergoing clinically indicated echocardiography were recruited for this study. Diagnosis of TC was based on the following criteria: (i) acute onset of apical and/or mid-ventricular wall-motion abnormalities of the left ventricle not confined to the vascular territory of a single major coronary artery, (ii) absence of severe coronary obstruction (>70%) or angiographic evidence of plaque rupture, (iii) new ECG abnormalities (either ST-segment elevation and/or T-wave inversion) or elevated cardiac troponin in the absence of phaechromocytoma and myocarditis. Depending on the additional presence of visually observed RV wall-motion abnormalities, patients were divided into two groups: fourteen patients with RV involvement (group 1) and fourteen without RV involvement (group 2).

Echocardiography

Echocardiography of both groups was performed within 48 h of diagnosis and upon follow-up, using a Vivid 7 machine (GE Ultrasound, Horten, Norway) with a 2,5 MHz phased-array transducer. Standard echocardiographic images were obtained at end-expiratory apnoea. 2D strain analysis was performed offline using custom 2D strain imaging software (EchoPac, GE Ultrasound). The endocardial borders were traced at the end-systolic frame of the 2D images. The interactive software then automatically tracked myocardial motion and divided each image into six segments. For each of the six segments numerical and graphical displays of deformation parameters were generated, reflecting the average value for tracking all acoustic markers in each segment [10]. Longitudinal RV peak systolic strain (RVPSS) was acquired in the myocardium of the RV free wall from the apical four-chamber view that was modified, if necessary, to include the RV free wall. LV longitudinal peak systolic strain was acquired from apical two-, three- and four-chamber views. RVPSS was calculated as the average RV peak systolic longitudinal strain values of the basal, mid and apical RV free wall. RV fractional area change (RVFAC) and tricuspid annular plane systolic excursion (TAPSE) were assessed in the four-chamber view. LV ejection fraction (LVEF) was determined using Simpson's method. LV global longitudinal strain (LVGLS) was assessed from 3 apical views.

Statistical analysis

Continuous variables are expressed as mean ± standard deviation. Continuous variables were compared using the two-sided Mann-Whitney U-test. A p-value <0.05 was considered statistically significant. Receiver operating characteristic (ROC) curves and Kendall-tau-b correlation coefficients were computed to assess the ability of RVPSS, RVFAC, TAPSE and LVGLS to predict RV involvement. Inter- and intraobserver correlation coefficients for strain measurements in our laboratory were 0.82 and 0.98, respectively [9].

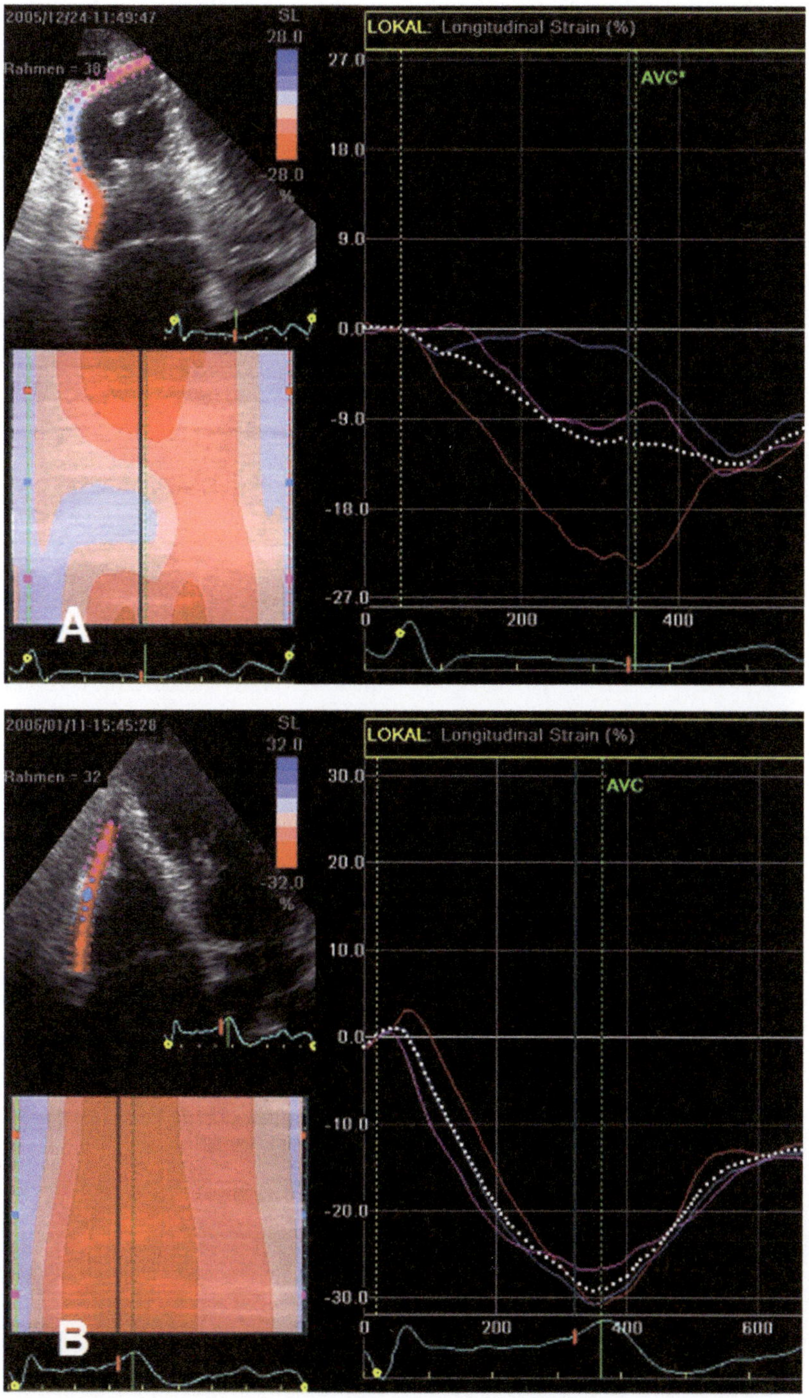

Figure 1. Right ventricular (RV) free wall systolic strain curves in a patient with RV involvement at baseline (A) and upon follow-up (B).

Results

The clinical and echocardiographic features of patients at initial presentation are shown in table 1. All patients were in sinus rhythm. Patients in both groups either had classical TC with apical involvement or mid-ventricular variant of TC, where apical wall-motion abnormalities are absent. None of the patients had the reverse variant of TC where LV dysfunction is confined to the base of the heart.

Follow-up examinations were performed in group 1 after 40±45 days and in group 2 after 68±170 days. Longitudinal peak systolic strain could be obtained in group 1 in 34 of 42 segments (81%) at baseline and in 32 of 42 segments (76%) upon follow-up (group 2, 35 of 42 segments (83%) at baseline and 30 of 42 segments (71%) upon follow-up). Figure 1 shows an example of RV free wall systolic strain in a patient with RV involvement at baseline (A) and upon follow-up (B). Table 2 shows regional RV strain values of both groups at baseline and upon follow-up.

Table 2. Right ventricular longitudinal strain (%) by segment in patients with Takotsubo cardiomyopathy with biventricular involvement (group 1) and only left ventricular involvement (group 2).

	group 1			group 2			
Segment	baseline	follow-up	p-value	baseline	follow-up	p-value	p-value**
apical free wall	−11.1±6.8	−22.1±8.5	**0.003**	−22.5±5.9	−26.1±8.3	0.244	**<0.001**
mid free wall	−13.5±11.4	−24.9±7.9	**0.020**	−25.3±6.5	−27.7±7.9	0.211	**0.005**
basal free wall	−16.6±14.1	−24.6±8.7	0.149	−25.5±6.9	−29.9±4.5	0.236	0.139

** group 1 compared to group 2 at baseline.

Regional longitudinal RV strain was significantly lower in apical and mid-ventricular segments at baseline in group 1 compared to group 2, and improved significantly in group 1 upon follow-up. RV strain was not significantly impaired in the basal segments at baseline.

RVPSS and RVFAC were significantly lower in group 1 compared to group 2 at baseline, and improved significantly in group 1 but not in group 2 upon follow-up (table 3). TAPSE improved significantly in group 1 upon follow-up but was not significantly different at baseline compared to group 2. Upon follow-up, no significant differences could be found between both groups with regard to all 3 parameters. Differences in RVPSS were predominantly based on lower strain values in apical and mid-ventricular segments.

The dot plots in figure 2 display the distribution of RVPSS, TAPSE, RVFAC and LVGLS among the 2 groups. All 4 parameters were significantly correlated with RV involvement (table 4). ROC curves of these parameters are shown in figure 3. RVPSS had the best discriminatory value for differentiating between the 2 groups. RVPSS>−19.1% was 85% sensitive and 71% specific for predicting RV involvement. Pleural effusion (PE) occurred exclusively in group 1 (n = 5). Within group 1, patients with PE had significantly lower RVPSS compared to patients without PE (−4.65±6.3 vs. −18.46±4.5, p = 0.003). A RVPSS value >−14.8% indicated the occurrence of PE with a sensitivity of 87% and a specificity of 80%. At baseline, LVEF and LVGLS were significantly lower in group 1 patients compared to group 2 patients (table 3). Both parameters improved significantly upon follow-up in both groups. No significant differences could be found between both groups upon follow-up.

Discussion

Assessment of RV function is one of the most challenging tasks in modern echocardiography. Subjective analysis is probably the most commonly used method for assessment of RV function. RV speckle tracking echocardiography (STE) is a novel method that allows quantitative assessment of RV function. Utility of RV STE both as a diagnostic and prognostic tool has been shown in various disease entities, including pulmonary hypertension (PH) [11], congenital heart disease [12,13], heart failure [14] and cardiomyopathies [15].

RV involvement is a well-known feature of TC. Initial experience was confined to single cases [4,5]. In 2006 Elesber et al. [6] reported on the Mayo Clinic experience in 25 consecutive patients. In their retrospective echocardiographic study, RV dysfunction was assessed visually and was found to be present in 8 of 25 patients. The authors found that RV dysfunction in TC indicated longer hospitalisation course, increased risk of hemodynamic instability, more severe congestive heart failure, and in some cases the requirement for intra-aortic balloon pump. They also found that the pattern of RV regional wall motion abnormalities was similar to the pattern of LV wall motion abnormalities.

Using cardiovascular magnetic resonance imaging Haghi et al. [16] were able to confirm most of these findings. RV involvement was present in roughly one-quarter of 34 patients and was associated with more depressed LV function. RV dysfunction was also indicative of extensive or bilateral pleural effusion.

The current study examined the utility of STE in the assessment of regional and global LV and RV function in TC. The importance of measuring RV longitudinal function is underlined by the fact that longitudinal shortening accounts for the majority of RV contraction in normal subjects and patients with PH [17].

Table 3. Right and left ventricular echocardiographic parameters.

Parameters	group 1	group 2	p-value
TAPSE baseline (mm)	14.8±4.1*	17.9±3.5***	0.050
TAPSE follow -up (mm)	20.2±5.7**	20.3±4.0****	p= 0.072 ** vs. *: p=0.010 **** vs. ***: p=0.128
RVFAC baseline (%)	30.7±9.3*	43.5±6.3***	p=0.001
RVFAC follow-up (%)	44.7±11.2**	39.6±7.3****	p=0.169 ** vs. *: p= 0.006 **** vs. ***: p= 0.880
RVPSS baseline (%)	−13.2±8.6*	−21.8±5.4***	p=0.001
RVPSS follow-up (%)	−24.1±6.6**	−26.0±7.2****	p=0.378 ** vs. *: p=0.002 **** vs. ****: p=0.252
LVGLS baseline (%)	−5.5±4.8*	−10.2±6.2***	p=0.040
LVGLS follow-up (%)	−14.1±2.8**	−18.1±2.6****	p=0.378 ** vs. *: p <0.001 **** vs. ***: p=0.001
Biplane ejection fraction (%) baseline	36±8 *	46±10 ***	p=0.006
Biplane ejection fraction (%) follow-up	55±9 **	57±6 ****	p=0.375 ** vs. *: p<0.001 **** vs.***: p=0.007

TAPSE: tricuspid annular plane systolic excursion, RVFAC: right ventricular fractional area change, RVPSS: right ventricular peak systolic strain, LVGLS: left ventricular global strain.
*-**** indicate the statistically compared subgroups for each parameter.

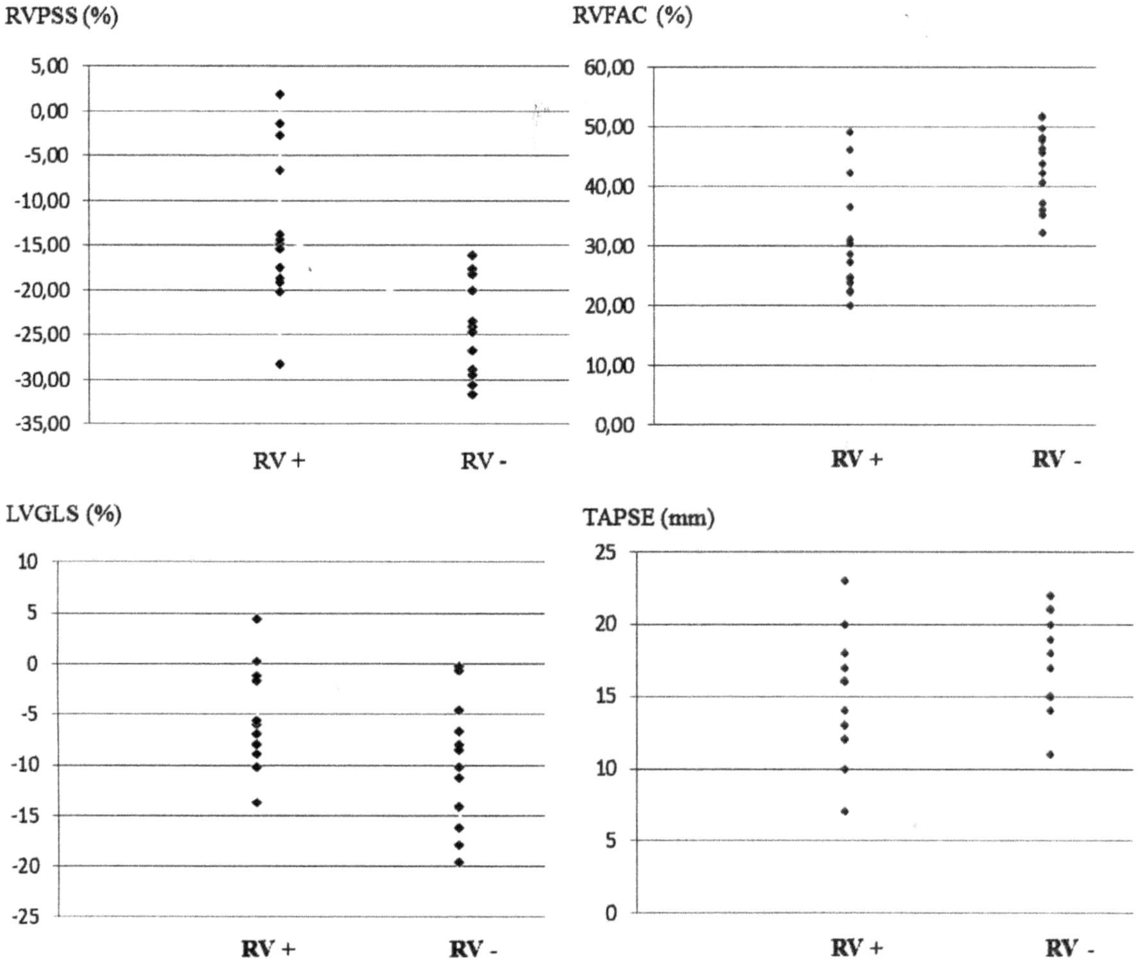

Figure 2. Distribution of RVPSS, TAPSE, RVFAC and LVGLS among patients with (RV+) and without (RV-) right ventricular involvement displayed by dotplots. RVPSS: right ventricular peak systolic strain, TAPSE: tricuspid annular plane systolic excursion, RVFAC: right ventricular fractional area change, LVGLS: left ventricular global strain.

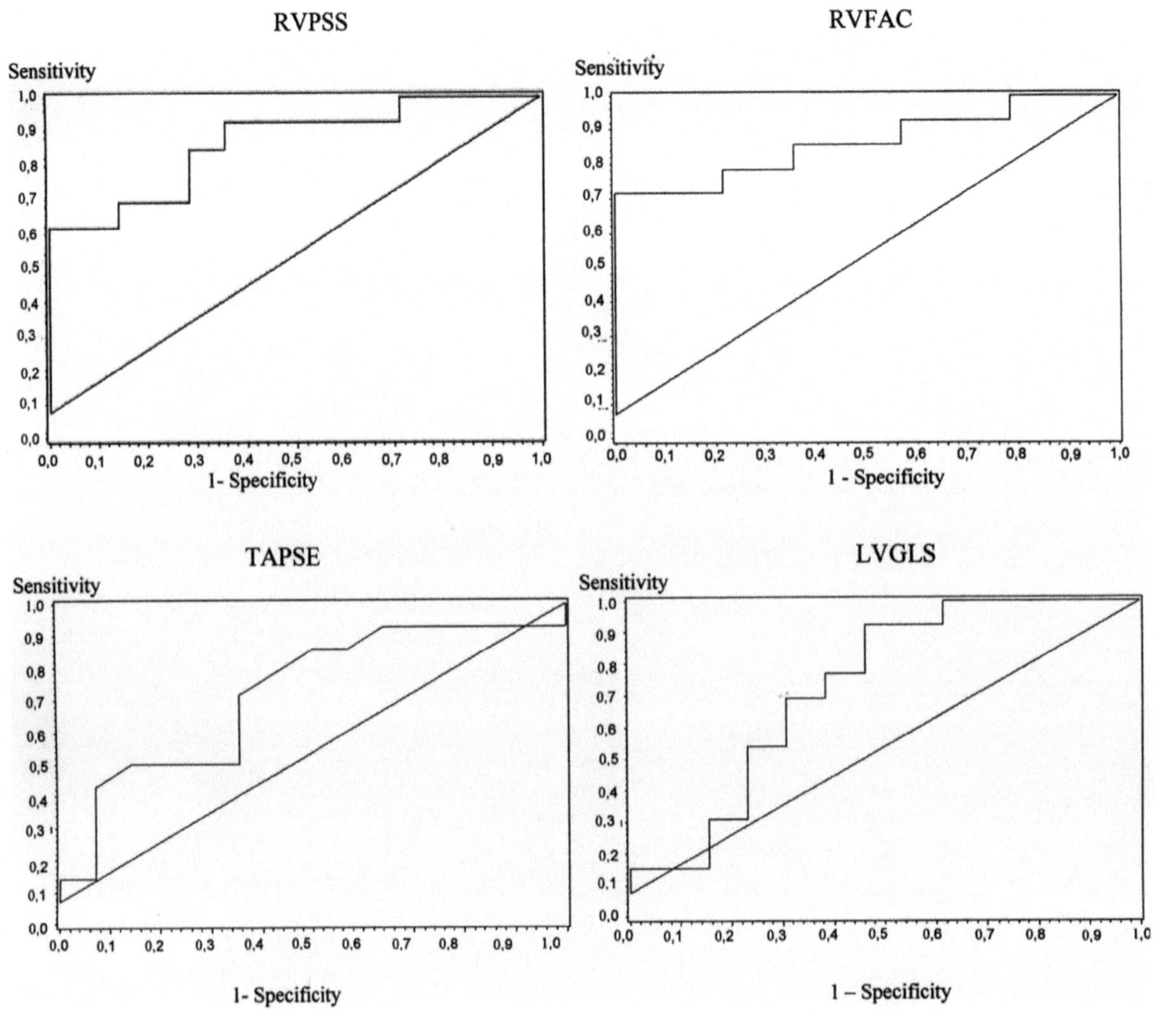

Figure 3. Correlation of RVPSS, RVFAC, TAPSE and LVGLS with occurrence of RV dysfunction displayed by receiver operating characteristic (ROC) curves. RVPSS: right ventricular peak systolic strain, TAPSE: tricuspid annular plane systolic excursion, RVFAC: right ventricular fractional area change, LVGLS: left ventricular global strain.

We were able to measure longitudinal strain in 78% of all segments. According to our results impaired global RV function in TC seems to be predominantly caused by mid-ventricular and apical RV free wall strain reduction. This is consistent with previous studies using visual estimation of regional wall motion during echocardiography [6] and cardiovascular magnetic resonance imaging [16] in TC.

Previous studies in patients with heart failure [18], chronic PH [19], arrhythmogenic right ventricular disease [20] and in patients referred for cardiac surgery [21] have found that strain imaging is more precise in the quantification of RV function than the global parameters RVFAC and TAPSE. The complex shape of the right ventricle and the monoplane measurement are one reason why RVFAC has to be used with caution. Although RVFAC values

Table 4. Correlation of RVPSS, TAPSE, RVFAC and LVGLS with occurrence of RV- involvement in TC using Kendall-Tau-b correlation coefficient.

	Kendall-Tau-b correlation coefficient	p-value
RVPSS	0.490	0.004
RVFAC	−0.499	0.003
TAPSE	−0.379	0.025
LVGLS	0.329	0.048

RV: right ventricular, TC: Takotsubo cardiomyopathy, RVPSS: right ventricular peak systolic strain, RVFAC: right ventricular fractional area change, TAPSE: tricuspid annular plane systolic excursion, LVGLS: left ventricular global strain.

were significantly different between patients with and without RV involvement in our study, the degree of overlap between both groups was high and no clinically useful cut-off value to separate between both groups could be established. More importantly, TAPSE which is believed to be a useful and simple tool for the assessment of RV function could not differentiate between patients with and without RV involvement. One reason for this observation could be that hypercontractility of basal segments, which is a well-known phenomenon during the acute phase of TC, could compensate for hypocontractility of the mid and apical segments, therefore, leading to similar values for TAPSE in both groups.

We found that RVPSS $>-19.1\%$ indicates RV involvement in patients with TC with a sensitivity of 85% and specificity of 71%. Previous studies have shown that RVPSS is superior to conventional parameters of RV function in various disease entities. For example, Teske et al. [22] found that a cut-off value of -18.1% in any RV segment could differentiate between patients with and without arrhythmogenic RV cardiomyopathy with a sensitivity and specificity of 91%. Ternacle et al. [21] observed that a cut-off value of -21% was an independent prognostic marker of mortality in patients referred for cardiac surgery. Guendouz et al. [18] found that in chronic heart failure patients with RVPSS $>-21\%$ were at greatest risk for worse outcome. Right heart failure is known to increase the risk of PE [24,25]. In our assessment, PE was found only in the group of patients with RV involvement. A RVPSS of $>-14.8\%$ was a good indicator for the occurrence of PE (sensitivity 87%, specificity 80%). Although RVPSS is one of the most reliable parameters of RV function quantification, one limitation of this parameter is the fact that only the RV free wall, which is known to only contribute 80% of the RV stroke volume [18], is analysed.

All patients with RV involvement also had LV involvement. Cases of isolated RV TC have been published (25–27] but were not observed in our series. Patients of the present study had classical (apical) or variant (mid-ventricular involvement) forms of TC. RV-involvement occurred in both forms of TC.

It has been described that patients with RV involvement have higher degrees of LVEF reduction and longer hospitalization compared to patients without RV involvement [6,7]. In our study RV involvement was associated with significantly lower LVEF and global LV strain which supports the hypothesis that these patients could have a more severe initial insult.

The pathophysiological mechanism underlying TC has not been clearly established. The biventricular involvement confirms the notion that TC is not a consequence of coronary artery occlusion [10,16]. Although entirely speculative, differences in the distribution and/or density of RV adrenoceptors could be a potential explanation for RV involvement in TC.

Limitations

There are limitations to this study that must be acknowledged. Because of the small number of patients the results should be regarded with caution. Some of the myocardial segments were uninterpretable due to signal noise. This was not always caused by poor acoustic windows. Tracking problems were particularly common in the LV and RV base.

Conclusion

We conclude that 1) RV function quantification can be performed in patients with TC using 2D strain echocardiography. 2) Patients with TC who have RV involvement have significant impairment of several parameters of regional and global RV function. This is predominantly caused by dysfunction of RV mid and apical segments. 3) Patients with RV involvement have significantly lower LVEF and lower LV global strain at baseline which might be caused by a more severe initial insult. 4) A RVPSS cut off value of $>-19.1\%$ can differentiate between patients with and without RV dysfunction in a clinically meaningful way. 5) Pleural effusion was only found in patients with RV involvement and a RVPSS value $>-14.8\%$ indicated the occurrence of PE with good sensitivity and specificity.

Author Contributions

Conceived and designed the experiments: FH KH DH TP CD FS. Performed the experiments: FH KH DH. Analyzed the data: FH KH DH JB. Contributed reagents/materials/analysis tools: MB FS. Wrote the paper: FH DH KH.

References

1. Dote K, Sato H, Tateishi H, Uchida T, Ishihara M (1991) Myocardial stunning due to simultaneous multivessel coronary spasms: a review of 5 cases. J Cardiol 21: 203–214.
2. Heggemann F, Weiss C, Hamm K, Kaden J, Süselbeck T, et al. (2009) Global and regional myocardial function quantification by two-dimensional strain in Takotsubo cardiomyopathy. Eur J Echocardiogr 10: 760–764.
3. Nyui N, Yamanaka O, Nakayama R, Sawano M, Kawai S (2000) 'Tako-Tsubo' transient ventricular dysfunction: a case report. Jpn Circ J 64: 715–719.
4. Nishikawa S, Ito K, Adachi Y, Katoh S, Azuma A, et al. (2004) Ampulla ('takotsubo') cardiomyopathy of both ventricles: evaluation of microcirculation disturbance using 99mTc-tetrofosmin myocardial single photon emission computed tomography and doppler guide wire. Circ J 68: 1076–1080.
5. Kurisu S, Inoue I, Kawagoe T, Ishihara M, Shimatani Y, et al. (2005) Takotsubo-like transient biventricular dysfunction with pressure gradients. Intern Med 44: 727–732.
6. Elesber AA, Prasad A, Bybee KA, Valeti U, Motiei A, et al. (2006) Transient cardiac apical ballooning syndrome: prevalence and clinical implications of right ventricular involvement. J Am Coll Cardiol 47: 1082–1083.
7. Haghi D, Athanasiadis A, Papavassiliu T, Suselbeck T, Fluechter S, et al. (2006) Right ventricular involvement in Takotsubo cardiomyopathy. Eur Heart J 27: 2433–2439.
8. Rudski LG, Wyman WL, Afilalo J, Hua L, Handschumacher MD, et al. (2010) Guidelines for the Echocardiographic Assessment of the Right Heart in Adults: A Report from the American Society of Echocardiography. J Am Soc Echocardiogr 23: 685–713
9. Jurcut R, Giusca S, La Gerche A, Vasile S, Ginghina C, et al. (2010) The echocardiographic assessment of the right ventricle: what to do in 2010 ? Eur J Echocardiogr 11: 81–96
10. Hanekom L, Cho GY, Leano R, Jeffriess L, Marwick TH (2007) Comparison of two-dimensional speckle and tissue Doppler strain measurement during dobutamine stress echocardiography: an angiographic correlation. Eur Heart J 28: 1765–1772.
11. Haeck ML, Scherptong RW, Marsan NA, Holman ER, Schalij MJ, et al. (2012) Prognostic value of right ventricular longitudinal peak systolic strain in patients with pulmonary hypertension. Circ Cardiovasc Imaging 5: 628–636.
12. Kempny A, Fernández-Jiménez R, Orwat S, Schuler P, Bunck AC, et al. (2012) Quantification of biventricular myocardial function using cardiac magnetic resonance feature tracking, endocardial border delineation and echocardiographic speckle tracking in patients with repaired tetralogy of Fallot and healthy controls. J Cardiovasc Magn Reson 14: 32.
13. Diller GP, Radojevic J, Kempny A, Alonso-Gonzalez R, Emmanouil L, et al. (2012) Systemic right ventricular longitudinal strain is reduced in adults with transposition of the great arteries, relates to subpulmonary ventricular function, and predicts adverse clinical outcome. Am Heart J 163: 859–866.
14. Cameli M, Bernazzali S, Lisi M, Tsioulpas C, Croccia MG, et al. (2012) Right ventricular longitudinal strain and right ventricular stroke work index in patients with severe heart failure: left ventricular assist device suitability for transplant candidates. Transplant Proc 44: 2013–2015.
15. Aneq MA, Engvall J, Brudin L, Nylander E (2012) Evaluation of right and left ventricular function using speckle tracking echocardiography in patients with arrhythmogenic right ventricular cardiomyopathy and their first degree relatives. Cardiovasc Ultrasound 10:37.
16. Haghi D, Fluechter S, Suselbeck T, Kaden JJ, Borggrefe M, et al. (2007) Cardiovascular magnetic resonance findings in typical versus atypical forms of the acute apical ballooning syndrome (Takotsubo cardiomyopathy). Int J Cardiol 120:205–211.

17. Brown SB, Raina A, Katz D, Szerlip M, Wiegers SE, et al. (2011) Longitudinal shortening accounts for the majority of right ventricular contraction and improves after pulmonary vasodilator therapy in normal subjects and patients with pulmonary arterial hypertension. Chest 140: 27–33.
18. Guendouz S, Rappeneau S, Nahum J, Dubois-Randé JL, Gueret P, et al. (2012) Prognostic significance and normal values of 2D strain to assess right ventricular systolic function in chronic heart failure. Circ J 76: 127–136.
19. Giusca S, Dambrauskaite V, Scheurwegs C, D'hooge J, Claus P, et al. (2010) Deformation imaging describes right ventricular function better than longitudinal displacement of the tricuspid ring. Heart 96: 281–288.
20. Teske PR, Cowley PD, Forget FR, Beheregaray LB (2009) Microsatellite markers for the roman, Chrysoblephus laticeps (Teleostei: Sparidae), an overexploited seabream from South Africa. Mol Ecol Resour 9: 1162–1164.
21. Ternacle J, Berry M, Cognet T, Kloeckner M, Damy T, et al. (2013) Prognostic Value of Right Ventricular Two-Dimensional Global Strain in Patients Referred for Cardiac Surgery. J Am Soc Echocardiogr 26: 721–726.
22. Teske AJ, Cox MG, De Boeck BW, Doevendans PA, Hauer RN, et al. (2009) Echocardiographic tissue deformation imaging quantifies abnormal regional right ventricular function in arrhythmogenic right ventricular dysplasia/cardiomyopathy. J Am Soc Echocardiogr 22: 920–927.
23. Natanzon AI, Kronzon I (2009) Pericardial and pleural effusions in congestive heart failure-anatomical, pathophysiologic, and clinical considerations. Am J Med Sci 338: 211–216.
24. Brixey AG, Light RW (2011) Pleural effusions occurring with right heart failure. Curr Opin Pulm Med 17: 226–231.
25. Burgdorf C, Hunold P, Radke PW, Schunkert H, Kurowski V (2011) Isolated right ventricular stress-induced ("Tako-Tsubo") cardiomyopathy. Clin Res Cardiol 100: 617–619.
26. Mrdovic I, Kostic J, Perunicic J, Asanin M, Vasiljevic Z, et al. (2010) Right ventricular takotsubo cardiomyopathy. J Am Coll Cardiol 55: 1751.
27. Stahli BE, Ruschitzka F, Enseleit F (2011) Isolated right ventricular ballooning syndrome: a new variant of transient cardiomyopathy. Eur Heart J 32: 1821.

Low-Dose Prospectively Electrocardiogram-Gated Axial Dual-Source CT Angiography in Patients with Pulsatile Bilateral Bidirectional Glenn Shunt: An Alternative Noninvasive Method for Postoperative Morphological Estimation

Xiaopeng Ji[1], Bin Zhao[1], Zhaoping Cheng[1], Biao Si[2], Zhiheng Wang[2], Yanhua Duan[1], Pei Nie[1], Haiou Li[1], Shifeng Yang[1], Hui Jiao[1], Ximing Wang[1]*

1 Shandong Medical Imaging Research Institute, Shandong University, Jinan, People's Republic of China, **2** Cardiovascular Institute of Jinan Military district, Jinan, People's Republic of China

Abstract

Objective: To explore the clinical value of low-dose prospectively electrocardiogram-gated axial dual-source CT angiography (low-dose PGA scanning, CTA) in patients with pulsatile bilateral bidirectional Glenn shunt (bBDG) as an alternative noninvasive method for postoperative morphological estimation.

Methods: Twenty patients with pulsatile bBDG (mean age 4.2±1.6 years) underwent both low-dose PGA scanning and conventional cardiac angiography (CCA) for the morphological changes. The morphological evaluation included the anatomy of superior vena cava (SVC) and pulmonary artery (PA), the anastomotic location, thrombosis, aorto-pulmonary collateral circulation, pulmonary arteriovenous malformations, etc. Objective and subjective image quality was assessed. Bland–Altman analysis and linear regression analyses were used to evaluate the correlation on measurements between CTA and CCA. Effective radiation dose of both modalities was calculated.

Results: The CT attenuation value of bilateral SVC and PA was higher than 300 HU. The average subjective image quality score was 4.05±0.69. The morphology of bilateral SVC and PA was displayed completely and intuitively by CTA images. There were 24 SVC above PA and 15 SVC beside PA. Thrombosis was found in 1 patient. Collateral vessels were detected in 13 patients. No pulmonary arteriovenous malformation was found in our study. A strong correlation ($R^2>0.8$, $P<0.001$) was observed between the measurements on CTA images and on CCA images. Bland–Altman analysis demonstrated a systematic overestimation of the measurements by CTA (the mean value of bias>0).The mean effective dose of CTA and CCA was 0.50±0.17 mSv and 4.85±1.34 mSv respectively.

Conclusion: CT angiography with a low-dose PGA scanning is an accurate and reliable noninvasive examination in the assessment of morphological changes in patients with pulsatile bBDG.

Editor: Rozemarijn Vliegenthart, University of Groningen, Netherlands

Funding: This study was supported by Provincial Natural Science Foundation of Shandong (ZR2012HM006); http://www.sdnsf.gov.cn/portal/. The funders had no role in study design, data collection and analysis, decision to publish, or preparation of the manuscript.

Competing Interests: The authors have declared that no competing interests exist.

* E-mail: wxming369@163.com

Introduction

Historically the Bidirectional Glenn shunt (BDG) was a palliative surgical procedure typically done in children with a single effective ventricle as an intermediate step before completion of a Fontan operation. The bilateral BDG (bBDG) is an end-to-side anastomosis between the bilateral superior vena cava (SVC) and the pulmonary artery (PA) respectively (Fig. 1A). Compared with the standard unilateral BDG, the bBDG has been found to be associated with a higher operative mortality, an increased risk of thrombus formation, and a lower conversion rate to the "Fontan-type" circulation [1,2]. The role and effect of pulsatile pulmonary blood flow at the time of BDG is controversial. Several studies show a modest increase in arterial oxygen saturations and pulmonary artery growth for patients with anterograde pulmonary blood flow after BDG procedure [3,4]. However, Ferns SJ, et al found that a higher postoperative complication rate was associated with pulsatile pulmonary blood flow [5]. Therefore, the postoperative estimation of bBDG procedure is extremely important.

There is no doubt that medical imaging plays a critical role in the postoperative estimation. Conventional cardiac angiography

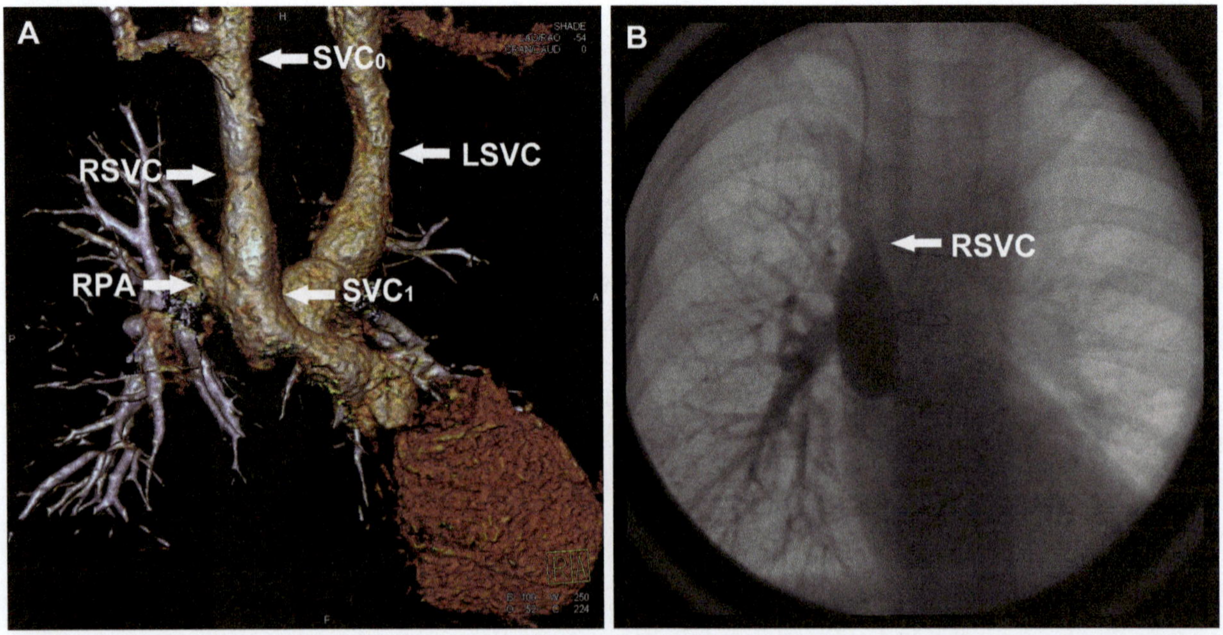

Figure 1. A 6-year-old boy underwent low-dose PGA scanning with 80 kV and 140 mAs/rot (effective dose, 0.77 mSv). A. Volume-rendered image (right lateral view) shows the morphologic measurements of SVC and the dilation of the proximal part of RSVC. **B.** CCA image confirms the dilation. *RSVC* right superior vena cava, *RPA* right pulmonary artery, *LSVC* left superior vena cava. SVC_1 the proximal end of SVC, SVC_0 the distal end of SVC.

(CCA), which is routinely performed after bBDG, gives an accurate estimation of the morphological and hemodynamic information. However, with the improvement in noninvasive imaging modalities, as well as the technical difficulty, expense, and ionizing radiation exposure (for instance, 4.6 mSv for diagnostic catheterization and 6.0 mSv for therapeutic catheterization [6–9]) of CCA, there has been increasing interest in noninvasive evaluation. Echocardiography, the primary noninvasive imaging modality, is often limited by poor acoustic windows due to a large body habitus or immediate postoperative status. Cardiovascular magnetic resonance (CMR) which has been verified to provide anatomic and functional information without ionizing radiation, has been incorporated into the postoperative evaluation of patients with bBDG [10]. However, CMR is resource-intensive, technically challenging, and requires general anaesthesia or deep sedation for most children to avoid movement and imaging distortion [10–12]. Anesthetics by gas or by continuous infusion must be maintained throughout the MRI study [13]. Therefore, the operational risks of general anesthesia or deep sedation must be considered for these patients during the long acquisition time of CMR [14].

Recently, multidetector computed tomography angiography (CTA) with high spatial resolution and reduced acquisition time has been validated as a precise examination in the evaluation of children with repaired congenital heart diseases (CHD), and only short time sedation (chloral hydrate) rather than general anesthesia was used in uncooperative patients [15–18]. Prospectively electrocardiogram-gated axial (PGA) technique has been widely used in children suffering from CHD with a low radiation dosage of 0.26–0.38 mSv in recent years [19–21]. To the best of our knowledge, no study published study has evaluated the low-dose PGA protocol in patients after pulsatile bBDG procedure. The goal of this prospective trial of low-dose prospectively electrocardiogram-gated axial dual-source CT angiography (low-dose PGA scanning, CTA) versus CCA in children after pulsatile bBDG procedure was to test the hypothesis that CTA can provide accurate morphological information with low radiation dose.

Materials and Methods

2.1 Ethics Statement

This study received approval from the Shandong Medical Imaging Research Institute ethics board. The possible adverse effects of contrast medium injection and radiation exposure as well as the complications of CCA were explained to all patients (the guardians of patients). Written informed consent was obtained from all patients (the guardians of patients) to prospectively enter this research.

2.2 Patients

Twenty children underwent pulsatile bBDG at a single institution. Both low-dose PGA scanning and CCA were performed in all patients (mean age 4.2±1.6 years, range 2–6 years; 15 males and 5 females; mean body weight 15.4±3.7 kg, range 10–21 kg) as a routine during a follow-up period of 6 to 12 months between April 2011 and July 2012.

2.3 Low-dose PGA scanning protocol

All examinations were performed on a first generation dual-source CT scanner (Siemens Somatom Definition, Siemens Healthcare, Forchheim, Germany). Younger children (≤15 kg) were sedated with oral chloral hydrate (50 mg/kg) [22] under the supervision of a pediatrician. Anesthesia was not given. Older children (>15 kg) usually responded well to verbal reassurance, and were usually relatively cooperative and good at breath holding. The scanning was performed in caudo-cranal direction from the bottom of the heart to the thoracic inlet.

CT parameters were as follows: 0.33 s gantry rotation time, 2×32×0.6 mm detector collimation, a slice collimation

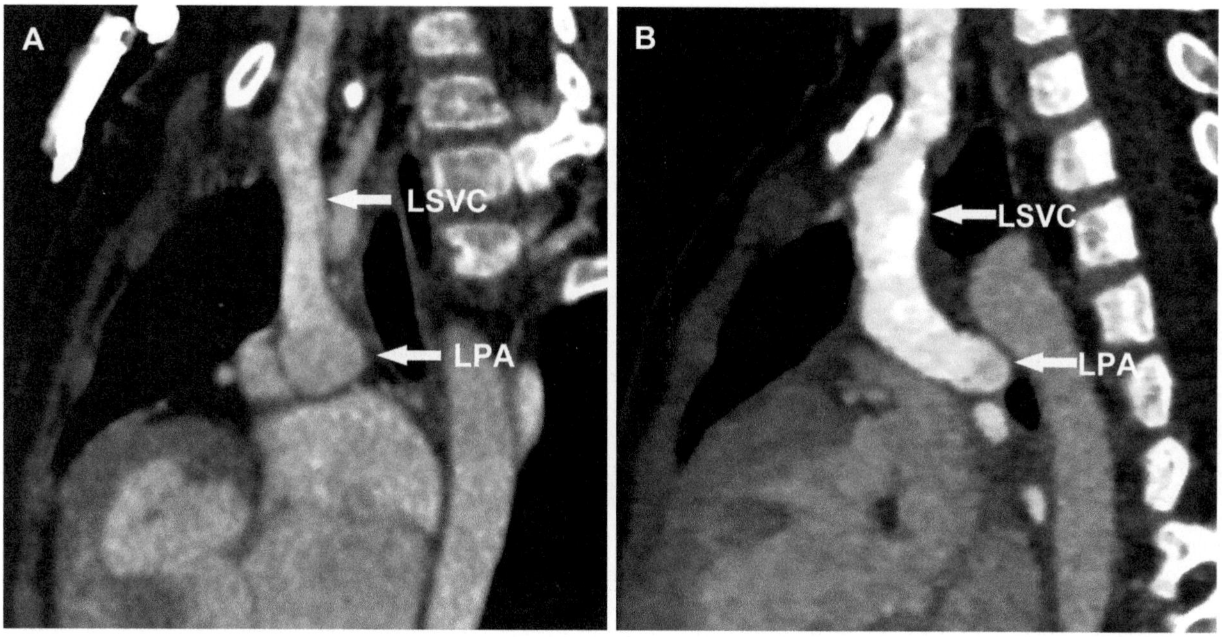

Figure 2. The anastomotic location between SVC and PA. A. Multiplanar reformation image shows that SVC was above PA when it located at ten to two o'clock of PA on the sagittal section. **B.** Multiplanar reformation image shows that SVC was beside PA at six to twelve o'clock of PA on the sagittal section. *LSVC* left superior vena cava, *LPA* left pulmonary artery.

2×64×0.6 mm by z-flying focal spot technique, 80 kV tube voltage and weight adapted setting for tube current (10 mAs/rot per kg up to 6 kg then 5 mAs/rot per kg up to 140 mAs/rot). We did not use β-blocker therapy to decrease the heart rate. The data acquisition window was set at 40% of the R-R interval.

Iodinated contrast medium (Schering Ultravist, Iopromide, 350 mg I/ml, Berlin, Germany) was injected via unilateral peripheral veins in the elbow or back of the hand at a volume of 2.0 ml/kg body weight with a saline chaser of 1.0 ml/kg body weight [19]. The delay between the start of injection and the start of data acquisition was set at 40 seconds. Injection rate was calculated at total injected volume divided by 30. For example, a 15 kg child with peripheral access would be injected with 30 ml of contrast medium and 15 ml saline at 1.5 ml/s.

2.4 CT data post-processing

Images were reconstructed with a slice thickness of 0.75 mm and increment of 0.5 mm using a medium smooth-tissue convolution kernel (B26f). All images were anonymous and transferred to an external workstation (Multiple Modality Workplace, Siemens Healthcare, Forchheim, Germany) for further analysis. In addition to the CT axial slices, Multiplanar reformation (MPR), maximum intensity projection (MIP) and volume rendering (VR) were used for image interpretation.

2.5 Assessment of image quality of CTA

As the postoperative changes of bilateral SVC and PA drawed pediatric cardiologists' attention, we paid great attention to the morphological evaluation of SVC and PA. Intraluminal attenuation and image noise of bilateral SVC and PA were assessed as objective image quality parameters. The magnitude and uniformity of arterial enhancement was measured using 1.0 cm^2 circular ROIs at different regions. The noise was defined as the standard deviation of the attenuation value.

Blinded to the results of CCA findings, two cardiac radiologists with more than 5 years' experience respectively interpreted the subjective image quality of great vessels (mainly bilateral SVC and PA) using a 5-grade scoring system (5, excellent; 4, good; 3, fair; 2, insufficient for complete evaluation; 1, not interpretable) [21]. Grades 3, 4 and 5 were considered sufficient for complete diagnosis. For any disagreement between the two observers, consensus agreement was achieved.

2.6 Postoperative morphological evaluation of CTA

2.6.1 Morphological measurements of SVC and PA. The diameters of the proximal (SVC_1) and distal (SVC_0) part of SVC, as well as the maximum diameter (SVC_{max}) were measured (Fig. 1A). As the proximal end of SVC was stitched with PA and impacted more obviously by blood flow, SVC_0 was chosen as the original diameter of SVC and the comparison between SVC_{max} and SVC_0 was as follows: $(SVC_{max} - SVC_0)/SVC_0 \times 100\%$. The dilation of SVC was observed visually according to VR image.

The diameters of the prebranching point (PA_0) of PA and the descending aorta at the diaphragm (DA) were measured, and McGoon ratio = $(LPA_0 + RPA_0)/DA$. The stenosis of PA was assessed visually according to VR image.

The measurements were carried out three times in the MPR images and the average value was adopted. If the section of measurement was not circular, the caliber was quantified using 2 perpendicular measurements of the diameter on the transverse section. The represented diameter was the root of the multiple of these 2 perpendicular measurements.

2.6.2 The anastomotic relationship between SVC and PA. The anastomotic location between SVC and PA was observed. We defined that SVC was above PA when it located at ten to two o'clock of PA on the sagittal section (Fig. 2A), while SVC was beside PA at six to twelve o'clock of PA (Fig. 2B).

2.6.3 Thrombosis, aorto-pulmonary collateral circulation and pulmonary arteriovenous malformations. We paid great attention to thrombosis which is one of the severe postoperative complications of this procedure [23,24]. An aorto-pulmonary collateral vessel (APC) was defined as one arising from the arterial circulation that had a discretely identifiable origin and perfused the pulmonary parenchyma [25]. APCs may form in patients postoperatively as a result of decreased pulmonary blood flow or pulmonary vein stenosis [26], and they were quantified by three indexes: the presence or absence of collateral vessels, the number of collateral vessels identified and the diameter of the proximal end of the most obvious collateral vessel (APC_{max}). Another potential complication is the development of pulmonary arteriovenous malformations (AVMs). Pulmonary AVMs are postulated to occur because the SVC blood lacks a humoral factor from the liver which is needed to prevent the development of AVMs in the lungs [27]. Therefore, whether pulmonary AVMs existed also interested us.

2.7 Conventional cardiac angiography

CCA was performed by means of a Phillips' machine (Allura CV20, Phillips Medical Systems, The Netherlands) using a 4-6 Fr catheter 2 or 3 days after low-dose PGA scanning in all patients. They were kept fasting for 3–4 hr prior to the procedure. The procedure was done under general anesthesia with Midazolam (0.1 mg/kg) and Ketamine (1–2 mg/kg). Groin was cleaned and local anesthesia was given. All children were restrained by tying them over the board so as to avoid unnecessary movements. Arterial and venous access was obtained after puncturing right or left femoral artery and vein as well as unilateral or bilateral internal jugular veins by Seldinger's technique. Heparin was given 80 units/kg at the beginning of the procedure. Angiographic pictures were recorded on the Phillips' machine. The contrast medium used for angiography was non-ionic (Schering Ultravist, Iopromide, 350 mg I/ml, Berlin, Germany) with total dose limited to 5 ml/kg, and the average amount of contrast enhancement was 4.6±0.3 ml/kg.

As for the morphological assessment, biplane anteroposterior and lateral projection aortography by internal jugular vein was performed to evaluate the anatomy of SVC and PA, the anastomotic location between SVC and PA as well as thrombosis and pulmonary AVMs. Anteroposterior, lateral and left anterior oblique projection aortography or selective angiography was performed to observe the amount of APCs and APC_{max}. With regard to the hemodynamic evaluation, the oxygen saturation of cardiac atrium, ventricle, the aorta and PA as well as the pressures of cardiac ventricle, aorta, main pulmonary artery, bilateral SVC and PA were measured. Since we focused on the morphological evaluation, the corresponding measurements of CCA were recorded and compared with those of low-dose PGA scanning while the hemodynamic data of CCA was not listed below.

2.8 Radiation dose estimations

The volume CT dose index and dose length product (DLP) were obtained from the information generated by the CT system and the effective radiation dose was calculated from the DLP as follows. The recorded DLP was multiplied by 2.3 to adapt it to the 16-cm phantom, because on the machine used for the study, the DLP for body surface area was given on a 32-cm phantom and 2.3 is scanner specific for pediatric examinations at 80 kV as provided by the manufacturer. The corrected DLP value was then multiplied by the infant-specific conversion coefficient given for a 16-cm phantom: 0.018 mSv/(mGy•cm) between 1 year and 6 years of age [28].

As for CCA, the dose-area product was displayed by the fluoroscopy system itself and the infant-specific coefficient 0.41 mSv/(Gy•cm^2) [29] was used to convert the dose-area product into the effective dose.

2.9 Statistics

Statistical analysis was performed by SPSS 17.0 software (SPSS, Chicago, IL, USA) and Microsoft Windows Excel 2007 (Microsoft Co., Redmond, Washington, USA). Results were expressed as means ± standard deviations for quantitative variables and as frequencies or percentages for categorical variables. Interobserver agreement on grades of subjective image quality was assessed by kappa statistics ($\kappa>0.81$, excellent agreement; $\kappa=0.61$–0.80, good agreement). With CCA results as the standard, linear regression analysis and Bland–Altman analysis were used to evaluate the correlation on measurements between CTA and CCA, and Pearson's correlation coefficient was calculated ($R^2>0.8$, strong correlation). $P<0.05$ was considered statistically significant.

Results

The CTA data of twenty children with pulsatile bBDG were successfully acquired. All patients were in sinus rhythm at the time of data acquisition. Mean heart rate was 98±11.7 bpm (range 77–119), mean heart-rate variability was 10.8±5.8 bpm (4–23). Data acquisition took place at every 2nd or 3rd heart beat (2nd: n = 15, 3rd: n = 3, 2nd and 3rd: n = 2). Mean scan length was 109.7±15.1 mm (85–136), resulting in a mean of 6±1 (5–8) slab acquisitions per examination. Mean scan time was 6.6±1.1 s (4.79–8.63).

3.1. Image quality of CTA

Objective image quality parameters are listed in Table 1. All examinations showed diagnostic image quality, with no examination rated non-diagnostic (5, n = 5; 4, n = 11; 3, n = 4). The average subjective image quality score was 4.05±0.69, and 4.15±0.67 for reader 1 and 4.00±0.73 for reader 2 respectively. Overall interobserver agreement on subjective image quality was good ($\kappa=0.76$, $P<0.05$). Artifacts due to respiratory motion were present in 6 examinations without impairing diagnostic quality.

3.2 Postoperative morphological evaluation

3.2.1 Morphological measurements of SVC and PA. The measurements were listed in Table 2. A strong correlation ($R^2>0.8$, $P<0.001$) was observed between the measurements on CTA images and on CCA images. Bland–Altman analysis demonstrated a systematic overestimation of the measurements by CTA (the mean value of bias>0) [14]. The McGoon ratio obtained by CTA and CCA was 1.99±0.48 mm (1.19–3.38) and 1.96±0.45 mm (1.12–3.24) respectively, and there was a strong correlation ($R^2=0.96$, $P<0.001$) (Fig. 3A). Bland–Altman analysis

Table 1. Objective image quality parameters.

	Attenuation(HU)	Image noise(HU)
RSVC	353.8±60.4	24.5±5.4
LSVC*	351.1±52.3	26.4±4.1
RPA	356.5±67.6	24.5±4.4
LPA	345.7±57.0	25.2±3.7

Notes: *RSVC* right superior vena cava, *LSVC* left superior vena cava, *RPA* right pulmonary artery, *LPA* left pulmonary artery. *LSVC was filled with thrombus in one patient, so LSVC was evaluated in nineteen patients.

Table 2. Morphological measurements of CTA and CCA.

	the diameters* (mm)		comparison between CTA and CCA	
	CTA	CCA	linear regression analyses(R^2)	Bland-Altman analysis(bias)(mm)
$RSVC_0$	10.5(9.6 to 11.3)	10.4(9.6 to 11.3)	0.89	0.11±0.60
$RSVC_{max}$	13.2(11.8 to 14.6)	13.0(11.6 to 14.4)	0.96	0.15±0.64
$RSVC_1$	12.5(11.2 to 13.7)	12.3(11.1 to 13.6)	0.95	0.14±0.63
$LSVC_0$**	9.4(8.6 to 10.1)	9.3(8.6 to 10.0)	0.89	0.12±0.52
$LSVC_{max}$**	10.5(9.5 to 11.5)	10.3(9.4 to 11.3)	0.92	0.16±0.57
$LSVC_1$**	10.1(9.1 to 11.2)	10.0(9.0 to 11.0)	0.94	0.13±0.53
RPA_0	10.6(9.5 to 11.7)	10.5(9.4 to 11.7)	0.95	0.11±0.53
LPA_0	9.2(8.2 to 10.2)	9.1(8.1 to 10.1)	0.93	0.13±0.55
DA	10.3(9.7 to 10.9)	10.2(9.5 to 10.8)	0.84	0.15±0.54

Notes: * The mean and 95% confidence interval were provided. **LSVC was filled with thrombus in one patient, so LSVC was evaluated in nineteen patients.

showed a systematic overestimation of the measurements by CTA (bias 0.032±0.10 mm) (Fig. 3B).

The comparison between SVC_{max} and SVC_0 was as follows: ≤10%, n = 14; 10%–20%, n = 11; ≥20%, n = 14. The dilation was observed in 14 SVC by both CTA and CCA, and the corresponding SVC_{max} was 20% larger than SVC_0 without exception. Therefore, we set ≥20% as the standard of dilation, and SVC_1 was 20% larger than SVC_0 in 10 of 14 dilated SVC. As for PA, 16 stenosis was found by CT and confirmed by CCA. There were 3 stenosis at the root (Fig. 4), 7 stenosis in the proximal part and 6 stenosis in the distal part of PA.

3.2.2 The anastomotic relationship between SVC and PA. There were 24 SVC above PA and 15 SVC beside PA found by both CT and CCA. Considering dilation of SVC, we observed that 50% (12/24) SVC above PA dilated while only 13.3% (2/15) SVC beside PA dilated.

3.2.3 Thrombosis, APCs and pulmonary AVMs. Thrombosis was found in 1 patient, locating in the whole course of LSVC as well as the proximal part of left internal jugular vein and left sub-clavian vein (Fig. 5A–C). The thrombus was removed by means of CCA a day later (Fig. 5D). A total of 33 APCs were identified by both CT and CCA among 13 patients (2 in 6 cases, 3 in 7 cases), and no APCs were identified in the remaining 7 patients (Fig. 6). The mean diameter of APC_{max} measured by CTA and CCA was 2.7±0.5 mm (2.1–3.6) and 2.5±0.4 mm (1.9–3.3) respectively, and there was a strong correlation (R^2 = 0.83, P<0.001). Bland–Altman analysis demonstrated a systematic overestimation of the measurements by CTA (bias 0.11±0.20 mm).There were no pulmonary AVMs in 20 patients.

3.3. Radiation dose estimates

The mean volume CT dose index was 1.08±0.25 mGy (0.77–1.82), and the mean DLP was 12.1±4.1 mGy•cm (6.6–21.6), resulting in a mean estimated effective dose of 0.50±0.17 mSv (0.27–0.89). The mean dose-area product of CCA was 11.82±3.27 Gy•cm^2 (7.49–16.39), resulting in an average effective dose of 4.85 ±1.34 mSv (3.07–6.72).

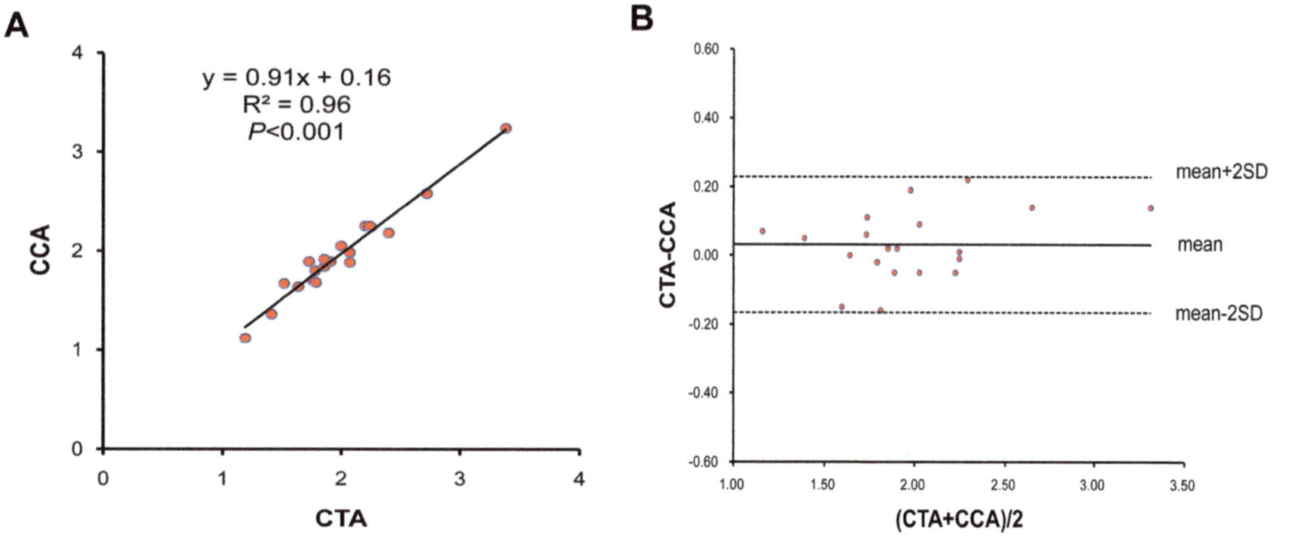

Figure 3. Correlation of McGoon ratio obtained by CTA and CCA. A. Two modalities showed a strong correlation. **B.** Bland–Altman plots illustrated bias and limits of agreement of McGoon ratio using CTA when compared with CCA.

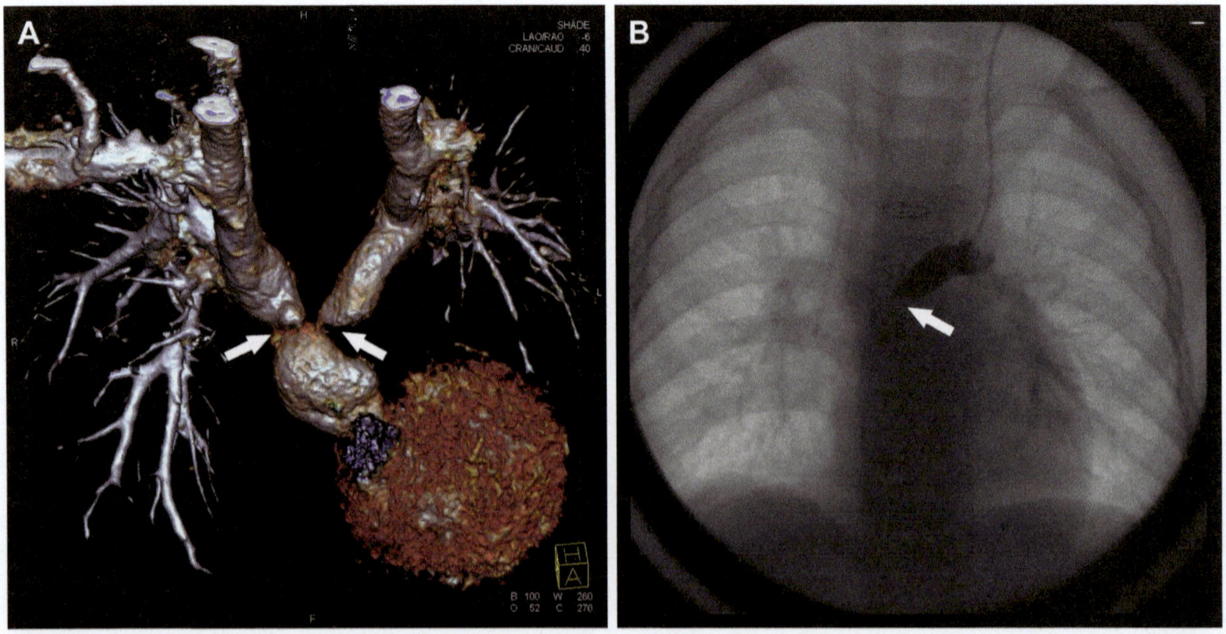

Figure 4. A 4.2-year-old boy underwent low-dose PGA scanning with 80 kV and 112 mAs/rot (effective dose, 0.46 mSv). A. Volume-rendered image shows severe stenosis (white arrow) in the root of bilateral PA. **B**. CCA image confirms the stenosis (white arrow) of LPA.

Discussion

4.1 The challenge of CT scanning

The patients after bBDG had bilateral SVC. Then it comes to a question whether bilateral cavopulmonary anastomoses can be shown at the same time when the iodinated contrast medium was injected via unilateral peripheral veins. As we know, the blood containing the iodinated contrast medium mainly flushes into the unilateral PA from ipsilateral SVC after the injection. If the scanning had been performed at this time, higher attenuation would have been achieved at the ipsilateral SVC and PA of the injection while the contralateral SVC and PA would have lower attenuation. Therefore the scanning was delayed until the contrast medium came to the arteries of neck and upper limb and refluxed through the veins. Then the bilateral SVC was expected to achieve the preferable attenuation.

4.2 Postoperative morphological evaluation

As the dilation of SVC implied the obstructed blood reflow or the unfavorable hemodynamics and the dilation sometimes developed into aneurysm (Fig. 7), much attention was paid to the measurement of SVC, and we found that the diameter of the proximal part of SVC was 20% larger than that of the distal part of SVC in 71.4% (10/14) dilated SVC. Therefore, the expansion of the proximal part of SVC reflected the dilation of SVC to some extent, and the proximal part of SVC should be detected by echocardiography in the follow-up in the event that the whole course of SVC is unable to be shown. With regard to PA, the stenosis of PA after pulsatile bBDG always draws the attention of pediatric cardiologists, and relief of stenosis by stent implantation is effective and can be realized safely to optimize pulmonary hemodynamics [30]. In our study, between the root and the anastomotic stoma of PA located ten stenosis (3 at the root, 7 in the proximal part), which may result from the surgery and made against the additional pulsatile pulmonary blood flow into the ipsilateral PA. The other 6 stenosis in the distal part of PA implied the pulmonary dysplasia.

To the best of our knowledge, there was no study discussing the anastomotic relationship between SVC and PA. We found that 50% SVC above PA dilated while only 13.3% SVC beside PA dilated. This phenomenon implied that SVC beside PA was less likely to dilate and the surgery may be optimized by anastomosing SVC beside PA. Thrombosis was one of the most severe complications in the patients after pulsatile bBDG [23,24]. CTA was able to display the thrombus and surrounding tissues so as to provide sufficient information for thrombectomy. APCs are common after BDG and Fontan procedures [25]. John K, et al reported that the presence of APCs was diagnosed in at least one postoperative catheterization in 36% patients (71/196) [25]. Our study found that 65% patients (13/20) had collateral vessels. The proportion was much higher than 36%, which showed the prevalence of APCs after bBDG.

4.3 Different Imaging modalites

Our study demonstrated a close correlation between quantitative measurements by low-dose PGA scanning and CCA, although a small systematic overestimation by low-dose PGA scanning was observed. This overestimation may be attributed to partial volume effects and motion artifact by CT. The dilation of SVC, stenosis of PA, the anastomotic location between SVC and PA as well as thrombosis and APCs were also observed by both modalities. However, compared with the two-dimension CCA images, it was more accessible for doctors to understand the morphological changes by means of three-dimension reformation of CT images.

On the other hand, the dose of contrast medium for low-dose PGA scanning (2 ml/kg) was less than half of that for CCA (4.6 ml/kg), and the radiation dosage of low-dose PGA scanning (0.50 mSv) was much lower than that of CCA (4.85 mSv). Besides the potential risk of a large amount of contrast and radiation exposure [6,9], other disadvantages of CCA include patient discomfort, bad availability, costs of hospital stay and a small but

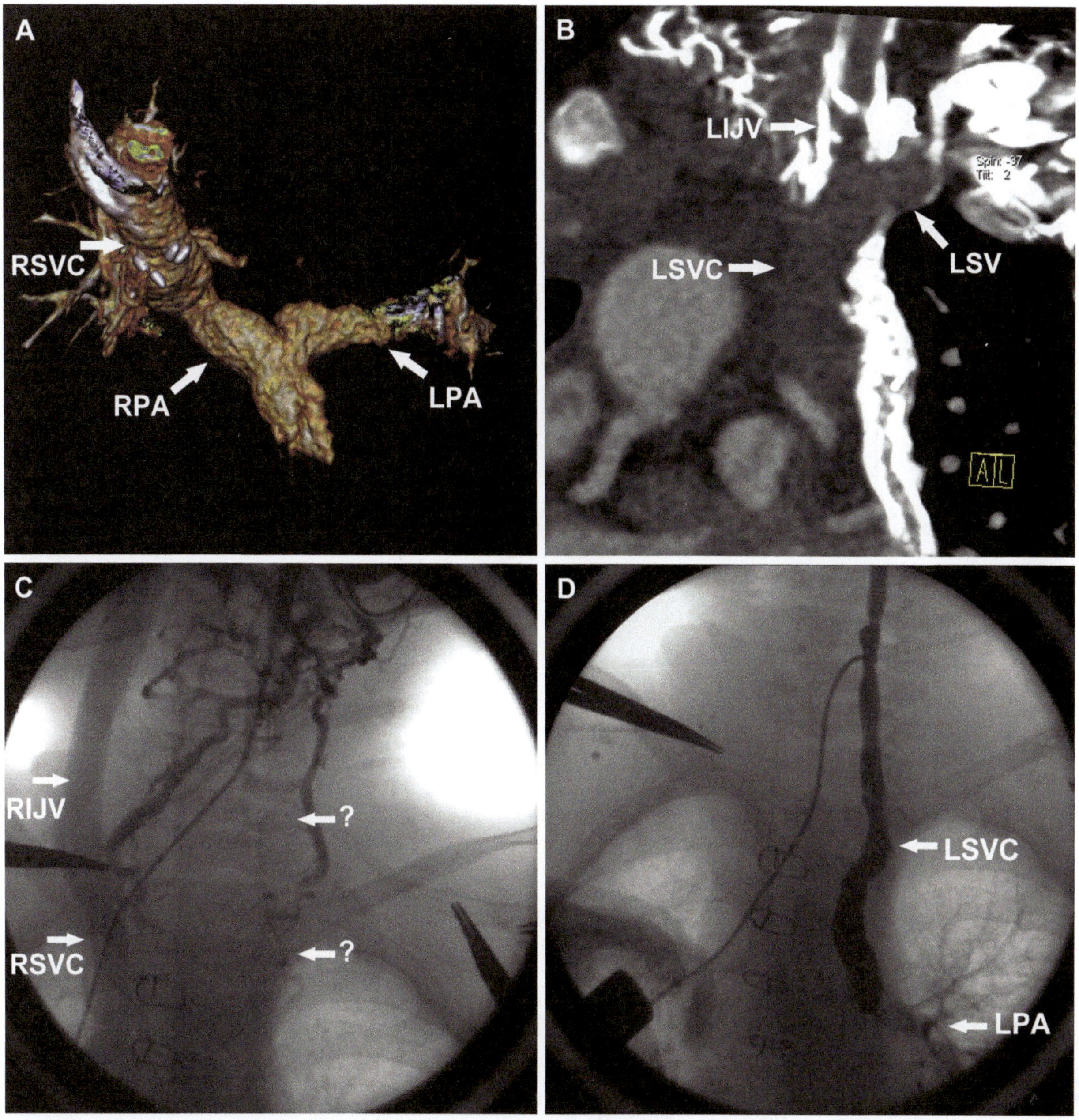

Figure 5. A 5-year-old boy underwent low-dose PGA scanning with 80 kV and 118 mAs/rot (effective dose, 0.48 mSv). A. Volume-rendered image shows the absence of LSVC. **B.** Multiplanar reformation image shows that thrombus was in the proximal part of left internal jugular vein, left subclavian vein and the whole course of LSVC. **C.** CCA image confirms the thrombus. **D.** CCA image shows the thrombus has been removed. *RSVC* right superior vena cava, *RPA* right pulmonary artery, *LPA* left pulmonary artery, *LSVC* left superior vena cava, *LIJV* left internal jugular vein, *RIJV* right internal jugular vein.

non-negligible risk of complications such as stroke, vessel dissection and pseudoaneurysm formation [6]. Therefore, except for the hemodynamic assessment, the diagnostic role CCA has largely been replaced by CT and other noninvasive imaging modalities.

Computed tomography scanners are widely available and easy to use in practice, and require shorter image acquisition time. With improvements in multi-detector technology, the spatial and temporal resolution of CT angiography has been dramatically improved to allow for imaging of even the most complex forms of CHD [16–21]. Up to now, there are four scanning modes for children with CHD, non-electrocardiogram-gated scanning, retrospectively electrocardiogram-gated technique, prospectively electrocardiogram-gated axial technique, and prospectively electrocardiogram-gated high-pitch spiral mode (HP mode). Non-electrocardiogram-gated imaging is usually used for the evaluation of extracardiac structural abnormalities [31,32]. Retrospectively electrocardiogram-gated CT angiography was superior over non-electrocardiogram-gated acquisition when morphological evaluation of rapidly moving intracardiac or paracardiac structures, including the ascending aorta, cardiac valves and coronary artery, was required [33,34]. However, high radiation due to its low pitch and overlapping data acquisition is still the major inherent

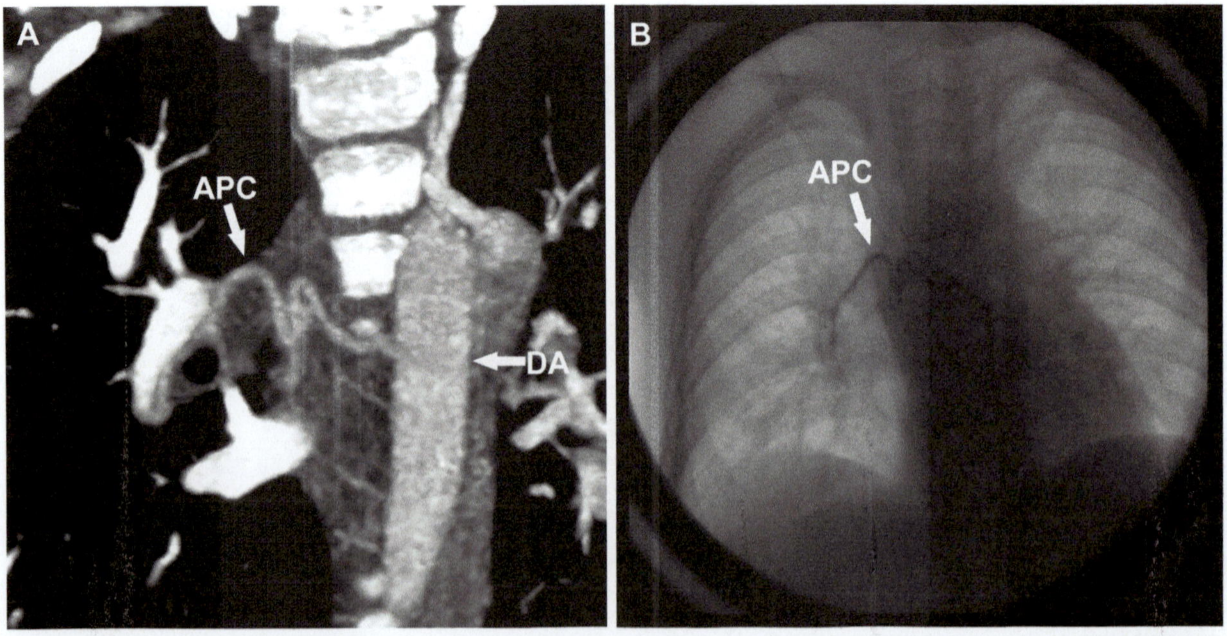

Figure 6. The same boy with Fig 4. A. maximum intensity projection image shows the existence of the collateral vessel. **B**. CCA image confirms the collateral vessel. *APC* aortopulmonary collateral vessel, *DA* descending aorta.

limitation, especially for children [16,35]. PGA technique, which has been widely used in children with CHD in recent years, usually provides adequate thoracic and coronary artery image quality in neonates, infants and young children with a low effective radiation [19–21], so we chose PGA technique as the evaluative method for patients after pulsatile bBDG. HP mode with a pitch of 3.4 provides high diagnostic accuracy and markedly reduces radiation dose, although image quality is mildly reduced [36]. Further studies may be conducted by means of HP mode if possible.

Echocardiography remains a first-line noninvasive imaging tool for evaluation of postoperative anatomy and ventricular function. However, echocardiography is operator-dependent and limited by the acoustic window, especially the post-surgical case with sternal wires and mediastinal scar tissue [8,15]. Cardiac MRI has also

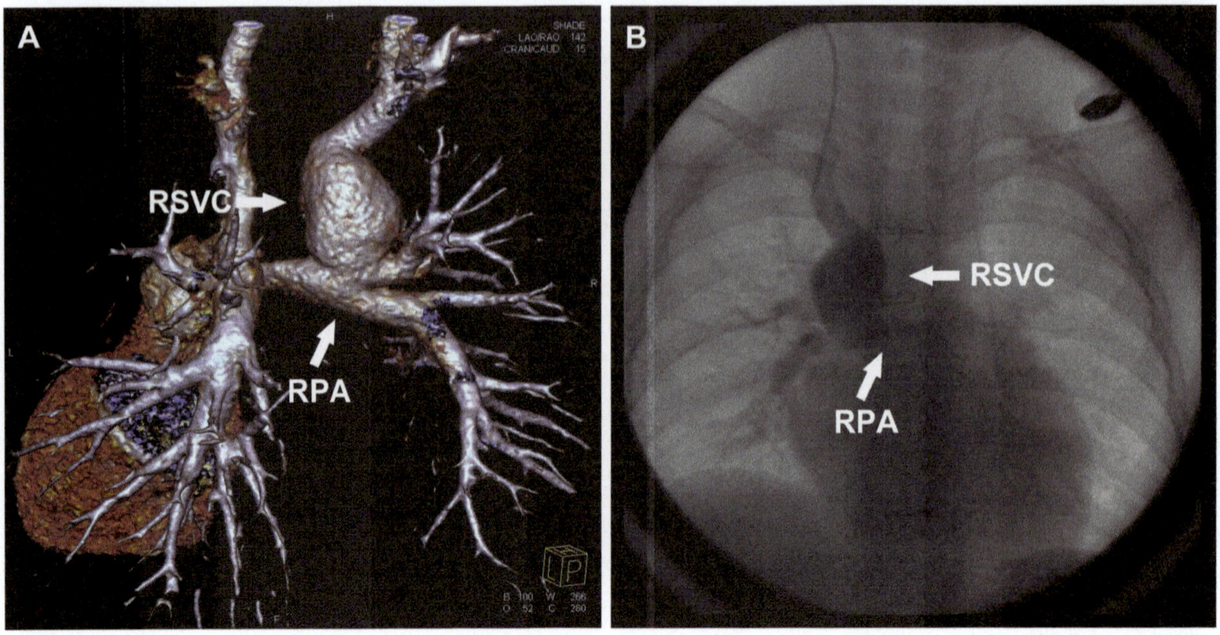

Figure 7. A 3.4-year-old boy underwent low-dose PGA scanning with 80 kV and 106 mAs/rot (effective dose, 0.44 mSv). A. Volume-rendered image (posterior view) shows the dilation of RSVC develops into aneurysm. **B**. CCA image (anterior view) confirms the aneurysm. *RSVC* right superior vena cava, *RPA* right pulmonary artery.

been incorporated into the postoperative evaluation of patients after bBDG over the past few years due to its rapid development. Recent studies have demonstrated the ability of various CMR techniques to accurately evaluate congenital cardiac valve morphology and extracardiac thoracic vessels [37–39]. As for flow measurement, phase-contrast MRI can quantify aorto-pulmonary collateral flow after bidirectional cavopulmonary connections [40] and a negative correlation was found between aorto-pulmonary collateral flow and the pulmonary artery index [41]. However, metallic implanted devices, such as stents and embolization coils may be associated with susceptibility artifacts, which can cause substantial limitation for MRI examinations. Furthermore, CMR is resource-intensive, technically challenging, and requires general anaesthesia or deep sedation for most children to avoid movement and imaging distortion [10–12]. Anesthetics by gas or by continuous infusion must be maintained throughout the MRI study [13]. Therefore, the operational risks of general anesthesia or deep sedation must be considered for these patients during the long acquisition time of CMR [14].

4.4 Limitation

Our study has several limitations. First of all, we included a relatively small group of patients as the number of the children repaired via pulsatile bBDG was relatively small. What's more, radiation is the inherent limitation of CT, and the HP mode of 128-slice dual-source CT may further lower the radiation dose.

Conclusion

CT angiography with a low-dose PGA scanning is an accurate and reliable noninvasive examination in the assessment of morphological changes in patients with pulsatile bBDG.

Author Contributions

Conceived and designed the experiments: BZ ZC BS XM. Performed the experiments: XJ ZW PN. Analyzed the data: XJ BS. Contributed reagents/materials/analysis tools: YD HL SY HJ. Wrote the paper: XJ ZC.

References

1. Iyer GKT, Van Arsdell GS, Dicke FP, McCrindle BW, Coles JG, et al. (2000) Are bilateral superior vena cavae a risk factor for single ventricle palliation? Ann Thorac Surg 70: 711–716.
2. Vida VL, Leon-Wyss J, Garcia F, Castaneda AR (2006) A Gore-Tex 'newinnominate' vein: a surgical option for complicated bilateral cavopulmonary shunts. Eur J Cardiothorac Surg 29: 112–113.
3. Gray RG, Altmann K, Mosca RS, Prakash A, Williams IA, et al. (2007) Persistent antegrade pulmonary blood flow post-glenn does not alter early post-Fontan outcomes in single-ventricle patients. Ann Thorac Surg 84: 888–893.
4. Demirtürk OS, Güvener M, Coşkun I, Yıldırım SV (2013) Results of additional pulsatile pulmonary blood flow with bidirectional glenn cavopulmonary anastomosis: positive effect on main pulmonary artery growth and less need for fontan conversion. Heart Surg Forum 16: e30–e34.
5. Ferns SJ, El Zein C, Multani K, Sajan I, Subramanian S, et al. (2013) Is additional pulsatile pulmonary blood flow beneficial to patients with bidirectional Glenn? J Thorac Cardiovasc Surg 145: 451–454.
6. Lee YW, Yang CC, Mok GS, Wu TH (2012) Infant cardiac CT angiography with 64-slice and 256-slice CT: comparison of radiation dose and image quality using a pediatric phantom. PLoS One 7: e49609. doi: 10.1371/journal.pone.0049609.
7. Bhalla S, Javidan-Nejad C, Bierhals AJ, Woodard PK, Gutierrez FR (2008) CT in the evaluation of congenital heart disease in children, adolescents, and young adults. Curr Treat Options Cardiovasc Med 10: 425–432.
8. Cook SC, Raman SV (2008) Multidetector computed tomography in the adolescent and young adult with congenital heart disease. J Cardiovasc Comput Tomogr 2: 36–49.
9. Feltes TF, Bacha E, Beekman RH 3rd, Cheatham JP, Feinstein JA, et al. (2011) Indications for Cardiac Catheterization and Intervention in Pediatric Cardiac Disease. Circulation 123: 2607–2652.
10. David W Brown, Andrew J Powell, Tal Geva (2010) Imaging complex congenital heart disease — functional single ventricle, the Glenn circulation and the Fontan circulation: A multimodality approach. Progress in Pediatric Cardiology 28: 45–58.
11. Schulte-Uentrop L, Goepfert MS (2010) Anaesthesia or sedation for MRI in children. Curr Opin Anaesthesiol 23:513–517.
12. Sreevastava DK, Setlur R (2008) Anaesthesia for Paediatric Cardiac MRI. MJAFI 64: 204–207.
13. Chan FP (2009) MR and CT imaging of the pediatric patient with structural heart disease. Semin Thorac Cardiovasc Surg Pediatr Card Surg Annu: 99–105. doi: 10.1053/j.pcsu.2009.01.009.
14. Hayabuchi Y, Inoue M, Watanabe N, Sakata M, Nabo MM, et al. (2010) Assessment of systemic-pulmonary collateral arteries in children with cyanotic congenital heart disease using multidetector-row computed tomography: comparison with conventional angiography. Int J Cardiol 138:266–271.
15. Spevak PJ, Johnson PT, Fishman EK (2008) Surgically corrected congenital heart disease: Utility of 64-MDCT. AJR Am J Roentgenol 191: 854–861.
16. Leschka S, Oechslin E, Husmann L, Desbiolles L, Marincek B, et al. (2007) Pre- and postoperative evaluation of congenital heart disease in children and adults with 64-section CT. Radiographics 27: 829–846.
17. Gaca AM, Jaggers JJ, Dudley LT, Bisset GS 3rd (2008) Repair of congenital heart disease: A primer—Part 1. Radiology 247: 617–631.
18. Gaca AM, Jaggers JJ, Dudley LT, Bisset GS 3rd (2008) Repair of congenital heart disease: A primer—Part 2. Radiology 248: 44–60.
19. Cheng ZP, Wang XM, Duan YH, Wu LB, Wu DW, et al. (2010) Low-dose prospective ECG-triggering dual-source CT angiography in infants and children with complex congenital heart disease: first experience. Eur Radiol 20: 2503–2511.
20. Pache G, Grohmann J, Bulla S, Arnold R, Stiller B, et al. (2011) Prospective electrocardiography-triggered CT angiography of the great thoracic vessels in infants and toddlers with congenital heart disease: Feasibility and image quality. Eur J Radiol 80: e440– e445.
21. Paul JF, Rohnean A, Elfassy E, Sigal-Cinqualbre A (2011) Radiation dose for thoracic and coronary step-and-shoot CT using a 128-slice dual-source machine in infants and small children with congenital heart disease. Pediatr Radiol 41: 244–249.
22. Tann OR, Muthurangu V, Young C, Owens CM (2010) Cardiovascular CT imaging in congenital heart disease. Progress in Pediatric Cardiology 28: 21–27.
23. Manlhiot C, Brandão LR, Kwok J, Kegel S, Menjak IB, et al. (2012) Thrombotic complications and thromboprophylaxis across all three stages of single ventricle heart palliation. J Pediatr 161: 513–519.
24. Procelewska M, Kolcz J, Januszewska K, Mroczek T, Malec E (2007) Coagulation abnormalities and liver function after hemi-Fontan and Fontan procedures - the importance of hemodynamics in the early postoperative period. Eur J Cardiothorac Surg 31: 866–872.
25. Triedman JK, Bridges ND, Mayer JE Jr, Lock JE (1993) Prevalence and risk factors for aortopulmonary collateral vessels after Fontan and bidirectional Glenn procedures. J Am Coll Cardiol 22: 207–215.
26. Krishnan US, Lamour JM, Hsu DT, Kichuk MR, Donnelly CM, et al.(2004) Management of aortopulmonary collaterals in children following cardiac transplantation for complex congenital heart disease. J Heart Lung Transplant 23: 564–569.
27. Srivastava D, Preminger T, Lock JE, Mandell V, Keane JF, et al. (1995) Hepatic venous blood and the development of pulmonary arteriovenous malformations in congenital heart disease. Circulation 92: 1217–1222.
28. Thomas KE, Wang B (2008) Age-specific effective doses for pediatric MSCT examinations at a large children's hospital using DLP conversion coefficients: a simple estimation method. Pediatr Radiol 38: 645–656.
29. Rassow J, Schmaltz AA, Hentrich F, Streffer C (2000) Effective doses to patients from paediatric cardiac catheterization. Br J Radiol 73:172–183.
30. Kretschmar O, Sglimbea A, Prêtre R, Knirsch W (2009) Pulmonary artery stent implantation in children with single ventricle malformation before and after completion of partial and total cavopulmonary connections. J Interv Cardiol 22: 285–290.
31. Tsai IC, Chen MC, Jan SL, Wang CC, Fu YC, et al. (2008) Neonatal cardiac multidetector row CT: why and how we do it. Pediatr Radiol 38: 438–451.
32. Shiraishi I, Kajiyama Y, Yamagishi M, Hamaoka K, Yagihara T (2012) The applications of non-ECG-gated MSCT angiography in children with congenital heart disease. Int J Cardiol. 156: 309–314.
33. Wang XM, Wu LB, Sun C, Liu C, Chao BT, et al. (2007) Clinical application of 64-slice spiral CT in the diagnosis of the tetralogy of Fallot. Eur J Radiol 64: 296–301.
34. Ben Saad M, Rohnean A, Sigal-Cinqualbre A, Adler G, Paul JF (2009) Evaluation of image quality and radiation dose of thoracic and coronary dual-source CT in 110 infants with congenital heart disease. Pediatr Radiol 39: 668–676.
35. Khatri S, Varma SK, Khatri P, Kumar RS (2008) Sixty-four-slice multidetector-row computed tomographic angiography for evaluating congenital heart disease. Pediatr Cardiol 29: 755–762.
36. Han BK, Lindberg J, Grant K, Schwartz RS, Lesser JR (2011) Accuracy and safety of high pitch computed tomography imaging in young children with complex congenital heart disease. Am J Cardiol 107: 1541–1546.

37. Benavidez O, Prakash A, Gauvreau K, Powell AJ, Geva T (2009) Diagnostic quality of steady state free precession imaging of cardiac valve morphology in pediatric/congenital heart disease. J Cardiovasc Magn Reson 11(Suppl 1): 115. Ref Type: Abstract.
38. Prakash A, Torres AJ, Printz BF, Prince MR, Nielsen JC (2007) Usefulness of magnetic resonance angiography in the evaluation of complex congenital heart disease in newborns and infants. Am J Cardiol 100: 715–721.
39. Browne LP, Krishnamurthy R, Chung T (2011) Preoperative and postoperative MR evaluation of congenital heart disease in children. Radiol Clin North Am 9: 1011–1024.
40. Grosse-Wortmann L, Al-Otay A, Yoo SJ (2009) Aortopulmonary collaterals after bidirectional cavopulmonary connection or Fontan completion: quantification with MRI. Circ Cardiovasc Imaging 2: 219–225.
41. Wang RP, Liang CH, Huang MP, Liu H, Deng QP, et al. (2012) Assessment of aortopulmonary collateral flow and pulmonary vascular growth using a 3.0 T magnetic resonance imaging system in patients who underwent bidirectional Glenn shunting. Eur J Cardiothorac Surg 41: e146–e153.

Permissions

All chapters in this book were first published in PLOS ONE, by The Public Library of Science; hereby published with permission under the Creative Commons Attribution License or equivalent. Every chapter published in this book has been scrutinized by our experts. Their significance has been extensively debated. The topics covered herein carry significant findings which will fuel the growth of the discipline. They may even be implemented as practical applications or may be referred to as a beginning point for another development.

The contributors of this book come from diverse backgrounds, making this book a truly international effort. This book will bring forth new frontiers with its revolutionizing research information and detailed analysis of the nascent developments around the world.

We would like to thank all the contributing authors for lending their expertise to make the book truly unique. They have played a crucial role in the development of this book. Without their invaluable contributions this book wouldn't have been possible. They have made vital efforts to compile up to date information on the varied aspects of this subject to make this book a valuable addition to the collection of many professionals and students.

This book was conceptualized with the vision of imparting up-to-date information and advanced data in this field. To ensure the same, a matchless editorial board was set up. Every individual on the board went through rigorous rounds of assessment to prove their worth. After which they invested a large part of their time researching and compiling the most relevant data for our readers.

The editorial board has been involved in producing this book since its inception. They have spent rigorous hours researching and exploring the diverse topics which have resulted in the successful publishing of this book. They have passed on their knowledge of decades through this book. To expedite this challenging task, the publisher supported the team at every step. A small team of assistant editors was also appointed to further simplify the editing procedure and attain best results for the readers.

Apart from the editorial board, the designing team has also invested a significant amount of their time in understanding the subject and creating the most relevant covers. They scrutinized every image to scout for the most suitable representation of the subject and create an appropriate cover for the book.

The publishing team has been an ardent support to the editorial, designing and production team. Their endless efforts to recruit the best for this project, has resulted in the accomplishment of this book. They are a veteran in the field of academics and their pool of knowledge is as vast as their experience in printing. Their expertise and guidance has proved useful at every step. Their uncompromising quality standards have made this book an exceptional effort. Their encouragement from time to time has been an inspiration for everyone.

The publisher and the editorial board hope that this book will prove to be a valuable piece of knowledge for researchers, students, practitioners and scholars across the globe.

List of Contributors

Michael Forsting and Thomas C. Lauenstein
Department of Diagnostic and Interventional Radiology and Neuroradiology, University Hospital Essen, Essen, Germany

Anja Fischer, Karsten Beiderwellen and Lale Umutlu
Department of Diagnostic and Interventional Radiology and Neuroradiology, University Hospital Essen, Essen, Germany
Erwin L. Hahn Institute for Magnetic Resonance Imaging, University Duisburg-Essen, Essen, Germany

Oliver Kraff and Stefan Maderwald
Erwin L. Hahn Institute for Magnetic Resonance Imaging, University Duisburg-Essen, Essen, Germany

Mark E. Ladd
Department of Diagnostic and Interventional Radiology and Neuroradiology, University Hospital Essen, Essen, Germany
Erwin L. Hahn Institute for Magnetic Resonance Imaging, University Duisburg-Essen, Essen, Germany
German Cancer Research Center (DKFZ), Heidelberg, Germany

Karsten H. Wrede and Philipp Dammann
Erwin L. Hahn Institute for Magnetic Resonance Imaging, University Duisburg-Essen, Essen, Germany
Department of Neurosurgery, University Hospital Essen, Essen, Germany

Christoph Mönninghoff
Department of Diagnostic and Interventional Radiology and Neuroradiology, University Hospital Essen, Essen, Germany

Sören Johst, Stefan Maderwald, Mark E. Ladd and Lale Umutlu
Erwin L. Hahn Institute for Magnetic Resonance Imaging, University Duisburg-Essen, Essen, Germany
Department of Diagnostic and Interventional Radiology and Neuroradiology, University Hospital Essen, Essen, Germany

I. Erol Sandalcioglu, Oliver Müller, Neriman Özkan and Ulrich Sure
Department of Neurosurgery, University Hospital Essen, Essen, Germany

Michael Forsting and Marc U. Schlamann
Erwin L. Hahn Institute for Magnetic Resonance Imaging, University Duisburg-Essen, Essen, Germany
Department of Diagnostic and Interventional Radiology and Neuroradiology, University Hospital Essen, Essen, Germany

Jan Hansmann, Henrik J. Michaely, André Luckscheiter, Stefan O. Schoenberg and Ulrike I. Attenberger
Institute of Clinical Radiology and Nuclear Medicine, University Medical Center Mannheim, Medical Faculty Mannheim - Heidelberg University, Mannheim, Germany

John N. Morelli
The Russel H. Morgan Department of Radiology and Radiological Science, The Johns Hopkins Hospital, Baltimore, Maryland, United States of America

Dietrich Beitzke, Richard Nolz, Sylvia Unterhumer, Christina Plank, Michael Weber, Rüdiger Schernthaner, Florian Wolf and Christian Loewe
Department of Biomedical Imaging and Image-guided Therapy, Division of Cardiovascular and Interventional Radiology, Medical University Vienna, Vienna, Austria

Veronika Schöpf
Department of Biomedical Imaging and Image-guided Therapy, Division of Neuroradiology and Musculoskeletal Radiology, Medical University Vienna, Vienna, Austria

Aad van der Lugt
Dept. of Radiology, Erasmus MC, Rotterdam, the Netherlands

Emilie M. M. Santos
Dept. of Radiology, Erasmus MC, Rotterdam, the Netherlands
Dept. of Medical Informatics, Erasmus MC, Rotterdam, the Netherlands
Dept. of Radiology, AMC, Amsterdam, the Netherlands
Dept. of Biomedical Engineering and Physics, AMC, Amsterdam, the Netherlands

Wiro J. Niessen
Dept. of Radiology, Erasmus MC, Rotterdam, the Netherlands
Dept. of Medical Informatics, Erasmus MC, Rotterdam, the Netherlands
Faculty of Applied Sciences, Delft University of Technology, Delft, the Netherlands

Henk A. Marquering
Dept. of Radiology, AMC, Amsterdam, the Netherlands
Dept. of Biomedical Engineering and Physics, AMC, Amsterdam, the Netherlands

Olvert A. Berkhemer and Charles B. Majoie
Dept. of Radiology, AMC, Amsterdam, the Netherlands

Wim H. van Zwam
Dept. of Radiology, Maastricht University Medical Centre, Maastricht, the Netherlands

Xinkai Qu, Weiyi Fang, Shaofeng Guan, Ruogu Li, Yingjia Xu, Min Zhang and Hua Liu
Department of Cardiology, Shanghai Chest Hospital, Shanghai Jiao Tong University, Shanghai, China

Kaizheng Gong
Department of Cardiology, The Second Clinical Medical School of Yangzhou University, Jiangsu Province, China

Jianding Ye and Yan Shen
Department of Radiology, Shanghai Chest Hospital, Shanghai Jiao Tong University, Shanghai, China

Wenhui Xie
Department of Nuclear medicine, Shanghai Chest Hospital, Shanghai Jiao Tong University, Shanghai, China

Pengli Zhou, Jianzhuang Ren., Xinwei Han, Gang Wu, Wenguang Zhang, Pengxu Ding and Yonghua Bi
Department of Interventional Radiology, The First Affiliated Hospital, Zhengzhou University, Zhengzhou, Henan Province, China

Tong-yi Xu, Xin Li, Lin Han and Zhi-yun Xu
Department of Cardiothoracic Surgery, Changhai Hospital, Second Military Medical University, Shanghai, China

Ben Zhang
Centre of Cardiovascular Surgery, Guangzhou General Hospital of Guangzhou Military Region, Guangzhou, China

Xiang Chen and Zhi-gang Zhang
Department of Cardiology, Changhai Hospital, Second Military Medical University, Shanghai, China

Eugene S. Mananga, Ali A. Bonab, Jinsong Ouyang and Georges El Fakhri
Center for Advanced Medical Imaging Sciences, Division of Nuclear Medicine and Molecular Imaging, Massachusetts General Hospital, Boston, Massachusetts, United States of America
Department of Radiology, Harvard Medical School, Boston, Massachusetts, United States of America

Joshua Schaefferkoetter
A*STAR-NUS Clinical Imaging and Research Centre (CIRC), Singapore, Singapore

Giancarlo Todiere, Andrea Barison, Annamaria Del Franco, Michele Emdin and Giovanni Donato Aquaro
Fondazione G. Monasterio Regione Toscana-National Research Council, Pisa, Italy

Lorena Pisciella, Elisabetta Zachara and Federica Re
Cardiologia 2 Azienda Ospedaliera San Camillo-Forlanini, Rome, Italy

Paolo Piaggi
Endocrinology Unit, University Hospital, Pisa, Italy

Alessandro Pingitore
Institute of Clinical Physiology, National Research Council, Pisa, Italy

Massimo Lombardi
Multimodality Imaging Section, San Donato, Milano, Italy

Rachael E. Moorin
Centre for Population Health Research, Curtin University, Perth, Western Australia, Australia
Centre for Health Services Research, School of Population Health, University of Western Australia, Perth Western Australia, Australia

David A. J. Gibson
Centre for Health Services Research, School of Population Health, University of Western Australia, Perth Western Australia, Australia

Rene K. Forsyth
Department of Medical Imaging Science, Curtin University, Perth, Western Australia, Australia

Richard Fox
School of Physics, University of Western Australia, Perth, Western Australia, Australia

Cong Han, Zheng-Shan Zhang, Wei-Zhong Yang, Lian Duan and Yi-Qin Han
Department of Neurosurgery, 307 Hospital, PLA, Beijing, China

Hui Feng
Department of Ultrasound, 302 Hospital, PLA, Beijing, China

Wei-Wei Liu
Consulting centre of biomedical statistics, academy of military medical sciences, PLA, Beijing, China

Jill J. F. Belch, Matthew A. Lambert, Andrew D. Morris and Allan D. Struthers
Division of Cardiovascular and Diabetes Medicine, Medical Research Institute, University of Dundee, Dundee, United Kingdom

Jonathan R. Weir-McCall and J. Graeme Houston
Division of Cardiovascular and Diabetes Medicine, Medical Research Institute, University of Dundee, Dundee, United Kingdom
NHS Tayside Clinical Radiology, Ninewells Hospital, Dundee, United Kingdom

Prasad Guntur Ramkumar
NHS Tayside Clinical Radiology, Ninewells Hospital, Dundee, United Kingdom

Faisel Khan
Vascular & Inflammatory Diseases Research Unit, Medical Research Institute, University of Dundee, Dundee, United Kingdom

Carly L. Adamson and Michael Gardner
University of Dundee, Ninewells Hospital & Medical School, Dundee, United Kingdom

Stephen J. Gandy
NHS Tayside Medical Physics, Ninewells Hospital, Dundee, United Kingdom

Petra Rauchhaus
Dundee epidemiological and biostatistics unit, University of Dundee, Dundee, United Kingdom

Yeyang Yu, Jin Jin, Feng Liu and Stuart Crozier
School of Information Technology and Electrical Engineering, the University of Queensland, St Lucia, Queensland, Australia

Li Qi, Chang Sheng Zhou, Yan E. Zhao, Long Jiang Zhang and Guang Ming Lu
Department of Medical Imaging, Jinling Hospital, Clinical School of South Medical University, Nanjing, Jiangsu, China

Felix G. Meinel
Department of Radiology and Radiological Science, Medical University of South Carolina, Charleston, South Carolina, United States of America

U. Joseph Schoepf
Department of Medical Imaging, Jinling Hospital, Clinical School of South Medical University, Nanjing, Jiangsu, China
Department of Radiology and Radiological Science, Medical University of South Carolina, Charleston, South Carolina, United States of America

Lea M. Alhilali, Arich R. Reynolds and Saeed Fakhran
Department of Radiology, University of Pittsburgh Medical Center, Pittsburgh, Pennsylvania, United States of America

Artur Klepaczko, Piotr Szczypiński, Grzegorz Dwojakowski, Michał Strzelecki and Andrzej Materka
Medical Electronics Division, Institute of Electronics, Lodz University of Technology, Lodz, Poland

Jian-wei Zhang, Qing Yang, Shi-wei Yang and Yu-jie Zhou
Department of Cardiology, Beijing Anzhen Hospital, Capital Medical University, Beijing Institute of Heart Lung and Blood Vessel Disease, The Key Laboratory of Remodeling-related Cardiovascular Disease, Ministry of Education, Beijing, China

Ling-jie He
Department of Emergency, Beijing Friendship Hospital, Capital Medical University, Beijing, China

Shu-jun Cao
Department of Cardiology, Beijing Daxing Hospital, Capital Medical University, Beijing, China

Florian Schwarz and Dominik Zinsser
Institute for Clinical Radiology, Hospital of the Ludwig Maximilian University of Munich, Munich, Germany

Maximilian F. Reiser and Hans C. Becker
Institute for Clinical Radiology, Hospital of the Ludwig Maximilian University of Munich, Munich, Germany
Medical Clinic I - Cardiology, Hospital of the Ludwig Maximilian University of Munich, Munich, Germany

Philipp Lange and Martin Greif
Medical Clinic I - Cardiology, Hospital of the Ludwig Maximilian University of Munich, Munich, Germany

Christian Kupatt
Medical Clinic I - Cardiology, Hospital of the Ludwig Maximilian University of Munich, Munich, Germany
DZHK (German Centre for Cardiovascular Research), Partner Site Munich Heart Alliance, Munich

Peter Boekstegers
HELIOS Klinikum Siegburg, HELIOS Kliniken GmbH, Siegburg, Germany

Christoph Schmitz
Department of Cardiac Surgery, Hospital of the Ludwig Maximilian University of Munich, Munich, Germany, Germany

Truls Råmunddal, Jacob Odenstedt, Dan Ioanes, Christian Dworeck, Oskar Angerås, Göran Matejka, Per Albertsson and Elmir Omerovic
Department of Cardiology, Sahlgrenska University Hospital, Gothenburg, Sweden

Loes Hoebers and Jose P. S. Henriques
Department of Cardiology, Academic Medical Center, Amsterdam, The Netherlands

Göran Olivecrona and Jan Harnek
Department of Coronary Heart Disease, Skåne University Hospital, Scania, Sweden

Ulf Jensen, Mikael Aasa and Risto Jussila
Department of Cardiology, Stockholm South General Hospital, Stockholm, Sweden

Stefan James and Bo Lagerqvist
Department of Medical Sciences, Uppsala University, Uppsala, Sweden

Gabriele Bonanno, Ruud B. van Heeswijk and Matthias Stuber
Department of Radiology, University Hospital (CHUV) and University of Lausanne (UNIL), Lausanne, VD, Switzerland
Center for Biomedical Imaging (CIBM), Lausanne, VD, Switzerland

Gilles Puy
Institute of Electrical Engineering, École Polytechnique Fédérale de Lausanne (EPFL), Lausanne, VD, Switzerland

Yves Wiaux
Department of Radiology, University Hospital (CHUV) and University of Lausanne (UNIL), Lausanne, VD, Switzerland
Center for Biomedical Imaging (CIBM), Lausanne, VD, Switzerland
Institute of Electrical Engineering, École Polytechnique Fédérale de Lausanne (EPFL), Lausanne, VD, Switzerland
Department of Radiology and Medical Informatics, University of Geneva (UniGE), Genève, GE, Switzerland
Institute of Sensors, Signals & Systems, Heriot Watt University, Edinburgh, United Kingdom

Davide Piccini
Department of Radiology, University Hospital (CHUV) and University of Lausanne (UNIL), Lausanne, VD, Switzerland
Center for Biomedical Imaging (CIBM), Lausanne, VD, Switzerland
Advanced Clinical Imaging Technology, Siemens Healthcare IM BM PI, Lausanne, Switzerland

Richard I. Aviv
Department of medical Imaging, University of Toronto, Division of Neuroradiology Sunnybrook Health Sciences Centre, Toronto, Ontario, Canada

Adam G. Kelly
Department of Neurology, University of Rochester, Rochester, New York, United States of America

Babak S. Jahromi
Department of Neurosurgery, University of Rochester, Rochester, New York, United States of America
Department of Imaging Sciences, University of Rochester, Rochester, New York, United States of America

Curtis G. Benesch
Department of Neurology, University of Rochester, Rochester, New York, United States of America
Department of Neurosurgery, University of Rochester, Rochester, New York, United States of America

Kate C. Young
Department of Neurology, University of Rochester, Rochester, New York, United States of America, Department of Neurosurgery, University of Rochester, Rochester, New York, United States of America, Department of Imaging Sciences, University of Rochester, Rochester, New York, United States of America

Kaylee E. Smith and Norman A. Michaud
Angiogenesis Laboratory, Department of Ophthalmology, Massachusetts Eye & Ear Infirmary, Boston, Massachusetts, United States of America,

Eiichi Hasegawa, Harry Sweigard, Deeba Husain, Demetrios G. Vavvas, Joan W. Miller and Kip M. Connor
Angiogenesis Laboratory, Department of Ophthalmology, Massachusetts Eye & Ear Infirmary, Boston, Massachusetts, United States of America

Ana M. Olivares
Schepens Eye Research Institute, Massachusetts Eye & Ear Infirmary, Boston, Massachusetts, United States of America

Bo Chang
The Jackson Laboratory, Bar Harbor, Maine, United States of America

Amy E. Birsner
Vascular Biology Program, Department of Surgery, Boston Children's Hospital, Harvard Medical School, Boston, Massachusetts, United States of America

Robert J. D'Amato
Department of Ophthalmology, Harvard Medical School, Boston, Massachusetts, United States of America
Vascular Biology Program, Department of Surgery, Boston Children's Hospital, Harvard Medical School, Boston, Massachusetts, United States of America

Yinan Han
Schepens Eye Research Institute, Massachusetts Eye & Ear Infirmary, Boston, Massachusetts, United States of America

Neena B. Haider
Department of Ophthalmology, Harvard Medical School, Boston, Massachusetts, United States of America
Schepens Eye Research Institute, Massachusetts Eye & Ear Infirmary, Boston, Massachusetts, United States of America

Pei Nie and Ximing Wang
Shandong Provincial Key Laboratory of Diagnosis and Treatment of Cardio-Cerebral Vascular Diseases, Shandong Medical Imaging Research Institute, Shandong University, Jinan, Shandong, China

Chunjuan Sun
Shandong Provincial Key Laboratory of Diagnosis and Treatment of Cardio-Cerebral Vascular Diseases, Shandong Medical Imaging Research Institute, Shandong University, Jinan, Shandong, China
Shandong Provincial Key Laboratory of Diagnosis and Treatment of Cardio-Cerebral Vascular Diseases, Shandong Medical Imaging Research Institute, Shandong University, Jinan, Shandong, China

Yinghua Pan, Hongbo Wang, Jian Li, Heng Ma and Futao Huo
Department of Radiology, Yuhuangding Hospital, Yantai, Shandong, China

Karsten H. Wrede and Philipp Dammann
Erwin L. Hahn Institute for Magnetic Resonance Imaging, University Duisburg-Essen, Essen, Germany
Department of Neurosurgery, University Hospital Essen, Essen, Germany

Neriman Özkan and Ulrich Sure
Department of Neurosurgery, University Hospital Essen, Essen, Germany

Sören Johst, Stefan Maderwald and Lale Umutlu
Erwin L. Hahn Institute for Magnetic Resonance Imaging, University Duisburg-Essen, Essen, Germany
Department of Diagnostic and Interventional Radiology and Neuroradiology, University Hospital Essen, Essen, Germany

Christoph Mönninghoff and Marc Schlamann
Department of Diagnostic and Interventional Radiology and Neuroradiology, University Hospital Essen, Essen, Germany

Markus Kraemer
Department of Neurology, Alfried Krupp von Bohlen und Halbach Hospital, Essen, Germany

Mark E. Ladd
Erwin L. Hahn Institute for Magnetic Resonance Imaging, University Duisburg-Essen, Essen, Germany
Department of Diagnostic and Interventional Radiology and Neuroradiology, University Hospital Essen, Essen, Germany
Division of Medical Physics in Radiology (E020), German Cancer Research Center (DKFZ), Heidelberg, Germany

Felix Heggemann, Florian Streitner, Christina Doesch, Theano Papavassiliu, Martin Borggrefe and Dariusch Haghi
First Medical Department, University Medical Center Mannheim, University of Heidelberg, Mannheim, Germany

Karsten Hamm
Department of Cardiology, Center of Cardiovascular Medicine, Bad Neustadt, Germany

Joachim Brade
Department of Biometrics and Statistics, University Medical Center Mannheim, University of Heidelberg, Mannheim, Germany

Xiaopeng Ji, Bin Zhao, Zhaoping Cheng, Yanhua Duan, Pei Nie, Haiou Li, Shifeng Yang, Hui Jiao and Ximing Wang
Shandong Medical Imaging Research Institute, Shandong University, Jinan, People's Republic of China

Biao Si and Zhiheng Wang
Cardiovascular Institute of Jinan Military district, Jinan, People's Republic of China

Index